PHARMACEUTICS

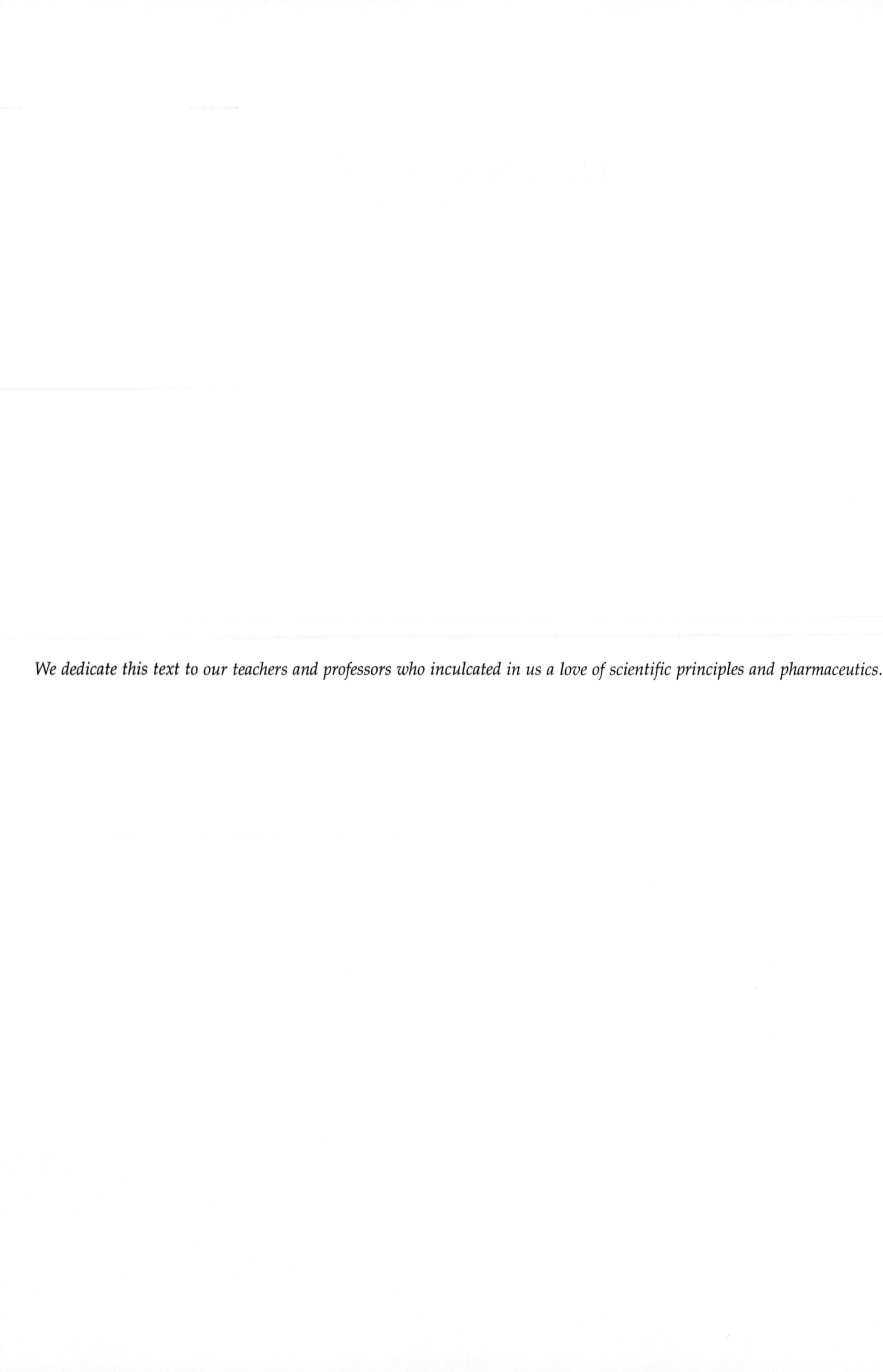

We dedicate this text to our teachers and professors who inculcated in us a love of scientific principles and pharmaceutics.

PHARMACEUTICS

Basic Principles and Application to Pharmacy Practice

Edited by

Alekha K. Dash, RPh, PhD
Creighton University, Nebraska, USA

Somnath Singh, PhD
Creighton University, Nebraska, USA

Justin Tolman, PharmD, PhD
Creighton University, Nebraska, USA

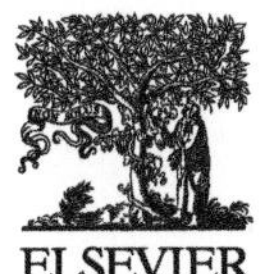

AMSTERDAM • BOSTON • HEIDELBERG • LONDON
NEW YORK • OXFORD • PARIS • SAN DIEGO
SAN FRANCISCO • SINGAPORE • SYDNEY • TOKYO
Academic Press is an imprint of Elsevier

Academic Press is an imprint of Elsevier
525 B Street, Suite 1800, San Diego, CA 92101-4495, USA
32 Jamestown Road, London NW1 7BY, UK
225 Wyman Street, Waltham, MA 02451, USA

British Library Cataloguing-in-Publication Data
A catalogue record for this book is available from the British Library

Library of Congress Cataloging-in-Publication Data
A catalog record for this book is available from the Library of Congress

ISBN: 978-0-12-386890-9

For information on all Academic Press publications
visit our website at http://store.elsevier.com/

Printed and bound in the United States of America

Transferred to Digital Printing in 2014

Contents

6. Biopolymers

SOMNATH SINGH AND JUSTIN TOLMAN

II

PRACTICAL ASPECTS OF PHARMACEUTICS

7. Drug, Dosage Form, and Drug Delivery Systems

ALEKHA K. DASH

8. Solid Dosage Forms

ALEKHA K. DASH

9. Liquid Dosage Forms

HARI R. DESU, AJIT S. NARANG, LAURA A. THOMA AND RAM I. MAHATO

10. Aerosol Dosage Forms

JUSTIN A. TOLMAN AND MEGAN HUSLIG

11. Semisolid Dosage Forms

SHAILENDRA KUMAR SINGH, KALPANA NAGPAL AND SANGITA SAINI

12. Special Dosage Forms and Drug Delivery Systems

SARAT K. MOHAPATRA AND ALEKHA K. DASH

III

BIOLOGICAL APPLICATIONS OF PHARMACEUTICS

13. Membrane Transport and Permeation

JUSTIN A. TOLMAN AND MARIA P. LAMBROS

14. Factors Affecting Drug Absorption and Disposition

CHONG-HUI GU, ANUJ KULDIPKUMAR AND HARSH CHAUHAN

15. Routes of Drug Administration

MOHSEN A. HEDAYA AND JUSTIN A. TOLMAN

16. Bioavailability and Bioequivalence

AJIT S. NARANG AND RAM I. MAHATO

Preface

Pharmaceutical education in the United States of America has been undergoing substantial changes over the past several decades to address changes in a pharmacist's role in the provision of pharmaceutical care. Pharmacy education has had a historical perspective that prepared student pharmacists to engage in pharmaceutical dispensing or pursue graduate pharmaceutical education focused on research. Any clinically-focused education was then obtained through post- baccalaureate training and experience. The currently evolving perspective of pharmacy education is focused on preparing student pharmacists as providers of clinical pharmaceutical care and as the medication expert in the healthcare system.

These evolutions have increased the need for pharmacy education to be solidly-grounded in scientific principles. Key domains of pharmaceutical knowledge include: medicinal chemistry and pharmacology for an understanding of drug molecule properties and mechanisms of action; pharmaceutics and biopharmaceutics to utilize physicochemical properties of drugs to develop a safe, effective and reliable drug product and their interactions with human physiology; pharmacokinetics and pharmacodynamics to explain drug movement and pharmacologic effects within systems; pharmacy practice to interpret the role of medications in the diagnosis, treatment, and prevention of disease; and social and administrative studies to evaluate health services and patient safety. Pharmaceutical education should substantively address all of these domains to provide scientific foundations for rational clinical decision making. Additionally, only pharmacy education can provide the scientific depth and breadth across these various levels of knowledge domains.

This textbook is intended to provide a basic scientific introduction to the fields of pharmaceutics and biopharmaceutics specifically tailored to meet the need of practice of Pharmacy. Current educational resources in these fields are principally focused on a historical perspective of pharmaceutical education. They either provide a mathematically rigorous and theoretical introduction to these fields or are briefly integrated into larger resources focused on other knowledge domains. *Pharmaceutics: Basic Principles and Application to Pharmacy Practice* will help pharmacy students gain the scientific foundation to understand drug physicochemical properties, practical aspects of dosage forms and drug delivery systems, and the biological applications of drug administration.

Alekha H. Dash
Justin Tolman
Somnath Singh

Pharmaceutics: Basic Principles and Application to Pharmacy Practice includes a companion website with a full color image bank and flip videos featuring difficult processes and procedures, as well as sample questions for students to test their knowledge. To access these resources, please visit booksite.elsevier.com/9780123868909.

Acknowledgments

We would like to thank all our family members for their unstinted support during the preparation of this text. We would also like to acknowledge the following individuals who have contributed to this book or supplemental materials:

Daniel Munt
Barbara Bittner
Dawn Trojanowski
Megan Huslig
Roger Liu
Katherine Smith

List of Contributors

Eman Atef School of Pharmacy-Boston, Massachusetts College of Pharmacy and Health Sciences, Boston, MA, USA

Harsh Chauhan College of Pharmacy, Creighton University, Omaha, NE, USA

Alekha K. Dash Department of Pharmacy Sciences, School of Pharmacy and Health Professions, Creighton University, Omaha, NE, USA

Vivek S. Dave St. John Fisher College, Wegmans School of Pharmacy, Rochester, NY USA

Hari R. Desu Department of Pharmaceutical Sciences, University of Tennessee Health Science Center, Memphis, TN, USA

Ramprakash Govindarajan Research and Development, GlaxoSmithKline, Research Triangle Park, North Carolina, USA

Chong-Hui Gu Vertex Pharmaceuticals, Inc., Cambridge, MA, USA

Mohsen A. Hedaya Department of Pharmaceutics, Faculty of Pharmacy, Kuwait University, Safat, Kuwait

Seon Hepburn University of Maryland, School of Pharmacy, Baltimore, MD, USA

Stephen W. Hoag University of Maryland, School of Pharmacy, Baltimore, MD, USA

Megan Huslig Affiliation to come

Sunil S. Jambhekar LECOM Bradenton, School of Pharmacy, Bradenton, FL, USA

Anuj Kuldipkumar Vertex Pharmaceuticals, Inc., Cambridge, MA, USA

Maria P. Lambros Department of Pharmaceutical Sciences, College of Pharmacy, Western University of Health Sciences, Pomona, CA, USA

Ram I. Mahato Department of Pharmaceutical Sciences, University of Tennessee Health Science Center, Memphis, TN, USA

Sarat K. Mohapatra Department of Pharmacy Sciences, School of Pharmacy and Health Professions, Creighton University, Omaha, NE, USA

Kalpana Nagpal Department of Pharmaceutical Sciences, G. J. University of Science and Technology, Hisar, India

Ajit S. Narang Drug Product Science and Technology, Bristol-Myers Squibb, Co., New Brunswick, NJ, USA

Sangita Saini PDM College of Pharmacy, Sarai Aurangabad, Bahadurgarh, Haryana, India

Shailendra Kumar Singh Department of Pharmaceutical Sciences, G. J. University of Science and Technology, Hisar, India

Somnath Singh Department of Pharmacy Sciences, School of Pharmacy and Health Professions, Creighton University, Omaha, NE, USA

Laura A. Thoma Department of Pharmaceutical Sciences, University of Tennessee Health Science Center, Memphis, TN, USA; Creighton University School of Pharmacy and Health Professions, Omaha, NE, USA

PART I

PHYSICAL PRINCIPLES AND PROPERTIES OF PHARMACEUTICS

CHAPTER

1

Introduction: Terminology, Basic Mathematical Skills, and Calculations

Eman Atef[1] *and Somnath Singh*[2]

[1]School of Pharmacy-Boston, Massachusetts College of Pharmacy and Health Sciences, Boston, MA, USA

[2]Pharmacy Sciences, School of Pharmacy and Health Professions, Creighton University, Omaha, NE, USA

CHAPTER OBJECTIVES

- Review the basic mathematics applicable in pharmacy.
- Apply the concept of significant figures in pharmacy.
- Apply basic calculus, logarithms, and antilogarithms to solve pharmaceutical problems.
- Apply basic statistics (mean, mode, median, and standard deviation) to interpret pharmaceutical data.
- Interpret a graph and straight-line trend of data to derive useful information.
- Review frequently used units and dimensions in pharmacy.

Keywords

- Basic mathematics review
- Basic statistics
- Dimensional analysis
- Graphical representations
- Logarithmic calculations
- Significant figures
- Units and dimensions

1.1. INTRODUCTION

How much drug should be prescribed to a newborn baby compared to an adult? How do different pathological conditions affect the prescribed dose? How is the drug therapeutic dose determined? How long is a drug stable and can be used without compromising its therapeutic efficacy? Why do some drugs expire within 1 month, whereas others expire after a couple of years? How do you interpret data reported in the literature to derive some useful and clinically significant information about the therapeutic outcomes of a drug that can be used to counsel a patient and answer some of the pertinent questions a pharmacist encounters daily? To answer such questions and more, the pharmacist must have adequate mathematical and statistical skills. Therefore, this chapter provides a basic introduction to pharmaceutical calculations, units, and basic statistics terms.

1.2. REVIEW OF BASIC MATHEMATICAL SKILLS

1.2.1 Integers

The numbers 0, 1, 2, 3, −1, −2, −3, and so on, are called integers or whole numbers, which can be either positive or negative and can be arranged in ascending order, as shown in Figure 1.1, where they increase as you move from left to right on the line. Therefore, a negative integer such as −3 is smaller than −2.

1.2.2 Zero and Infinity

Mathematical operations involving zero and infinity do not work in the usual way, which sometimes is the reason for errors in pharmaceutical calculations. The following examples and key concepts illustrate the

Pharmaceutics. DOI: http://dx.doi.org/10.1016/B978-0-12-386890-9.00001-7

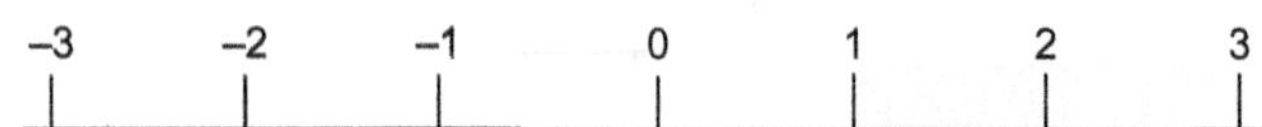

FIGURE 1.1 Ascending order of integers from left to right.

special rules governing the role of zero and infinity in mathematical operations:

- Any number multiplied by zero equals zero, e.g., $12 \times 0 = 0$. This result is unusual because generally multiplication of any number x by y results in a number that is different from either x or y, except when y is equal to 1, which results in no change in x. Otherwise, x increases if y is a positive integer (i.e., a whole number) greater than 1 and decreases if y is a fraction or an integer lower than 1. In the following examples, x is always 12:
  $12 \times 1 = 12$ (i.e., no change in the value of x if $y = 1$).
  $12 \times 3 = 36$ (i.e., the value of x increases from 12 to 36 if $y = 3$).
  $12 \times -3 = -36$ (i.e., the value of x decreases from 12 to -36 if $y = -3$)
  $12 \times -\frac{1}{3} = -4$ (i.e., the value of x decreases from 12 to -4 if $y = -\frac{1}{3}$ which is a negative fraction
  $12 \times \frac{1}{3} = 4$ (i.e., the value of x decreases from 12 to 4 if $y = \frac{1}{3}$ which is a positive fraction)
- Any number multiplied by infinity (∞) equals infinity, e.g., $12 \times \infty = \infty$. This is also unusual following the discussion provided for "multiplication by zero."
- Any number divided by zero is mathematically undefined; e.g.,$12/0$ = Undefined. This result is unusual because generally division of any number x by y results in a number z, which provides x when multiplied by y. For example, dividing 12 by 4 results in 3, which is correct because 3 multiplied by 4 provides the original number 12. However, 12 divided by 0 cannot result in a specific number that can provide 12 when multiplied by 0. Therefore, the outcome of 12 divided by 0 is undefined.
- Any number divided by infinity is mathematically undefined; e.g.,$12/\infty$ = Undefined. This result is also unusual following the discussion provided for "division by zero" because any number multiplied by ∞ would result in ∞; it cannot ever provide the original number, 12.

1.2.3 Rule of Indices

A number with a power or exponent such as 12^7 is called an indice, where 12 is called the base and 7 is the exponent. Mathematical problems involving indices with a common base are solved easily by applying the following rules:

- Exponents are added when multiplying indices, e.g.,

$$12^7 \times 12^5 = 12^{(7+5)} = 12^{12}$$
$$12^7 \times 12^5 \times 12^{-3} = 12^{(7+5-3)} = 12^9$$

- The exponent of the divisor is subtracted from the exponent of the dividend when dividing one indice by another, e.g.,

$$12^5 \div 12^3 = 12^{(5-3)} = 12^2$$
$$12^3 \div 12^5 = 12^{(3-5)} = 12^{-2}$$
$$(12^9 \times 12^3) \div (12^4 \times 12^2) = 12^{((9+3)-(4+2))} = 12^6$$

- Multiple exponents of a base are multiplied, e.g.,

$$(12^5)^3 = 12^{(5\times 3)} = 12^{15}$$
$$(12^{-5})^3 = 12^{(-5\times 3)} = 12^{-15}$$
$$\sqrt{12^6} = 12^{6\times\frac{1}{2}} = 12^3$$
$$\sqrt[3]{12^6} = 12^{6\times\frac{1}{3}} = 12^2$$

- An indice having a negative exponent is equal to its inverse with a positive exponent, e.g.,

$$12^{-3} = \frac{1}{12^3}$$

$$\left(\frac{5}{12}\right)^{-3} = \left(\frac{12}{5}\right)^3 = \left(\frac{12\times 12\times 12}{5\times 5\times 5}\right) = \frac{1728}{125} = 13.82$$

- An indice having a fraction as its exponent is equal to its root with a power equal to the denominator of the fraction followed by an exponent equal to the numerator of the fraction, e.g.,

$$(64)^{\frac{2}{5}} = \left(\sqrt[5]{64}\right)^2 = \left(\sqrt[5]{2\times 2\times 2\times 2\times 2\times 2}\right)^2 = (2)^2 = 4$$

- Any indice having zero as an exponent is equal to 1, e.g.,
  $12^0 = 1$
  $100^0 = 1$
- All the rules governing mathematical operations involving indices can be summarized as shown here, assuming x as a base:

$$x^y \times x^z = x^{y+z}$$
$$\frac{x^y}{x^z} = x^{y-z}$$
$$(x^y)^z = x^{yz}$$
$$x^{-y} = \frac{1}{x^y}$$
$$x^{\frac{y}{z}} = (\sqrt[z]{x})^y$$
$$x^0 = 1$$

1.2.4 Scientific or Exponential Notation

Pharmacists often encounter extremely large or small numbers, which creates a challenge when doing simple mathematical operations involving such numbers. For example, the normal range of testosterone level in men (16–30 years old) is 72–148 pg/mL (i.e., 0.000,000,000,072–0.000,000,000,148 g/mL) [1], and the number of skin cells in humans is 110,000,000,000 [2]. Therefore, scientific notation is used to handle such large or small numbers, using exponential notation or the power of 10. Thus, the testosterone level can be conveniently expressed as 7.2×10^{-11} to 1.48×10^{-10} g/mL. Similarly, the number of skin cells can be represented by 1.1×10^{11}. The number expressed by scientific notation is called the scientific number.

Generally, only one figure appears before the decimal point in the first part of scientific notation; it is called the coefficient. When multiplying or dividing two scientific numbers, the exponents are added or subtracted respectively, as shown below:

Multiplication of scientific numbers:

$(1.1 \times 10^{-11}) \times (7.2 \times 10^{10}) = 7.92 \times 10^{-1}$; where the exponents, −11 and 10, have been added.
$(1.1 \times 10^{11}) \times (7.2 \times 10^{10}) = 7.92 \times 10^{21}$; where the exponents, 11 and 10, are added.

Division of scientific numbers:

$(1.1 \times 10^{11}) \div (7.2 \times 10^{-11}) = 0.15 \times 10^{22}$ or 1.5×10^{21}; where exponent −11 is subtracted from exponent 11.
$(1.1 \times 10^{11}) \div (7.2 \times 10^{7}) = 0.15 \times 10^{4}$ or 1.5×10^{3}; where exponent 7 is subtracted from exponent 11.

Addition or subtraction of scientific numbers can be easily carried by following the two steps shown below:

Step 1: The exponent of each number must be same as shown in example below where (7.2×10^{9}) has been converted to (0.072 × 1011).
Step 2: The coefficients are added or subtracted depending on the problem.

Addition of scientific numbers:

$(1.1 \times 10^{11}) + (7.2 \times 10^{9}) = (1.1 \times 10^{11}) + (.072 \times 10^{11}) = (1.1 + .072) \times 10^{11}$ or 1.17×10^{11}; where the decimal point in coefficient 7.2 is moved left by two positions to make exponents in both the scientific numbers equal to 11.

Alternatively, 1.1×10^{11} can be converted to 110.0×10^{9} to make the exponents in both the scientific numbers equal to 9 as shown below:

$(1.1 \times 10^{11}) + (7.2 \times 10^{9}) = (110.0 \times 10^{9}) + (7.2 \times 10^{9}) = (110.0 + 7.2) \times 10^{9}$ or $117.2 \times 10^{9} = 1.17 \times 10^{11}$

Subtraction of scientific numbers:

$(1.1 \times 10^{11}) - (7.2 \times 10^{9}) = (1.1 \times 10^{11}) - (.072 \times 10^{11}) = (1.1 - .072) \times 10^{11}$ or $1.028 \times 10^{11} = 1.03 \times 10^{11}$

1.2.5 Logarithms and Antilogarithms

Exponential data often are used in pharmacy calculations; e.g., the acidity constant, *Ka*, of acetaminophen is 3.09×10^{-10}, [3] which is used for developing its stable formulation. Performing mathematical calculations using such exponentials is not convenient. Furthermore, in many instances such as accelerated stability studies of drugs, it is difficult to find any correlation between exponential data. Another example is of data generated out of first-order rate kinetic studies. In such situations, using logarithms is helpful because it linearizes the data. Using logarithms makes calculations such as multiplication or division involving exponentials easy because it converts them into easy-to-handle simple addition or subtraction problems. A logarithm is the power to which a base must be raised to obtain a number. Therefore, there are two kinds of logarithms on the basis of differences in the base: the *common logarithm* (log), where the base is 10, and *natural logarithm* (ln), where the base is *e* (where $e = 2.7182818\ldots$). The following examples clarify this concept:

- **Using $\log_{10}$("log to the base 10"):**
  $\log_{10}1000 = 3$ (i.e., log of 1000 to the base 10 is 3) is equivalent to $10^3 = 1000$ where 10 is the base, 3 is the logarithm (i.e., the exponent or power), and 1000 is the number.
- **Using natural log ($\log_e$ or ln):**
  $\ln 100 = 4.6052$ (i.e., log of 100 to the base *e* is 4.6052) is equivalent to $e^{4.6052} = 100$ or $2.7183^{4.6052} = 100$ where *e* or 2.7183 is the base, 4.6052 is the logarithm (i.e., the exponent or power), and 100 is the number.

Anytime something, *c*, changes at a rate proportional to *c*, it is represented by a natural logarithmic equation, e.g., the equation representing the first-order rate kinetics as shown next.

The first-order reaction is represented by $dc/c = -k_1dt$, where *c* is the concentration of the reactant at any time, *t* and k_1 is the proportionality constant. Integration of this equation between concentration C_0 at time $t = 0$ and concentration C_t at time $t = t$ results in the following equation using natural log:

$$lnC_t = lnC_0 - k_1t$$

Therefore, it is essential to know the interconversion from a common logarithm to a natural logarithm and vice versa, which can be derived as shown next.

TABLE 1.1 Rules for Logarithmic Mathematical Operations

Common Logarithm	Natural Logarithm
$log\ xy = log\ x + log\ y$	$ln\ xy = ln\ x + ln\ y$
$log\ \frac{x}{y} = log\ x - log\ y$	$ln\ \frac{x}{y} = ln\ x - ln\ y$
$log\ x^y = y\ log\ x$	$ln\ x^y = y\ ln\ x$
$log\ \sqrt[y]{x} = log\ x^{\frac{1}{y}} = \frac{1}{y}\ log\ x$	$ln\ \sqrt[y]{x} = ln\ x^{\frac{1}{y}} = \frac{1}{y}\ ln\ x$

Assume that the ratio of a natural and common log of the same number is x, i.e.

$$\frac{ln10}{\log 10} = x$$

Since ln 10 = 2.303 and log 10 = 1, the ratio $x = 2.303$.

Therefore, for any number y,

$$\mathbf{ln}\ y = \mathbf{2.303}\ \mathbf{log}\ y$$

Sometimes the logarithm (or ln) of a number is available, but you need to find the number itself, which can be done by finding the antilogarithm of a logarithmic number. Therefore, the antilogarithm is also called the inverse logarithm. The following examples illustrate this concept:

$$\log x = 2; x = \text{antilog of } 2 = 100$$
$$\text{because } 10^2 = 100$$
$$\log x = -2; x = \text{antilog}\ (-2) = 0.01$$
$$\text{because } 10^{-2} = 0.01$$

The natural logarithm also works in the same way:

$$\ln x = 2.303;\ \text{so},\ x = \text{antiln}\ (2.303) = 10$$

The rules governing logarithmic calculation are shown in Table 1.1.

1.2.6 Accepted Errors and Significant Figures

All numbers can be categorized as either exact or inexact numbers:

- **Exact numbers:** Any numbers that can be determined with complete certainty; e.g., there are 110 students in a class, 12 eggs in one dozen eggs, 7 days in a week, 12 months in a year, etc. All these numbers can be figured out without any doubt.
- **Inexact numbers:** Numbers associated with any measurement are not exact because accuracy depends on the sensitivity of the instrument used in said measurement. You can increase the precision of the measurement by carefully following the standard operating procedure or by selecting a more sensitive instrument.

Let's start by defining and differentiating two terms that often are interchanged mistakenly: accuracy and precision.

Accuracy refers to how closely measured values agree with the correct value, whereas *precision* refers to how closely an individual measurement agrees with another. Precision is correlated to reproducibility of a measurement and is indicated by standard deviation of multiple repeated measurements. Obviously, a higher standard deviation indicates a lower precision of measurements. Therefore, a measurement can be of high precision but of low accuracy. For example, 100 grams of a drug are weighed using a balance having +10% errors due to a manufacturing defect. Thus, you can weigh out 100 grams multiple times with 99.99% precision (i.e., each 100 grams weighed out does not differ from another by more than 0.01 gram), but the weight accuracy is 90% due to the systematic error.

In another example, if an assay method reports 495 mg of ampicillin in a 500 mg capsule of ampicillin, the measurement accuracy is 99% [(495/500) × 100], i.e., a 1% error. If the assay is repeated 5 times for the same sample of ampicillin capsule and each time the result is 495 mg of ampicillin, the precision of the experimental method is 100%. Thus, precision indicates the repeatability of an experimental method. If the same error or mistake is repeated during each experiment, the result may be precise but inaccurate.

1.2.6.1 *Measurement Accuracy*

All measurements have a degree of uncertainty because no device can provide absolutely perfect measurement with absolute zero error. The error can be predicted from but not limited to, for example, the process used to prepare the dosage form, the sensitivity of the utilized balance or measuring devices, or the number of significant figures.

1.2.6.1.1 BASED ON THE OFFICIAL COMPENDIA

The U.S. Pharmacopeia [6] states that

> Unless otherwise specified, when a substance is weighed for an assay, the uncertainty should not exceed 0.1% of the reading.

Also according to the USP,

> Measurement uncertainty is satisfactory if 3 times the standard deviation of not less than 10 replicates weighings divided by the amount weighed, does not exceed 0.001.

Another commonly used parameter is the relative standard deviation (RSD), which equals to *Standard deviation/Mean* × 100.

For example, if the weight of 100 mg of active pharmaceutical ingredient (API) is taken 10 times ($n = 10$) and the following weights were recorded

0.1001 g, 0.1002 g, 0.0999 g, 0.1003 g, 0.1003 g,
0.1002 g, 0.1001 g, 0.1001 g, 0.1003 g, 0.1003 g

you can determine the average weight, standard deviation, and relative standard deviations for these measurements as follows:

Average weight (Mean weight)

$$= \frac{0.1001\,g + 0.1002\,g + 0.0999\,g + 0.1003\,g + 0.1003\,g + 0.1002\,g + 0.1001\,g + 0.1001\,g + 0.1003\,g + 0.1003\,g}{10}$$

$$= \frac{1.0018\,g}{10} = 0.10018\,g$$

Standard deviation $(SD) = \sqrt{Variance} = \sqrt{(\text{The average of the } \textbf{squared} \text{ differences from the Mean})}$

Difference from the Mean	Squared Differences
(0.1001 − 0.10018)	$(-0.00008)^2$
(0.1002 − 0.10018)	$(0.00002)^2$
(0.0999 − 0.10018)	$(-0.00028)^2$
(0.1003 − 0.10018)	$(0.00012)^2$
(0.1003 − 0.10018)	$(0.00012)^2$
(0.1002 − 0.10018)	$(0.00002)^2$
(0.1001 − 0.10018)	$(-0.00008)^2$
(0.1001 − 0.10018)	$(-0.00008)^2$
(0.1003 − 0.10018)	$(0.00012)^2$
(0.1003 − 0.10018)	$(0.00012)^2$

Average of the squared differences

$$= \frac{[(-0.00008)^2 + \cdots + (-0.00012)^2]}{10} = 1.56 \times 10^{-8}$$

The standard deviation $(SD) = \sqrt{1.56 \times 10^{-8}} = 0.000125$

Relative standard deviation (RSD)

$$= \frac{SD}{Mean} \times 100 = \frac{0.000125}{0.10018} \times 100 = 0.125\%$$

Since 3×0.000125 (i.e., $3 \times \text{SD}) = 0.000375$ and $0.000375 < 0.001$, the preceding measurement uncertainty is acceptable according to the USP.

1.2.6.1.2 COMPOUNDING PRESCRIPTIONS AND INDUSTRIAL MANUFACTURING

Based on the USP, a maximum error of $\pm 5\%$ is acceptable in compounding prescriptions [4]. Unless otherwise indicated, especially relatively potent prescriptions may require higher accuracy.

On the other hand, a maximum error of $\pm 1\%$ is acceptable in pharmaceutical industrial measurements.

1.2.6.1.3 THE SENSITIVITY OF THE UTILIZED BALANCE

The sensitivity (i.e., the lowest weight detected) of a balance is an important and crucial parameter, enabling pharmacists to decide on which balance to use to fulfill the needed accuracy. The following examples illustrate this concept.

A powder weight is found to be 13.2 g using a balance with sensitivity = 0.1 g. In other words, you may be somewhat uncertain about that last digit; it could be a 2, 1, or 3.

On the other hand, a measurement done to the closest hundredth of a gram indicates the following: 13.21 g can be 13.22 g or 13.20 g.

Thus, the former balance should be used if accuracy of a tenth of a gram is required. However, if a drug is highly potent and has a narrow therapeutic window, such as digoxin or warfarin, a higher order of accuracy could be needed. Therefore, a balance with a sensitivity of a thousandth of a gram should be preferred to using a balance with sensitivity only up to a tenth or hundredth of a gram.

The sensitivity is also called resolution, which depends on types of balances, which include the following:

- Precision top pan balances have 0.001 g resolution.
- Analytical balances have 0.1 mg or 0.01 mg resolution.
- Semi-micro balances have 0.001 mg or 0.002 mg resolution.
- Micro balances have at least 0.0001 mg resolution.

1.2.6.1.4 SIGNIFICANT FIGURES

The number of significant figures is simply the number of figures that are known with some degree of reliability. The number 13.2 is said to have three significant figures. The number 13.20 is said to have four significant figures.

Therefore, the number of significant figures in a measurement is the number of digits that are known with certainty, plus the last one that is not absolutely certain but rather an approximate (inexact) number. For example, 13.2 g has three significant figures: 0.2 is the last and thus an inexact number; it could be a 0.249 or 0.15. Both are rounded to 0.2. For simplicity, you can indicate the tolerance as 13.2 ± 0.05. A mass of 13.20 g indicates an uncertainty of 0.00 g, so the expected weight would be any value in the range of $13.20\text{ g} \pm 0.005\text{ g}$. Thus, any measuring instrument such as a balance with greater sensitivity would provide measured value having a greater number of significant figures. Table 1.2 summarizes the rules helpful in deciding the number of significant figures in a measured value.

The potential ambiguity in the last rule can be avoided through the use of standard exponential, or "scientific," notation. For example, depending on whether two or three significant figures are correct, you could write 120 g as follows:

$$1.2 \times 10^2 \text{ g (two significant figures)}$$

or

$$12.0 \times 10 \text{ g (three significant figures)}$$

1.2.6.1.5 DETERMINING SIGNIFICANT FIGURES IN MATHEMATICAL OPERATIONS

1.2.6.1.5.1 ADDITION AND SUBTRACTION When measured quantities are used in addition or subtraction, the uncertainty is determined by the absolute uncertainty in the least precise measurement (not by the number of significant figures). Sometimes this is considered to be the number of digits after the decimal point.

Now consider these numbers:

78956.23 m
11.875 m

Addition of the preceding two numbers provides 78968.105 m, but the sum should be reported as 78968.10 m because there are two digits after the decimal point in 78956.23 m, which is less precise than 11.875 m.

1.2.6.1.5.2 MULTIPLICATION AND DIVISION When experimental quantities are multiplied or divided, the number of significant figures in the result is determined by the quantity with the least number of significant figures. If, for example, a density calculation is made in which 27.124 grams is divided by 2.1 mL, the density should be reported as 13 g/mL, not as 13.562 g/mL because the number of significant figures in 2.1 is two.

1.2.6.1.5.3 LOGARITHMIC CALCULATIONS In logarithmic calculations, the same number of significant figures is retained in the mantissa as there are in the original number; e.g., a 10-digit calculator would show that $\log 579 = 2.762678564$. Since the original number (579) contains three significant figures, the result should be reported as 2.763; i.e., the mantissa also should contain three significant figures. Likewise, when you are taking antilogarithms, the resulting number should have as many significant figures as the mantissa in the logarithm (so the antilog of $1.579 = 37.9$, not 37.931). For any log, the number to the left of the decimal point is called the *characteristic*, and the number to the right of the decimal point is called the *mantissa*.

Caution: The concept of significant figure should be applied with caution while dispensing a pharmaceutical prescription. The minimum weight or volume of each ingredient in a pharmaceutical formula or prescription should be large enough that the error introduced is not greater than 5% (5 in 100); i.e., pharmaceutical calculations incorporating three digits after decimal point are of acceptable precision [4]. While applying the concept of significant figures, you should know that some of the values could never be

TABLE 1.2 Rules for Determining Number of Significant Figures

Measured Values	Number of Significant Figures	Rules
12.786 g	5	All nonzero digits are significant.
12.078 g	5	Zero is significant if flanked by nonzero digits.
0.02 g	1	Zero immediately after a decimal point but before a nonzero digit is not significant where it merely indicates its position.
0.20 g	2	Zero after a decimal point is significant if preceded by a nonzero digit.
120 g	2 or 3	Zero at the end of a number and not preceded by a decimal point is not necessarily significant. If sensitivity of the balance is 10 g, the number of significant figures would be two. Similarly, the number of significant figures would be three if sensitivity of the balance is 1 g.

approximate because they are exact. The question of significant figures arises only when there is approximation in a measurement. For example, if a pharmacist combines five unit dose packages of a liquid that are 4.5 ml each, the total volume obtained would be ($5 \times 4.5 = 22.5$) 22.5 mL, which should be rounded off to two significant figures, not one. The reason is that the only inexact number, 4.5 mL, contains only two significant figures; and 5, which contains one significant figure, is an exact number. So, now the question is whether 22.5 should be reported as 22 or 23. Actually, it should be reported as 23 mL. The following rules should help when deciding to round up or down.

1.2.6.1.5.4 RULES FOR ROUNDING OFF NUMBERS The rules for rounding off are based on whether the digit to be dropped is equal to or greater than 5, as well as the digits flanking that digit. The following examples illustrate rules for rounding off numbers up to the required significant figures such as two:

- The last digit to be retained is increased by one if the digit to be dropped is greater than 5; e.g., 17.9 is rounded up to18 because the digit to be dropped, 9, is greater than 5.
- The last digit to be retained is left unaltered if the digit to be dropped is less than 5; e.g., 17.4 is rounded down to 17 because the digit to be dropped, 4, is less than 5.
- If 5 is the digit to be dropped but is followed by nonzero digit(s), the last remaining digit is increased by one; e.g., 17.512 is rounded up to 18 because digits 1 and 2 follow 5 and are not zero.
- If 5 is the digit to be dropped and is followed by zero only or no other digits, the last remaining digit should be rounded up or down depending on whether it is an even number or odd number. The last remaining digit is increased by one if it is an odd digit or left unaltered if it is an even digit; e.g., 17.5 is rounded up to 18 because the last remaining digit, 7, is an odd digit, but 18.5 is rounded down to 18 because the last remaining digit is an even digit.

1.2.7 Significant Difference

Conclusions can frequently be drawn about significant differences by looking at the standard deviation or standard error bars in case of clear overlapping. But sometimes the following points should be considered:

- Clinical significance versus statistical significance
- Comparison between treatments and treatments versus control

The effect of three antipyretic drugs in Figure 1.2 is used to clarify the preceding two points. Compared to the control group, the three tested antipyretic drugs resulted in a statistically significant drop in the patients' temperature, $p < 0.05$. But Antipyretic 1, although statistically significant from the control, may be insignificant because a drop of less than 1°C is not enough to create a clinically important effect. Although Antipyretics 2 and 3 are not significantly different, they are both statistically different from the control group; i.e., both are effective medications.

1.2.8 Samples and Measure of Centrality

Collecting, managing, and interpreting sample data are important responsibilities for pharmacists. Samples are generally small numbers of observations or data taken from a comparatively large population with clearly defined parameters [5]. For example, all the hypertensive patients having systolic blood pressure greater than 170 mmHg are a population, but 150 such patients selected for a clinical trial study of a hypertensive drug constitute a sample. Such a study generates a large amount of data based on experimental design of the study. One hundred twenty patients selected for the study may be divided in different groups being administered different dosages of the hypertensive drug under study. One group may be administered placebo, whereas another group may get the hypertensive drug under current clinical practice. The blood pressure change could be different in different groups or even in different subjects in the same group. Thus, reporting the conclusion of the study requires a summary number(s) because the original raw data are not communicable.

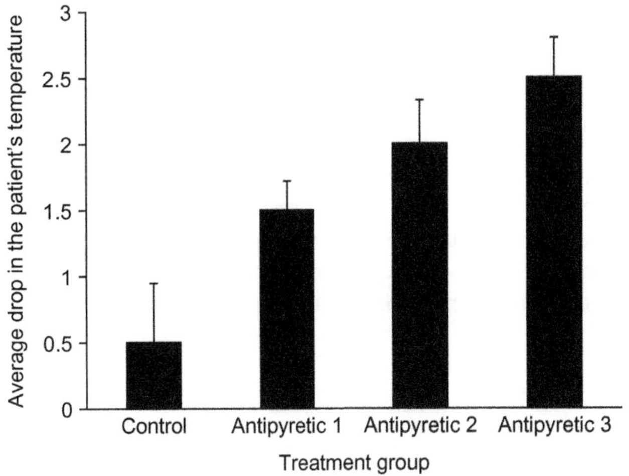

FIGURE 1.2 Average drop in the patients' body temperature following treatment with antipyretic.

One of the most useful approaches is using some sort of summary number or numbers, which are good indicators of centrality of sampling observations or data. The three measures of central tendency used in pharmacy are mean, median, and mode. Calculating mean is discussed in the Section 1.2.6.1.1. Following sections describe how to calculate median and mode using the same example used for calculating mean.

1.2.8.1 *Calculating Median*

The median is the middle data of observations arranged in ascending or descending order. Thus, half of the data or observation would be greater than the median, but the other half would be less than it.

If the weights of 100 mg of active pharmaceutical ingredient (API) are taken 10 times ($n = 10$) and these weightings are

0.1001 g, 0.1002 g, 0.0999 g, 0.1003 g, 0.1003 g,
0.1002 g, 0.1001 g, 0.1001 g, 0.1003 g, 0.1003 g

you can arrange the preceding data in ascending order as follows:

0.0999 g, 0.1001 g, 0.1001 g, 0.1001 g, 0.1002 g,
0.1002 g, 0.1003 g, 0.1003 g, 0.1003 g, 0.1003 g

Therefore, the median is the mean of the fifth (i.e., 0.1002) and sixth (i.e., 0.1002) data, which is equal to 0.1002. Obviously, median is the mean of two middle data in case of an even number of observations or data, but in the case of an odd number of observations, it would be the middle datum.

It is evident that median is not influenced by any extreme data because it would be the same in the preceding example whether the first datum is any number less than 0.0999 g or the tenth datum is greater than 0.1003. On contrast, mean or average is significantly influenced by any extreme data.

1.2.8.2 *Calculating Mode*

Mode is simply the data that occur most of the time and, therefore, generally is used for a large set of observations or data. In the preceding example, mode is equal to 0.1003. Sometimes, the frequency of two numbers could be equal in a data set, in which case the data are termed bimodal.

1.2.9 Dimensional Analysis

Dimensional analysis is a mathematical method, also known as the unit factor method, that utilizes the units and ratios between them in calculating a desired quantity with the required unit.

To use the dimensional analysis method, you have to know the relations between different units, as in these examples: 1 kg = 2.2 lb, 1 ft = 12 inches, 1 g = 1000 milligrams, 1 day = 24 hours.

Examples:

1. The recommended amoxicillin dose for severe infection is 25 mg/kg/day in divided doses every 12 hours. How many milliliters of amoxicillin can be given to a 66 lb patient per 12 hours, knowing that the oral suspension has 125 mg per 5 mL?

   To solve this problem using dimensional analysis, you should recognize the given parameters with the correct units and the unit required in the final answer.

   You need the final answer unit to be in mL/12 hours. And you have to utilize the given patient and drug information as well as your knowledge of ratios between different units to solve this problem.

   The following relations are needed to solve the problem:

   1 kg = 2.2 lb; 1 day is 24 hours.

The number of mL/12 hours

$$= \frac{25\ mg}{kg \times day} \times \frac{1\ kg}{2.2\ lb} \times 66\ lb \times \frac{5\ mL}{125\ mg}$$

$$\times \frac{1\ day}{2(12\ h)} = \text{-----}\frac{mL}{12\ h}$$

   In the preceding formula, all the units that are undesired in the final answer will cancel each other, and you end up with a final answer in the desired unit, i.e., the number of milliliters every 12 hours. (The correct answer is 15 mL/12 hours.)

   It is worth mentioning that the use of dimensional analysis is not the only way to solve this problem. The problem can be solved using multiple sets of proportions and can be performed stepwise.

2. The digoxin dose of a premature baby is 20 microgram/kg once a day. The available elixir is 0.05 mg/mL. How many milliliters should be given to a 5.5 lb baby per day?

   Remember that

   1 kg = 2.2 lb; 1 mg = 1000 microgram.

$$\text{The number of milliliters per day} = \frac{20\ microgram}{kg/day}$$

$$\times \frac{1\ kg}{2.2\ lb} \times 5.5\ lb \times \frac{1\ mg}{1000\ micrograms}$$

$$\times \frac{1\ mL}{0.05\ mg} = \text{-----}mL/day$$

   (The correct answer is 1 mL/12 hours.)

3. A drug provides 10,000 units/250 mg tablet. How many total units does the patient get by administering 4 tablets per day for 10 days?
   Key: The 250 mg is the total tablet weight. This is a distracting number and has nothing to do with your calculation.
   (The correct answer is 400,000 units/10 days.)
4. The recommended dose of a drug is 10 mg/kg/day (the drug is given every 6 hours). How many mL/6 hours should be prescribed to 60 lb child? The available suspension is 150 mg/tsp.
   (The correct answer is 2.3 mL/6 hours.)

1.3. GRAPHICAL REPRESENTATION

A graph is simply a visual representation showing the relationship between two or more variables. It shows how one variable (a dependent variable) changes with alteration in another variable (an independent variable). A graph consists of four quadrants in which the abscissa or ordinate is negative or positive, as shown in Table 1.3.

Looking at the theoretical and measured value changes with time in Table 1.4, you might find it difficult to observe the relationship between the two variables. However, when you look at the graph in Figure 1.3, the relationship becomes quite apparent. Thus, the graph is a better tool to present data in a clear, visual manner.

TABLE 1.3 Quadrants on a Cartesian Graph

Quadrant II (− x, + y)	Quadrant I (+ x, + y)
Quadrant III (− x, − y)	Quadrant IV (+ x, − y)

TABLE 1.4 Theoretical and Measured Value Changes with Time

Time	Measured Value	Theoretical Value
0	− 4.6	−5
1	− 3.4	−3
2	− 0.6	−1
3	0.8	1
4	3.4	3
5	4.4	5

1.3.1 Interpreting Graphs

When you attend a lecture, your initial comprehension is high. However, as the lecture progresses, your comprehension typically decreases with time. This information may be presented graphically as a two-dimensional graph

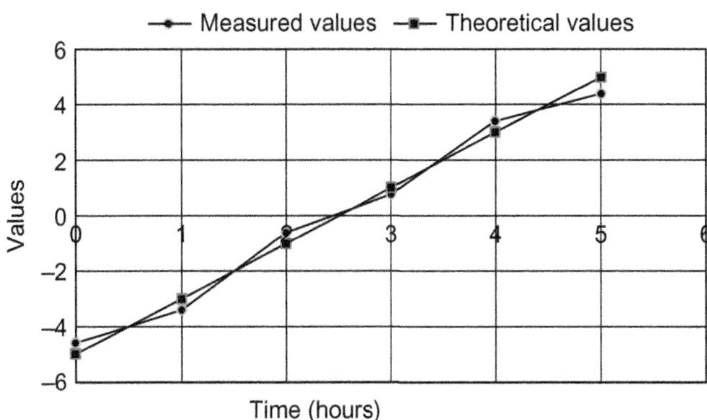

FIGURE 1.3 Graphical representation of the theoretical and measured values changes with time.

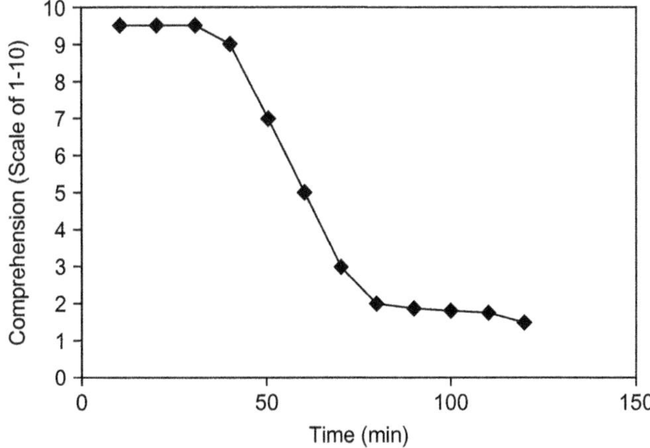

FIGURE 1.4 Graph representation of the comprehension of the students versus time.

consisting of a dependent variable (comprehension) and an independent variable (time).

The magnitude of the independent variable is usually measured along the x-axis, or the horizontal scale. The dependent variable is measured along the y-axis, or the vertical scale. See Figure 1.4.

The graph in this figure enables you to see quickly that for the initial time of about 30 minutes, the comprehension is high at approximately 9.5, and it gradually falls to about 2.0 after about 60 minutes, or 1 hour. It is evident that graphs are useful in providing a visual representation of data.

1.3.2 Straight-Line Graphs (Simple Linear Regression)

A graph is a straight line (linear) only if the equation from which it is derived has the following form:

$$y = mx + b$$

TABLE 1.5 Osmolality and Molality of Solution of Nicotinamide

Molality, mmol/kg	Osmolality, mOsmol/kg
25	23.9
50	48.2
75	71.9
100	93.2
125	122.5
150	143.7
175	168.1
200	191.2
225	215.2
250	231.1
275	262.9
300	286.9

where y is the dependent variable, x is the independent variable, m is the slope of the straight line $= \Delta y/\Delta x$, and b is the y intercept (when $x = 0$).

Example:

The data in Table 1.5 represent the osmolality and molality of solution of nicotinamide.

1. Find the linear relationship between the molality and osmolality of nicotinamide solutions.
2. What is the predicted value of osmolality when the molality of the solution is 255 mmol/kg?
3. Calculate the correlation coefficient for the linear relationship that exists between the osmolality and molality of solutions of nicotinamide.

Answers:

1. Microsoft Excel was used to plot a graph using the following data (see Figure 1.5).

   Using Excel functions, you can find out that the linear relationship between molality and osmolality can be described using the straight-line equation as $y = (0.9483x) + 0.8045$; i.e., Osmolality $= (0.9483 \times$ Molality$) + 0.8045$ at low concentrations.
2. Substitute the molality term with 255 in the preceding equation:

   Osmolality $= (0.9483 \times 255) + 0.8045 =$ 242.6 mOsmol/kg.
3. The correlation coefficient, r, is the square root of R^2 shown in the plot of molality and osmolality in Figure 1.5. So,

   Correlation coefficient, $r = \sqrt{R^2} = \sqrt{0.99951} = 0.9995$.

Note: The coefficient of correlation value, r, points to the strength of the relationship between the x and y

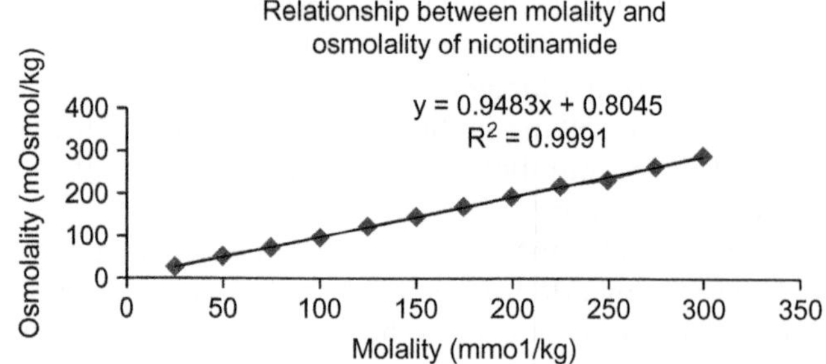

FIGURE 1.5 Graphical representation of the relationship between osmolality and the molality of solution of nicotinamide.

variables, which can range between -1 and $+1$. If the value of r is zero, this means there is no relationship between the two variables. If $r = -1$ or $+1$, there is perfect negative or positive linear correlation, respectively. In science generally, an acceptable value for r must be at least 0.70. Values below 0.70 reflect weak correlation.

The square of r is known as the coefficient of determination (represented by R^2 in Figure 1.5), which tells how much of the variability in the dependent variable y is explained by x, the independent variable. An R^2 of 0.60 means that 60% of the variability in y is explained by x and 40% of the variability in y could be due to other factors.

1.4. DIMENSIONS AND UNITS

Matter is anything that has weight and occupies space. Based on this broad definition, anything you see, feel, or interact with—such as computers, tables, coffee mugs, tablets, capsules, and solutions—constitutes matter. To define the properties of matter—amount, composition, position in space and time, and more—you need quantitative tools called *dimensions* and *units*. How heavy is your laptop? If you said "5 pounds," you have just used the unit of weight to define the heaviness of a substance that constitutes matter.

Why do you need to study dimensions and units? The pharmacist, being the drug expert on the healthcare team, is responsible for formulating, dispensing, and evaluating drugs and dosage forms for optimal therapeutic efficacy. A few examples in which this knowledge will help practicing pharmacists include (1) effectively formulating tablets, capsules, powders, solutions, ointments, or other dosage forms to meet therapeutic objectives; (2) performing dosage adjustments for patients based on the patients' weight, age, or body surface area; (3) determining the amount of active ingredient in a dosage form; and (4) determining the rate of infusion of a parenteral dosage form.

1.4.1 The Three Fundamental Dimensions

The properties of matter are usually expressed through the use of three fundamental dimensions: length, mass, and time. Each of these properties is assigned a definite unit and a reference standard. In the metric system, these units are assigned the centimeter (cm), the gram (g), and the second (sec); accordingly, it is called the cgs system.

The International Union of Pure and Applied Chemistry (IUPAC) introduced a System International, or SI, unit system to establish an internationally uniform set of units. Although physical pharmacy uses cgs units for most calculations, SI units are appearing with increasing frequency in textbooks.

1.4.2 Units Based on Length

Length and area: The SI unit for length is the meter. Other commonly used prefixes are listed in Table 1.6. In addition to the units here, many textbooks prefer using angstrom units (Å, equal to 10^{-10} meters or 10^{-8} cm) to express microscopic distances. The prefixes shown in the table may also be used to represent other dimensions such as mass and time. For example, 10^{-9} seconds is termed as a nanosecond.

The units of area are cm^2 or m^2 in cgs and SI systems, respectively. Therefore, area is represented as the square of length.

Volume: Volume is also derived from units based on length, and uses units in cm^3, also represented as cubic centimeter or cc (or m^3 in the SI system). Volume is also frequently defined in terms of the liter, with 1 liter or 1 L being equal to 1000.027 cm^3. The frequently used unit for volume in physical pharmacy is the milliliter, or mL, which is roughly equal to 1 cm^3 or mL.

TABLE 1.6 Common Multiples and Their Prefixes and Symbols

Multiple	Prefix	Symbol
10^{12}	Tera	T
10^{9}	Giga	G
10^{6}	Mega	M
10^{3}	Kilo	K
10^{-2}	Centi	c
10^{-3}	Milli	m
10^{-6}	Micro	m
10^{-9}	Nano	n
10^{-12}	Pico	p

1.4.3 Units Based On Mass

Mass and weight: The SI unit of mass is the kilogram, or the Kg. The cgs unit of mass is the gram, which is 1/1000 of the kilogram. Mass is often expressed as the "weight" of a substance, which is actually a force, and is discussed under "Derived Dimensions" in Section 1.4.4.

Example:

The concentration of a drug in a patient's blood was reported to be 15 mcg(microgram)/mL. Total volume of the blood in the same patient was 5 liters. Answer the following questions based on the information provided in this case study.

1. Identify the amount, volume, and concentration terms from this example.
2. What is the total amount of drug in the patient's blood?
3. Is there any relationship among concentration, volume, and amount? If so, identify it.

Answers:

1. In this example, 15 mcg is an amount term, 1 ml and 5 liters are volume terms, and 15 mcg/mL is a concentration unit.
2. Total amount of drug in the blood = Concentration × Total Volume:
   $= 15$ mcg/mL × 5000 mL = 75000 mcg
   $= 75$ mg
3. Yes, a relationship exists:
   Amount = Concentration × Volume.

1.4.4 Derived Dimensions

Four derived dimensions are usually discussed in pharmacy calculations. They include (1) density and specific gravity; (2) force; (3) pressure; and (4) work, energy, and heat.

1.4.4.1 Density and Specific Gravity

The pharmacist uses the quantities density and specific gravity for interconversions between mass and volume. Density is a derived quantity and combines the units of mass and volume:

Density = mass/volume

The units of a derived quantity can be obtained by substituting the units for the individual fundamental units. This process is called dimensional analysis. For example, the units of mass and volume in the cgs system are g and cm^3. So the units of density in the cgs system are g/cm^3.

The specific gravity of a substance is the ratio of its density to that of water, at a constant temperature.

Note that, being a ratio of two similar quantities, the specific gravity is not described by a unit:

Specific gravity = density of a substance/density of water

For the same reason, any quantity expressed as a ratio is always dimensionless.

The density of the drug, excipients, and dosage form are important for the following reasons:

1. During manufacturing, mixing solids with similar densities ensures complete mixing and minimizes the solid segregation (i.e., demixing).
2. Knowing the density of a dosage form helps in predicting the final volume occupied by the prescription.
3. Knowing the density of a substance can allow the conversion of percentage (w/w) to % (w/v) and vice versa.

Example:

Knowing that concentrated hydrochloric acid has 36% (w/w), (specific gravity 1.179), can you calculate the percentage w/v?

Answer:

Here, 36% (w/w) = 36 grams in 100 grams, based on the density the 100 grams occupies:

$$\frac{100\ grams}{1.179\ grams/mL} = 84.8\ mL$$

To calculate the % (w/v), you set a proportion:

$$\frac{36\,grams}{84.8\,mL} = \frac{x\,grams}{100\,mL} > x = 42.5 \rightarrow 36\%(w/w) = 42.5\%(w/v)$$

Example 2:

Calculate the volume occupied by the container volume of 21.2 grams of a toothpaste if the density = 0.94.

Answer:

$$\frac{21.2\ grams}{0.94\ \frac{gram}{mL}} = 22.6\ mL$$

1.4.4.2 *Force*

The force exerted on a body is equal to its mass multiplied by the acceleration achieved as a result of that force:

Force = mass × acceleration

Now can you derive the units of force in the cgs system, given that the units of acceleration are cm/s^2 in the cgs system? Also, can you derive the units in the SI system?

The weight of a body is equal to the force exerted on that body due to gravity. The weight of a substance with a mass of 1 g is therefore equal to

Weight = 1 g × 981 cm/sec^2 = 981 g cm/sec^2, or 981 dynes

However, it is a common practice to express weight in the units of mass (g) for convenience.

1.4.4.3 *Pressure*

Pressure is the force applied per unit area and is expressed as dynes per cm^2. Its cgs units are

(g cm/sec^2)/cm^2 = g/(cm sec^2).

1.4.4.4 *Work, Energy, and Heat*

When you apply a force on a body and move it for a certain distance, you do work. Work is defined as force × distance, and its cgs units are dynes cm, or ergs. Another commonly used unit for work is joules (J), which is equal to 10^7 ergs, and is the SI unit of work. Energy is the capacity to do work and has the same unit as work.

Heat and work are equivalent forms of energy, and their units are interchangeable. The cgs unit of heat is the calorie and is equal to 4.184 J.

1.5. CONCLUSIONS

This chapter reviewed the basic mathematical concepts frequently used in the practice of pharmacy and introduced the basic concepts of graphical data representation, interpretation, and analysis for finding linear regression. Moreover, the system of units, their interconversion, and dimensional analysis are invaluable in pharmacy calculations. We hope that the concepts presented in this chapter will help students in interpreting literature data more efficiently and that they will find it a handy tool while doing calculations for dispensing prescriptions.

CASE STUDIES

Case 1.1

The USP monograph states, "Pravastatin sodium contains not less than 90.0 percent and not more than 110.0 percent of the labeled amount of pravastatin sodium ($C_{23}H_{35}NaO_7$)." The chemical analysis of a pravastatin sodium 80 mg tablet found it to contain 71.9 mg of the chemical. Does it comply with the USP standard?

Approach: No, it does not comply with the USP standard because 71.9 mg is 89.9% of the labeled amount. The USP standard is not less than 90.0%, which means 90.1% or 90.2% is an acceptable amount, but not 89.9%.

Case 1.2

A physician in a hospital wrote a prescription for 342.45 mg of theophylline in 250 ml of 5% dextrose solution. The pharmacy department of the hospital compounded an intravenous solution containing 340 mg of theophylline per 250 ml 5% dextrose solution. The prescribing physician thought that his prescription was not accurately dispensed and returned the compounded theophylline admixture. How would you resolve this situation?

Approach: The computer program used in calculation of dose generates data consisting of three or more digits after the decimal point, which happened in this instance. If the pharmacy department dispensed 340 mg of the drug instead of 342.45 mg, that amount is acceptable because the error introduced is well below the acceptable limit of 5%. The compounding pharmacist should resolve this issue by patiently and professionally explaining the concept of significant figures and the realistic precision expected during measurement of ingredient(s) for intravenous fluids.

Case 1.3

A prescription with a dose of 2 mg/kg was written for a 66 lb patient. The pharmacy technician calculated the dose and forgot the right conversion (1 kg = 2.2 lb). Instead, the technician used a wrong conversion factor of 1 kg = 2 lb. As the pharmacist in charge, you are supposed to inform the technician regarding her mistake and find out whether the error is within the acceptable limit of ±5%.

Approach: You know that 66 lb should be 66/2.2 = 30 kg.

The actual dose = 30 × 2 = 60 kg × mg/kg = 60 mg.

The wrong dose calculated by the technician = 66/2.0 = 33 kg. The calculated dose = 33 × 2 = 66 mg.

% Error = (66 − 60)/60 × 100 = (6/60) × 100 = 10%

This error is higher than 5% of the allowed limit and is *not* an acceptable calculation.

References

[1] <http://www.hgh-pro.com/hormones.html> Normal hormone level, [accessed on 01.06.2013].

[2] <http://bionumbers.hms.harvard.edu/search.aspx?task=searchbyamaz> Amazing BioNumbers, [accessed on 01.06.2013].

[3] Ma JKH, Hadzija BW. Basic physical pharmacy. Burlington, MA, USA: Jones & Bartlett Learning; 2013. p. 53

[4] Brecht EA. Pharmaceutical measurements. In: Sprowls JB, Dittert LW, editors. Sprowls' American pharmacy: an introduction to pharmaceutical techniques and dosage forms. 7th ed. Philadelphia: Lippincott; 2008. p. 511. 1974, digitized 2008

[5] Bolton S. *Pharmaceutical statistics: practical and clinical applications.* 2nd ed. New York: Marcel Dekker, Inc.; 1990.

[6] United States Pharmacopenia 36 General Chapter 41: Weights and Balances, p. 53.

CHAPTER

2

Physical States and Thermodynamic Principles in Pharmaceutics

Vivek S. Dave[1], *Seon Hepburn*[2] *and Stephen W. Hoag*[2]
[1]St. John Fisher College, Wegmans School of Pharmacy, Rochester, NY USA
[2]University of Maryland, School of Pharmacy, Baltimore, MD, USA

CHAPTER OBJECTIVES

- Define atoms, molecules, elements, and compounds, and discuss their roles in the composition of matter.
- Explain the binding forces between molecules.
- Define gaseous state and describe the kinetic theory of gas.
- Analyze various gas laws and interpret the liquefaction of gases.
- Discuss supercritical fluids and apply this discussion in explaining aerosols and the implantable infusion pump.
- Define the liquid state and explain vapor pressure and boiling of a liquid.
- Apply the Clausius–Clapeyron equation, Raoult's law, and Henry's law for explaining the behavior and properties of a liquid state.
- Define solid state and discuss amorphous and crystalline solids.
- Interpret the significance of polymorphism, dissolution, wetting, and solid dispersion in pharmacy.
- Define the basic terminology used in thermodynamics.
- Discuss laws of thermodynamics and their application in explaining protein stability and spontaneity of the transport phenomenon.

Keywords

- First law of thermodynamics
- Gas
- Liquid
- Physical states of matter
- Second law of thermodynamics
- Solid
- Thermodynamics

2.1. INTRODUCTION

This chapter is divided into two parts: the first part deals with the nature of matter, and the second part deals with the thermodynamics of pharmaceutical systems. The goal of this chapter is to introduce the scientific principles you need to understand how and why pharmaceutical dosage forms work and what kinds of problems a dispensing pharmacist can encounter when working with pharmaceutical products and how to solve these problems.

2.2. COMPOSITION OF MATTER

Matter can be defined as anything that has a mass and a volume. The mass of matter is generally determined by its inertia or its resistance to change in acceleration when in motion or at rest. One common way

Pharmaceutics. DOI: http://dx.doi.org/10.1016/B978-0-12-386890-9.00002-9

of defining this is to consider the acceleration when an external force is applied to a mass. The acceleration of matter is described by Newton's second law of motion and expressed by

$$F = ma \tag{2.1}$$

Thus, a greater mass will have a slower acceleration for the same applied force. The volume of matter is determined by the space it occupies in three dimensions. Almost all matter is composed of atoms, also called atomic matter. There are forces between the atoms and molecules that make up matter, and the nature of these forces dictate some of the important properties of matter.

One of the most important concepts is to understand the state of matter and the properties associated with each state. When dispensing tablets or capsules, the things you have to worry about are very different from that when you are dispensing a solution, emulsion, or suspension. Because every prescription should have storage conditions listed on the packaging, this knowledge will affect how you label every prescription. For example, everyone knows tablets and capsules should not be stored in the same bathroom where the patient likes to take hot and steamy showers, but how about cough syrup? The goal of the following sections is to give you the scientific principles to answer these questions so that you can better counsel patients and advise physicians. The key concepts you need to understand are the states of matter, the properties associated with each state, and where these properties come from.

2.3. FORCES OF ATTRACTION AND REPULSION

Molecules interact with each other via the forces of *attraction* and *repulsion*. Attractive forces are of two types: *cohesive* forces and *adhesive* forces. The forces of attraction between molecules of the same substance are known as *cohesive* forces. The forces of attraction between the molecules of different substances are known as *adhesive* forces. The forces that act on molecules to push them apart are known as *repulsive* forces.

Consider two atoms that start far apart and come together. As they approach each other, a combination of attractive and repulsive forces act on the two atoms. The attractive forces act to pull the molecules closer. Attractive forces (F_A) are inversely proportional to the distance separating the molecules (r), as shown by the relationship

$$F_A \propto \frac{1}{r^n} \tag{2.2}$$

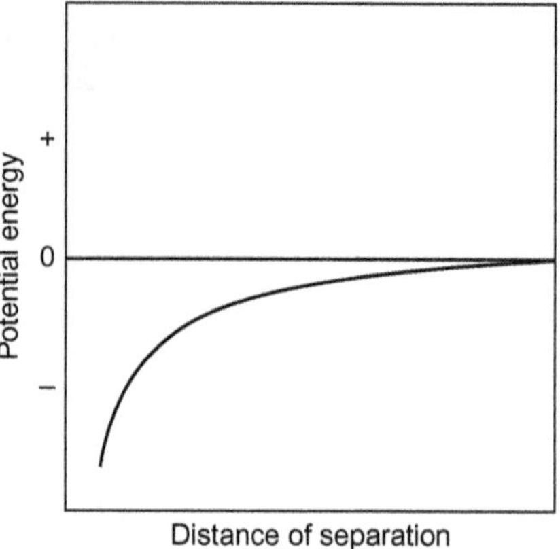

FIGURE 2.1 Potential energy diagram as a function of separation distance for attractive forces.

where n varies with the type of atoms/molecules [1]. For example, n typically equals ≈ 6, but for some gases such as nitrogen $n \approx 7$. These forces arise from the Van der Waals or dispersion forces, which are described later. Using Eq. 2.2, one can represent the force of attraction between atoms/molecules as a function of the distance between them using a potential energy diagram, as shown in Figure 2.1. As the attractive forces increase, the potential energy becomes increasingly negative. From this curve, you can see several important characteristics. First, as the atoms or molecules get close together, the attractive forces increase very rapidly; and second, the magnitude of the attractive forces act over a range of atomic distances, and it requires close proximity for the forces to affect molecular behavior.

If the overlap of the electron cloud is small, the long-range component of attractive forces is significant. Conversely, when the molecules come close enough that their electron clouds interact, the short-range component of the attractive forces dominate (see Figure 2.2).

However, as you bring the atoms or molecules very close together, the electron clouds start to overlap, which leads to very strong repulsive forces. The repulsive forces (F_R) are proportional to an exponential relationship with the reciprocal of the distance separating the molecules (r) as follows:

$$F_R \propto e^{1/r} \tag{2.3}$$

For repulsive forces, an exponential function changes more rapidly on the potential energy diagram (see Figure 2.3). As the repulsive forces increase, the potential energy becomes increasingly positive. Compared to repulsive forces, attractive forces act over a longer distance.

The total force on two atoms or molecules as a function of distance is given by the sum of the attractive

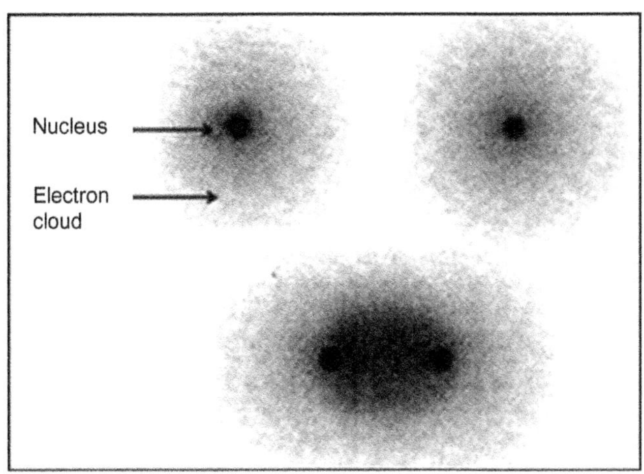

FIGURE 2.2 Overlapping electron clouds.

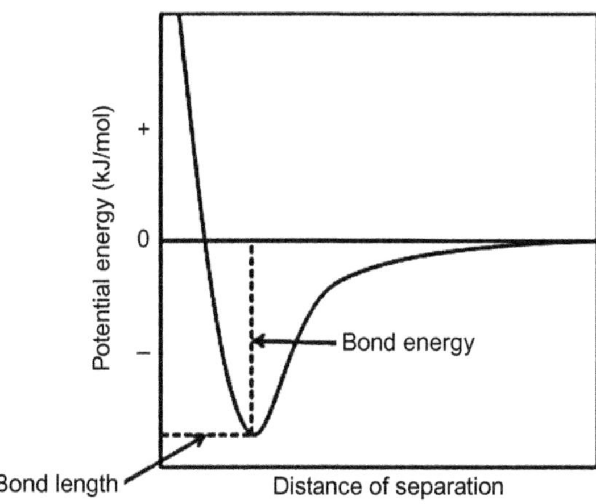

FIGURE 2.4 The total potential energy diagram of two atoms or molecules.

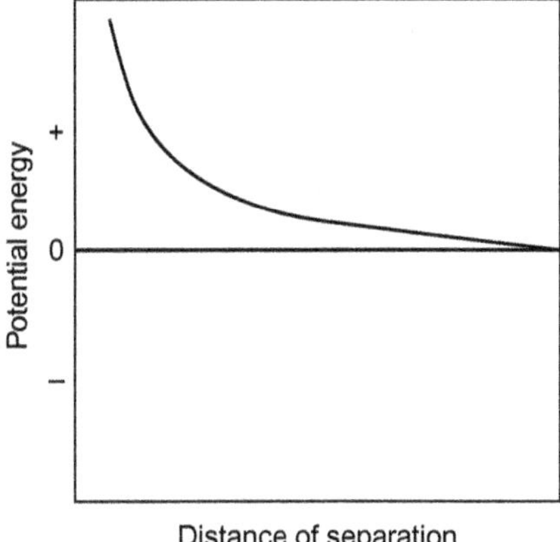

FIGURE 2.3 Potential energy diagram for repulsive forces.

and repulsive forces; this sum is given in Figure 2.4. As two distant molecules approach each other, the energy changes are gradual and attractive to a point of minimum energy; this minimum in potential is the equilibrium or average bond length, which is the balance point between attractive and repulsive forces. After the minimum as the molecules come closer together, the energy starts rising rapidly, and repulsive forces dominate. The distance where the attractive and repulsive forces balance each other is the *collision diameter*.

It is important to distinguish between *intramolecular* and *intermolecular* bonds. *Intramolecular* bonds are forces of attraction between the atoms that hold an individual molecule together (e.g., covalent or ionic bonds). *Intermolecular* bonds are forces of attractions between a molecule and its neighboring molecule. All molecules exhibit intermolecular bonding to a certain degree. Most of these attractions are relatively weak in nature. The common types of intermolecular attractive forces can be divided in several classes. They include electrostatic forces, polarization forces, dispersion forces, and hydrogen bonding [2]. The sum of the electrostatic, polarization, and dispersion forces is often called the Van der Waals forces. Each of these classes is described in the following text.

Before discussing these forces, we need to introduce the concept of a dipole. A *dipole* is a charge separated over a range. For example, HCl has a permanent dipole:

$$\overset{\delta^+}{\mathrm{H}} - \overset{\delta^-}{\mathrm{Cl}}$$

Because H is much less electronegative than Cl, the electrons are predominantly around the Cl atom, which creates a permanent negative charge. Also, the H is electron deficient, so it has a permanent positive charge, which is separated by the bond length. Dipoles can be permanent or transient. The degree of charge separation can be quantified by calculating the dipole moment; interested readers can check out references [3] and [4].

2.3.1 Electrostatic Forces

The class of electrostatic forces includes the interactions between charged atoms and molecules such as ion-ion, ion-permanent dipole, and permanent dipole–permanent dipole. These interaction forces can be intra- and intermolecular.

One example of electrostatic interactions is an *ionic bond*, which is a type of chemical bond formed through an electrostatic attraction between two oppositely charged ions. Ionic bonds are formed between a cation, which is usually a metal, and an anion, which is usually a nonmetal. The larger the difference in electronegativity between the two atoms involved in a bond, the more ionic (polar) the bond is. An ionic bond is formed when the atom of an element (metal), whose ionization energy is low, loses an electron(s) to become a cation, and the other atom (nonmetal), with a higher electron affinity, accepts the electron(s) and becomes an anion. An ionic bond is a relatively strong bond with the bond energy > 5 kcal/mole, e.g., sodium chloride.

Ion-dipole bonds are forces that originate from the electrostatic interactions between an ion and a neutral molecule containing a permanent dipole. These interactions commonly occur when solutions of ionic compounds are dissolved in polar liquids—for example, NaCl dissolving in water. The interactions occur when a positive ion attracts the partially negative end of a neutral polar molecule or vice versa. Ion-dipole attractions become stronger as either the charge on the ion increases or as the magnitude of the dipole of the polar molecule increases. Ion-dipole interactions are relatively strong and relatively insensitive to temperature and distance. When an organic base is added to an acidic medium, an ionic salt may be formed that, if dissociable, will have increased water solubility owing to ion-dipole bonding.

Dipole-dipole forces are the forces that originate from the interaction of permanent dipoles. For example, the interaction of a Cl atom with the H of an adjacent HCl molecule looks like this:

$$\overset{\delta^+}{H} — \overset{\delta^-}{Cl} \cdots\cdots \overset{\delta^+}{H} — \overset{\delta^-}{Cl}$$

These are also known as "Keesom" forces, named after Willem Hendrik Keesom. Of the Van der Waals forces, these are relatively strong forces with the energy of attraction ~1–7 kcal/mole.

2.3.2 Polarization and Dispersion Forces

The polarization class includes the interactions between dipoles induced in a molecule by an electric field from a nearby permanent dipole, ionized molecule, or ion. The dipole-induced dipole interaction, also known as "Debye Forces," is named after Peter J. W. Debye. Dispersion forces include the interactions between atoms and molecules even if they are charge neutral and don't have permanent dipoles. Dispersion forces are electrodynamic in nature and occur when charge separation occurs in a molecule due to the random motion of elections, and this transient charge induces a dipole in an adjacent molecule. These forces, called Van der Waals forces (dispersion forces), are also known as "London forces," named after a German–American physicist Fritz London, who came up with this theory.

Polarization forces originate as a result of temporary dipoles induced in a molecule by a permanent dipole in a neighboring polar or charged molecule. As a dipole approaches a molecule, the charge attracts the opposite charge and repels the same charge, which results in the polarization of the adjacent molecule, and this polarization leads to an electrostatic interaction between the two molecules:

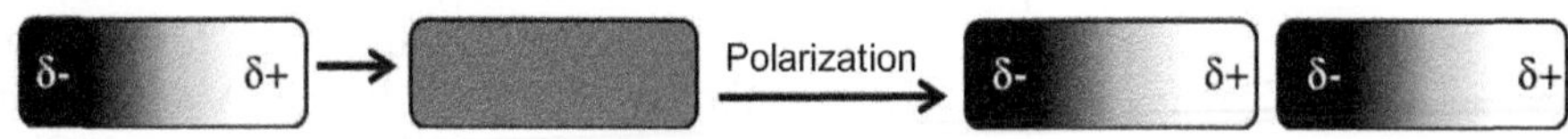

These interactions are relatively weak with the energy of attraction ~1–3 kcal/mole.

Van der Waals forces originate from *temporary dipole fluctuations*, which affect electron distributions in adjacent molecules. The attraction between the molecules is electrical in nature. In an electrically symmetrical molecule like hydrogen, there doesn't seem to be any electrical distortion to produce positive or negative parts, but that's only true on average.

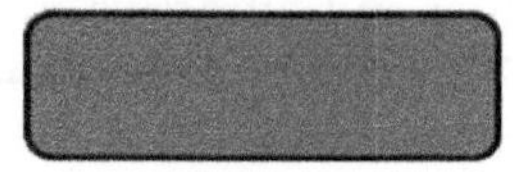

The preceding diagram represents a small symmetrical molecule of hydrogen (H_2). The even shading shows that on average there is no electrical distortion or polarization. But the electrons are mobile, and at any given moment, they might position themselves toward one end of the molecule, making that end δ−. The other end will be temporarily devoid of electrons and become δ+. A moment later the electrons may well move to the other end, reversing the polarity of the molecule, as illustrated here:

This constant motion of the electrons in the molecule results in rapidly fluctuating dipoles even in the most symmetrical molecule. Imagine a molecule that has a temporary polarity being approached by a molecule that happens to be entirely nonpolar just at that moment:

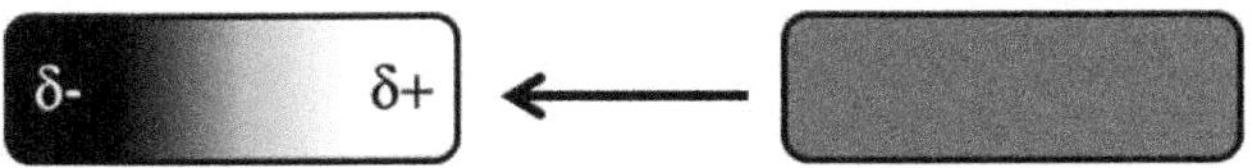

As the molecule on the right approaches, its electrons tend to be attracted by the slightly positive end of the molecule on the left. This sets up an induced dipole in the neighboring molecule, which is oriented in such a way that the δ+ end of one is attracted to the δ− end of the other:

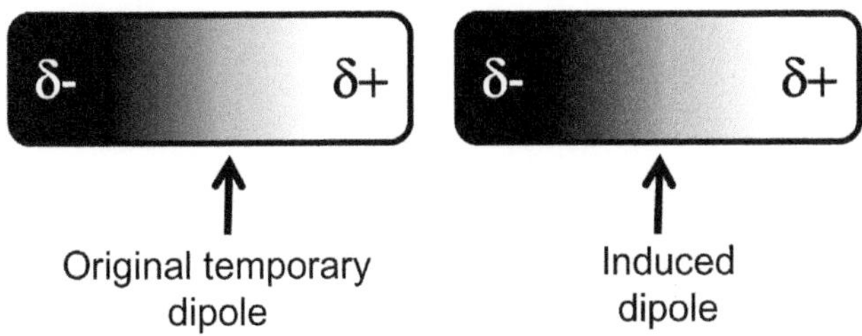

A moment later the electrons in the left molecule may move up the other end. In doing so, they repel the electrons in the molecule at the right:

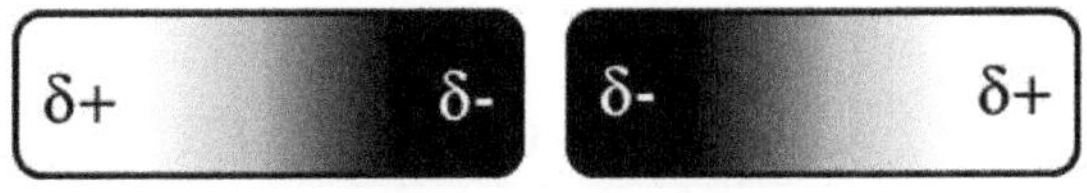

For groups of molecules, these random fluctuations result in attractive forces that hold the molecules together:

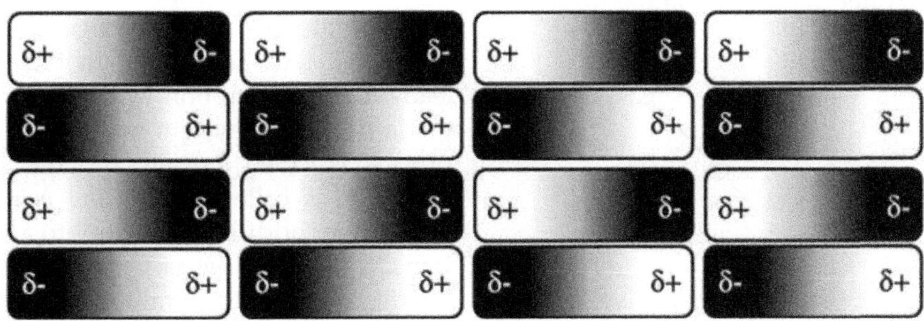

These forces between molecules are much weaker than the covalent bonds within molecules. It is difficult to give an exact value, because the extent of the attraction varies considerably with the size of the molecule and its shape. Some of the main characteristics of these forces are as follows:

- Van der Waals forces are extremely weak; i.e., the typical bond energies range from 0.5 to 1.0 kcal/mole for each atom involved.
- They are temperature dependent; i.e., with increasing temperatures, the attractive forces diminish significantly.
- They occur at very short distances; i.e., they require tight packing of molecules.
- Steric factors influence the attraction; e.g., branching in molecules significantly decreases attraction.
- These forces commonly occur in lipophilic materials and are relatively less significant in aqueous systems.

Despite being relatively weak in nature, Van der Waals forces may play an important role in pharmaceutical systems. An important implication of these forces is observed in the "flocculation" and "deflocculation" phenomena commonly observed in pharmaceutical suspensions [5]. The presence of Van der Waals forces between the suspended particles results in the formation of loose agglomerates, or "floccules," which rapidly settle down upon standing but are easily redispersible upon shaking. Conversely, if the repulsive forces predominate, the suspended particles do not flocculate but remain as discrete entities. These particles are slower to settle on standing; however, once settled, they form a relatively denser mass in a process commonly known as "caking," which is difficult to redisperse.

2.3.3 Hydrogen Bonds

Hydrogen bonds are stronger and an important form of dipole-dipole interactions. Hydrogen bonding originates when at least one dipole contains electropositive hydrogen. The bond exhibits an electrostatic attraction of a hydrogen atom for a strongly electronegative atom such as oxygen, nitrogen, fluoride. Because hydrogen atoms are so small, they can get very close to the

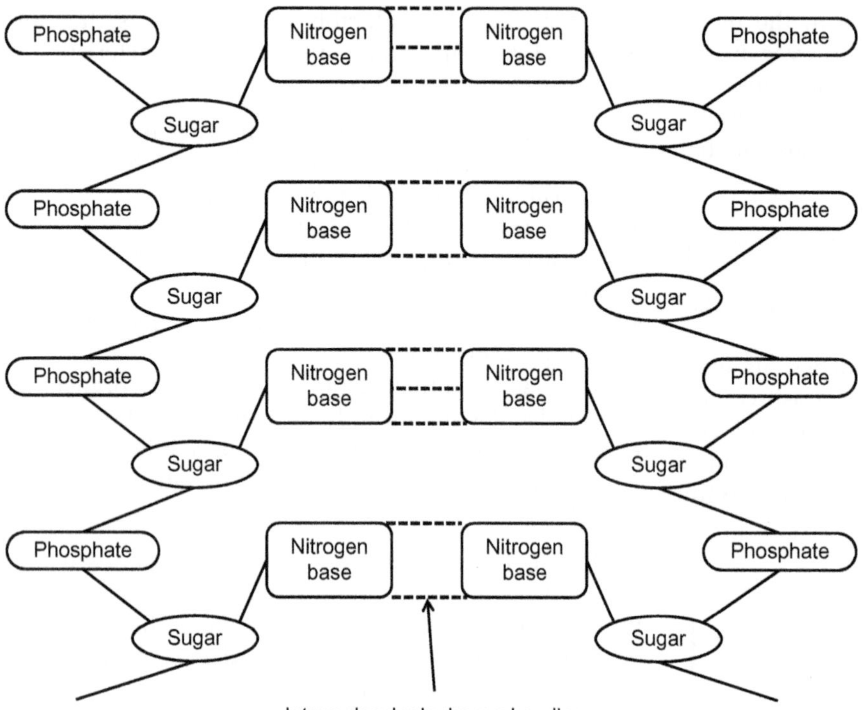

FIGURE 2.5 Hydrogen bonding between DNA standards.

electronegative atom; and in strong hydrogen bonds, the hydrogen bond is partly covalent in nature, as the electron of the hydrogen atom is delocalized to the electronegative atom. Hydrogen bonds can be inter- or intramolecular in nature. A common example of intermolecular hydrogen bonding is that observed between water molecules as discussed in the following paragraphs.

An example of intramolecular hydrogen bonding is a DNA molecule, where the nitrogen bases from the two strands are joined by intramolecular hydrogen bonds (see Figure 2.5). The hydrogen bonding between nitrogen bases is critical to DNA structure and is important to DNA translation and replication.

For an example of intermolecular hydrogen bonding, consider two or more water molecules coming together:

The δ^+ hydrogen of one molecule is strongly attracted to the lone pair of electrons on the oxygen of other molecule. It is not a covalent bond, but the attraction is significantly stronger than a typical dipole-dipole interaction. Hydrogen bonds have about a 1/10th of the strength of an average covalent bond, and are being constantly broken and reformed in water. The energy of hydrogen bonding is 1.0–10 kcal/mole for each interaction. Each water molecule can potentially form four hydrogen bonds with surrounding water molecules. This is why the boiling point of water is high for its molecular size.

2.4. STATES OF MATTER

The three primary states or phases of matter are *gases*, *liquids*, and *solids* (see Figure 2.6). In the solid state, molecules, atoms, and ions are held in close proximity by *intermolecular*, *interatomic*, and *ionic* forces. Atoms exhibit *restricted oscillations* in a fixed position within a solid. With an increase in temperature, the atoms acquire sufficient energy to overcome the forces that hold them in the solid lattice, which leads to the disruption of the ordered arrangement of the lattice as the system moves into a liquid state. This process is called *melting*, and the temperature of this transition is called the *melting point* of the substance. The further addition of energy to a liquid results in the transition into a *gaseous* state. This process is called *boiling*, and the temperature of this transition is called the *boiling point*.

Occasionally, some solids (particularly those with high vapor pressures, e.g., carbon dioxide) can pass directly from the solid to the gaseous state without melting. This process is called *sublimation*. The reverse

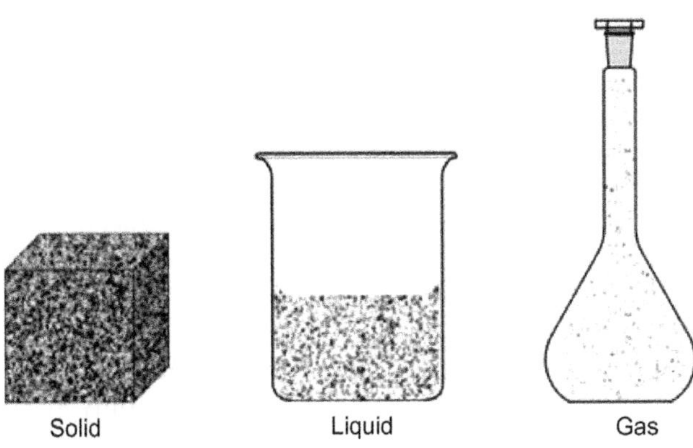

FIGURE 2.6 The different states of matter.

process, i.e., from gaseous to solid state, is called *deposition*. Note that a *phase* is defined as a homogeneous physically distinct portion of a system that is separated from the other portions of the system by bounding surfaces. For example, ice in water is an example of two phases—a solid and a liquid. You can also have phases of the same state; for example, you can have an oil and water emulsion in which you have two phases—an oil phase and a water phase—both in the liquid state. These concepts are discussed in more detail later in Section 2.5 on thermodynamics.

Under certain conditions, substances can exhibit an in-between phase known as *mesophase* (Greek: *mesos* = middle) as shown in the phase diagram in Figure 2.7. Commonly observed mesophase states include *liquid crystals* and *supercritical fluids*. *Liquid crystals* are a state of matter that has properties between those of a conventional liquid and those of a solid crystal. *Supercritical fluids* occur when a substance is at a temperature and pressure above their *critical point* or at the *triple point* because there are three phases in equilibrium at this point. When a material is in the supercritical fluid state, there is not a distinct liquid or gas phase, and the system has properties of both gas and liquid. One unique property of supercritical fluids is that gases like CO_2 can have properties similar to a solvent, and the solvent properties can be varied by changing the pressure and temperature. Because of this unique solvent property that can be varied, supercritical fluids have found significant importance in the pharmaceutical industry. For example, the selective extraction of pharmaceutical actives from biological sources is efficiently carried out using this approach.

2.4.1 Gaseous State

In the gaseous state, the attractive forces between the atoms or molecules are not sufficient to hold the modules in close contact, and the molecules are free to randomly move about in three dimensions (see Figure 2.6). Matter in gaseous state has the following general properties:

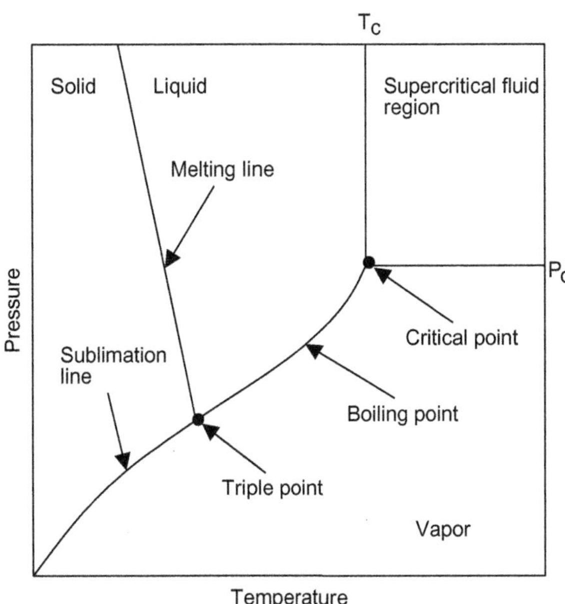

FIGURE 2.7 A typical phase diagram of a closed system in equilibrium.

- Molecules exhibiting rapid motion due to higher kinetic energy
- Molecules having weaker intermolecular forces
- Devoid of regular shape
- Capable of filling all the space in an enclosed system
- Compressible upon application of external pressure
- Mostly invisible to the human eye

The properties of matter in gaseous state can be described by the ideal gas law. The *ideal gas law* describes the behavior of an ideal gas as a function of temperature, pressure, volume, and amount of gas. The ideal gas law is derived from a combination of gas laws formulated by Boyle, Charles, and Gay-Lussac. The main assumptions in the ideal gas law derivation are

- The gas molecules are hard spheres with no intermolecular interactions between the molecules.
- Collisions between the molecules are perfectly elastic; i.e., there is no energy loss between the molecules of gas during collisions.

Boyle's law states that for one mole of an ideal gas at fixed temperature, the product of *pressure* (P) and *volume* (V) is a constant, which can be described by

$$PV = k \tag{2.4}$$

Gay-Lussac's and *Charles's laws* state that the volume and absolute *temperature* (T) of a given mass of gas at constant pressure are directly proportional, as given by the following relationship:

$$V \propto T \tag{2.5}$$

$$V = kT \tag{2.6}$$

Combining both laws gives

$$\frac{P_1V_1}{T_1} = \frac{P_2V_2}{T_2} \tag{2.7}$$

From the preceding equation, one can assume that PV/T is constant and can be mathematically expressed as

$$\frac{PV}{T} = R \quad \text{or} \quad PV = RT \tag{2.8}$$

where R is the constant value for an ideal gas. However, this equation assumes there is *only* one mole of gas. For n moles of an ideal gas, the equation becomes

$$PV = nRT \tag{2.9}$$

This equation is known as the *ideal gas law*. The constant R in the equation of state is also known as the *molar gas constant*; and for an ideal gas, its value is calculated to be $8.314\ \text{J K}^{-1}\text{mol}^{-1}$, $0.08206\ \text{L atm K}^{-1}\text{mol}^{-1}$, or $1.986\ \text{cal K}^{-1}\text{mol}^{-1}$. Since it relates the specific conditions or state (pressure, volume, and temperature of a given mass of gas), it is also called the *equation of state* of an ideal gas; see Section 2.5 on thermodynamics for more discussion about state equations. Because *real gases* do interact and exchange energy during collisions, they deviate from this law at higher pressures, i.e., when the concentration of gas molecules becomes higher and the closer proximity of gas molecules increase the chances of molecules interacting.

The ideal gas law can be used to determine the molecular weight of a gas by expressing n in terms of mass and molecular weight (M_W). Thus, when g/M_W (gram/molecular weight) is substituted for n and the equation is rearranged, the molecular weight can be calculated as

$$M_W = \frac{gRT}{PV} \tag{2.10}$$

The ideal gas law, just described, is a macroscopic law that only depends on macroscopic properties such as pressure, volume, and temperature. An alternative approach is to derive the macroscopic behavior of ideal gases from atomic/molecular properties. This theory is often called the *kinetic molecular theory*. The theory is based on postulates about the movement of atoms or molecules, and uses statistical concepts to calculate macroscopic behavior of gases and other materials. The important postulates of the theory include the following:

- A gas consists of a collection of particles that are in continuous, random motion, in straight lines and following Newton's laws.
- In a confined space, the volume of gas molecules is negligible compared to the total volume of the space (this can happen only at low pressures and high temperatures).
- The particles of gas move with complete independence, without much interaction (only at low pressures).
- Collisions between molecules are perfectly elastic; i.e., there is no exchange of energy during collisions.
- In addition to potential energy, particles have *kinetic energy*, which is responsible for their rapid, random motion.

The *kinetic molecular theory* states that the average kinetic energy of a mole of gas molecules is proportional to absolute temperature:

$$(1/2)M_Wv^2 = (3/2)kT \tag{2.11}$$

where the proportionality constant k is called the Boltzmann constant and is calculated by dividing the gas constant (R) by Avogadro's constant (N_A). The temperature T is the absolute temperature in K. Rearranging the equation to calculate the linear velocity (v) in m/s gives

$$v = \sqrt{\frac{3RT}{M_W}} \tag{2.12}$$

For a system of molecules, if you average all the individual molecular energies as given by Eq. 2.11, there is a distribution of energies. This distribution is called the Maxwell–Boltzmann distribution and is pictured in Figure 2.8. This figure illustrates several important concepts that help you better understand pharmaceutical systems. In particular, there is a wide range of molecular energies with no molecules having zero energy, and there is no upper limit to the energy a molecule can have, but the Maxwell–Boltzmann distribution drops off exponentially as the energy increases, so there are very few molecules at the high end of the distribution. Also, as the temperature increases, the entire distribution shifts to a higher average energy level.

The Maxwell–Boltzmann distribution is at the heart of the Arrhenius equation and accelerated stability testing of active pharmaceutical ingredients (APIs) and drug products performed by virtually all pharmaceutical companies. These concepts are covered in more detail in Chapter 5. For example, when a chemical reaction occurs, i.e., an API breaks down, the

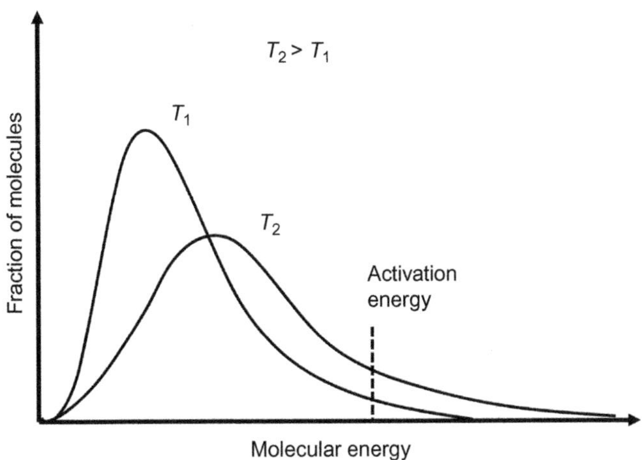

FIGURE 2.8 Maxwell–Boltzmann distribution of molecular energies.

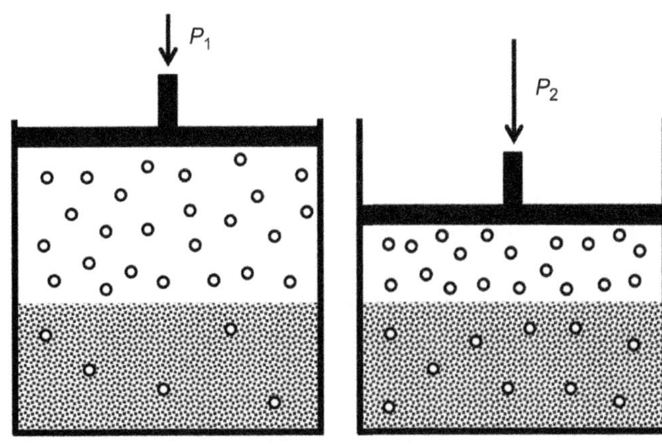

FIGURE 2.9 Illustration of Henry's law showing that as the pressure increases, the gas concentration in the liquid also increases.

molecules that are reacting must have enough energy to overcome the activation energy. As you can see in Figure 2.8, as the temperature increases, more molecules have sufficient energy to react; thus, you can test drug products at higher temperatures and extrapolate the results to lower temperatures. Also, this helps to explain why some drugs such as ampicillin suspensions need to be stored in the refrigerator. At lower temperatures far fewer molecules have enough energy to react, so the product will be more stable at cooler temperatures.

To this point, we have been describing a single pure gas, but these concepts can be extended to mixtures of gases. In a mixture of gases, each gas will contribute to the total pressure, and this individual contribution of a gas is called the *partial pressure*. From these partial pressures, the total pressure can be calculated using *Dalton's law of partial pressures*, which was developed by John Dalton in 1801. Dalton's law states that "the total pressure exerted by the mixture of non-reactive gases is equal to the sum of the partial pressures of individual gases." The partial pressure is equal to the pressure a gas would exert if that gas alone occupied the whole volume of the mixture; in other words, the gases act independently of each other, and each gas contributes to the total pressure. The total pressure of a mixture of gases can be calculated by adding the partial pressures:

$$P_{\text{total}} = P_1 + P_2 + \cdots\cdots\cdots + P_n \tag{2.13}$$

where $P_1, P_2, \cdots\cdots\cdots P_n$ are the partial pressures of each component, mathematically expressed as a summation:

$$P_{\text{total}} = \sum_{i=1}^{n} P_i \tag{2.14}$$

2.4.1.1 *Solubility of Gases in Liquids*

Most gases are soluble in liquids to some degree. The term *solubility* is a technical term that describes how much one phase, such as a liquid, can hold of another material that is in equilibrium with a different phase. For example, to make children's cough syrup, you would dissolve a drug such as dextromethorphan into the syrup, and the solubility would be the maximum amount of dextromethorphan the liquid could hold when the dextromethorphan precipitated and formed a solid phase that was in equilibrium with the liquid. Gases also exhibit similar properties when in equilibrium with a liquid phase. The solubility of gases in a liquid can be expressed using *Henry's law* of gas solubility formulated by William Henry in 1803. Henry's Law states that "at a constant temperature, the amount of a given gas that dissolves in a given type and volume of liquid is directly proportional to the partial pressure of that gas in equilibrium with that liquid." Henry's law can be mathematically expressed (at constant temperature) as

$$P_i = k_H C \tag{2.15}$$

where P_i is the partial pressure of the solute in the gas above the solution, c is the concentration of the solute, and k_H is a constant with the dimensions of pressure divided by concentration. The constant, known as the Henry's law constant, depends on the solute, the solvent, and the temperature. In other words, as you increase the pressure, the gas molecules move from the vapor phase into the liquid phase (see Figure 2.9).

2.4.2 Liquid State

In the liquid state, the attractive forces between the atoms or molecules are strong enough to hold the modules in close contact, but not strong enough to hold them in a fixed position like in a solid. The molecules are free to randomly move about in three dimensions (see Figure 2.6). Matter in liquid state has the following general properties:

- Liquids in general have a defined albeit flexible volume; i.e., liquids conveniently take the shape of the container in which they are held.
- Liquids differ from gases in having higher densities and viscosities, and not being as compressible.
- Molecules in liquids also typically have lower kinetic energy compared to those in gases.
- Liquids respond to temperature changes and may transition to a different state, i.e., solid or gas, depending on the magnitude and direction of such change.
- Liquids tend to flow readily in response to external forces, and the flow behavior is influenced by internal/external resistance, e.g., friction and viscosity.

2.4.2.1 *Vapor Pressure*

An important property of liquids is vapor pressure, and vapor pressure is a characteristic property of a material. *Vapor pressure* or *equilibrium vapor pressure* is defined as the pressure exerted by a vapor in equilibrium with a liquid at a given temperature in a closed system. Solids can also have vapor pressures, but they are much lower than liquids. The vapor pressure is the macroscopic expression of a molecule's tendency to escape from the liquid (or a solid), and this is related to the rate of evaporation of a liquid. Volatile substances are materials with a relatively higher vapor pressure at room temperature.

Because vapor pressure is a measure of a molecule's escaping tendency from a liquid or solid, it depends on temperature but does not depend on the amount of liquid, atmospheric pressure, or presence of other vapors. Molecules in the liquid state have a wide range of kinetic energies (see Figure 2.8), and only the molecules with the highest energy will escape into the gaseous phase. Also, some of the molecules in the gaseous phase that collide with the liquid will remain in the liquid state; this process is called *condensation*. If a liquid is placed in a closed vacuum chamber at constant temperature, initially the liquid will rapidly evaporate. As the amount of vaporized liquid in the gaseous state increases, the rate of condensation will increase until the rate of condensation and vaporization are equal, i.e., are in a state of equilibrium. This equilibrium vapor pressure is known as the *saturation vapor pressure* above a liquid. The vapor pressure of a liquid is proportional to the temperature of the system, and one way it can be measured is with a mercury manometer. In this case, the units are mm Hg.

The relationship between vapor pressure and the absolute temperature of a liquid is expressed by the *Clausius–Clapeyron equation*:

$$In\left(\frac{VP_2}{VP_1}\right) = \frac{-\Delta H_v}{2.3R}\left(\frac{1}{T_2T_1}\right) \quad (2.16)$$

where VP_1 and VP_2 are the equilibrium vapor pressures of a liquid at temperatures T_1 and T_2, respectively; and ΔH_v is the heat of vaporization. The heat, or enthalpy, is discussed in more detail in Section 2.5 on thermodynamics. This equation can also be expressed as

$$VP_2 = VP_1e^{\frac{-\Delta H_v}{2.3R}\left(\frac{1}{T_2T_1}\right)} \quad (2.17)$$

Figure 2.10 shows the relationship between the vapor pressure of a liquid and its temperature for several different liquids. As you can see in Figure 2.10 and Eq. 2.17, this relationship is exponential, and the vapor pressure increases much faster than the temperature. Note that in the equation and graphs we assume that ΔH_v is independent of temperature. The Clausius–Clapeyron equation is useful to scientists because you can calculate the enthalpy of vaporization from a plot of the log of *VP vs T*. (Recall that with logs if you get rid of the negative sign in Eq. 2.16, the *T* moves to the numerator.) For example, if the vapor pressure of water at room temperature is ~20 mm Hg, when heated to 100°C the vapor pressure increases to 760 mm Hg and water vaporizes. The heat of

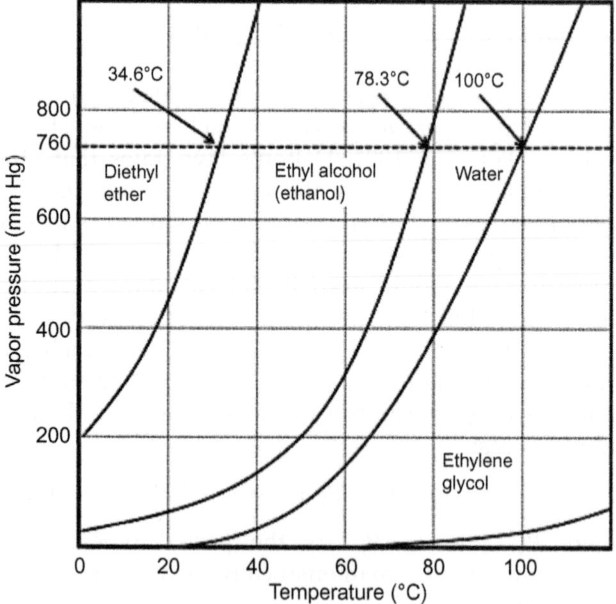

FIGURE 2.10 Interrelationship between the temperature and vapor pressure of common liquids.

vaporization (ΔH_v) of water at 100° is 9720 cal/mole. The Clausius–Clapeyron equation is also useful because it can help you to understand the behavior of liquids. For liquids with a positive enthalpy of vaporization (which is true for virtually all liquids), as the temperature increases, the vapor pressure will increase exponentially until the boiling point is reached.

The *boiling point* is the temperature at which the vapor pressure of a liquid equals the atmospheric pressure. At this point the molecules in the liquid have enough energy to escape into the vapor phase, and because these molecules have the same pressure as the external vapor phase, when they escape, the gas bubbles that are formed do not collapse because they have the same pressure as the external pressure. From a molecular point of view, the gas molecules escape into the vapor phase because they have enough energy to overcome the attractive forces of the liquid. One consequence of this process is the lower the external pressure above a liquid, the lower the boiling point.

The vapor pressure of a system in equilibrium with a multicomponent solution is an important parameter that can be predicted from the composition of the liquid phase. The method for these calculations was developed in 1882 by François-Marie Raoult and is known as *Raoult's law*, which states that "at equilibrium, the vapor pressure of an ideal solution is dependent on the vapor pressure of each chemical component and the mole fraction of the component present in the solution." It can be mathematically expressed as

$$P = P_A^* x_A + P_B^* x_B + \cdots\cdots\cdots + P_i^* x_i \quad (2.18)$$

The individual vapor pressure of each component can be given as

$$P_i = P_i^* x_i \quad (2.19)$$

where P_i is the partial pressure of the ith component, P^*_i is the vapor pressure of the pure component i, and x_i is the mole fraction of component i. This law assumes an ideal solution in which the intermolecular forces are the same for all molecules.

Vapor pressure is an important colligative property in pharmaceutical products. A classic example is that of nitroglycerine, which has a vapor pressure of ~0.00025 mm at 20° and ~0.30 mm at 93°. Because of the high vapor pressure, nitroglycerine has a tendency to diffuse out of tablets and vaporize. This results in a significant loss of the drug and consequently the potency of the product. To lower the vapor pressure and volatility, nitroglycerin is commonly formulated along with macromolecules such as polyethylene glycol (PEG), polyvinylpyrrolidone (PVP), and microcrystalline cellulose (MCC); also, nitroglycerine tablets are stored in air-tight packaging. Because of the high volatility of nitroglycerine, it is important to counsel patients not to remove the tablets from the packaging until they actually use the tablets.

2.4.3 Phase Equilibria and the Phase Rule

The three phases (solids, liquids, and gaseous) are generally considered individually. However, in most systems, the phases coexist, e.g., a glass of ice water. The amount of each phase present depends on several variables such as temperature, pressure, type of system (e.g., enclosed), composition. Changes in any of these variables may influence the equilibrium of all the phases. To understand and describe the state of each phase, and its relationship to the other phases, you can use the phase rule. The *phase rule* was developed by J. Willard Gibbs in 1870. The rule can be used to determine the least number of *intensive variables* (see the thermodynamic section for a definition) that can be changed without changing the equilibrium state of the system. This critical number of variables that can be varied is called the *degrees of freedom F*; the Gibbs phase rule is given by

$$F = C - P + 2 \quad (2.20)$$

where C is the number of components and P is the number of phases. At first glance, this equation seems very odd, but a few examples should illustrate the equation and the insights it can give to pharmaceutical systems. For example, a system containing water and its vapor is a two-phase system. A mixture of ice, water, and water vapor is a three-phase system. The term *component* is defined as a distinct chemical substance in the system. For example, a mixture of ice, water, and water vapor is a one-component system, i.e., H_2O. A mixture of ethanol and water is a two-component system.

To illustrate the phase rule, consider a closed gaseous system of pure water vapor. For this system, you can calculate the degrees of freedom, $F = 1 - 1 + 2 = 2$. This answer makes sense if you look at the ideal gas law (Eq. 2.9); you can see that if you know any two variables T, P, or V, you know the third variable and can completely describe the state of the system. Recall a closed system means that there is no mass exchange with the environment and n can't change; however, according to the phase rule, you don't need to assume that n is constant, but then the argument becomes more complex and beyond the scope of this discussion. The two degrees of freedom means two variables are needed to describe this system; i.e., you must fix two variables, such as T and P, to know the state of the system. Also, you know that two variables can change, and the equilibrium will be still of the same character as long as another phase does not form.

Another example would be ice and water in equilibrium. The degrees of freedom would be $F = 1 - 2 + 2 = 1$. When there are two phases present, you have a more constrained system, and you need only one variable such as T or P to be able to describe the state of the system. At the triple point of water (see Figure 2.7), three phases are present, hence $F = 0$ (from Figure 2.7). This makes sense because there is only one triple point for a substance; i.e., at the triple point of a single component system, there is only one T and P where all phases can coexist in equilibrium.

An example of a two-component system is an ointment that can be applied to the skin. If a small amount of betamethasone is incorporated into an ointment base such as petrolatum, initially there would be a single phase system, but as the amount of betamethasone increased, eventually its solubility would be reached, and it would precipitate in the petrolatum, forming two phases. The degrees of freedom would be as follows:

$$\textbf{1 phase: } F = 2 - 1 + 2 = 3$$
$$\textbf{2 phases: } F = 2 - 2 + 2 = 2$$

Thus, for the single-phase ointment, the system could be completely described by T, P, and composition; and for the two-phase ointment, you would need only two variables such as T and P. In a clinical setting, the patient's skin is a constant temperature, and the atmospheric pressure doesn't vary much. Therefore, in the single-phase ointment base, the betamethasone concentration could vary; whereas in the two-phase system, there are zero degrees of freedom, and the betamethasone concentration can't vary as long as two phases are present. When it comes to diffusion, the release rate of a system with a fixed API concentration is very different from a system in which the API concentration can vary. See Chapter 5 for details.

2.4.4 Solid State

In a solid state, the attractive forces between atoms or molecules are sufficient to hold the molecules in close contact and often in a particular location within a crystal lattice (see Figure 2.6). As a consequence of these interactions, matter in solid state has the following general properties:

- When a force is applied to a solid, it has a fixed shape; i.e., it will not deform or flow without limit like a liquid or gas that can flow without limit.
- They are nearly incompressible.
- They have strong intermolecular forces and very little kinetic energy.

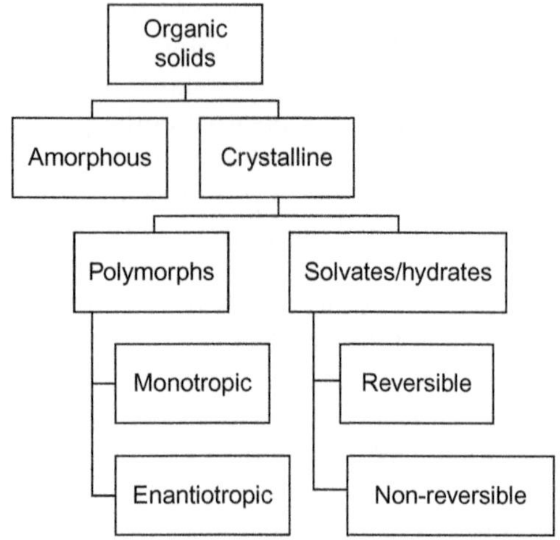

FIGURE 2.11 Classification of organic solids based on atomic/molecular morphology.

- Atoms in a solid vibrate about a fixed position and have very little translational motion.
- They are characterized by shape, size, and melting point and a few have sublimation points.
- Pharmaceutically relevant characteristics include surface energy, hardness, elastic properties, and compactability.

Organic solids can be broadly classified by the system; see Figure 2.11.

2.4.4.1 *Crystalline Solids*

Crystalline solids are substances whose constituent atoms, molecules, or ions are arranged in an ordered three-dimensional pattern. A key aspect of the ordered structure of a crystalline solid is the *unit cell*, which is the basic repeating structure of the crystal. The unit cell is the smallest group of atoms that form the basic building blocks of the crystal, and this building block is repeated to build up the crystal into a macroscopic structure. The nature of the unit cell is very important because different unit cells have different properties such as solubility, stability, and compressibility; these properties are very important for drug delivery and pharmaceutical manufacturing. In addition, the macroscopic crystals can have different geometric shapes such as plates, needles, blades (like a sword blade), prisms, and blocks. These different external shapes are called the *crystal habit*.

The unit cells of a crystal can be composed of atoms (e.g., diamond, graphite), molecules (e.g., solid carbon dioxide), or ions (sodium chloride). An important property of crystalline solids is that they have fixed melting points. For organic compounds, the molecules are often held together by Van Der Waal's forces and hydrogen bonding. These compounds exhibit relatively weak binding and low melting points. Ionic and

- **Cubic**
  - a = b = c
  - $\alpha = \beta = \gamma = 90^\circ$
- **Trigonal (rhombohedral)**
  - a = b = c
  - $\alpha = \beta = \gamma \neq 90^\circ$
- **Tetragonal**
  - a = b ≠ c
  - $\alpha = \beta = \gamma = 90^\circ$
- **Orthorhombic**
  - a ≠ b ≠ c
  - $\alpha = \beta = \gamma = 90^\circ$
- **Hexagonal**
  - a = b ≠ c
  - $\alpha = \beta = 90^\circ$
  - $\gamma = 120^\circ$
- **Monoclinic**
  - a ≠ b ≠ c
  - $a = \gamma = 90^\circ$
  - $\beta \neq 90^\circ$
- **Triclinic**
  - a ≠ b ≠ c
  - $\alpha \neq \beta \neq \gamma \neq 90^\circ$

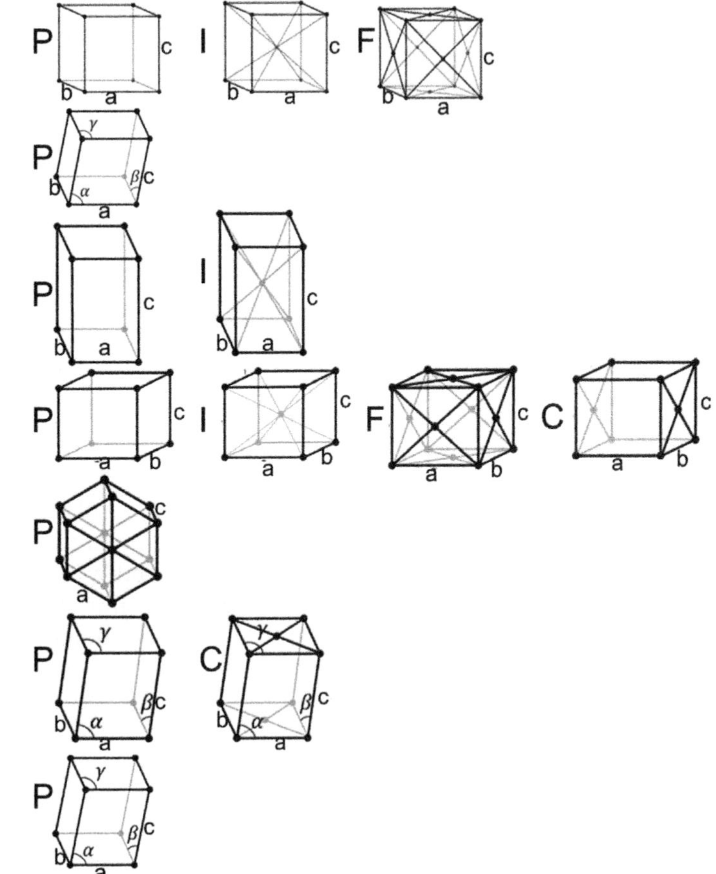

Seven crystal classes → 14 Bravais Lattices
Four types of unit cells → P = Primitive, I = Body Centered, F = Face Centered, C = Side Centered

FIGURE 2.12 The possible unit cell arrangements.

atomic crystals in general are hard and brittle and have higher melting points.

Based on the symmetry of the atomic, molecular, or ionic arrangements in the unit cell, these arrangements can be divided into seven major categories; see Figure 2.12. The key differences between the different categories are whether the unit cell is cubic or rectangular and whether the angles are 90°, acute, or obtuse (see Figure 2.12). In addition, the unit cells can be primitive (do not contain any internal atoms); body centered (contain an internal atom/molecule in the middle of the cell); face centered (contain one atom/molecule in the middle of each face); or side centered, also called base centered, (contain one atom/molecule in the center of two opposite faces) (refer to Figure 2.12).

Cubic (isometric) crystalline solids are those containing a unit cell in the shape of a cube. This is one of the most common and simplest shapes found in nature. The key dimensional characteristics are $a = b = c$ and $\alpha = \beta = \gamma = 90^\circ$. A common example of a cubic crystalline solid is sodium chloride (common table salt).

Trigonal (rhombohedral) crystals have the key dimensional characteristics $a = b = c$ and $\alpha = \beta \neq \gamma \neq 90^\circ$.

Tetragonal crystal systems can be thought of as cubic crystals stretched in one direction. The key characteristics are $a = b \neq c$ and $\alpha = \beta = \gamma = 90^\circ$. These tetragonal crystals can be either primitive or body centered. A common example of a cubic crystalline solid is urea.

Orthorhombic crystals do not have equal sides. The key dimensional characteristics are $a \neq \mathrm{b} \neq \mathrm{c}$ and $\alpha = \beta = \gamma = 90^\circ$. Orthorhombic crystals can be primitive, body centered, face centered, or side centered.

Hexagonal crystals, as the name suggests, have a hexagonal crystal lattice, and its component atoms, ions, or molecules are arranged in the shape of a hexagon. Iodoform, a disinfectant, is an example of solid that exists in hexagonal crystalline form. *Monoclinic* crystals have the component atoms, molecules, or ions form a rectangular prism with a parallelogram as its base. The key dimensional characteristics are $a \neq b \neq c$ and $\alpha = \beta = 90°$ and $\gamma \neq 90°$. They exist in two forms: primitive and base centered. Sucrose, a sugar, exists in monoclinic crystalline form. *Triclinic* crystals are arranged so that the length and the angles formed in the lattice are unequal, and it comes only in the primitive form. The key dimensional characteristics are $a \neq b \neq c$ and $\alpha \neq \beta \neq \gamma \neq 90°$. A common example of a solid existing as a triclinic crystal is boric acid.

2.4.4.2 Polymorphism and Pseudopolymorphism

Polymorphism is the ability of a solid material to exist in more than one form or crystal structure; i.e., one molecule can exist in two or more different unit cell types. Some elements may exist in more than one crystalline form, and these elements are said to be *allotropic*. For example, carbon exists in two allotropic forms: diamond and graphite. When polymorphism exists as a result of difference in crystal packing, it is called *packing polymorphism*. Polymorphism resulting from different conformers of the same molecule is called *conformational polymorphism*. Typical characteristics observed in different polymorphic forms of a compound include the following:

- Polymorphs have different thermodynamic stabilities and often different chemical stabilities.
- They can have different hygroscopicities, i.e., different propensities to absorb moisture from the atmosphere, which can indirectly affect stability.
- They may spontaneously convert from a metastable form to a more stable form.
- They generally exhibit different melting points and different enthalpies of melting; see Section 2.5 on thermodynamics for a discussion of enthalpy.
- They exhibit different X-ray diffraction patterns.
- Although they are chemically identical, they may have significantly different solubilities.
- The crystals can have different mechanical properties, which can result in different manufacturing properties such as compactability when making tablets, different propensities for particle milling, and different propensities to stick to metal machine parts.

During API production, one of the main reasons that different polymorphic forms are created is changes in the conditions used during the crystallization process. The following factors are known to cause polymorphic changes during crystallization:

- Solvent types (the packing of crystal may be different in polar and nonpolar solvents)
- Some impurities that inhibit the growth of certain polymorphic forms, which can favor the growth of a metastable polymorph
- The rate of crystallization, which can be affected by the degree of supersaturation from which a material is crystallized (generally, the higher a concentration is above the solubility, the more likely it is to create a metastable polymorph)
- Temperature at which crystallization is carried out
- Change in stirring hydrodynamics

Polymorphs can be categorized into two types, monotropes and enantiotropes, depending on their stability over a range of temperatures and pressures below the melting point. Because most pharmaceutical systems are studied at atmospheric pressure, for this discussion we will assume pressure is constant. If one of the polymorphs is the most stable over a certain temperature range, while the other polymorph is the most stable over a different temperature range below the melting point, then the substance is said to be *enantiotropic*. On the other hand, if one polymorph form is always the most stable for all temperatures below the melting point, with all the other polymorphs being less stable, then this substance is said to be *monotropic*. Knowing if a substance is enantiotropic or monotropic is very important to drug companies; if manufacturers have to heat the material during tablet coating, for example, they want to make sure that it doesn't undergo a phase transformation that will result in a less stable polymorphic form at room temperature.

Regarding *pseudopolymorphs*, during the production of pharmaceutical ingredients, they are often crystallized out of different types of solvents. During this process, occasionally solvent molecules are incorporated into the crystal lattice in a fixed stoichiometric ratio. This creates a *co-crystal*, which is termed a *solvate*, and when the solvent is water, this is termed a *hydrate*. For example, lamivudine methanol solvate (anti HIV-1) is a solid compound containing methanol and water molecules combined in a definite ratio as an integral part of the crystal structure. However, because of concerns with toxicity of many organic solvents, generally solvates are not preferred. An example of a hydrate is scopolamine HBr trihydrate USP, which has one HBr and three molecules of water associated with each scopolamine molecule (see Figure 2.13). All the previous discussion about polymorphs, such as different melting points, solubilities, and hygroscopicities, directly applies to solvates and hydrates, thus the term

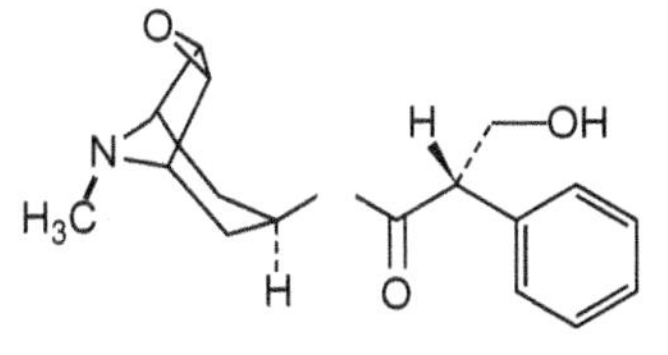

FIGURE 2.13 Structure of scopolamine HBr trihydrate.

pseudopolymorph. When you are working with an API, it is very important to know if it will form a hydrate. For example, during the process of granulation used to make granules that can be compressed into tablets, you have to add water and then remove the water. If the API forms a hydrate during granulation or loses a hydrate during drying, the properties of the API can completely change, and this could affect drug release rate via changes in solubility and stability. Plus, many other important properties of the API could change, which could lead to product to failure.

2.4.4.3 *Polymorphism in Pharmaceutical Drugs*

Most commercially available drugs are developed in the crystalline form. However, many of the drug molecules can exist in different crystal polymorphic forms. Thus, the study of polymorphism and crystallization of pharmaceutical compounds is highly important. Nowadays, research on polymorphism (polymorph screening and characterization) and material properties of active drug compounds and excipients is an integral part of the preformulation phase of drug development. The knowledge of solid-state properties in an early stage of drug development helps avoid manufacturing problems and optimize a drug's clinical performance. Drugs that were previously known to exist only in a single form are now shown to have various polymorphic forms. This has prompted pharmaceutical companies to more extensively investigate crystal polymorphism in order to optimize the physical properties of a pharmaceutical solid early in drug development. Since most drugs can exist in more than one polymorphic or pseudopolymorphic form, the importance of polymorphism in the drug development paradigm is well known and well established. To illustrate this, some classic examples are discussed here.

Acetaminophen is a widely used antipyretic (fever suppressant) and analgesic (pain killer). This drug has been shown to exist in two polymorphic forms: monoclinic Form-I (P21/n), which is marketed, and orthorhombic Form-II (Pbca) [6]. Similarly, Famotidine, a histamine H_2 receptor antagonist, is also found to exist in two different polymorphic forms: metastable polymorph B and stable polymorph A [7–10]. Piroxicam, a nonsteroidal anti-inflammatory drug (NSAID), exists in three forms: I, II and III [11,12].

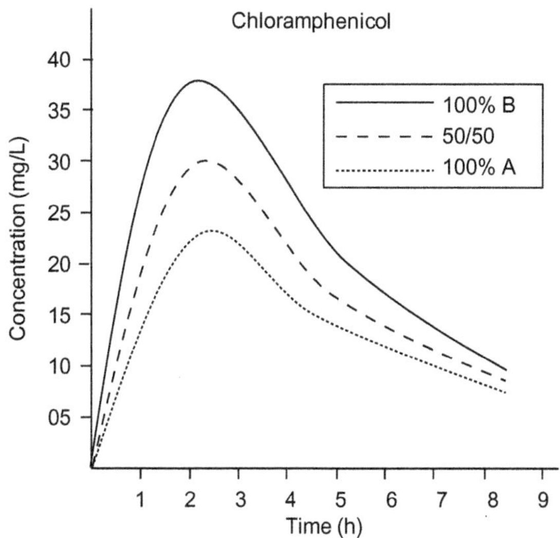

FIGURE 2.14 Hypothetical plasma profiles of polymorphs A and B of chloramphenicol from oral solid formulations.

Another important example is Ritonavir. It is a novel protease inhibitor for human immunodeficiency virus (HIV). This drug was launched in 1996 and distributed for about 18 months without issues. Later batches of the drug revealed unacceptable dissolution profiles and precipitation issues. After detailed investigations, it was found that the problem was due to conversion of the drug to a new thermodynamically more stable and less soluble polymorph Form-II. Surprisingly, multiple attempts to formulate Form-I thereafter turned out very difficult (perhaps the exact conditions could not be reproduced). The drug is now often quoted as a prime example in pharmaceutical industries to highlight the importance of polymorphism [13].

Norfloxacin is a synthetic broad-spectrum antibacterial drug for the treatment of prostate and urinary tract infections. This drug exists in two anhydrous polymorphs (A and B), an amorphous form, and several hydrate forms [14,15]. Of the two anhydrous polymorphs, Form B is the most stable at room temperature. However, the commercially used norfloxacin is Form A, which is metastable at room temperature.

As polymorphs exhibit different solubilities, for slightly soluble drugs, this may significantly influence the rate of dissolution. A classic example is that of chloramphenicol palmitate. Chloramphenicol exists as two major polymorphs (polymorph A and polymorph B) [16,17]. Figure 2.14 shows a hypothetical plasma profile of polymorphs of chloramphenicol from oral solid formulations. As a result of polymorphism, one polymorph may show better therapeutic efficacy than another polymorph of the same drug.

All these examples clearly show the importance of selecting a desired polymorphic form of a drug early on to prevent any undesired effects in the later stages of development. Usually, the most thermodynamically stable form of a drug is preferred in commercial formulations, as the metastable form may transform to other more stable forms. However, it is universally known that the metastable form has higher solubility than the stable form and that the metastable form converts into the stable form, the rate of which depends on the activation energy required for the transition (see Figure 2.8). Thus, whenever possible, metastable forms that have a higher solubility and can survive for years without changing to a more stable form are selected for formulation development. Such selection process requires careful evaluation of both thermodynamic parameters (tendency toward formation of stable polymorphs) and kinetic parameters (the rate of transformation) during product development.

2.4.4.4 Amorphous Solids

Amorphous (Greek: *a* = without, *morphé* = shape) or noncrystalline solids are solids that lack the long-range order characteristic of a crystal; i.e., they have no unit cells. They may also be considered to behave like supercooled liquids in which the molecules are arranged in a random manner as in the liquid state. They tend to flow over time, when subjected to sufficient pressure. They do not have definite melting points. Amorphous solids as well as cubic crystals are usually *isotropic;* i.e., they exhibit similar properties in all directions. Crystalline solids other than cubic are *anisotropic;* i.e., they have different properties (conductance, refractive index, etc.) in various directions along the crystal lattice. Visual differentiation between amorphous and crystalline solids is difficult. Some substances may be partially crystalline—for example, petrolatum, beeswax. The amorphous or crystalline characteristics of a solid pharmaceutical agent can influence therapeutic activity. For example, Novobiocin acid (antibiotic against *staphylococcus*) exists in both crystalline and amorphous forms. The crystalline form is poorly absorbed and exhibits no pharmacological activity, whereas the amorphous form is readily absorbed and therapeutically active.

Although amorphous solids do not have a long-range order, they are not completely random at the molecular level. At the molecular level, they may contain a short-range order and partial crystallinity. Due to their thermodynamic instability relative to crystalline solids, they may undergo partial or complete, spontaneous, or gradual conversion into a crystalline form and may even exhibit polymorphism. Many pharmaceutical materials, particularly pharmaceutical excipients, exist as multicomponent systems; i.e., they contain a ratio of amorphous and crystalline forms.

Solid-state characterization of pharmaceutical materials is an important preformulation activity and is routinely carried out during the drug-development process. Common analytical techniques used for solid-state characterization of drugs and excipients are briefly summarized here:

- Powder X-ray diffractometry (PXRD) is the most widely used technique and considered a "gold" standard for phase identification.
- Single crystal X-ray diffraction (XRD) is used to understand in-depth the structure of the crystal.
- Differential scanning calorimetry (DSC) is used to understand phase transitions and multicomponent interactions.
- Thermo gravimetric analysis (TGA) is used to analyze the stoichiometry of solvates/hydrates quantitatively.
- Infrared spectroscopy (IR) is used as a complementary tool for identification of phases, including types of water in crystals.
- Near infrared (NIR), Raman, and solid-state NMR are other techniques used to complement the characterization of pharmaceutical solids.

Using the preceding techniques, pharmaceutical solids can undergo the following phase transitions:

1. Polymorphic transitions—Interconversion between various polymorphic forms
2. Hydration/dehydration—Interconversion between hydrates and anhydrous forms of crystals
3. Vitrification and amorphous crystallization—Interconversion between the amorphous phase and crystalline polymorphs

2.4.5 The Supercritical Fluid State

A *supercritical fluid* is a mesophase formed from the gaseous state in which the gas is held under a combination of temperatures and pressures that exceed the critical point of a substance (see Figure 2.15). A gas that is brought above its *critical temperature* T_c will still behave as a gas irrespective of the applied pressure. The *critical pressure* P_c is the minimum pressure required to liquefy a gas at a given temperature.

As the pressure is raised higher, the density of the gas can increase without a significant increase in the viscosity, and the ability of the supercritical fluid to dissolve compounds increases. Gases have little or no ability to dissolve a compound under ambient conditions, but in the supercritical range, they can completely dissolve the compound. For example, CO_2 held at the same temperature can dissolve different chemical classes from a natural product source when pressure is increased. The addition of a particular gas or a solvent can improve the solubilization process. Thus, supercritical fluids have found use in botanical extraction, crystallization, and the preparation of micro- and nano-particle formulations. The following are some of the advantages of supercritical fluids for extraction over traditional methods:

- Supercritical fluids allow for lower-temperature extractions and purifications of compounds. This can significantly improve the stability profiles of compounds by preventing thermal degradation.
- Volatility under ambient conditions presents its own set of issues with the use of traditional solvents, e.g., solvent leakage. Such issues are nonproblematic with supercritical fluid extractions.
- Supercritical fluid extraction exhibits relatively higher selectivity of extracted compounds. This avoids multiple purification steps.

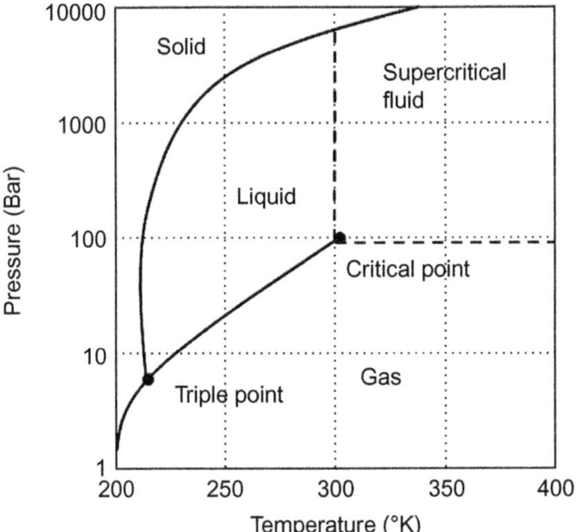

FIGURE 2.15 Carbon dioxide pressure-temperature phase diagram.

- There is usually a lower long-term consumption of energy, thus reducing overhead costs.
- The viscosity of supercritical fluids is typically lower than conventional solvents. This significantly eases the handling, processing, and equipment requirements.
- There is a reduced need for hazardous solvents for extraction. This helps avoid expensive and risky waste disposal. For example, CO_2 can be released directly into the atmosphere.

As shown in Figure 2.16, the SFE process consists of following general steps:

1. The system contains a pump for the carbon dioxide, a pressure cell to contain the sample, a pressure chamber, and a collecting vessel.
2. The carbon dioxide gas is converted to liquid and pumped to a heating zone, where it is heated to supercritical conditions.
3. It is then passed through the extraction vessel, where it rapidly diffuses into the solid matrix and dissolves the material to be extracted.
4. The dissolved material is carried from the extraction cell into a separator at lower pressure.
5. The extracted material is collected.
6. The carbon dioxide is then cooled, recompressed, or discharged to the atmosphere.

2.5. THERMODYNAMICS

Thermodynamics is the study of energy and how energy is converted between different forms. Based on postulates or laws, the theory of thermodynamics can tell which transformations are permissible and the final equilibrium state of many different types of

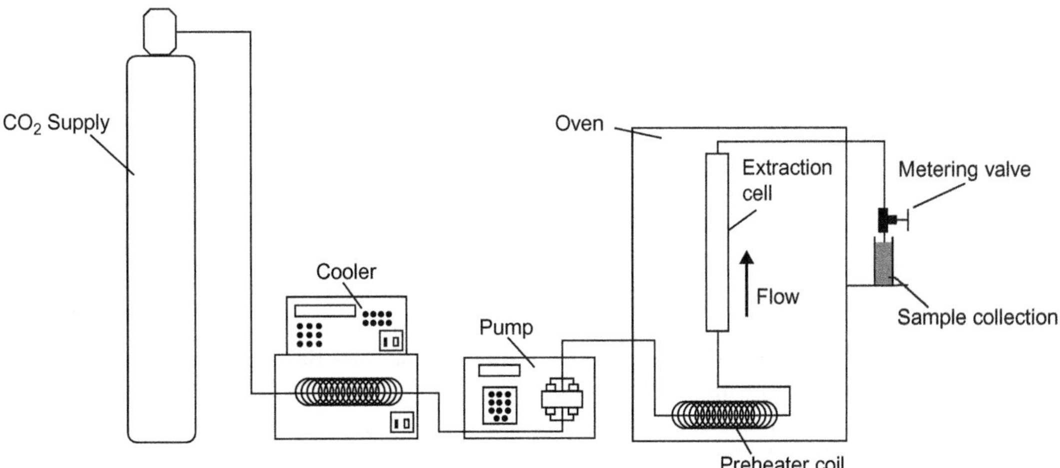

FIGURE 2.16 Schematic diagram of the supercritical fluid extraction (SFE). *(Figure adapted from http://en.wikipedia.org/wiki/File:SFEschematic.jpg)*

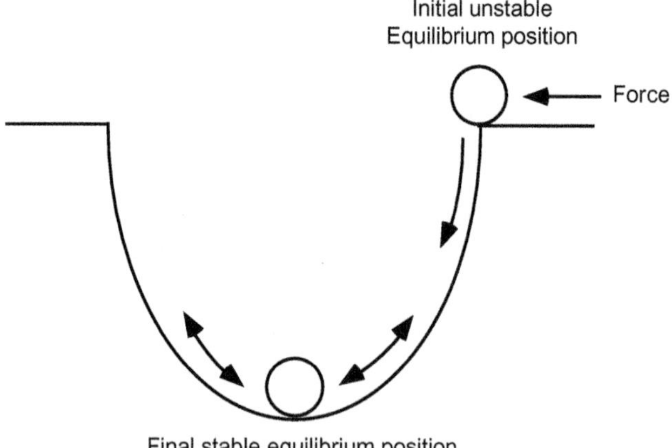

FIGURE 2.17 Energy well showing energy conversion.

systems important to pharmacy. Perhaps these aspects can best be illustrated by a simple example [18]. Figure 2.17 shows what would happen if a ball that was resting on the edge of a bowl, with a defined amount of gravitational potential energy, was pushed into the bowl. When the ball is pushed, it will roll down the sides of the bowl and oscillate back and forth, conserving both potential and kinetic energy, but eventually the ball will come to rest on the bottom of the bowl. In this simple example, the ball is resting in an unstable equilibrium position, and with a slight perturbation of the system, the ball rolls into the bowl. At this point, the gravitational potential energy of the ball is converted to kinetic energy (the energy of motion). Eventually, the ball will stop at the bottom of the bowl in a stable equilibrium position. What happened to the potential and kinetic energy of the ball? It was converted to heat through friction with the bowl and air. Thus, in going from an unstable equilibrium to a stable equilibrium, the ball has converted its gravitational potential energy first to kinetic energy and finally to heat. This simple example illustrates many of the attributes of thermodynamics. In other words, thermodynamics seeks to answer questions such as the following: What is the final equilibrium state of a system is that state stable or unstable? In what manner is heat converted to work and vice versa? What restrictions are placed on the conversion of energy from one form to another? Thermodynamics tries to answer these questions and much more.

While the preceding example may not be relevant to pharmacy, there are many examples in which thermodynamics is very important. For example, consider the process of life itself, in which sunlight hits a plant and through photosynthesis is converted to stored chemical energy in the plant carbohydrates. A cow can eat these plant carbohydrates and convert them into milk lactose, which you finally eat in a bowl of breakfast cereal (for some readers, the photon may have impinged on a coffee plant, giving it the energy necessary to synthesize caffeine). Finally, this gives you the energy needed to read this chapter. In this example, the energy of nuclear fusion in the sun is converted to a photon, which is converted into stored chemical energy and then converted into lactose by a cow, and finally burned up through the process of respiration. All of these energy transfers are governed by the laws of thermodynamics. Other examples in which thermodynamics are important to the understanding of pharmacy include drug receptor interactions; active, passive, and facilitated drug transport (i.e., drug adsorption); phase equilibrium; emulsion stability; and the temperature dependence of chemical reactions and drug solubility phenomena. In short, every process involves the exchange of energy, and hence, all processes are dictated by the laws of thermodynamics. Thermodynamics is a universal theory of wide applicability. By understanding this material, you can conceptually use thermodynamic principles to understand factors important to drug delivery and drug product stability.

2.5.1 Macroscopic vs. Microscopic Thermodynamics

All matter is made up of atoms that are constantly undergoing complex motions. The actual description of all these complex motions is done in the field of statistical mechanics. Thanks to the work of Gibbs, Boltzmann, and Maxwell [24], the theory of statistical mechanics has been able to derive satisfactory descriptions of these atomic-level motions for simple systems. They have shown that these hidden modes of atomic motion act as a repository for energy and help to define temperature, the transformation of energy, and other macroscopic properties such as heat capacity, solubility, volume, and length. However, the utilization of these microscopic theories requires a molecular description, which adds a layer of complexity and is not always available. With thermodynamics, however, you can summarize much of this information with simpler macroscopic observations. Often, these descriptions are material independent. For example, recall that 12 grams of carbon consists of Avogadro's number N_A of atoms ($N_A = 6.02217 \times 10^{23}$ atoms), which in thermodynamics is designated as 12 grams of the isotope ^{12}C. Because there are so many molecules, the average properties of these molecules are very reproducible and can be quantitated in such a manner that the macroscopic descriptions work very well. However, it is worthwhile to remember the atomic-level foundation of these macroscopic observations.

2.6. BASIC CONCEPTS AND DEFINITIONS

Before beginning a discussion of thermodynamics, we need to describe some of the vocabulary and concepts commonly used in the study of thermodynamics.

2.6.1 Thermodynamic Systems and Equations of State

A *thermodynamic system* is a set of objects that are being studied or described. By definition, this set of objects is typically separated from the rest of the environment by boundary, and the *environment* is usually defined as everything else in the universe. In this system, if there is no exchange of matter with the environment, the system is *closed;* and if there is exchange of matter with the environment, the system is *open*. The condition or mode of being of a system is known as the *thermodynamic state* of the system. The state of the system can be described by an *equation of state* (not to be confused with things that are a function of state or a state function; see the following text), which is a mathematical equation that describes the condition of the system in terms of *measurable* properties of that system [19]. One implication of this definition is that the selection of measurable properties or variables by which the system can be adequately described is a key element of thermodynamics. For example, n moles of a pure gas in a piston (in this case, the gas in the piston is the thermodynamic system; see Figure 2.18) can be described by a mathematical function of pressure (P), volume (V), and temperature (T):

$$f(n, P, T) = V \tag{2.21}$$

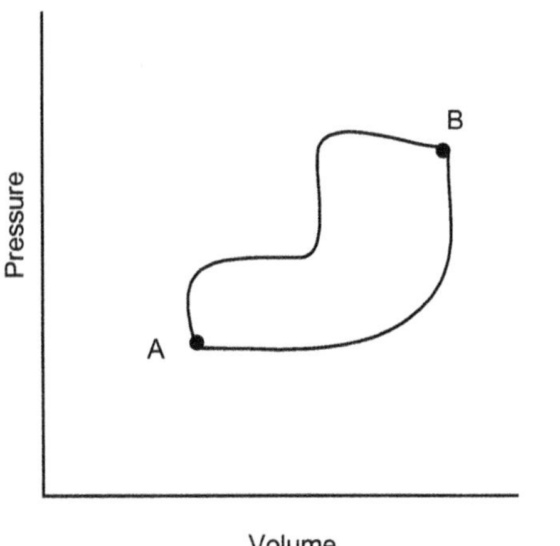

FIGURE 2.18 Cyclic path of an ideal gas undergoing a thermodynamic process.

For an ideal gas, the state equation is the well-known ideal gas law, discussed previously; thus, for a given amount of an ideal gas, the state variables are temperature, pressure, and volume:

$$V = \frac{nRT}{P} \tag{2.22}$$

The variables or properties that are used in the state equations can be divided into two categories. First, *intensive* properties are those that are independent of the amount of material present—for example, temperature, pressure, and density. The second, *extensive* properties are those that are dependent on the amount of material present—for example, volume, energy, and mass or number of moles. Some people like to think of intensive and extensive properties as intensity and capacity factors, respectively. The reason is that often the multiplication of an intensity times a capacity factor leads to a type of energy; for example, pressure times a change in volume is related to the mechanical work done (see following text) [20].

Another example of a system is a chemically defined *homogenous* liquid such as Scotch (Scotch is drink that contains approximately 40%–50% ethyl alcohol by volume). In this system, the state equation must include pressure, volume, temperature, and additional variables to account for the composition of the system. For example, how much water was added to the drink? If the system is *Scotch on the rocks* (a term referring to the serving of scotch with ice), the state equation must include pressure, volume, temperature, composition, and more variables necessary to account for the multiple phases present. In this example, we have two phases (Scotch and ice), which create an *inhomogeneous system*, where a *phase* is defined as an homogenous physically distinct portion of a system that is separated from other portions of the system by bounding surfaces.

One of the most important states of matter is the *state of equilibrium*, which is when the system is left to its own, none of its measurable properties will change. In other words, the macroscopic state of the system is time invariant and will not change unless perturbed by a rise in temperature or a change in pressure, for example. The equilibrium can be a *stable equilibrium*, which means that if the system is perturbed, it has a natural tendency to return to the original equilibrium position. In the previous example, this corresponds to the ball resting on the bottom of the bowl. The equilibrium state could also be an *unstable equilibrium*, which means that if the system is perturbed, the system will try to seek a new, more stable equilibrium position. In the previous example, this corresponds to the ball resting on the top of the bowl. As you can imagine, the type of equilibrium is very important to drug product stability, and determining thermodynamic stability is a major component of drug development research.

2.6.2 Thermodynamic Processes

When the state of a system undergoes a macroscopic change from one time to another, the system undergoes a *thermodynamic process* or just a *process* during that time period. For example, if the piston in Figure 2.18 increases in temperature or pressure, a thermodynamic process has occurred to cause this change. There are many different types of processes; the differences have primarily to do with the manner in which the process was conducted and the boundary between the system and the environment. If the boundary of a system is perfectly insulating and there is no heat exchange with the environment, a process occurring under these conditions is said to be *adiabatic*. An *isothermal process* is one in which the boundary can conduct heat and the process is done in such a manner that the environment and system are always at the same temperature. *Isobaric* and *isochoric* processes are carried out under constant pressure and volume, respectively.

2.6.3 Reversible and Irreversible Processes

A *reversible process* is one that is always at equilibrium during the entire process. In theory, a reversible process can be achieved by making each step an infinitesimal step (see Appendix 2.1), which gives the system time to adjust to its new equilibrium state. For example, if the gas in the piston shown in Figure 2.18 were expanded reversibly, then the piston would move at a rate slow enough so that no air currents or other dissipative or irreversible processes occurred. By always being in equilibrium, no temperature or pressure gradients occur within the system, and consequently, the process can be truly reversed by infinitesimally changing the forces. For example, instead of allowing the cylinder to expand, an infinitesimal change in the force would cause the gas to compress. If the cylinder is allowed to expand rapidly, then not every step is at equilibrium, and the process is said to be *irreversible*. During an irreversible process, air currents and other irreversible events can occur in the piston, which prevents the true reversal of the process. Because reversible processes occur in such a manner that each step is at equilibrium, the process is uniquely defined, and for most substances, the state of equilibrium is a unique state for a given set of conditions. Therefore, equilibrium processes provide a unique standard by which all other processes can be compared.

2.6.4 Functions of State and Exact Differentials

If a property or function of a system depends only on the initial and final states of the system, that property is called a *function of state* or *state function*. In other words, the change in a property depends only on the state of the system, and not on the process by which it got to that state or the path it took to get to that point. For example, the gravitational potential energy of a ball dropped from the second story of a pharmacy school would depend only on the height from which it was dropped, and not on how it got to the second floor. If the ball were carried to the seventh floor and then down to the second floor and dropped, it would have the same energy when it hit the ground as if it were carried directly to the second floor and dropped. Even though the amount of work done to the ball to get it to the second floor was very different for each case, the ball would still have the same gravitational potential energy and hence the same energy when it hit the ground.

Consequently, the change in a state function only depends on the difference between the initial and the final state. For example, the difference in pressure P of an ideal gas going from an initial state A to a final state B, the change can be given by:

$$\Delta P = P_B - P_A$$

No matter how the system goes from A to B, the difference is always the same (see Figure 2.18). This change can be computed by the total derivative; see Appendix 2.1 for an explanation:

$$\mathrm{d}P = \left(\frac{\partial P}{\partial V}\right)_T \mathrm{d}V + \left(\frac{\partial P}{\partial T}\right)_V \mathrm{d}T \tag{2.23}$$

If the derivatives $\partial P/\partial V$ and $\partial P/\partial T$ have the property

$$\frac{\partial}{\partial T}\left(\frac{\partial P}{\partial V}\right)_T = \frac{\partial}{\partial V}\left(\frac{\partial P}{\partial V}\right)_V \tag{2.24}$$

then P is said to be an *exact differential*. If a state function is an exact differential, then the change depends only on the initial and final states of the system (see Appendix 2.1).

Another property of state functions that meet the condition given by Eq. 2.24 is that the change in the property for a closed cyclic path is zero, which can be written as

$$\oint \mathrm{d}P = 0 \tag{2.25}$$

where the loop around the integral sign indicates that the integral is taken over a closed cyclic path (see Figure 2.18).

2.7. THE FIRST LAW OF THERMODYNAMICS

2.7.1 Conservation of Energy

The first law of thermodynamics is a statement of the conservation of energy. When you are trying to understand the principles involved with the conservation of energy, it is hard to understand where the law came from and why the law is formulated in this manner. In a way, the first law makes sense, but the only real justification for the first law is that no one has ever found a contrary example; i.e., for some reason unknown to humanity, this is the way nature appears to behave. For a fascinating historical review of how the first law came into being, see Moore [21]. While we don't know why, the first law gives a description for how nature behaves, and the application of the principles of conservation of energy gives us a powerful tool for understanding pharmaceutical systems. As with any conservation law, it tells us that the total amount of stuff is constant; therefore, application of a conservation law entails keeping track of where the stuff ends up. The following explanation was taken from a lecture given by Richard Feynman in 1963 and is an excellent description of the formulation of the first law [22]. Additional thoughts were also taken from reference [3].

> Imagine a child perhaps, "Dennis the Menace," who has blocks which are absolutely indestructible, and cannot be divided into pieces. Each is the same as the other. Let us suppose that he has 28 blocks. His mother puts him with his 28 blocks into a room at the beginning of the day. At the end of the day, being curious, she counts the blocks very carefully, and discovers a phenomenal law—no matter what he does with the blocks, there are always 28 remaining! This continues for a number of days, until one day there are only 27 blocks, but a little investigating shows that there is one under the rug—she must look everywhere to be sure that the number of blocks has not changed. One day, however, the number appears to change—there are only 26 blocks. Careful investigation indicates that the window was open, and upon looking outside, the other two blocks are found. Another day, careful count indicates that there are 30 blocks! This causes considerable consternation, until it is realized that Bruce came to visit, bringing his blocks with him, and he left a few at Dennis' house. After she has disposed of the extra blocks, she closed the window, does not let Bruce in, and then everything is going along all right, until one time she counts and finds only 25 blocks. However, there is a box in the room, a toy box, and the mother goes to open the toy box, but the boy says "NO, do not open my toy box," and screams. Mother is not allowed to open the toy box. Being extremely curious, and somewhat ingenious, she invents a scheme! She knows that a block weighs three ounces, so she weighs the box at a time when she sees 28 blocks, and it weighs 16 ounces. The next time she wishes to check, she weighs the box again, she subtracts 16 ounces and divides by three. She discovers the following:

$$\begin{pmatrix} \textit{number of} \\ \textit{blocks seen} \end{pmatrix} + \frac{\textit{weight of box} - 16 \textit{ ounces}}{3 \textit{ ounces}} = \textit{constant} \tag{2.26}$$

> There then appear to be some new deviations, but careful study indicates that the dirty water in the bathtub is changing its level. The child is throwing blocks into the water, and she cannot see them because it is so dirty, but she can find out how many blocks are in the water by adding another term to her formula. Since the original height of the water was 6 inches and each block raises the water a quarter of an inch, this new formula would be:

$$\begin{pmatrix} \textit{number of} \\ \textit{blocks seen} \end{pmatrix} + \frac{(\textit{weight of box}) - 16 \textit{ ounces}}{3 \textit{ ounces}} + \frac{(\textit{height of water}) - 6 \textit{ inches}}{1/4 \textit{ inch}} = \textit{constant} \tag{2.27}$$

> In the gradual increase in the complexity of her world, she finds a whole series of terms representing ways of calculating how many blocks are in places where she is not allowed to look. As a result, she finds a complex formula, a quantity which *has to be computed*, which always stays the same in her situation.

Now let's examine the analogies between the preceding example and the conservation of energy. This example illustrates that you must carefully keep track of all these transformations when energy enters or leaves a system. With energy, there are many different forms; they include heat energy, radiant energy, kinetic energy, chemical energy, surface energy, gravitational energy, electrical energy, elastic energy, nuclear energy, and mass energy. Thermodynamic processes can convert energy between these different forms, and a separate accounting or equation is needed for each type of conversion. While there is a lot known about how energy behaves, to be honest, no one really knows what energy is, so it's important to keep in mind that a description, no matter how complex or detailed, is not an explanation. Fortunately, accurate descriptions are enough to gain great insight into the behavior of pharmaceutical system and pass examinations on this subject.

Unfortunately, unlike Dennis's mother who counted the 28 blocks, you have no way to determine the total amount of energy present. However, when a thermodynamic process occurs, the total amount of heat and work transferred between the system and environment can be measured. For example, if heat energy is added or removed from a system (i.e., heating or cooling), the result is either a rise or fall in temperature, which can be measured and used to calculate the heat energy exchanged. When a rubber band is stretched, the force applied and the displacement of the rubber band can be measured and used to calculate the work done to the rubber band. In summary, the question becomes this: How is the first law of thermodynamics formulated when the total amount of energy present is unknown, but the amount of heat and work exchange between the system and environment can be measured?

If you return to the story of Dennis, because the number of blocks is conserved (i.e., the number of blocks always equals 28 and this never changes), the summation of all the changes that can occur will always equal zero. For example, if you don't know the total number of blocks and want to account for the exchange of blocks between the room and the toy box, you can measure the change in weight of the toy box and Eq. 2.26 therefore becomes

$$\begin{pmatrix} \textit{change in number of} \\ \textit{blocks seen} \end{pmatrix} + \frac{\textit{weight of box before} - \textit{weight of box after}}{3\ \textit{ounces}} = 0 \qquad (2.28)$$

In addition, because an infinite number of things could happen to the blocks when they leave the system, it is not practical for Dennis's mother to search the environment for the blocks every time the number of blocks that she sees changes. Thus, as a practical necessity, you can only keep track of the blocks as they enter or leave the room, in effect ignoring what happens to the blocks when they enter the environment. Therefore, when you focus only on the system and changes within Eq. 2.28, becomes

$$\begin{pmatrix} \textit{change in number of} \\ \textit{blocks seen} \end{pmatrix} + \frac{\textit{weight of box before} - \textit{weight of box after}}{3\ \textit{ounces}} \pm \textit{No. going through window} \pm \textit{No. Bruce brings} = 0 \qquad (2.29)$$

Notice the change in the system is expressed in terms of the number that enter or leave the system and *not* changes in the number going through the window or brought over by Bruce. Because the total number of blocks is conserved, the law of conservation should account for the system and environment; however, the environment is so immensely complicated that, in reality, this is impossible. Hence, the analysis can be simplified by focusing only on the system and what crosses its boundaries. In effect, the last two terms in Eq. 2.29 can account for changes in the environment that affect the number of blocks in the room.

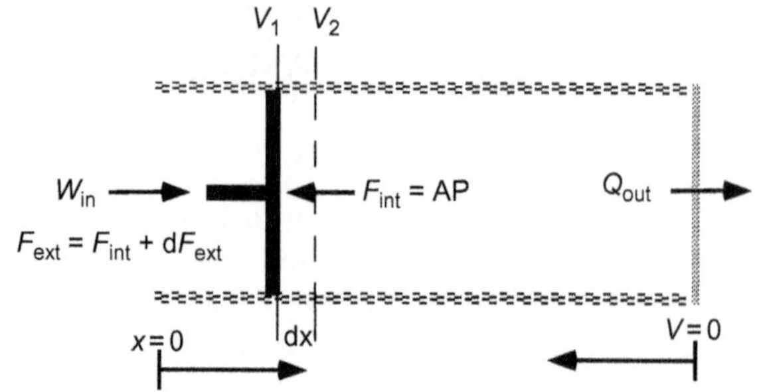

FIGURE 2.19 A friction-less piston of cross-sectional area A being compressed.

Now let's apply the preceding principles to the conservation of energy. The change in the energy of a system can be calculated by summing the total work and heat added or removed from the system. In other words, the change in energy can expressed as

$$\Delta U = Q + W \qquad (2.30)$$

where the symbol Δ stands for "the change in," Q is the amount of heat exchanged, and W is the amount of work done. The term ΔU is the change in energy of the system, and the energy associated with changes in work and heat is called the *internal energy* (see Figure 2.19).

2.7.2 Work

Work is defined as the transfer of energy from one physical system to another. This transfer can be done by many different mechanisms such as mechanical, chemical, electrical, but for this chapter, only mechanical work is considered. For a more complete discussion, see reference [18]. *Mechanical work* is the transfer of energy *via* the application of mechanical force to a system; in other words, mechanical work is force times distance. In calculus notation, which is used to calculate the work for a thermodynamic process such as the Carnot cycle, you use the integral of force with respect to distance as in

$$W = F \times dx \text{ for a thermodynamic process } W = \int_{x_1}^{x_2} F dx \qquad (2.31)$$

where work has units of ergs or Joules, F is the force in units of dynes or Newtons, and x is distance. When you are working with gases (see Figure 2.19), it is useful to calculate the work done in terms of pressure and volume. For the gas in the piston to be compressed, the external pressure must be greater than the internal pressure. However, for the compression to be reversible, the system must always be in a state of equilibrium, which can occur only if there is an infinitesimal difference between the inside and outside pressures. Therefore, when calculating the work, you can assume the infinitesimal pressure difference is zero $dF_{ext} \cong 0$ (see Figure 2.19), which implies the external force equals the internal force. Because the pressure (P) is force per unit area ($P = F/A$), the work to move the cylinder a distance dx is given by

$$W = F(x_2 - x_1) = Fdx = PAdx \quad (2.32)$$

As an arbitrary convention, work done on a system is defined as positive. In Eq. 2.32, P is positive, and because $x_2 > x_1$, dx is positive; however, when a gas is compressed, it takes up less volume, i.e., $V_2 < V_1$, which makes dV negative. Therefore, to maintain this arbitrary sign convention, pressure-volume work is defined with a negative sign outside the integral (note that $V = A\,x$):

$$W = \int_{x_1}^{x_2} PAdx = -\int_{V_1}^{V_2} PdV \quad (2.33)$$

2.7.3 Heat

Heat is a form of energy associated with the microscopic or hidden modes of atomic motion. In other words, when heat is added to a system, its internal energy increases, which, on the atomic level, results in increased molecular motion. Heat can be transferred by conduction in solids and liquids, convection in fluids, and radiation in empty space. Heat is an extensive property that is dependent on the amount of material present—not to be confused with temperature, which is an intensive property independent of the amount of material present. Again, as an arbitrary sign convention, heat absorbed by a system is considered positive.

2.7.4 Sign Convention

The sign convention used in Eq. 2.30 was chosen arbitrarily; however, the choice needs to be standardized; otherwise, great confusion can result. All the sign convention does is tell which way the energy is going, i.e., either into or out of the system. From the point of view of the system, this sign convention considers all energy going into the system positive and all energy leaving the system as negative (see Figure 2.20). Also, for consistency with this convention, pressure-volume work adds a negative sign to the equation (see Eq. 2.33). While this convention is widely used, especially in more recent texts, many books define work with the opposite sign. This convention is based on the historic roots of thermodynamics in which steam/heat engines took in heat and gave out work; hence, both the input of heat and the output of work were positive.

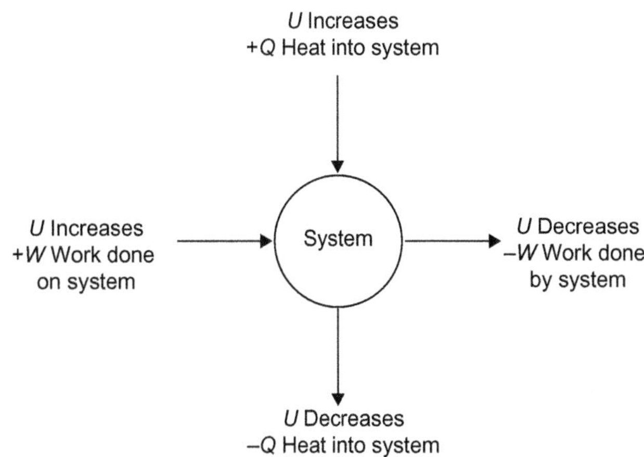

FIGURE 2.20 Sign convention from the point of view of a thermodynamics system.

2.8. ENTHALPY AND HEAT CAPACITY

In pharmacy, processes such as the melting of a suppository base, the dissolution of a solid in a liquid, the mixing of two miscible liquids, and chemical reactions are carried out at room pressure, which is virtually constant. For this important case, the first law shown in Eq. 2.30 at constant pressure can be used to calculate the heat evolved or absorbed by a process:

$$\Delta U = U_2 - U_1 = Q_p + W = Q_p - P(V_2 - V_1) \quad (2.34)$$

This equation can be rewritten as follows:

$$Q_p = (U_2 + PV_2) - (U_1 + PV_1) \quad (2.35)$$

The P subscript is written to indicate that the expression assumes P is constant; this notation is used throughout the chapter. The expression $U + PV$ is given the special name *enthalpy*, or *heat content*. In this new notation, Eq. 2.35 becomes

$$Q_p = (H_2 - H_1)_p = \Delta H_p \quad (2.36)$$

The enthalpy is an extensive property that gives the amount of heat exchanged for a process occurring at constant pressure (note this definition excludes non-PdV forms of work). In addition, the enthalpy is a state function because U, P, and V are all state functions. For processes that don't occur at constant pressure, the enthalpy may not equal the heat absorbed or evolved for that process. A process that absorbs energy is *endothermic*—for example, ice melting. If the process gives off energy, it is *exothermic*, such as the freezing of water or combustion reactions.

As mentioned previously, the amount of heat exchanged can't be directly measured, but changes in a system such as temperature along with the heat capacity can be used to determine the amount of heat transferred. Assuming no phase transitions, the *heat capacity* is defined as the proportionality constant between change in temperature that occurs when a body undergoes heat exchange with the environment:

$$Q = C(T_2 - T_1) \tag{2.37}$$

The heat capacity is an extensive property, i.e., dependent on the amount of material present. The *specific heat* or *specific heat capacity* is defined as the heat capacity per unit gram of material, and the *molar heat capacity* is the heat capacity per mole of material. Because the heat capacity can change with temperature, more exact definitions determine the heat capacity for infinitesimal changes in temperature:

$$C = \frac{\partial Q}{\partial T} \tag{2.38}$$

If you aren't familiar with the symbol ∂, refer to Appendix 2.1. For a constant pressure, the change in enthalpy for a change in temperature can be given by inserting Eq. 2.36 into Eq. 2.38 to give

$$\left(\frac{\partial H}{\partial T}\right)_P = C_P \tag{2.39}$$

Thus, the enthalpy can also be calculated by integrating Eq. 2.39 as follows:

$$\Delta H = H_2 - H_1 = \int_{T_1}^{T_2} C_P dT \tag{2.40}$$

2.8.1 Phase Changes

Phase changes are very important to pharmacy; for example, the vaporization of a liquid propellant in a metered-dose inhaler (MDI) is critical to particle size generation and hence therapeutic efficacy. In addition, phase changes can drastically affect dosage form stability, and understanding when a phase change can occur and how they affect stability is very important to drug development. A phase change is typically accompanied by an abrupt change in the properties of a material—for example, the melting of ice to form water.

Equation 2.40 gives the enthalpy change over a temperature range in which no phase transitions are occurring. However, when there is a phase change, such as going from a solid to a liquid or a liquid to a gas, the system absorbs or emits heat energy during the transition. If the process is done reversibly, i.e., at equilibrium, the temperature and pressure are constant during the transition. The thermodynamic process for the melting of ice in the Scotch and water example can be written as

$$\text{Phase(ice)} \Leftrightarrow \text{Phase(liquid)} \tag{2.41}$$

where the change in enthalpy for the melting or freezing of ice at a transition temperature T^* is given by

$$\begin{aligned} H_{T^*}(\text{liquid}) - H_{T^*}(\text{ice}) &= H_{T^*}(\text{ice}) - H_{T^*}(\text{liquid}) \\ &= \Delta H_{T^*}(\text{ice} \rightarrow \text{liquid}) = Q_{P,T^*} \end{aligned} \tag{2.42}$$

By analogy to Eq. 2.39, the enthalpy in the differential form is as follows:

$$\left(\frac{\partial \Delta H_{T^*}}{\partial T}\right)_P = C_P(liquid) - C_P(ice) \tag{2.43}$$

Equation 2.43 can be integrated to yield the following:

$$\Delta H_T - \Delta H_{T^*} = \int_{T^*}^{T} C_P(liquid) - C_P(ice) dT \tag{2.44}$$

The heat given off or absorbed in a phase change that occurs at constant temperature and pressure is sometimes called the *latent heat*, which is the amount of energy required to reorder the atoms when they change state.

2.8.2 Hess's Law

A unique property of the enthalpy is that it's a state function, which means that the change in enthalpy is path independent and depends only on the initial and final states of the system. Understanding this property can be very useful when you are trying to determine hard-to-measure changes. For example, the enthalpy of sublimation would be difficult to measure because the rate of sublimation is very slow. Therefore, you can use the fact that the enthalpy is a state function and calculate the enthalpy of sublimation by adding the enthalpies of vaporization and fusion (melting), which are more easily measured. However, there is only one difficulty with this approach: the enthalpies of fusion and vaporization are measured at their transition temperatures, which, for standard conditions, are 0°C and 100°C, respectively. Thus, Eq. 2.40 can be used to determine the heat that must be added or removed from the system due to a change in temperature.

To illustrate the calculation of ΔH_{sub} for water, you can use the scheme shown in Figure 2.21. Literature values for the enthalpy of fusion at 0°C/273 K $\Delta H_{fus} = 6.01$ kJ/mol and vaporization at 100°C/373 K $\Delta H_{vap} = 40.7$ kJ/mol and the heat capacities for liquid $C_p = 75.5$ J/K mol

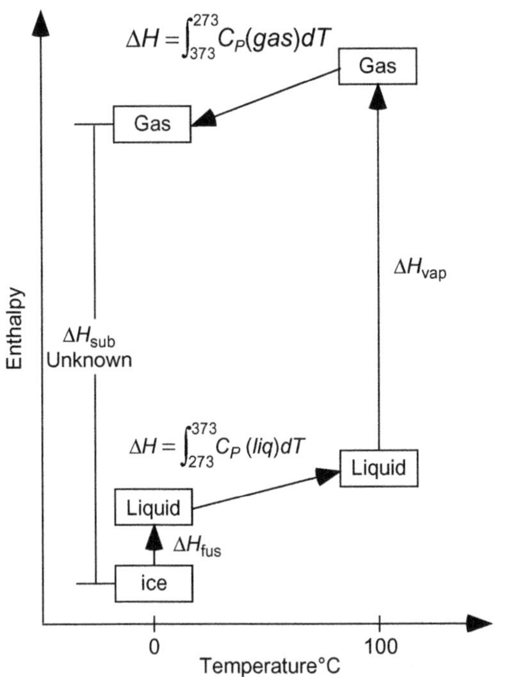

FIGURE 2.21 Schematic for calculating the enthalpy of sublimation at 0°C.

and gaseous $C_p = 30.5$ J/K mol + 10.3 T J/K^2 mol water are given in reference [4]. Based on Figure 2.21, the calculation of ΔH_{sub} at 0°C is given by

$$\begin{aligned}\Delta H_{sub} &= \Delta H_{fus}^{273} + \int_{273}^{373} C_P^{liq} dT + \Delta H_{vap}^{373} + \int_{373}^{273} C_P^{gas} dT \\ \Delta H_{sub} &= 6.01 \text{ kJ/mol} \\ &\quad +0.0755 \text{ kJ/K mol} \times (373 - 273)\text{K} \\ &\quad +40.7 \text{ kJ/mol} + 0.0305 \text{ kJ/K mol } (273 - 373)\text{K} \\ &\quad +0.0103 \text{ kJ/K}^2 \text{ mol } (273^2 - 373^2)\text{K}^2 \\ \Delta H_{sub} &= 50.2 \text{ kJ/mol}\end{aligned} \tag{2.45}$$

This method of determining the enthalpy of a process by adding the enthalpies of different possible paths is called *Hess's law* of heat summation. Hess's law can also be applied to chemical reactions. Using Hess's law, you can calculate the heat of a reaction from the measurement of other reactions. As the preceding example shows, when comparing the heats of reaction, it is important to have well-defined standard states so that all comparisons are done at comparable pressures and temperatures. Because phase transitions are dictated by material properties, they occur at well-defined points that can be used as a standard state for comparison. However, with chemical reactions, these easily defined standard states often do not exist. One convenient standard state is room temperature and pressure, which have been defined as 298.15 K and 1 atm, respectively. Under these conditions, the standard enthalpy of formation (ΔH°_f) can be calculated. The standard enthalpy of formation is defined as the ΔH of the reaction by which a compound is formed from its elements—for example, the formation of water

$$H_2 + \tfrac{1}{2} O_2 \rightarrow H_2O\,(l) \quad \Delta H^\circ_{298} = 285.8 \text{ kJ/mol}$$

By summing standard heats of formation for products and reactants, you can calculate the heat of a reaction by taking the difference of these sums:

$$\Delta H_{reaction} = \sum \Delta H_{products} - \sum \Delta H_{reactants} \tag{2.46}$$

2.9. THE SECOND LAW OF THERMODYNAMICS

The first law of thermodynamics states that energy is conserved and, for any thermodynamic process that converts energy from one form to another, the total energy in the universe remains constant. The second law of thermodynamics tells what types of conversions are possible. For example, in the previous example of the ball oscillating in the bowl, it was concluded that frictional forces between the air and bowl converted the kinetic and gravitational potential energy of the ball into heat. You could reasonably ask whether it would be possible to somehow convert this heat energy back into kinetic energy. Based on the first law, you know that the energy is there as heat, but can this heat be converted back into kinetic energy? While intuition may lead you to believe that this would not be possible, how do you know it is not a lack of intuition that prevents you from converting this energy back into kinetic? In other words, the second law specifies what is possible and puts stipulations on how heat can be removed from one source to another. The second law states that energy in the form of heat or work can't be extracted from a system unless there is a lower temperature heat reservoir available. Thus, for the ball example that was done at room temperature, the system can be considered approximately isothermal; hence, the second law states that the heat energy can't be removed from an isothermal system without putting energy into the system, i.e., doing a lot of work on the system. Along with the statement of the second law comes the definition of entropy.

These concepts are abstract and difficult to grasp; therefore, the goal of this chapter is to introduce these ideas. To really understand them, you need to consult more extensive references such as [3] and [21].

2.9.1 Carnot Cycle and Reversable Heat Engine Efficiency

The second law of thermodynamics can be stated as follows: "It is impossible to devise an engine which, working in a cycle, shall produce no other change other than the extraction of heat from a reservoir and the performance of an equal amount of work" [21]. To understand this statement, let's look at the Carnot cycle. The Carnot cycle is based on an ideal heat engine operating reversibly between hot and cold heat reservoirs at temperatures T_2 and T_1 with $T_2 > T_1$ (see Figures 2.22 and 2.23). A *heat engine* is an engine that converts heat into mechanical work, and the material undergoing the cyclic process is called the *working substance*, which for the Carnot cycle is typically an ideal gas.

The Carnot cycle, which consists of four reversible processes, is shown in Figures 2.22 and 2.23. Starting at point 1, the working substance, which has a state of P_1, V_1, and T_2, expands isothermally until it reaches point 2. During this expansion, Q_2 units of heat are transferred from the hot reservoir to the working substance. Starting at point 2, the engine then expands adiabatically until the temperature reaches T_1 at point 3. At this point, the working substance is isothermally compressed, returning Q_1 units of heat to the low-temperature reservoir at temperature T_1. At point 4, the working substance is adiabatically compressed until it reaches the starting point 1, thus completing a full cycle, and the working substance is returned to its initial state of P_1, V_1, and T_2.

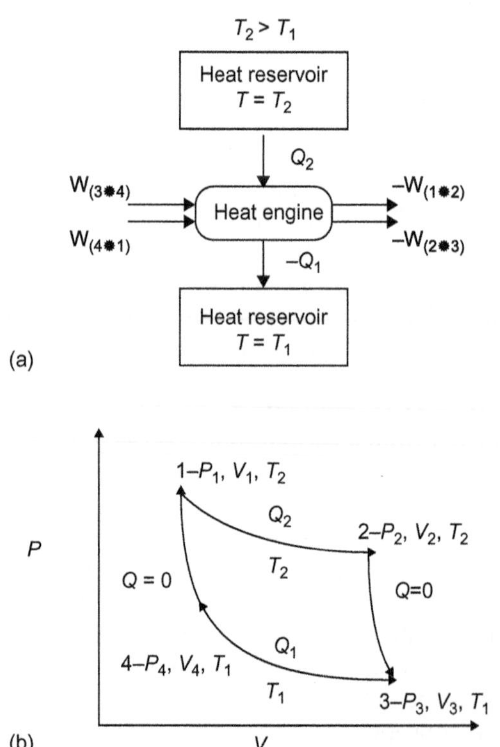

FIGURE 2.22 Diagram of a heat engine as that used in the Carnot cycle.

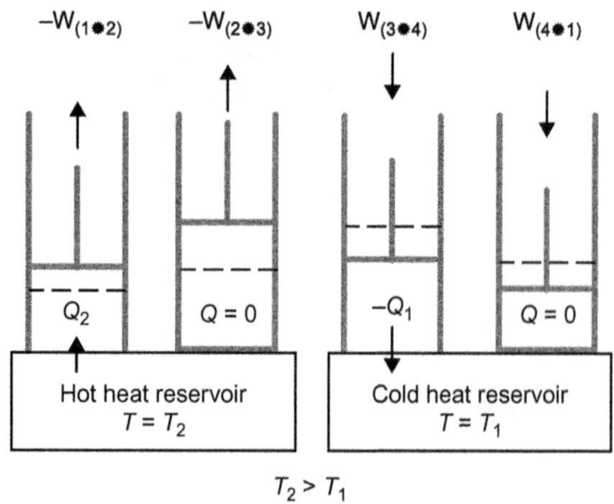

FIGURE 2.23 Carnot cycle for an ideal gas.

The change in internal energy for the working substance, which goes from state 1 to 3, is given by

$$\int_1^3 dU = U_3 - U_1 = Q_2 + \int_1^2 dW + \int_1^3 dW$$
$$- Q_2 - \int_{V_1}^{V_2} PdV - \int_{V_2}^{V_3} PdV \tag{2.47}$$

and the change in internal energy for the compression of the gas is given by

$$\int_3^1 dU = U_1 - U_3 = Q_1 + \int_3^4 dW + \int_4^1 dW$$
$$= Q_1 + \int_{V_3}^{V_4} PdV + \int_{V_4}^{V_1} PdV \tag{2.48}$$

The change in internal energy is zero because the internal energy is a state function independent of path and only dependent on the initial and final state of the system. Thus, using the first law Eq. 2.30, you can add Eq. 2.47 and Eq. 2.48 to yield

$$Q_2 + Q_1 = -W = \int_{V_1}^{V_2} PdV + \int_{V_2}^{V_3} PdV + \int_{V_3}^{V_4} PdV + \int_{V_4}^{V_1} PdV \tag{2.49}$$

When you are working with reversible heat engines operating in a cycle, which absorb heat from a reservoir at one temperature and then return heat back to lower temperature reservoir and do work, it is often useful to express the work done in terms of heat and temperatures.

For an ideal gas, you can compute the preceding integrals; again, we do not make reference to any particular substance, but for brevity we will demonstrate using an ideal gas (for more details, see reference [22]).

TABLE 2.1 Carnot Cycle of one mole of an Ideal Gas

Path	Work	Heat
1→2	$-RT_2 \ln\frac{V_2}{V_1}$	$Q_2 = RT_2 \ln\frac{V_2}{V_1}$
2→3	$C_v \times (T_1 - T_2)$	0
3→4	$-RT_1 \ln\frac{V_4}{V_3}$	$Q_1 = -RT_1 \ln\frac{V_4}{V_3}$
4→1	$C_v \times (T_2 - T_1)$	0

As would be expected for heat engines, it is convenient to express the work, etc., in terms of temperature and the amount of heat absorbed or emitted. For an ideal gas, the internal energy is dependent only on the temperature and the number of molecules. As such for the isothermal steps, the change in internal energy is zero, and the work done is equal to the heat absorbed. Thus,

$$Q_2 = \int_1^2 PdV = \int_{V_1}^{V_2} \frac{nRT_2}{V} dV = nRT_2 \ln\frac{V_2}{V_1} \tag{2.50}$$

and by analogy, the heat transfer for the isothermal compression can be given by

$$Q_1 = nRT_2 \ln\frac{V_3}{V_4} \tag{2.51}$$

The work and heat transferred for the individual paths are summarized in Table 2.1. To eliminate the V's, you need to express them in terms of the T's. To do this, you can use the results from the kinetic theory of gases; thus, you know that

$$TV^{\gamma-1} = \text{Constant} \tag{2.52}$$

where γ is the ratio of heat capacities (the explanation is beyond the scope of this chapter, but you can see reference [23]). Thus, you can apply this to your system to have

$$T_2V_2^{\gamma-1} = T_1V_3^{\gamma-1} \tag{2.53}$$

And for the other compression path, you have

$$T_2V_1^{\gamma-1} = T_1V_4^{\gamma-1} \tag{2.54}$$

If you divide Eq. 2.53 by Eq. 2.54, you find that $V_2/V_1 = V_3/V_4$. If this is the case, then the ln in Eq. 2.50 must equal the ln in Eq. 2.51, and this yields

$$\frac{Q_1}{T_1} = \frac{Q_2}{T_2} \tag{2.55}$$

This is the relationship that relates temperature to heat transferred in the Carnot cycle. While the results are based on an ideal gas here, it can be shown that this is a general equation that can be applied to any substance [22]. This equation can be used to define a temperature scale and the entropy, which are discussed in the next section.

2.9.2 Entropy and Temperature

As shown in the preceding section, the term dQ/T is a state function of special importance; in fact, it is called the entropy. This state function was first introduced by Clausius in 1850, and he named it the *entropy*.

$$dS = \frac{dQ}{T} \tag{2.56}$$

This expression was derived for the Carnot cycle, but it can be shown that for any reversible cyclic process, this expression is valid, and because it is a state function for any cyclic process, the total of all the steps must equal zero (see Eq. 2.25).

$$\sum_i \frac{dQ_i}{T} = \oint \frac{dQ_{rev}}{T} = 0 \tag{2.57}$$

Note dQ_{rev} is used to indicate this is true for a reversible process only. In addition, it can be shown that for any reversible process, the entropy change is zero, and for an irreversible process, the entropy change must be greater than zero [3], i.e., $dS > 0$. Also, the change in entropy for any process can be calculated by

$$S_2 - S_1 = \int_1^2 \frac{dQ}{T} \tag{2.58}$$

The entropy is very important because it tells whether a system will spontaneously change. Consider the case of a heat reservoir at temperature T_2 that is slowly losing heat to the environment at temperature T_1, where $T_2 > T_1$. If the temperature difference is infinitesimally small, then the process is reversible. The entropy changes in the reservoir and environment are, respectively,

$$dS_2 = -\frac{dQ_{rev}}{T_2} \text{ and } dS_1 = \frac{dQ_{rev}}{T_1} \tag{2.59}$$

The total change in entropy is the sum of the entropy changes:

$$dS = dS_1 + dS_2 = -\frac{dQ_{rev}}{T_2} + \frac{dQ_{rev}}{T_1} = dQ_{rev}\left(\frac{1}{T_1} - \frac{1}{T_2}\right) \tag{2.60}$$

Because $T_2 > T_1$, dS is positive. In other words, spontaneous processes occur only if the entropy change is positive. While the preceding example is very specific, this statement has been proven with general applicability [22]. In summary, the entropy change of a reversible process is zero, and for an irreversible process, the entropy change is always positive:

$$dS = dS_{sys} + dS_{env} \geq 0 \quad (2.61)$$

This statement is one of the more profound statements in science, and much research has been done on the subject and its implications are far reaching. On a molecular level, the entropy is related to the degree of molecular randomness. Based on statistical mechanics, it has been shown that the entropy is directly correlated with the degree of randomness the molecules in a system have. For example, in a gas, the molecules are not as restricted as in a solid or liquid, and thus have a higher degree of entropy. In another example using drug diffusion, the second law would predict that drugs diffuse throughout the body because the degree of randomness of the drug molecule increases as they spread out. Hence, the second law predicts that diffusion occurs spontaneously because the entropy increases as the drug molecules go from high concentration to low concentration.

2.10. THE THIRD LAW OF THERMODYNAMICS

One of the most popular statements of the third law of thermodynamics was given by Lewis and Randall in 1923:

> If the entropy of each element in some crystalline state be taken as zero at the absolute zero of temperature, every substance has a finite positive entropy; but at the absolute zero of temperature the entropy may become zero, and does so become in the case of perfect crystalline substances [21].

The consequences of the third law are that an absolute value for the entropy can be calculated, based on absolute zero as a reference point. Given this definition, the absolute entropy can be written as

$$S^{poly} = S_0^{poly} + \int_0^T \frac{C_P}{T} dT \quad (2.62)$$

where S^{poly} is the entropy of the polymorphic/crystalline form at absolute zero. If the substance is a perfect crystal, then $S^{poly} = 0$; however, most materials do not have perfect crystalline forms. The imperfect crystals have some disorder and, hence, entropy associated with their crystalline structure even at absolute zero. The one liquid that has a zero entropy at absolute zero is liquid He, which becomes a perfect superfluid at this temperature. For a more detailed discussion of the third law, see reference [21].

2.11. FREE ENERGY AND THERMODYNAMIC FUNCTIONS

Often when doing thermodynamic calculations, it is useful to define certain thermodynamic functions that have useful properties, summarize complex data, contain variables that are measurable, and can be controlled through experiments. As shown by Eq. 2.61, the entropy must increase for a process to be spontaneous. To express this in terms useful to pharmacy, the first and second laws (Eqs. 2.30, 2.56, and 2.61) can be equated as follows:

$$TdS \geq dQ = dU - dW \quad (2.63)$$

Equation 2.63 can be simplified for the special cases of constant temperature because $TdS = d(TS)$. Recall the product rule from calculus: $d(TS) = dTS + TdS = TdS$ and $dT = 0$ (see Appendix 2.1).

$$-d(U - TS) \geq -dW \quad (2.64)$$

Because U, T, and S are state functions,

$$A = U - TS \quad (2.65)$$

defines a new state function called the *Helmholtz free energy*, which, for constant temperature, gives the maximum work that can be done by a system during a reversible isothermal process. In other words (recall that multiplication by -1 flips $>$ to $<$):

$$dA_T \leq dW \quad (2.66)$$

Therefore, the Helmholtz free energy is less than or equal to the maximum work that can be done by a system. The equal sign applies if the process is reversible, and the less than sign applies if the process is irreversible. If the only work considered is pressure volume work and if this work is zero, then Eq. 2.66 reduces to $dA_T \leq 0$, which gives the condition for a constant T and V process to be spontaneous, and the Helmholtz free energy equals zero at equilibrium.

Now let's look at the case of constant temperature and pressure, which is very important for pharmacy. If no-pressure volume work is included, Eq. 2.63 can be written in the form

$$TdS \geq dQ = dU - dW'' + PdV \quad (2.67)$$

where dW'' is the no-pressure volume work. At constant pressure, $PdV = d(PV)$ [see Appendix 2.1], and at constant temperature, $TdS = d(TS)$ yields an expression that contains the enthalpy:

$$-d(U + PV - TS) = d(H - TS) \geq -dW'' \quad 2.68)$$

Again, because H, T, and S are state functions $H - TS$ is also a state function called the *Gibbs free energy:*

$$G = H - TS \quad (2.69)$$

Thus, at constant temperature and pressure (recall that multiplication by -1 flips $>$ to $<$),

$$dG_{T,P} \leq dW'' \quad (2.70)$$

and if only pressure volume work is considered, $dG_{T,P} \leq 0$, where the equal sign applies for reversible processes, the less than sign applies for irreversible processes, and the Gibbs free energy equals zero at equilibrium. Any process in which $dG_{T,P}$ is negative will proceed spontaneously. In summary, A and G are criteria for the spontaneity of a process, which sets them apart from U and H.

2.11.1 Total Differentials of Free Energy Functions

As you will see later in the chapter, sometimes it can be useful to express the thermodynamic functions as total differentials; therefore, these forms are derived. For example, to determine dG (the definition of enthalpy), you insert Eq. 2.36 into Eq. 2.69 and apply the chain rule of calculus (see Appendix 2.1); consequently, you can write dG as follows:

$$dG = dU + PdV + VdP - TdS - SdT \quad (2.71)$$

By substituting in the first law (Eq. 2.30) for the internal energy, you get

$$dG = dQ + dW + PdV + VdP - TdS - SdT \quad (2.72)$$

If the thermodynamic process is reversible, $dQ = TdS$, and if the only work is pressure-volume work, $dW = -PdV$. You can substitute these conditions into Eq. 2.72, which, after you cancel terms, yields the following:

$$dG = VdP - SdT \quad (2.73)$$

By analogy, the same type of relationship can be found for the Helmholtz free energy, enthalpy, and internal energy. The results are given in Table 2.2.

From the differential forms, many useful relationships can be derived. For example, the total derivative (Eq. 2.23, see also Appendix 2.1) of the Gibbs free energy (Eq. 2.69) with respect to temperature and pressure has the following form:

$$dG = \left(\frac{\partial G}{\partial P}\right)_T dP + \left(\frac{\partial G}{\partial T}\right)_P dT \quad (2.74)$$

By comparison with Table 2.1, the values of the partial derivatives of G can be found as follows:

$$\left(\frac{\partial G}{\partial P}\right)_T = V \quad \left(\frac{\partial G}{\partial T}\right)_P = -S \quad (2.75a)$$

By analogy, the other derivatives can be found by comparison with Table 2.1 as follows:

$$\left(\frac{\partial U}{\partial P}\right)_S = -P \quad \left(\frac{\partial U}{\partial S}\right)_V = T \quad (2.75b)$$

$$\left(\frac{\partial H}{\partial P}\right)_S = V \quad \left(\frac{\partial H}{\partial S}\right)_P = T \quad (2.75c)$$

$$\left(\frac{\partial A}{\partial V}\right)_T = -P \quad \left(\frac{\partial A}{\partial T}\right)_V = -S \quad (2.75d)$$

Because U, H, A, and G are all state functions, their differential form must satisfy Eq. 2.24 (see Appendix 2.1) by applying this relationship to functions listed in Table 2.1. Useful relationships between the partial derivative can be found; they are known as Maxwell's equations:

$$\left(\frac{\partial T}{\partial V}\right)_S = -\left(\frac{\partial P}{\partial S}\right)_V \quad (2.76a)$$

$$\left(\frac{\partial T}{\partial P}\right)_S = -\left(\frac{\partial V}{\partial S}\right)_P \quad (2.76b)$$

$$\left(\frac{\partial P}{\partial T}\right)_V = \left(\frac{\partial S}{\partial V}\right)_T \quad (2.76c)$$

$$\left(\frac{\partial V}{\partial T}\right)_P = -\left(\frac{\partial S}{\partial P}\right)_T \quad (2.76d)$$

TABLE 2.2 Summary of Thermodynamic Functions and Their Differential Forms

Function	State Variables	Definition	Differential Form
Internal energy	S, V	$U = Q + W$	$dU = TdS - PdV$
Enthalpy	S, P	$H = U + PV$	$dH = VdP + TdS$
Helmholtz free energy	T, V	$A = U + TS$	$dA = -PdV - SdT$
Gibbs free energy	T, P	$G = H + TS$	$dG = VdP - SdT$
Entropy	T, V	$S = Q/T$	

2.11.2 Gibbs Free Energy

To understand how pressure influences the Gibbs free energy, you can use Eq. 2.75a to better understand this important property and how it changes. First, look at pressure:

$$\Delta G = G_2 - G_1 = \int_1^2 VdP \quad (2.77)$$

To use this equation, you need to know how P and V are interrelated, i.e., how V varies with P. For an ideal gas, this can be easily done using the $PV = nRT$

relationship. This equation then can be inserted into Eq. 2.77 to yield the following:

$$\Delta G = G_2 - G_1 = \int_1^2 nRT\frac{dP}{P} = nRT\ln\frac{P_2}{P_1} \tag{2.78}$$

Using the preceding equations, you can determine many useful relationships.

2.12. CHEMICAL EQUILIBRIUM

Previously, we discussed the properties of the free energy functions and gave some information on how they relate to conditions of equilibrium. By knowing the sign and magnitude of ΔG, you know whether a process will occur spontaneously and if it is at equilibrium. Now let's examine how they relate to chemical equilibrium.

A chemical reaction in a closed system can be represented by

$$\nu_a A + \nu_b B \leftrightarrow \nu_c C + \nu_d D \tag{2.79}$$

where ν_a, ν_b, ν_c, and ν_d are the stoichiometric coefficients of the chemical reactants A and B and products C and D, respectively. For this reaction or any similar type of reaction, the total Gibbs free energy is the sum of the individual Gibbs free energies times their stoichiometric coefficients:

$$\Delta G = (\nu_c G_C + \nu_d G_D) - (\nu_a G_A + \nu_b G_B) \tag{2.80}$$

As discussed earlier, the Gibbs free energies for the reactants or products can be expressed by $G_i = G_i^o + RT\ln a_i$ or $G_i = G_i^o + RT\ln f_i$ for liquids or solids, respectively. Depending on the system, Eq. 2.78 can be substituted into Eq. 2.80, yielding

$$\begin{aligned}\Delta G = \nu_c(G_c^o + RT\ln a_c) + \nu_d(G_d^o + RT\ln a_d)\\ - \nu_a(G_a^o + RT\ln a_a) - \nu_b(G_b^o + RT\ln a_b)\end{aligned} \tag{2.81}$$

By separating the terms, you can write Eq. 2.81 as

$$\Delta G = \Delta G^o + RT\ln\frac{a_c^{\nu_c}a_d^{\nu_d}}{a_a^{\nu_a}a_b^{\nu_b}} \tag{2.82}$$

where $\Delta G^0 = \nu_c G_c^o + \nu_d G_d^o - \nu_a G_a^o - \nu_b G_b^o$. It is interesting to note that if the reaction has run to equilibrium, then $\Delta G = 0$ and Eq. 2.82 equals 0:

$$0 = \Delta G^o + RT\ln\left(\frac{a_c^{\nu_c}a_d^{\nu_d}}{a_a^{\nu_a}a_b^{\nu_b}}\right)_{eq} \tag{2.83}$$

The logarithm is equal to the equilibrium constant if the whole system is at standard temperature and pressure (i.e., are at the same conditions as ΔG^o was determined):

$$K_{eq} = \frac{a_c^{\nu_c}a_d^{\nu_d}}{a_a^{\nu_a}a_b^{\nu_b}} \tag{2.84}$$

At these conditions you can get the following well-known equation:

$$\Delta G^o = -RT\ln K_{eq} \tag{2.85}$$

2.12.1 Temperature Dependence

What happens if you or your patients leave a product in the car on a hot summer day? How will the heat affect physical and chemical stability of that product? To analyze this issue, you can look at how temperature influences chemical equilibrium. To begin, you can rewrite Eq. 2.85 as follows:

$$\text{In } K_{eq} = \frac{\Delta G^o}{RT} \tag{2.86}$$

By taking the derivative with respect to time of each side, you can rewrite Eq. 2.86 as follows:

$$\frac{\partial \ln K_{eq}}{\partial T} = \frac{1}{R}\frac{(\Delta G^o/T)}{\partial T} \tag{2.87}$$

Using the quotient rule (see Appendix 2.1), taking the deviation of the right side yields the following:

$$\frac{\partial \ln K_{eq}}{\partial T} = \frac{1}{RT^2}\left(T\frac{\partial \Delta G^o}{\partial T} - \Delta G^o\right) \tag{2.88}$$

At this point, it is useful to recall $\partial\Delta G^\circ/\partial T = -S$ and $\Delta G^\circ = H^\circ - TS$. As such,

$$\frac{\partial \ln K_{eq}}{\partial T} = \frac{\Delta H^o}{RT^2} \tag{2.89}$$

This is the van't Hoff equation, which can be used to assess the effect of temperature.

2.13. OPEN SYSTEMS

The preceding analyses have been restricted to closed systems, but it would be useful to know how the addition of a material affects the thermodynamics of a system. For example, what happens when salt is added to an IV bag? There are many other important examples where understanding how the exchange of mass affects a system. This subject is very broad, so this discussion is restricted to analysis of Gibbs free energy, which is the most important case.

To begin, you can ask how the basic equation of change for Gibbs free energy (Eq. 2.74) can be modified to account for the change of mass with the environment (in this case Eq. 2.74) to take the form

$$\begin{aligned}dG = \left(\frac{\partial G}{\partial P}\right)_{T,n_1,n_2} dP + \left(\frac{\partial G}{\partial T}\right)_{P,n_1,n_2} dT + \left(\frac{\partial G}{\partial n_1}\right)_{P,T,n_2} dn_1\\ + \left(\frac{\partial G}{\partial n_2}\right)_{P,T,n_1} dn_2 + \ldots\end{aligned} \tag{2.90}$$

where the term

$$\left(\frac{\partial G}{\partial n_1}\right)_{P,T,n_2} = \mu_1 \quad (2.91)$$

is given the name *chemical potential* or *partial molar free energy* and is used to assess how the addition of mass to a system affects Gibbs free energy. Also, the differential form of Gibbs free energy (Eq. 2.73) can also be modified to include the exchange of mass; in this case, it becomes

$$dG = VdP - SdT + \mu_1 dn_1 + \mu_2 dn_2 \quad (2.92)$$

If temperature and pressure are held constant, then Eq. 2.92 can be rewritten as follows:

$$dG_{TP} = \mu_1 dn_1 + \mu_2 dn_2 \quad (2.93)$$

It can be shown that the chemical potential or partial molar free energy has conditions for equilibrium of $dG = 0$. These relationships are very useful when you are analyzing pharmaceutical systems.

2.14. CONCLUSIONS

This chapter describes the various states of matter and laws governing their behavior, which are useful in designing drug, dosage form, and drug delivery systems; selecting proper storage conditions for drugs; as well as selecting their optimum formulation and administration strategies. Thermodynamics is based on three laws, and these laws have never been proved directly. However, various inferences have been deduced in the form of different mathematical equations from these laws, and the results have been found to be in close agreement with the observations. The concepts of thermodynamics help in appreciating the energy changes associated with various active biological processes and their applications in developing stable, effective, and reliable dosage forms.

CASE STUDIES

Case 2.1

There are some combination products for insulin for better management of diabetes because their onset of action, peak glycemic effect, and duration of effect are better than rapid-acting or short-acting or intermediate-acting insulin.

Question: Why do combination insulins behave differently than other insulin products?

Approach: The following three combination insulin products are listed in Lexicomp 2013 [25]:

1. Insulin aspartate porotamine suspension and insulin aspartate solution (70:30)
2. Insulin lispro protamine suspension and insulin lispro solution (75:25)
3. Insulin NPH suspension and insulin regular solution (70:30)

Human insulin is able to exist in a solid state as both amorphous and crystalline forms. The amorphous form of insulin dissolves quickly, becomes biologically available faster than the crystalline form, and thereby exhibits rapid action. In the preceding example of insulin combination products, the solid state form of it in solution is amorphous.

In contrast, the crystalline form of insulin goes into solution at a slower rate than its amorphous counterpart and hence becomes bioavailable later and exhibits effects for a longer duration of time. The solid state of insulin in suspension in the preceding examples is in crystalline form.

Thus, the mixture of insulin in amorphous and crystalline forms explains the unique efficacy profile of combination insulin products rather than other insulin products. The amorphous portion provides a quick release and absorption, followed by the slow release of the crystalline form.

Case Study 2.2

It is essential not to overheat cocoa butter, which is used as a suppository base during the preparation of the suppository by fusion method. Such suppositories must be stored in the refrigerator. Why?

Theobroma oil, or cocoa butter, melts to a large degree over a narrow temperature range of 34°C–36°C. It exists in four polymorphic forms: the unstable gamma form melting at 18°C, the alpha form melting at 22°C, the beta prime form melting at 28°C, and the stable beta form melting at 34.5°C. If theobroma oil is heated to the point at which it is completely liquefied (about 35°C), the nuclei of the stable beta crystals are destroyed, and the mass does not crystallize until it is supercooled to about 15°C. Otherwise, the crystals that form are the metastable gamma, alpha, and beta prime forms, and the suppositories melt at 23–24°C or at ordinary room temperature.

Therefore, the proper method of preparation involves melting cocoa butter at the lowest possible temperature, about 34°C. The mass is sufficiently fluid to pour, yet the crystal nuclei of the stable form are not lost. When the mass is chilled in a mold, a stable suppository—consisting of beta crystals and melting at 34.5°C—is produced. These suppositories are stored in a refrigerator to preserve their stable beta polymorphic state.

Case Study 2.3

Question: The concentration of urea in plasma and urine are 0.006 M and 0.345 M, respectively. Calculate the free energy in transporting 0.01 mole of urea from plasma to urine. Is this transport process spontaneous; i.e., would it happen on its own? How many ATP molecules would be consumed in providing energy for this transport process?

Approach: Thermodynamic principles can be used to answer this question. The Gibbs free energy equation, shown here, is the major deciding factor of spontaneous or nonspontaneous process:

$$\text{Free energy}, \Delta G = nRT \times In\frac{c_2}{c_1}$$

where c is the concentration.

From the question, let's see what we have already:

n = The number of moles to be transported = 0.01 mole
R = Gas constant = 1.987 cal/mole/K
T = Here, the transport of urea is inside the body, where the temperature = 37°C = 273 + 37 = 310/K
C_2 = 0.345 M
C_1 = 0.006 M (Always consider the concentration C_1 from where the transport is being initiated.)

Therefore, free energy

$$\Delta G = 0.01 \text{ mole} \times 1.987 \frac{\text{Cal}}{\text{mole} \times K} \times 310\ K \times \text{In}\frac{0.345\ M}{0.006\ M} = 24.96\ \text{Cal}$$

Since the value of free energy change is positive, the transport of urea from plasma or blood to urine would not be automatic but would require expenditure of energy equivalent to 24.96 calories, which most probably would be provided by hydrolysis of ATP. The hydrolysis of ATP releases 7.3 Kcals of energy in addition to producing ADP and inorganic phosphate as shown here:

$$\text{ATP} \rightarrow \text{ADP} + (P)_i + 7.3\ \text{Kcals}$$

There are 6.023×10^{23} (Avogadro's number) ATP molecules in one mole of ATP.

Therefore, 7300 cals (i.e., 7.3 Kcals) energy is produced by 6.023×10^{23} ATP molecules. Hence, 24.96 cals would be produced by

$$\frac{6.023 \times 10^{23}\ \text{molecules}}{7300\ \text{cals}} \times 24.96\ \text{cal} = 2.059 \times 10^{21}\ \text{ATP molecules}$$

APPENDIX 2.1 CALCULUS REVIEW

Partial Derivatives

A derivative is the instantaneous rate of change of a function, given by the slope of a tangent line to a curve described by the function of interest. When you have functions of more than one variable, the symbol ∂ is used to indicate partial derivatives should be used. When you are computing a partial derivative, all of the other variables are treated like constants, and then rules of differentiation are applied to the variable of interest. For example, let $f(x, y)$ be a function of x and y; then by the definitions of a partial derivative, the rate of change of $f(x, y)$, with respect to x and y are given by Eqs. 2.94 and 2.95, respectively:

$$\left(\frac{\partial f}{\partial y}\right)_y = \lim_{\Delta x \to 0} \frac{f(x + \Delta x, y) - f(x, y)}{\Delta x} \tag{2.94}$$

$$\left(\frac{\partial f}{\partial y}\right)_x = \lim_{\Delta y \to 0} \frac{f(x, y + \Delta y) - f(x, y)}{\Delta y} \tag{2.95}$$

However, the definition of a derivative based on limits is primarily used for theoretical investigation (see following text). When you are computing derivatives, the standard rules of differentiation given in any calculus textbook are used. For example, the equation for an ideal gas is $PV = \text{n}RT$. To know how pressure varies with temperature and volume change, you can solve the equation for P; in functional notation, it can be written as $P = f(V, T) = \text{n}RT/V$. The partial derivatives take partial derivatives:

$$\frac{\partial P}{\partial T} = \frac{\partial f}{\partial T} = \frac{\partial}{\partial T}\left(\frac{nRT}{V}\right) = \frac{nR}{V} \tag{2.96}$$

$$\frac{\partial P}{\partial V} = \frac{\partial f}{\partial V} = \frac{\partial}{\partial V}\left(\frac{nRT}{V}\right) = \frac{-nRT}{V^2} \tag{2.97}$$

Product Rule

The product rule is used to calculate the derivative for the product of two functions, where the $'$ is standard calculus notation for the derivative with respect to the variable of interest:

$$(fg)' = f'g + g'f \tag{2.98}$$

Chain Rule

The chain rule is used to compute the derivative of a function of a function:

$$f(g(x))' = \frac{df}{dg} \cdot \frac{dg}{dx} \tag{2.99}$$

Quotient Rule

The quotient rule for derivatives follows, and it can be derived by applying the chain rule and the product rule to a quotient:

$$\left(\frac{f}{g}\right)' = \frac{f'g - g'f}{g^2} \tag{2.100}$$

Total Derivatives

Often in thermodynamics, you need to calculate change Δf of the function $f(x, y)$ when both x and y are varying. For infinitesimally small changes, the total derivative is given by

$$\Delta f = f(x + \Delta x, y + \Delta y) - f(x, y) \tag{2.101}$$

$$\Delta f = \underbrace{f(x+\Delta x, y+\Delta y) - f(x, y+\Delta y)} + \underbrace{f(x, y+\Delta y) - f(x,y)}$$

$$\Delta f = \quad \Delta x\left(\frac{\partial f}{\partial x}\right)_y \quad + \quad \Delta y\left(\frac{\partial f}{\partial y}\right)_x \tag{2.102}$$

For example, the total derivative of P, written as $\mathrm{d}P$, is given by the following equation:

$$\mathrm{d}P = \left(\frac{\partial P}{\partial V}\right)_T \mathrm{d}V + \left(\frac{\partial P}{\partial T}\right)_V \mathrm{d}T \tag{2.103}$$

The total derivative has a lot of significance in thermodynamics because it gives information about exact differentials, which are path independent.

Abbreviations

a	Acceleration
A	Helmholtz free energy
API	Active pharmaceutical ingredient
c	Concentration
C	Heat capacity; C_p and C_V are the heat capacities at constant pressure and volume, respectively
C (phase equilibria)	Number of components in a system
$\delta+$	Positive charge
$\delta-$	Negative charge
F	Force [units: dyne (dyn) = gm cm sec^{-2} or Newton (N) = kg m sec^{-2}]
F_A	Attractive forces
F_R	Repulsive forces
F (phase equilibria)	Degrees of freedom
g	Weight in grams of gas
G	Gibbs free energy
H	Enthalpy
ΔH°_f	Standard enthalpy of formation
ΔH_v	Heat of vaporization
KE	Kinetic energy
m	Mass
M_W	Molecular weight of gas
n	Number of moles
P	Pressure (units: Pascal (Pa) = N m^2)
P_c	Critical pressure
P_i	Partial pressure
P (phase equilibria)	Number of phases
Q	Heat
r	Distance separating the molecules
R	Gas constant values in different unit systems: 8.3143 JK^{-1} mol^{-1}, 8.3143 × 10^{-7} erg K^{-1} mol^{-1}, 1.98762 cal K^{-1} mol^{-1}, and 0.0821 liter atm K^{-1} mole^{-1}
S	Entropy (J/°K)
T	Temperature
T^*	Temperature of a phase transition
T_C	Critical temperature
V	Volume
VP	Equilibrium vapor pressure
U	Internal energy (Joule N m, erg dyne cm)
W	Work [units: erg = dyne cm or Joule (J) = N m]
X	Mole fraction
x	Distance

References

[1] Sandmann BJ. Intermolecular forces and states of matter. In: Amiji MM, Sandmann BJ, editors. Applied physical pharmacy. New York: McGraw Hill; 2003. p. 27–45.

[2] Israelachvili JN. Intermolecular and surface forces. 3rd ed. San Diego: Academic Press; 2011.

[3] Van Ness H. Understanding thermodynamics. New York: McGraw-Hill; 1969. p. 103.

[4] Vemulapalli GK. Physical chemistry. Englewood Cliffs, NJ: Prentice Hall; 1993. p. 991.

[5] Hadkar UB. Physical pharmacy. Pune India: Nirali Prakashan; 2007.

[6] Perlovich GL, Volkova T, Bauer-Brandl A. Polymorphism of paracetamol. J Therm Anal Calorim 2007;89(3):767–74.
[7] Lu J, Wang X-J, Yang X, Ching C-B. Characterization and selective crystallization of famotidine polymorphs. J Pharm Sci 2007;96(9):2457–68.
[8] Lu J, Wang X-J, Yang X, Ching C-B. Polymorphism and crystallization of famotidine. Cryst Growth Des 2007;7(9):1590–8.
[9] Nagaraju R, Prathusha AP, Chandra-Bose PS, Kaza R, Bharathi K. Preparation and evaluation of famotidine polymorphs. Curr Drug Discov Technol 2010;7(2):106–16.
[10] Német Z, Kis GC, Pokol G, Demeter Á. Quantitative determination of famotidine polymorphs: X-ray powder diffractometric and Raman spectrometric study. J Pharm Biomed Anal 2009;49 (2):338–46.
[11] Sheth AR, Bates S, Muller FX, Grant DJW. Polymorphism in Piroxicam. Cryst Growth Des 2004;4(6):1091–8.
[12] Vrečer F, Srčič S, Šmid-Korbar J. Investigation of piroxicam polymorphism. Int J Pharm 1991;68(1–3):35–41.
[13] Bauer J, Spanton S, Henry R, Quick J, Dziki W, Porter W, et al. Ritonavir: an extraordinary example of conformational polymorphism. Pharm Res 2001;18(6):859–66.
[14] Barbas R, Martí F, Prohens R, Puigjaner C. Polymorphism of norfloxacin: evidence of the enantiotropic relationship between polymorphs A and B. Cryst Growth Des 2006;6(6):1463–7.
[15] Šuštar B, Bukovec N, Bukovec P. Polymorphism and stability of norfloxacin, (1-ethyl-6-fluoro-1,4-dihydro-4-oxo-7-(1-piperazinil) -3-quinolinocarboxylic acid. J Therm Anal Calorim 1993;40 (2):475–81.
[16] Aguiar AJ, Krc J, Kinkel AW, Samyn JC. Effect of polymorphism on the absorption of chloramphenicol from chloramphenicol palmitate. J Pharm Sci 1967;56(7):847–53.
[17] Aguiar AJ, Zelmer JE. Dissolution behavior of polymorphs of chloramphenicol palmitate and mefenamic acid. J Pharm Sci 1969;58(8):983–7.
[18] Callen HB. Thermodynamics and an introduction to thermostatistics. 2nd ed. New York: John Wiley & Sons; 1985.
[19] Fermi E. Thermodynamics. New York: Dover; 1936.
[20] Sinko PJ, Singh Y. Martin's physical pharmacy and pharmaceutical sciences: physical chemical and biopharmaceutical principles in the pharmaceutical sciences. 6th ed. Philadelphia: Lippincott Williams & Wilkins; 2011.
[21] Moore WJ. Physical chemistry. 4th ed. Englewood Cliffs, NJ: Prentice-Hall Inc; 1972.
[22] Feynman RP, Leighton RB, Sands M. The Feynman lectures on physics. Reading MA: Addison-Wesley Publishing Co.; 1963.
[23] Glasstone S. Physical chemistry. Princeton, NJ: D. Van Nostrand Co. Inc; 1946.
[24] Atkins PW. Physical Chemistry. 2nd ed. San Francisco: W.H. Freeman and Co.; 1982.
[25] Creighton University Health Sciences Online. Available from: <http://online.lexi.com.cuhsl.creighton.edu/lco/action/search?q=Insulin&t=name> [accessed 18.08.2013].

CHAPTER

3

Physical Properties, Their Determination, and Importance in Pharmaceutics

Somnath Singh and Alekha K. Dash

Department of Pharmacy Sciences, Creighton University, Omaha, NE, USA

CHAPTER OBJECTIVES

- Define surface and interfacial tension, adsorption and absorption, and surfactant working at the interface.
- Explain the working principles behind the measurement of surface tension and the extent of adsorption at the interface.
- Describe the properties of liquid interfaces and compare the forces of molecular attraction at interfaces with the bulk liquid.
- Discuss the types of surfactants and their pharmaceutical and clinical applications.
- Define and discuss various colligative properties.
- Define viscosity, fluidity, and kinematic viscosity, as well as mathematical expressions for these terms.
- Compare and contrast Newtonian and non-Newtonian liquids and their flow characteristics.
- Explain the methods used to measure viscosity of liquids and semisolids.
- Describe the application of rheology in pharmacy.
- Define spectroscopy and the electromagnetic radiation spectrum in terms of wavelength, wavenumber, frequency, and energy.
- Compare and contrast the energy requirement for vibrational, translational, and rotational transition.
- Discuss the working principles behind ultraviolet, visible, infrared, fluorescence, nuclear magnetic resonance, and mass spectroscopy and their applications.

Keywords

- Adsorption
- Colligative properties
- Interfacial tension
- Physical properties
- Rheology
- Spectroscopy
- Surface tension
- Surfactant

3.1. INTRODUCTION

Successful development of any dosage forms or drug delivery systems for a new drug requires that some fundamental physical and chemical properties of the drug molecule are known before proceeding to formulation development. In order to arrive at the target site in the appropriate form, the drug molecule has to travel from the site of administration and overcome many hurdles and barriers. As an example, for an orally administered drug, the molecule has to overcome many hurdles that include dissolving in gastrointestinal (GI) fluid, surviving a range of gastric pH (1.5–8.0), surviving intestinal enzymes, crossing many membranes, surviving liver metabolism, avoiding excretion by kidneys, partitioning into the targeted organ, and avoiding partition into undesired sites.

Some of the properties or tests that are necessary in the early stage of formulation development may include simple UV spectroscopy or HPLC assays for the drug molecules, aqueous solubility, p*Ka*, partition coefficient, moisture adsorption properties, dissolution, melting point, solution and solid-state stability, microscopic properties, bulk density, flow property, and compression properties. In a dosage form, besides the

Pharmaceutics. DOI: http://dx.doi.org/10.1016/B978-0-12-386890-9.00003-0

active pharmaceutical ingredient (API), many more inactive materials are present, which can greatly affect the overall property of the dosage form. It is also equally important to have a rational formulation. One must have a good understanding of the physicochemical properties of excipients and their influence on the overall formulation. Some of the physical properties just outlined are described in other chapters.

This chapter focuses on some of surface properties, flow properties, colligative properties, as well as some of the fundamentals of spectroscopy essential for dosage form design. Identity, purity, quality, and quality assurance are the four important aspects of dosage form design to ensure a product is safe, effective, and reliable. Various analytical tests are necessary for identification of drugs; they include FTIR, NMR, TLC, DSC, X-ray, and UV spectroscopy. To confirm purity, it is essential to determine the melting point by DSC; moisture content by Karl–Fisher titrimetry; and organic, inorganic, and heavy metal impurities. Finally, for quality assurance, various assay procedures including spectroscopy, HPLC, and other analytical methods are beneficial.

3.2. SURFACE AND INTERFACIAL TENSION

3.2.1 Interfaces

When two phases exist together, the boundary between the two phases is called an interface. For example, the surface of a tablet is the interface between a solid phase (tablet) and a gaseous phase (air). Similarly, if we mix two immiscible liquids such as olive oil and water, a boundary exists between the oil and water, and it may also be called the oil-water interface. Then the following question arises: Why is the study of interfaces important in pharmacy? The study of interfaces between solids and liquids is important in the formulation of pharmaceutical suspensions. The study of interfaces between two immiscible liquids also is important in formulating pharmaceutical emulsions. In addition to their importance in the formation and stability of suspensions and emulsions, the interfacial phenomenon is important in governing drug absorption and penetration through biological membranes.

3.2.2 Liquid Interfaces

In a beaker containing some water, the surface of the water is truly an air-water interface. Let's consider the forces that act on liquid molecules in the bulk region and compare them with the forces at the surface (see Figure 3.1).

Consider a water molecule that is present in the bulk. It is surrounded by water molecules in all directions. The intermolecular forces of attraction are therefore the same in all directions. In contrast, however, a water molecule at the surface is surrounded by water molecules on the sides and below, but by air molecules on the top. As the attractive forces between water-water molecules are greater than that of water-air molecules, water molecules at the surface experience a net inward pull. These molecules are therefore constantly under "tension." Because nobody, including liquids, likes to be under constant tension, liquids tend to minimize their total "tension" by minimizing the area of the total surface. Because a sphere has a minimum surface area–to–volume ratio, drops of most liquids, including water, assume a spherical shape when suspended in a vacuum. Although raindrops should also ideally assume a spherical shape, they are distorted due to the influence of wind and gravity.

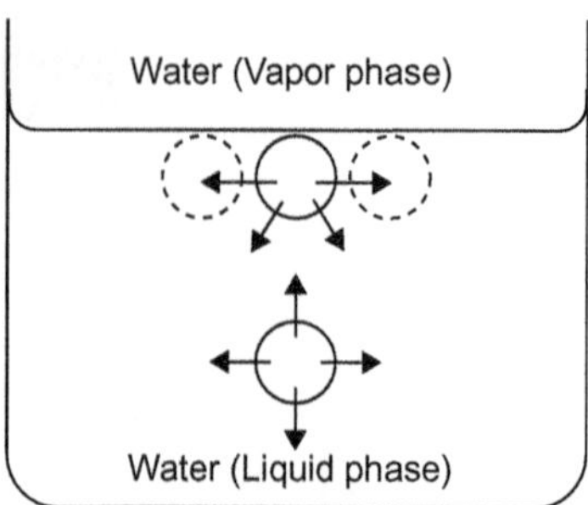

FIGURE 3.1 Schematic representation of molecular mechanism of surface tension.

You may recall that the force of attraction between like molecules (for example, water-water) is called the force of cohesion. Similarly, the force of attraction between unlike molecules (for example, water-air, water-glass, or water-olive oil) is called the force of adhesion. The term surface tension is used when one of the surfaces in contact is air. However, the interfacial tension term is used when both surfaces are immiscible liquids. Since, the adhesive forces between two immiscible liquid phases forming the interface are greater than that of between liquid and air interface, the surface tension is generally higher than the interfacial tension. There is no interfacial tension between two completely miscible liquids.

3.2.3 The Definition of Surface and Interfacial Tension

The surface tension at any temperature is the force per unit length (dynes/cm) that has to be applied parallel to the surface to counterbalance the net inward pull of a liquid at the liquid-air interface. Similarly, interfacial tension is the tension at the interface of two immiscible liquids.

3.2.4 Effect of Temperature

The surface tension of any liquid or the interfacial tension of any liquid-liquid system has to be reported

TABLE 3.1 Surface Tension of Water at Various Temperatures

Temperature (°C)	Surface Tension (dynes/cm)
0	76.5
20	72.8
30	71.2
75	63.5
100	58.0

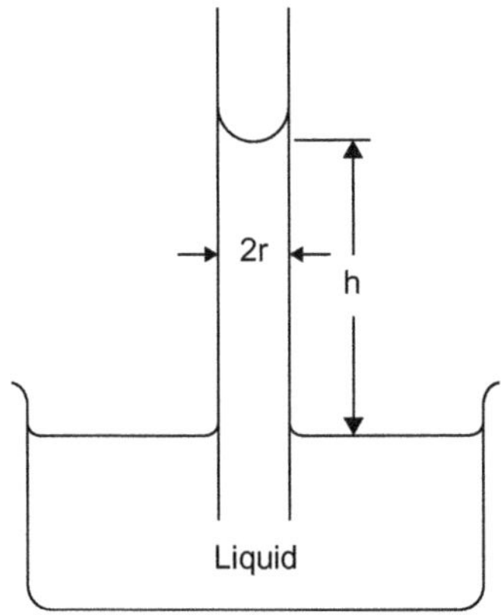

FIGURE 3.2 Determination of surface tension by the capillary rise method.

at a particular temperature. The tension in both cases varies significantly with temperature. Note, for example, the effect of temperature on the surface tension of water in Table 3.1.

3.2.5 Measurement of Surface Tension

Numerous methods are used to measure surface and interfacial tension. However, a simple method of practical importance is the capillary rise method.

When a capillary tube is placed in water in a beaker, the water rises in the capillary tube to a level higher than the liquid surface (see Figure 3.2). Water rises in the capillary tube because the forces of adhesion between water and the wall of the glass capillary (glass) are greater than the cohesive forces between the water-water molecules. This may not be the case for all liquids. For example, in the case of mercury, placing a capillary tube at the surface will show a fall in the level of the liquid because the cohesive forces between mercury-mercury molecules are stronger than the adhesive forces between mercury-glass. However, most liquids behave similar to water, which is considered for the rest of this discussion.

If a capillary tube of radius, r, is placed on the surface of a liquid, and the liquid rises to a height, h, in the capillary tube, then the surface tension of the liquid, γ, at the temperature of the measurement is given by Eq. 3.1.

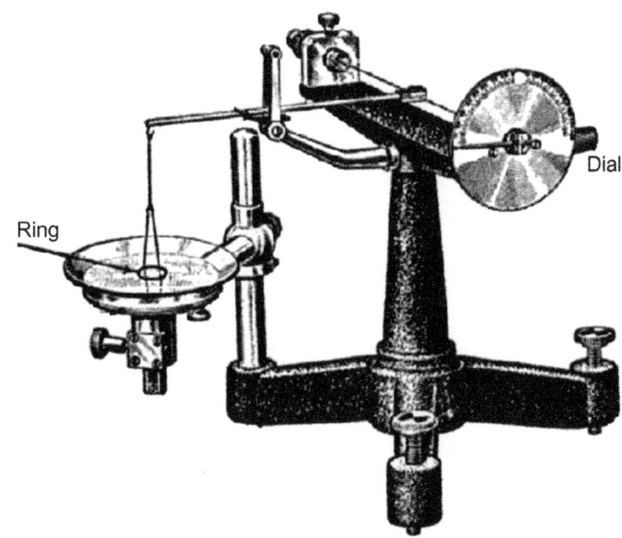

FIGURE 3.3 Tensiometer operating on DuNoüy ring method [1].

$$\gamma = \frac{1}{2} rh\rho g \quad (3.1)$$

where γ is the surface tension, r is the inner radius of the capillary tube, h is the height to which the liquid rises in the capillary tube, ρ is the density of the liquid, and g is the acceleration due to gravity (981 cm/sec^2)

3.2.6 Measurement of Interfacial Tension

In the DuNoüy ring method, the DuNoüy tensiometer (see Figure 3.3) is used to measure surface and interfacial tensions. The principle behind this method is based on the fact that the force required to detach a platinum-iridium ring immersed at the surface or interface is proportional to the surface or interfacial tension. The force required to detach the ring in this manner is provided by a torsion wire and recorded in dynes on a calibrated dial.

3.3. ADSORPTION

3.3.1 Adsorption and Absorption

Adsorption is primarily a surface phenomenon, whereas absorption occurs through the entire bulk of a substance. In the following sections, we are concerned primarily with the adsorption in liquids and solids. Adsorption of a poison onto an activated carbon surface is an example of a surface phenomenon, whereas passive diffusion of a drug molecule from an oral tablet via the GI tract membrane is called an absorption phenomenon.

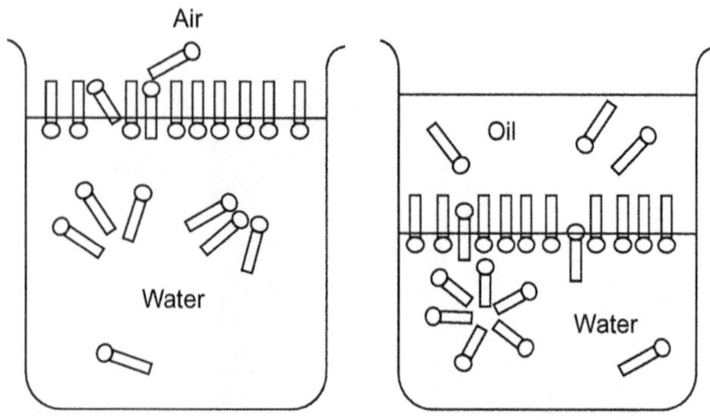

FIGURE 3.4 (A) Diagrammatic representation of accumulation of surfactants at the air-water interface and (B) formation of micelles in an aqueous medium.

3.3.2 Adsorption at Liquid Interfaces

3.3.2.1 *Surface Active Molecules or Surfactants*

Molecules or ions that are adsorbed at surfaces or interfaces and dramatically reduce surface tension of the liquid in which they are dispersed are called surface active agents, surfactants, or amphiphiles. For surface activity to be present in a molecule, the molecule must contain a hydrophilic (water-loving) group and also a lipophilic (oil-loving) group on the same molecule. When this molecule is added to a beaker of water, it orients itself at the surface of the water in such a manner that the hydrophilic group faces the bulk of water and the lipophilic group faces the air (see Figure 3.4A).

3.3.2.2 *The Critical Micelle Concentration (CMC)*

We now know that surfactants are preferentially adsorbed at the water-air interface. If we keep adding more and more surfactant to the water, there comes a time when the surface becomes completely saturated with the surfactant. There is no space available on the surface to occupy that position. The surfactant molecules then start entering the bulk water, but to minimize interfacial energy, they orient themselves in a manner so that all the hydrophilic groups face the bulk water, whereas the lipophilic groups face each other (see Figure 3.4B). These regular structures in the bulk liquid consisting of groups of molecules in a specific orientation are called micelles, whereas the individual molecules present at the surface are called monomers. Micelles have a hydrophilic surface and a lipophilic core that can be used to entrap and solubilize lipophilic substances. The diameter of the micelles is generally of the order of 50 Å. The size may vary with the size of the individual monomers and the solvent used.

The concentration above which the monomers of surfactant start associating to form micelles is called the critical micelle concentration, or the CMC. Until the CMC is reached, the surface properties of the liquid, such as the surface and interfacial tension and the vapor pressure, are affected. However, at concentrations above the CMC, the bulk properties of the liquid, such as density and conductivity, are affected.

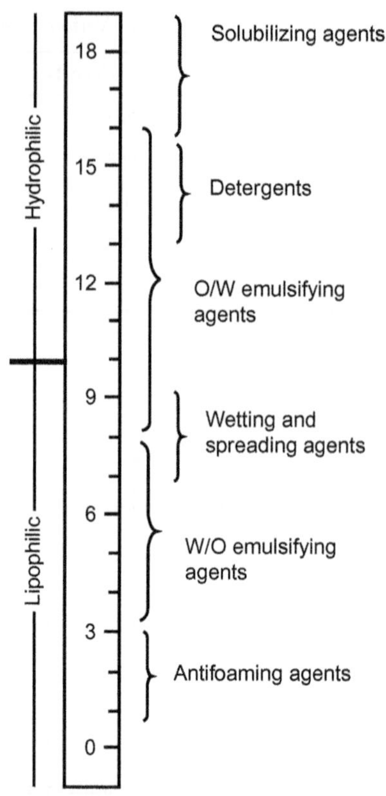

FIGURE 3.5 Hydrophilic-lipophilic-balance (HLB) scale.

3.3.3 Surface Active Agents in Pharmacy

This lipophilic core of micelles can be used to solubilize drug molecules in solutions and suspensions. The core can also be used to solubilize droplets of oil that is ordinarily immiscible in water. It is therefore evident that surfactants have a variety of uses in the manufacture of pharmaceutical solutions, suspensions, and emulsions. They are discussed in detail in the next section devoted to surfactants.

3.3.4 The Hydrophilic-Lipophilic-Balance (HLB) Scale

The surface activity of surfactants can be measured by their hydrophilic-lipophilic-balance (HLB) scale. The HLB value ranges from 0 to 20 on an arbitrary scale, as shown in the Figure 3.5.

The higher the HLB value of a surface active agent, the more hydrophilic it is, which determines its usefulness for a specific purpose. For example, spans or sorbitan esters, have low HLB values of 1.8–8.6 and therefore are useful for preparing water-in-oil (w/o) emulsions; whereas Tweens, or polyoxyethylene derivatives of spans, have high HLB values of 9.6–16.7 and are therefore useful for making oil-in-water (o/w) emulsions. However, a mixture of surfactants (with different HLB values) can be selected and preferred over a single surfactant with the required HLB value. The following example clarifies this concept.

Example:

The required HLB (RHLB) value for making an o/w emulsion is 10.9. Calculate the amounts of Tween 20 (HLB value = 16.7) and Span 80 (HLB value = 4.3) for making 2 g of the required emulsifiers.

Solution:

The formula for calculating the weight fraction of Tween 20 (surfactant with the higher HLB value) is as follows:

$$\textit{The weight fraction of Tween } 20 = \frac{RHLB - HTB\ low}{HLB\ high - HLB\ low}$$

$$\textit{The weight fraction of Tween } 20 = \frac{10.9 - 4.3}{16.7 - 4.3} = 0.53$$

Obviously, the weight fraction of Span 80 = 1 − 0.53 = 0.47. Therefore, the amount of Tween 20 = 2 g × 0.53 = 1.06 g, and the amount of Span 80 = 2 − 1.06 = 0.94 g or 2 g × 0.47 = 0.94 g.

3.3.5 Adsorption at Solid Interfaces

Adsorption onto solid surfaces can occur from gases or liquids. The principles of solid-gas absorption are used in the removal of objectionable odors from rooms or food, operation of gas masks, and measurement of dimensions of particles in a powder. The principles of solid-liquid adsorption are used in decolorizing solutions, adsorption chromatography, detergency, and wetting.

3.3.6 The Solid-Gas Interface

The adsorption of a gas by a solid depends on the physical and chemical nature of both the adsorbent (the material used to adsorb the gas) and the adsorbate (the substance being adsorbed). On this basis, the solid-gas adsorption may be classified as physical or chemical:

- **Physical adsorption:** This adsorption occurs due to the Van der Waal's forces of attraction, and can be reversed by increasing temperature or reducing pressure. The process by which a physically adsorbed gas is removed is called desorption.
- **Chemical adsorption:** This adsorption occurs due to attachment of the adsorbate to the adsorbent by chemical bonds. Typically, only one layer (monolayer) of adsorbate is attached. This process is irreversible.

3.3.7 Quantitative Measurement of Physical Adsorption

Physical adsorption can be measured by using the Freundlich adsorption isotherms or Langmuir adsorption isotherms.

3.3.7.1 Freundlich Adsorption Isotherms

The measurement of physical adsorption consists of a balance contained within a vacuum. A known amount of solid, previously degassed, is placed into the pan, and known amounts of gas are introduced into the vacuum chamber. If the weight of the solid used at the beginning of the experiment is W_s grams, then the increase in weight of the solid on introducing gas occurs due to adsorption of the gas on the solid surface. The relation between the amount of gas adsorbed and the pressure of the gas was given by Freundlich, as shown in Eq. 3.2:

$$\frac{W_g}{W_s} = kp^{1/n} \tag{3.2}$$

where W_g is the amount of gas adsorbed, p is the partial pressure of the gas, and k and $1/n$ are empirical constants. Converting Eq. 3.2 to logarithmic form, we obtain Eq. 3.3:

$$log\frac{W_g}{W_s} = \log k + \frac{1}{n}\log p \tag{3.3}$$

If $\log(W_g/W_s)$ is plotted as a function of log p, the slope of the straight line is $1/n$, and the antilog of the y-intercept is the constant, k.

3.3.7.2 Langmuir Adsorption Isotherms

Langmuir adsorption isotherms are based on the hypothesis that adsorption occurs as a monolayer. According to Langmuir, adsorption can be quantitated using Eq. 3.4:

$$\frac{p}{m_g} = \frac{1}{bm_{gs}} + \frac{p}{m_{gs}} \tag{3.4}$$

where p is pressure of the gas; m_{gs} is the amount of gas adsorbed per gram of adsorbent, i.e., $m_g = W_g/W$; and b is a constant. In case of adsorption of drug from its aqueous solution onto a solid surface, the term p in Eq. 3.4 could be substituted with c, i.e., the equilibrium concentration of drug. Both Freundlich and Langmuir adsorption isotherms have been used in characterizing the adsorption properties of solids; however, the former provides better results with lower concentration of adsorbate, whereas the latter one provides better results with a greater concentration.

3.3.8 The Solid-Liquid Interface

Numerous drugs such as dyes, alkaloids, fatty acids, and even inorganic acids and bases may be adsorbed from solution onto solids such as charcoal and alumina. The adsorption of solute molecules from solution may be treated in a manner analogous to the adsorption of molecules at the solid-gas interface. For example, the adsorption of strychnine, atropine, and quinine from aqueous solutions by many clays may be expressed by using the Langmuir adsorption isotherm discussed previously.

Activated charcoal is commonly employed as an antidote in poisoning by sulfonylureas such as tolbutamide, acetohexamide, and also acetaminophen and acetylcysteine. The adsorption by activated charcoal not only prevents bioabsorption by the gastrointestinal tract, but also causes elimination of drugs from the tissues into the GI tract by a process known as gastrointestinal dialysis. In this process, the adsorbing charcoal sets up a concentration gradient that favors diffusion of drugs from the systemic circulation into the GI tract.

3.3.9 Surface Active Agents

Surfactants or surface active agents or amphiphiles are chemical compounds that tend to accumulate at the boundary (i.e., interface) between two phases. Therefore, they are adsorbed at the various interfaces existing between solids and/or liquids, resulting in changing the nature of interfaces. This has huge significance in pharmacy, such as in the formation of emulsions or suspensions and solubilization of poorly soluble drugs via entrapment in the micelles.

3.3.9.1 *Classification*

On the basis of their charge, surfactants may be classified as anionic, cationic, amphoteric, or nonionic:

- *Anionic surfactants:* These surfactants contain carboxylate, sulfonate, or sulfate groups. Examples include sodium stearate, sodium dodecyl sulfate, and sodium lauryl sulfate.
- *Cationic surfactants:* These surfactants contain amine salts or quaternary ammonium salts. One example is cetrimonium bromide.
- *Amphoteric surfactants:* These surfactants contain carboxylate or phosphate groups as the anion and amino or quaternary ammonium groups as the cation. The former group, consisting of carboxylate anions and amine cations, are called polypeptides or proteins, and the latter group, consisting of phosphate anions and quaternary ammonium cations, are called natural phospholipids such as lecithins and cephalins.
- *Nonionic surfactants:* These surfactants do not have any charge. Examples include sorbitan esters (Spans®), polysorbates (Tweens®), and poloxamer (Pluronics®). Spans are mixtures of partial esters of sorbitol and its mono- and di-anhydrides with oleic acid. They are generally insoluble in water and have low hydrophilic-lipophilic-balance (HLB) values. Therefore, they are used for making water-in-oil emulsions and wetting a substance. Tweens differ from Spans in the sense that they are condensed with varying moles of ethylene oxide instead of oleic acid; hence, they have high HLB values, are soluble in water, and are used for making oil-in-water emulsions.

Pluronics are block copolymers of hydrophilic poly (oxyethylene) (POE) and hydrophobic poly(oxypropylene) (POP) represented by the general formula POE_n-POP_m-POE_n, where n and m represent the number of OE and OP, respectively. Table 3.2 shows the structures and the hydrophilic and hydrophobic components of some of the most frequently used surfactants.

3.3.10 Surface Activity of Drugs

Some drugs that are amphipathic in nature show surface activity that may influence their therapeutic activity. They differ from a surfactant in the sense that their hydrophobic groups are much more complex. Generally, the surface activity is increased due to the nature of the functional groups present on the hydrophobic moiety of these drugs. The decrease in CMC and increase in surface activity is found for the Br^- functional group containing antihistaminic drug brompheniramine in comparison to those in pheniramine [2]. Figure 3.6 shows the structures of some drugs whose pharmacological properties can be explained by their surface activity.

3.3.10.1 *Formation of Film at the Interface and its Application*

Surfactants are localized as monolayer films at the interface of water-air due to their amphiphilic nature. If the surfactant added is soluble or partially soluble in water, it forms a soluble layer at the interface which is in equilibrium with surfactant molecules in the bulk; otherwise, it forms an insoluble layer that is obviously not in equilibrium with those in the bulk region. An insoluble film or monolayer on the water surface can be conveniently obtained by injecting an organic solution of surfactant such as stearic acid in an organic solvent. An organic solvent would evaporate into air due

TABLE 3.2 Classification of Surfactants

Types and Examples	Structures	Hydrophobic Moiety	Hydrophilic Moiety
ANIONIC SURFACTANTS			
Sodium dodecyl sulfate	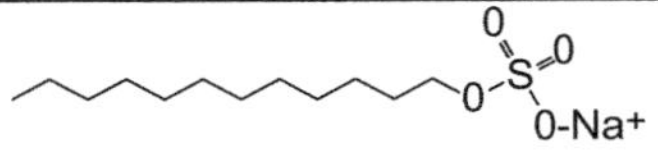		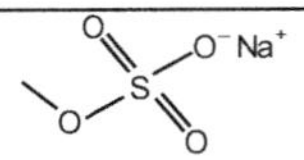
Sodium stearate	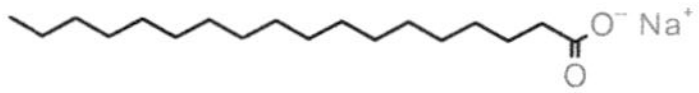		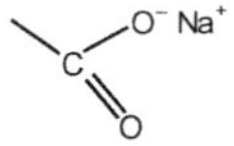
Sodium palmitate	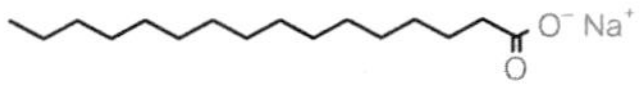		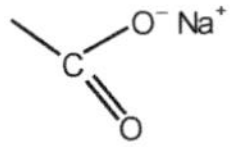
Sodium cholate	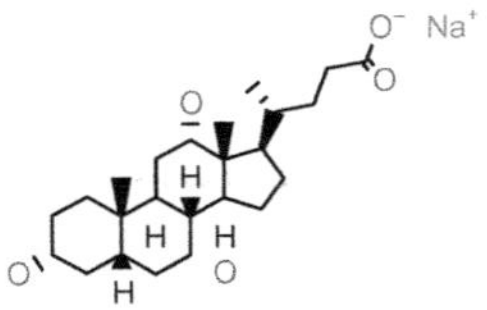	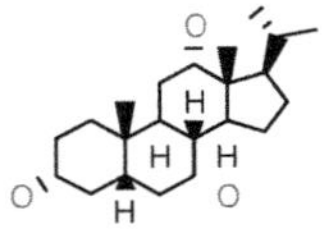	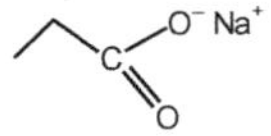
CATIONIC SURFACTANTS			
Cetyl trimethyl ammonium bromide (CETAB) or Hexadecyl trimethyl ammonium bromide (HTAB)	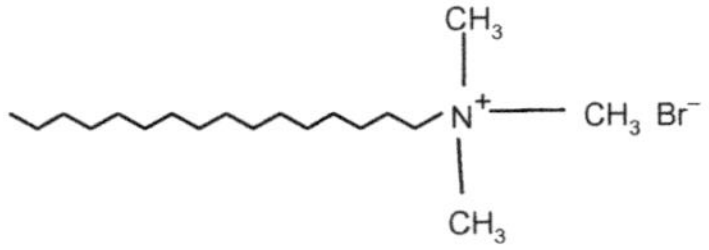		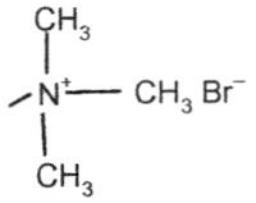
Benzalkonium or dodecyl dimethyl benzylammonium chloride	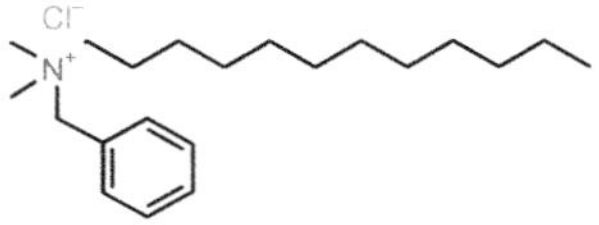	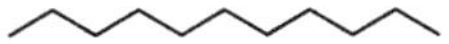	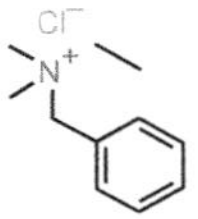
AMPHOTERIC SURFACTANTS			
Lecithin	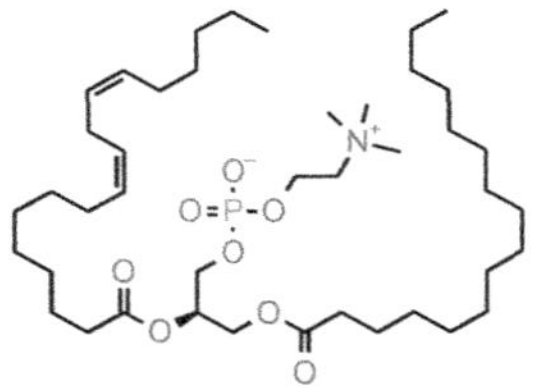	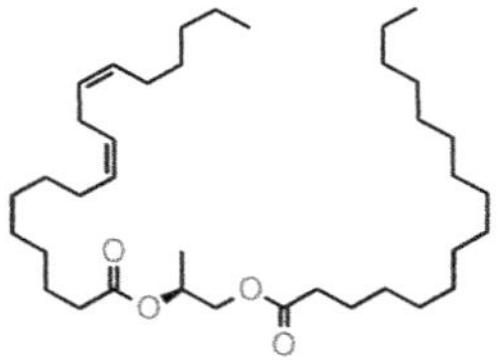	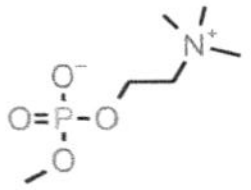

(Continued)

TABLE 3.2 (Continued)

Types and Examples	Structures	Hydrophobic Moiety	Hydrophilic Moiety
NONIONIC SURFACTANTS			
Spans	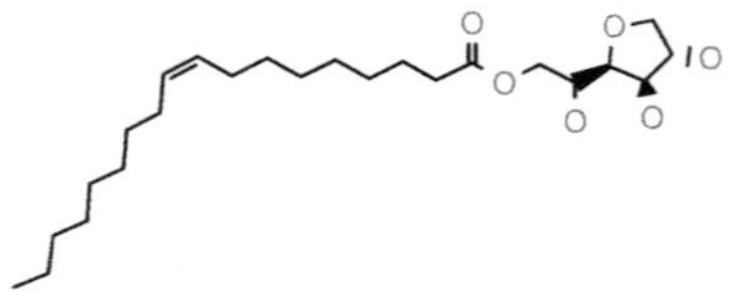		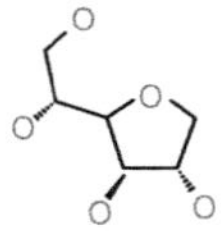
Tween 80	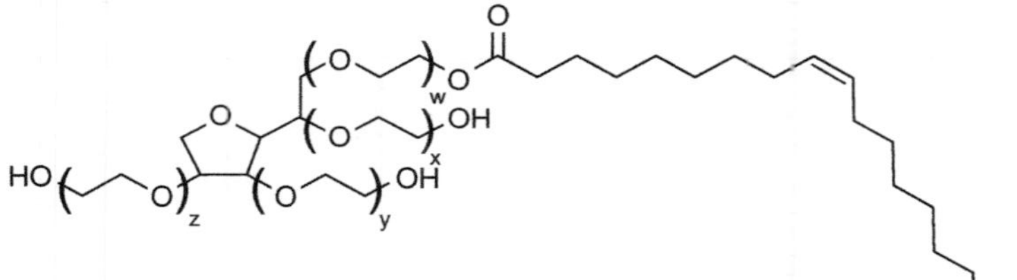 HO OH OH w x y z O w + x + y + z = 20	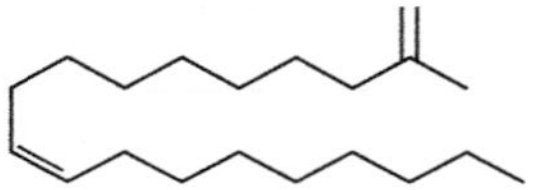	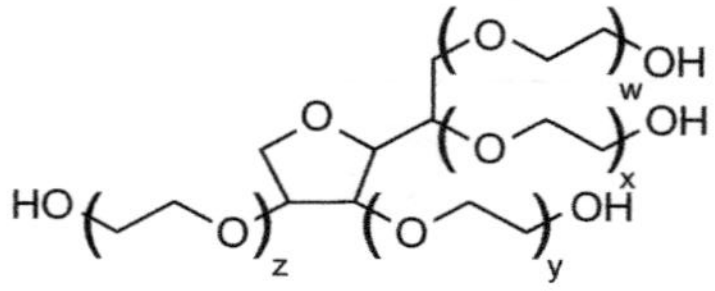 HO OH OH OH w x y z O w + x + y + z = 20
Pluronic F127 (n = 100, m = 65)	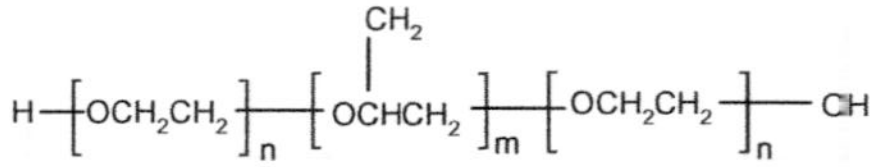 H OCH2CH2 n CH2 OCHCH2 m OCH2CH2 n CH	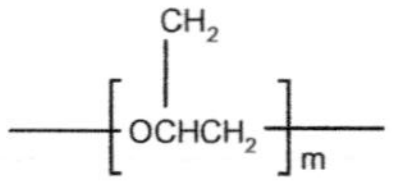 CH2 OCHCH2 m	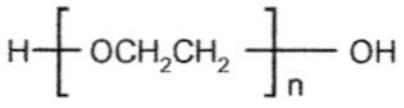 H OCH2CH2 n OH

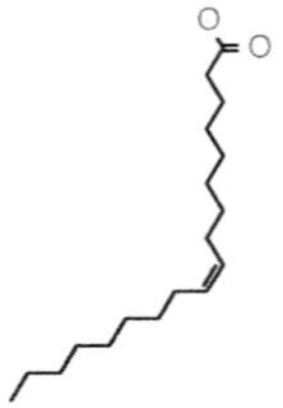

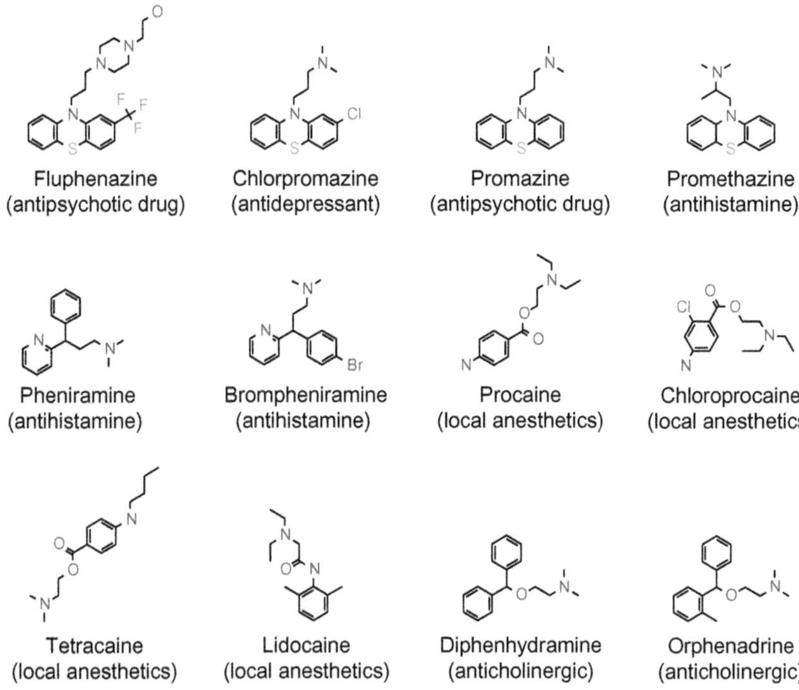

FIGURE 3.6 Structures of some of the drugs owing their activity to their surface activity.

to its volatile nature, thereby leaving surfactant on the water surface as an insoluble monolayer of film.

Monolayers are useful models that could be used for investigating properties of polymers used as packaging materials. The permeability of packaging material to gas or liquid contained therein or its adsorption onto packaging material is important for protecting drug quality. The permeability of the packaging material or the rate of evaporation of drug through it can be easily determined from the increase in mass of a desiccant suspended over the monolayer of the packaging material, or from the decrease in weight of a Petri dish containing the drug solution over which the monolayer of packaging material is spread.

Monolayer models can also be used for screening polymers or their blends for their potential use as enteric and film-coating materials for solid dosage forms. Monolayers of cellulose acetate butyrate or stearate are not affected by pH changes from 3 to 6.5 due to the formation of highly compact condensed films that cannot be degraded either in stomach or intestine; therefore, they are not suitable for enteric coating. However, cellulose acetate phthalate forms a condensed monolayer film at pH 3 but not at pH 6.5 and therefore is a suitable material for enteric coating purposes.

Example:

When 1 mL of a 0.009% (w/v) solution of stearic acid (Mol. Wt. 284.3) dissolved in a volatile organic solvent is placed on the surface of water in a trough, the solvent evaporates, leaving the stearic acid spread over the surface as an insoluble monolayer film. If the surface area occupied by the film is 420 cm^2, calculate the area occupied by each molecule of stearic acid in the film.

Solution:

Here you need to know that 1 mole of a substance contains 6.022×10^{23} molecules, and you need to calculate the number of moles present in 1 mL of 0.009% (w/v) of stearic acid, which is occupying an area equal to 420 cm^2. The question asks for the area occupied by 1 molecule, which you can calculate by dividing 420 cm^2 by the number of molecules in 1 mL of 0.009% (w/v) stearic acid, as follows:

$$1 \text{ mL of } 0.009\% \text{ (w/v) stearic acid} = 0.00009 \text{ g}$$
$$= 3.16 \times 10^{-7} \text{moles (i.e., } 0.00009 \text{ g}/284.3 \text{ g/mole)}$$

Therefore, the number of molecules in 1 mL of 0.009% (w/v) stearic acid $= 3.16 \times 10^{-7}$ moles $\times 6.022 \times 10^{23}$ molecules/mole $= 1.91 \times 10^{17}$ molecules. Consequently, the area occupied by one molecule $= 420$ cm^2/ 1.91×10^{17} molecules $= 219.89 \times 10^{-17}$ cm^2/molecule.

3.3.11 Factors Affecting Adsorption at Monolayer Surface Film

3.3.11.1 Solubility of the Adsorbate

The solubility of the solute (i.e., adsorbate) is inversely related to its adsorption. The bond between adsorbate and the solvent must be broken for adsorption to happen. Greater solubility means a stronger bond between the adsorbate and the solvent. Therefore, the greater solubility of adsorbate results in

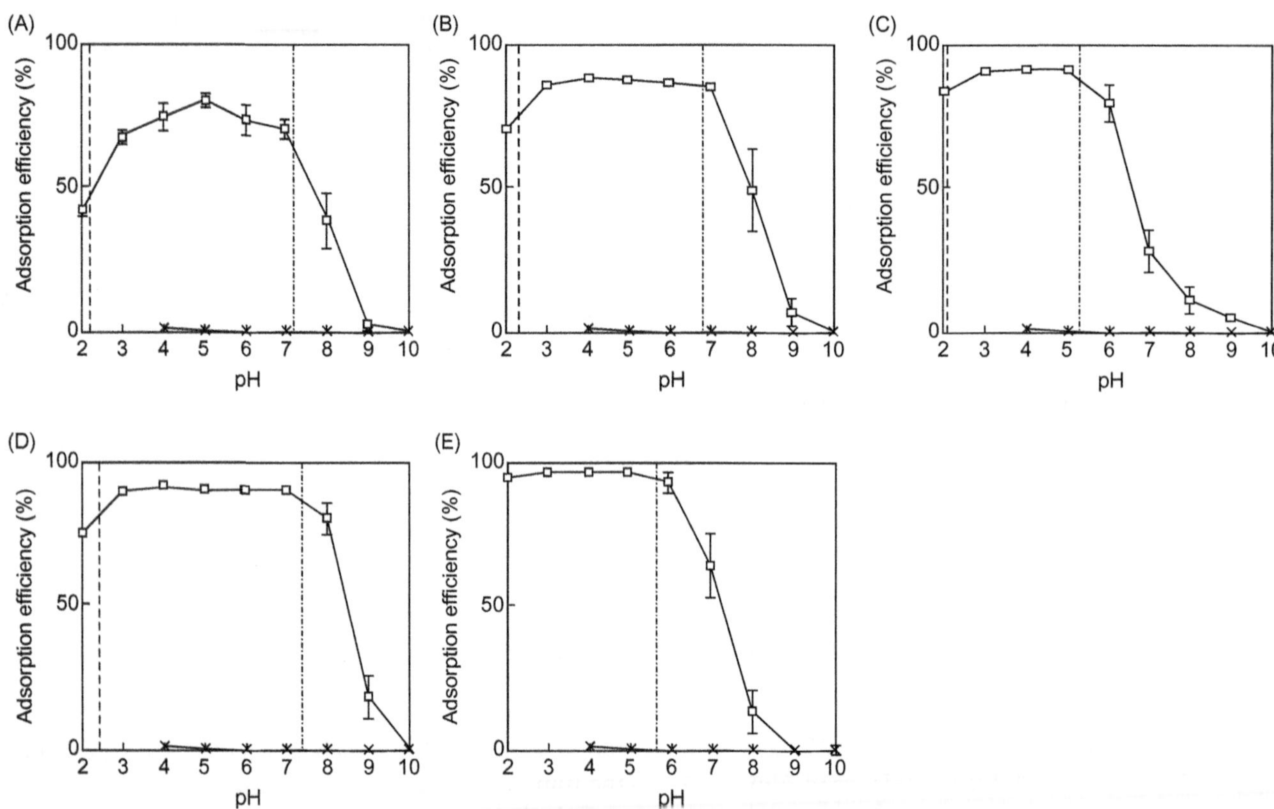

FIGURE 3.7 Relationship between pH and the adsorption efficiency of sulfa drugs on HSZ-385 (squares), A-type zeolite (crosses), and F-type zeolite (triangles): (A) sulfathiazole, (B) sulfamerazine, (C) sulfamethizole, (D) sulfadimidine, and (E) sulfamethoxazole. The $pK_{a,1}$ and $pK_{a,2}$ values for each sulfa drug are displayed as dashed and dash-dotted lines, respectively [3].

less adsorption. As an example, when iodine (an adsorbent) is dissolved in three solvents like carbon tetrachloride, chloroform and carbon disulfide and further exposed to activated charcoal (adsorbent), the adsorption of iodine to carbon surface is higher in the carbon disulphide as compared to the other two solvents because iodine is less soluble in this solvent.

3.3.11.2 *pH of the Solvent*

The pH of an aqueous solution of weak acids or weak bases can affect its solubility. The pH favoring un-ionization decreases the aqueous solubility of a drug, which in turn increases its adsorption. The adsorption efficiency (i.e., the ratio of the amount of sulfa drug adsorbed onto zeolites to the initial amount of sulfa drug) of different sulfa drugs (see Figure 3.7) is maximum at a pH range from pK_1 through pK_2 when they exist as un-ionized neutral molecules, which are the least soluble in comparison to their ionized forms.

3.3.11.3 *Nature of the Adsorbent*

The adsorbent is the material on which adsorption occurs. The greater the surface area of the adsorbent, the greater would be the adsorption. Therefore, adsorbents having pores and fine particles would adsorb more. Adsorbent clay such as bentonite, attapulgite, and kaoline has charged sites too, which also facilitate the adsorption of oppositely charged particles. This is the basis of how bentonite detox works in its application of treating diarrhea. Some adsorbents such as magnesium trisilicate, which is used as antacid, adsorb digoxin. Therefore, a simultaneous administration of digoxin and antacid should be avoided. Use of activated charcoal in detoxication of some orally ingested poison is another application of adsorption in clinical practice.

3.3.11.4 *Temperature*

Adsorption is generally an exothermic process, so an increase in temperature favors the opposite phenomenon: desorption. This technique is used to prepare activated carbon from carbon at a high temperature (600°C–900°C).

3.4. SOLUBILIZATION

Surfactants form micelles when their concentration is greater than the critical micelle concentration

(CMC). Solubilization is the process of increasing aqueous solubility of a drug through the presence of a surfactant at or above its CMC. Formation of micelles helps in solubilizing a water-insoluble substance by incorporation into micelles. It is affected by the factors described in the following sections.

3.4.1 Nature of the Surfactant

Generally, the longer the hydrophobic chain of a surfactant, the larger would be the micelles' size, resulting in greater solubilization. The solubility of phenobarbital increases more in Tween 80 than in Tween 20, which contains 12 carbon chain long hydrophobic moiety versus 18 carbon chain length in Tween 80. Although increased chain length of hydrophilic moiety results in an overall increase in solubility, the mechanism involved is different from the size of the hydrophobic chain length. An increase in chain length of hydrophilic moiety results in a decrease in micellar size, but the number of micelles per unit volume of the liquid increases. Therefore, even if drug molecules solubilized per micelle decrease due to a decrease in size, overall solubility increases due to an increase in number. For example, solubility of dexamethasone increases in n-alkyl polyoxyethylene with an increase in oxyethylene number while keeping the alkyl length constant at 16 carbon long.

3.4.2 Nature of the Solubilisate

There is no simple correlation between the physical properties of the solubilisate and solubilization. As a general rule, a decrease in alkyl chain length, unsaturation in comparison to saturation, and cyclization of solubilisate can affect solubilization. There could be specific rules for a particular category of drug; e.g., the solubility of steroidal hormones increases with the presence of more polar groups at the 17th carbon, and the reported order of solubility is progesterone < testosterone < deoxycorticosterone, where the C_{17} substituents are $-COCH_3$, $-OH$, and $-COCH_2OH$, respectively.

3.4.3 Effect of Temperature

Generally, an increase in temperature increases micellar size, and thus increases solubilization. This increase is particularly pronounced with nonionic surfactants. However, this situation becomes more complicated when aqueous solubility of the solubilisate increases with an increase in temperature in the surfactant solution.

3.4.4 Application of Solubilization

Micellar solubilization has been used extensively for the formulation and delivery of insoluble drugs. Following are some examples:

- Phenolic compounds (cresol, chlorocresol, chloroxylenol, and thymol) are solubilized in water with help from soap, which makes possible their use as a disinfectant. Iodine is solubilized in Iodophor (Povidone-Iodine) by using polyvinylpyrrolidone, which releases iodine when diluted with water. Iodophor is superior to an iodine-iodide solution because less of it is lost through the sublimation process.
- Many steroidal ophthalmic solutions (e.g., dexamethasone, fluocinolone, fluorometholone, difluprednate, loteprednol, prednisolone, and triamcinolone) are prepared using the surfactants polysorbate or polyoxyethylene sorbitan esters (Tween®) of fatty acids. These water-insoluble steroidal drugs can be solubilized in oily solvents but are not acceptable for ophthalmic use due to their cloudy nature.
- Water-insoluble vitamins such as vitamin A, D, E, and K are solubilized by adding polysorbate 20 or 80 for preparing parenteral formulations.
- The nonionic surfactant Cremophor EL has been used in the solubilization of a wide variety of hydrophobic drugs. They include anesthetics, photosensitizers, sedatives, immunosuppressive agents, and anticancer drugs such as paclitaxel, for which development was suspended for many years due to its solubilization problem.
- In addition to solubilization, micelles are also useful in developing a long-circulating drug delivery system. Polymeric micelles formed from polyethylene oxide (PEO)–polypropylene oxide (PPO) diblock copolymer have been found to prevent opsonization and subsequent recognition by the macrophages of the reticuloendothelial system, thereby allowing the micelles to circulate longer and deliver drugs in a sustained manner at the desired site.

Students interested in a greater understanding of the process of solubilization and its application should refer to reference [4], which provides comprehensive mechanistic details of its various uses.

3.5. RHEOLOGY

The term *rheology* is derived from the Greek *rheo* (flow) and *logos* (science). Rheology is the science that studies the flow of liquids and deformation of solids. Rheology is involved in the mixing and flow of materials, their packaging into containers, and their removal prior to use, whether this is achieved by pouring from a bottle, extrusion from a tube, or passage through a syringe needle. The rheology of a particular product, which can range in consistency from a fluid to a semisolid to a solid, can affect its patient acceptability, physical stability, and even biological availability.

3.5.1 Viscosity and Fluidity

Viscosity is the resistance offered by a liquid or a fluid to flow. The greater the resistance, the higher is the viscosity. For example, the viscosity of a toothpaste is significantly higher than a mouthwash. Viscosity is denoted by the symbol η. Another term also commonly used in rheology is *fluidity*. Fluidity is the ease with which a liquid or a fluid flows, and is defined as the reciprocal of viscosity. Fluidity is denoted by the symbol Φ and expressed by Eq. 3.5:

$$\Phi = \frac{1}{\eta} \tag{3.5}$$

3.5.2 Newtonian Versus Non-Newtonian Fluid

Fluids that flow according to Newton's law of flow are called Newtonian systems, whereas those that do not comply are called non-Newtonian systems. Water for injection is a Newtonian fluid, but zinc oxide paste and ointment are examples of non-Newtonian fluids.

For Newtonian liquids, let's consider a cube of liquid with the surface area of each side equal to A, as shown in Figure 3.8. For convenience, let's imagine this cube to consist of parallel plates of liquid stacked on one another. If we apply a force equal to F on the top plate, it starts moving with a velocity v. The plate below this top plate, however, does not move as fast as the top plate, and its velocity is lower than v.

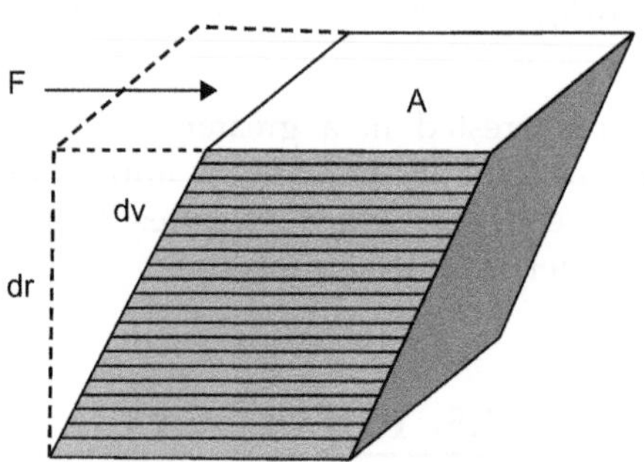

FIGURE 3.8 Diagrammatic representation of the shearing force required to produce a definite velocity gradient between the parallel planes of a block of materials.

The velocity of the plates decreases further with distance from the top plate, and the plate on the base does not move at all. We therefore see that the velocity of flow is a function of distance, and mathematically, we represent this as dv/dr, as shown in Figure 3.8. The term dv/dr is the velocity gradient, or the rate of shear, and is often represented by V_g.

For Newtonian fluids, the force, F, applied per unit area, A (shearing stress, or P) is proportional to V_g, which is represented by Eq. 3.6:

$$\frac{F}{A} \propto \frac{dv}{dr}$$

$$\frac{F}{A} = \eta \frac{dv}{dr} \quad \text{or} \quad p = \eta V_g \tag{3.6}$$

η is the coefficient of viscosity, or simply the viscosity. For Newtonian liquids, as the P is directly proportional to V_g, a plot of V_g versus P gives a straight line that passes through the origin, as shown in Figure 3.9A.

3.5.3 Common Units of Viscosity

The unit of viscosity is the poise, and its CGS units are g/cm.sec.

The poise is sometimes considered large for many fluids, and it is more common to represent viscosity by the centipoises, or cp, which is equal to 0.01 poise.

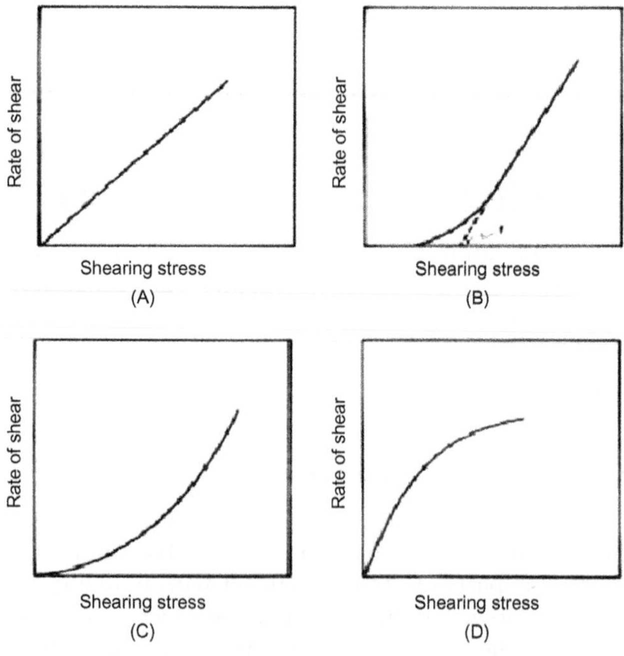

FIGURE 3.9 Various kinds of flow patterns: (A) Newtonian flow, (B) plastic flow, (C) pseudoplastic flow, and (D) Dilatant flow.

Another commonly used term to represent viscosity of liquids is kinematic viscosity, which is equal to the viscosity normalized to its density at a particular temperature, as shown in Eq. 3.7:

$$\text{Kinematic viscosity} = \frac{\eta}{\rho} \tag{3.7}$$

The units of kinematic viscosity are stoke (s) and centistokes (cs).

3.5.4 Effect of Temperature on the Viscosity of a Fluid

The viscosity of fluids is affected by temperature. Therefore, whenever the viscosity of a fluid is reported, the temperature at which it was determined should be provided. While the viscosity of a gas increases with temperature, for liquids, it decreases with temperature. The dependence of viscosity on temperature is given by the Arrhenius equation, as shown in Eq. 3.8:

$$\eta = Ae^{E_v/RT} \tag{3.8}$$

where A is a constant depending on molecular weight and molar volume of the liquid, E_v is the activation energy required to initiate flow, R is the gas constant, and T is the absolute temperature.

Non-Newtonian liquids do not follow Newton's equation of flow. Liquid and solid heterogeneous dispersions such as colloidal solutions, emulsions, liquid suspensions, ointments, and similar products are some examples of this class. The main types of non-Newtonian flow, as shown in Figure 3.9, are plastic flow, simple pseudoplastic, dilatant, and thixotropic:

- *Plastic flow*: A liquid that exhibits plastic flow does not flow until the applied shearing stress exceeds a minimum value (called yield value or yield strength of the plastic material). Below the yield value, the material behaves as an elastic solid; and above the yield value, as a Newtonian liquid (Figure 3.9B). Plastic flow is generally exhibited by concentrated suspensions.
- *Pseudoplastic flow*: A liquid that flows more readily with increased shearing stress exhibits pseudoplastic flow (Figure 3.9C). Such liquids become thinner on the application of stress. Polymers in solution generally exhibit pseudoplastic flow. No yield value is exhibited by these systems.
- *Dilatant flow (shear thickening)*: The flow pattern exhibited by dilatant liquids is opposite to that of the pseudoplastic liquids. In this case, the liquids become thicker, or flow with increased resistance with the application of stress (Figure 3.9D). This property is generally exhibited by concentrated suspensions (more than 50% w/v).
- *Thixotropic*: Thixotropy is a special characteristic that is exhibited by shear thinning systems, such as pseudoplastic and plastic liquids When shear is applied to these materials, the resistance to flow progressively decreases. If the shear is removed, one would expect the liquids to regain their original viscosity. Thixotropic substances, however, remain in their "thinned" state, even after the shear is removed, for an extended period of time, which is represented by the area demarked by upward and downward curve shown in Figure 3.10.

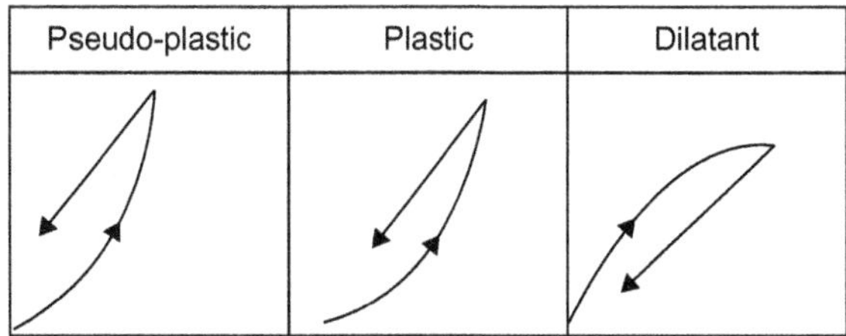

FIGURE 3.10 Thixotropic flow pattern.

Thixotropic behavior is useful for many pharmaceutical preparations. For example, during the formulation of a drug suspension, a suspending agent is added to make the suspension more viscous to avoid the settling of drug particles. However, if the suspension is too viscous, it may not flow from the bottle containing the suspension. However, if the suspension is thixotropic, it would remain viscous in the bottle, thereby minimizing sedimentation. However, if the bottle is shaken vigorously, the shear resulting from the shaking will cause the suspension to thin down and remain in that state for long enough to facilitate pouring and dispensing from the bottle.

3.5.5 Measurement of Viscosity

The measurement of viscosity is called viscometry, and numerous viscometers are available for measuring the viscosity of Newtonian and non-Newtonian liquids. The viscometers can be divided into two categories:

1. Those that operate at a single rate of shear. These viscometers are useful for determining the viscosity of Newtonian liquids because the viscosity is a constant function of the rate of shear. Examples include capillary viscometers such as the Ostwald viscometer (Figure 3.11). These viscometers may be used for liquids that flow relatively easily because the measurement is based on the flow of the liquid through a capillary tube.

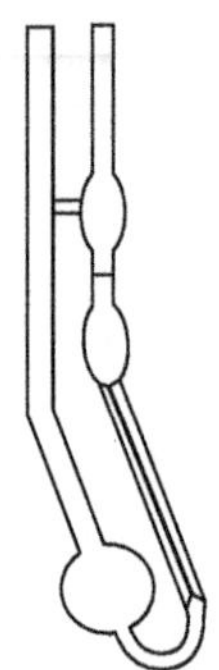

FIGURE 3.11 A diagrammatic representation of an Ostwald viscometer.

2. Those that operate at multiple rates of shear. These viscometers are useful for non-Newtonian fluids and may also be used for semisolid substances such as gels and pastes. Examples include the cup and bob viscometer and the cone and plate viscometer. A cone and plate viscometer is shown in Figure 3.12.

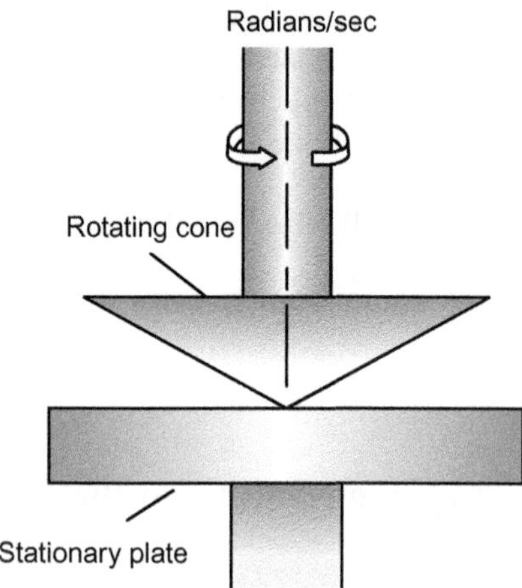

FIGURE 3.12 Constant shear rate condition in a cone and plate viscometer.

3.5.6 Applications of Rheology in Pharmacy

Rheology affects many significant pharmaceutical issues such as mixing and preparation of dosage forms, particle-size reduction of a drug through the use of shear, removal of medicines before use by pouring from a bottle or extruding from tubes or passaging through hypodermic needles, physical stability of a drug in a dispersed system, flow of powders from hoppers to die during tablet manufacturing, release of a drug from its dosage form, etc.

3.5.7 Clinical Rheology

3.5.7.1 *Plasma Viscosity and Blood Viscoelasticity*

Blood is not a fluid in the ordinary sense. It is a fluidized suspension of elastic cells whose flow profile is regulated by its viscoelastic properties. Many blood parameters such as plasma viscosity, red blood cell deformability, aggregation, and hematocrit influence the viscoelastic characteristics of blood. Major shifts in the viscoelasticity of blood have been found to be associated with pathological conditions such as myocardial infarction, peripheral vascular disease, cancer, and diabetes.

3.5.7.2 *Viscosity and Viscoelasticity*

If flow is constant with time, the ratio of shear stress to shear rate is the viscosity. When flows change with time, such as blood flow in human circulation, the liquid generally demonstrates both a viscous and an elastic effect, both of which determine the stress-to-strain rate relationship. Such liquids are called viscoelastic.

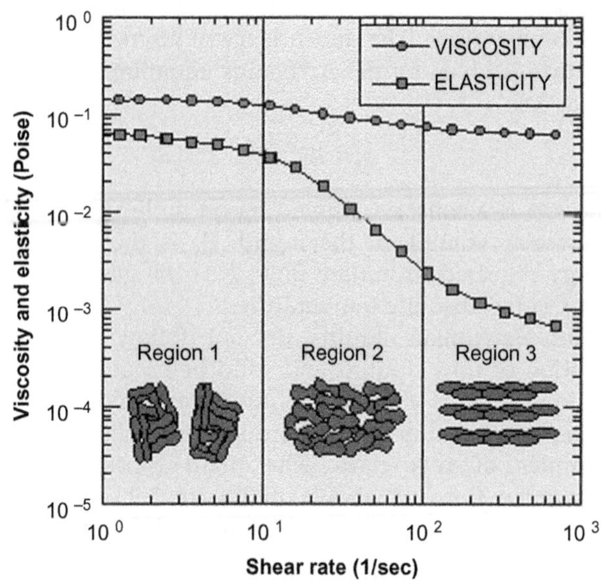

FIGURE 3.13 The dependence of normal human blood viscoelasticity at 2 Hz (i.e., about human pulse rate) and 22°C on shear rate. *(Adapted from reference [5]).*

Blood plasma normally shows viscosity only, whereas whole blood is both viscous and elastic.

3.5.7.3 *Origin of Blood Viscoelasticity*

Red blood cells (RBCs) are not rigid but elastic, which provides viscoelasticity to blood. When red cells are at rest, they tend to aggregate and stack together in a space-efficient manner, as shown in Figure 3.13 marked by region 1. In order for blood to flow freely, these aggregates are required to be disaggregated and deformed elastically. As blood flow further proceeds, RBCs slide over each other continuously and elastically. Thus, blood flow is better characterized by both viscosity and elasticity than viscosity alone. The failure of RBCs either to disaggregate or deform (or both) results in impaired perfusion of the capillary beds and in turn surrounding tissues. Since the viscoelasticity of blood is mainly determined by the disaggregation and deformability of RBCs, any factor or condition influencing viscoelasticity of blood would eventually affect its flow pattern too.

Figure 3.13 shows that as the shear rate increases in region 1, the viscoelasticity gradually decreases due to expected decrease in aggregate size. As the shear rate increases further in region 2, the applied forces deform the cells even further, resulting in some sort of orientation. Finally, the increased shear rate in region 3 orients the cells in a parallel laminar sheet most suitable for easy flow of the blood, which is indicated by a decrease in both viscosity and elasticity; however, the decrease in elasticity is much more pronounced. Therefore, any condition causing a decrease in deformability of RBCs would produce dilatant viscoelasticity marked by elevated viscosity and elasticity in the high shear rate of region 3.

Any alteration in plasma composition brought about by changes in osmotic pressure, pH, concentration of fibrinogen and other plasma proteins, clinically introduced blood volume expanders, and any pathological condition causing change in hematocrit value can have major effects on blood viscoelasticity [5].

3.6. COLLIGATIVE PROPERTIES

The physical properties of solutions may be classified as additive, constitutive, or colligative:

- *Additive properties:* These properties depend on the sum of properties of constituents in a solution. For example, the mass of a solute in a solution is an additive property because it is a sum of the mass of constituent molecules.
- *Constitutive properties:* These properties depend on the arrangement of the atoms within a molecule and also the number and kinds of atoms within a molecule. Examples include refraction of light, electrical properties, surface and interfacial characteristics, and solubility. The solubility of the same substance existing in different crystalline forms could be different although all the forms represent the same substance chemically.
- *Colligative properties*: These properties depend mainly on the number of particles in a solution and are not affected by the nature of the chemical species. The colligative properties of solutions are osmotic pressure, vapor pressure lowering, freezing point depression, and boiling point elevation. For example, the osmotic pressure generated by 1 million molecules of urea in 100 mL of water is the same as that generated by 1 million particles of sucrose or naphthalene.

When a nonvolatile component, e.g., salt, is combined with a volatile solvent, such as water, the vapor pressure above the solution is provided solely by the solvent. However, the nonvolatile solute decreases the vapor pressure of the solvent, and the decrease in vapor pressure is proportional to the number of molecules of the solute, and not on the identity of the solute. As a result, the solution properties that are affected include lowering of vapor pressure, depression of freezing point, elevation of boiling point, and osmotic pressure. These properties are called colligative properties (from the Greek, meaning "collected together") as they depend on the number rather than the nature of the constituents.

3.6.1 Vapor Pressure Lowering and Elevation of Boiling Point

The normal boiling point of a solvent is the temperature at which its vapor pressure equals the external pressure or atmospheric pressure, which is equal to 760 mm of Hg. As the addition of a nonvolatile solute lowers the vapor pressure, the vapor pressure of such a solution at the normal boiling temperature is less than 760 mm of Hg. Therefore, more heat is required so that the vapor pressure can approach the value of the external pressure. In other words, an elevation of the boiling point is observed. It has also been observed that the ratio of the elevation in boiling point, $T_{solu} - T_{solv}$, or ΔT_b, to the vapor pressure lowering, $p_{solv} - p_{solu}$, or Δp is approximately a constant; i.e.,

$$\frac{\Delta T_b}{\Delta p} = k \tag{3.9}$$

or

$$\Delta T_b = k\Delta p \tag{3.10}$$

where k is a constant; T_{solu} and T_{solv} are the boiling points of solution and pure solvent, respectively; and p_{solu} and p_{solv} are vapor pressures of solution and pure solvent, respectively. Since the pure vapor pressure, p_{solv}, for any solvent is a constant, we can consider elevation in the boiling point, ΔT_b, to be proportional to $\Delta p/p_{solv}$, the relative lowering of vapor pressure. By Raoult's law, the relative lowering of vapor pressure is equal to the mole fraction of the solute, X_{solute}. Therefore,

$$\Delta T_b = k' X_{solute} \tag{3.11}$$

where k' is another constant. In dilute solutions, the mole fraction is proportional to the molality, m, of the solute. As a result, Eq. 3.11 reduces to

$$\Delta T_b = k_b m \tag{3.12}$$

where k_b is known as the molal elevation constant, or the *ebullioscopic* constant, which has a characteristic value for each solvent.

3.6.2 Depression of Freezing Point

The addition of a nonvolatile solute also causes depression of the freezing point of the pure solvent. Therefore, the freezing point of a solution is always lower than that of the pure solvent. This is the principle used to manufacture antifreeze solutions for winter or even the use of salt on icy roads in the winter. In the case of antifreeze, which are water-based solutions, they do not freeze at 0°C, but freeze at significantly lower temperatures. An equation similar to that shown previously is used to quantitate this decrease in freezing point, as shown in Eq. 3.13:

$$\Delta T_f = k_f m \tag{3.13}$$

Here, ΔT_f is the depression in the freezing point, and k_f is called the molal depression constant, or the *cryoscopic constant.* This concept is used for adjusting the tonicity of parenterals.

3.6.3 Osmosis and Osmotic Pressure

If a volume of pure solvent and solution containing a nonvolatile solute, e.g., sucrose solution, is separated by a semipermeable membrane, there occurs a flow of the solvent from the pure solvent to the solution, as indicated by an increase in the level of solution in the right compartment in Figure 3.14A, called osmosis. The pressure applied by the increased level of the liquid column in the right compartment (Figure 3.14A) is called osmotic pressure, which is a pressure just sufficient to stop the process of osmosis. Obviously, water would move in the opposite direction if pressure were applied over the solution (Figure 3.14B), a process called reverse osmosis, which is used in purifying water or desalinating sea water.

The phenomenon of osmosis can be explained at a molecular level assuming the dissolved solute (e.g., sucrose) molecules are interacting with the solvent (e.g., water) molecules. The water molecules in the left compartment containing fewer solute molecules are more mobile than those in the more concentrated right compartment. These two compartments are separated by a semipermeable membrane that permits only water to pass through itself. Consequently, the solute molecules

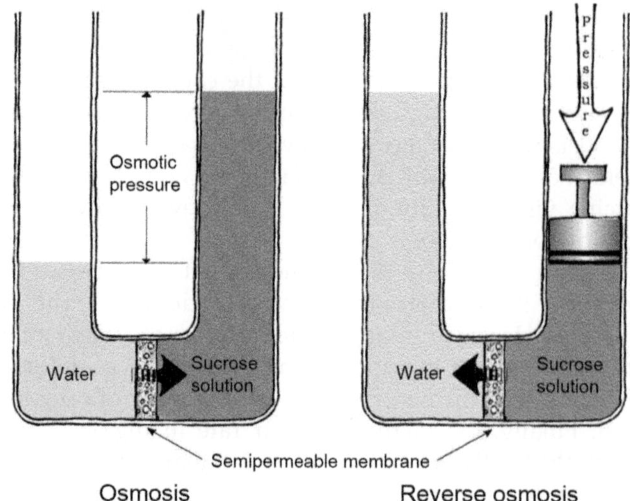

FIGURE 3.14 Diagrammatic representation of osmosis and reverse osmosis.

cannot redistribute themselves between the compartments because their movement is restricted by the semipermeable membrane. However, solvent molecules can pass through the membrane; and consequently, they would flow predominantly from the compartment containing less solute to the one containing more solute, resulting in an increase in level of solution. The increased column of solution over that of solvent would create a pressure termed as osmotic pressure.

In fact, no membrane is perfectly semipermeable; e.g., the membrane surrounding mammalian red blood cells does allow the passage of some solute particles. Thus, when two solutions are separated by a semipermeable membrane and there is no net movement of solvent across the membrane, the two solutions are said to be *isotonic* with respect to that membrane.

- Hypotonic solutions have a lower concentration of ions and undissociated molecules than blood serum. When in contact with red blood cells, liquid passes into the cells, causing them to swell and burst (hemolysis).
- Hypertonic solutions have a higher concentration of ions and undissociated molecules than blood serum. When in contact with red blood cells, liquid passes out of the cells, causing them to shrink and become crenated.

Two solutions are said to be iso-osmotic if they have the same osmotic pressure. Solutions that are iso-osmotic with blood serum or tissue fluids are not always isotonic. This happens when the cell membrane is permeable to one or more solutes as well as to the solvent. Cell membranes are not perfectly semipermeable because otherwise no nutrients or waste products would diffuse through them and the cell would die.

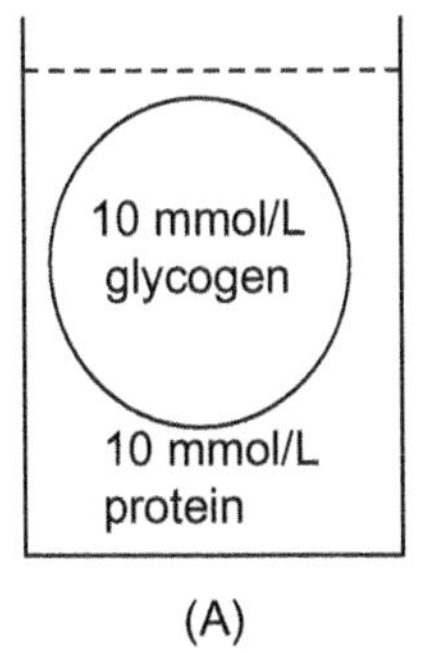

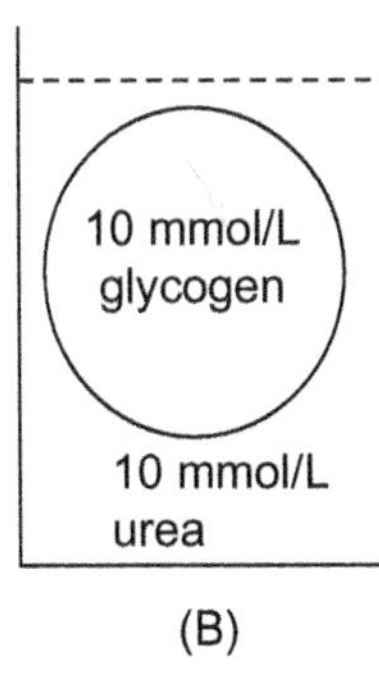

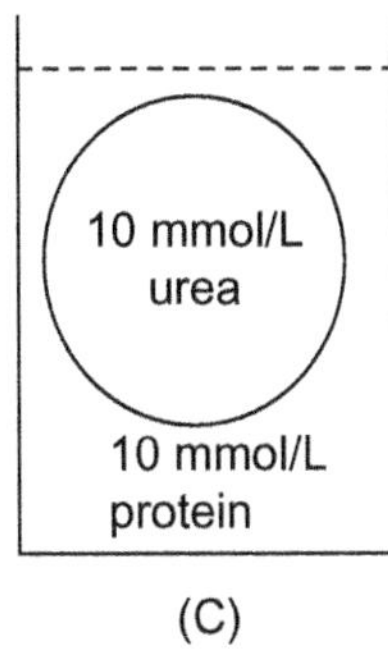

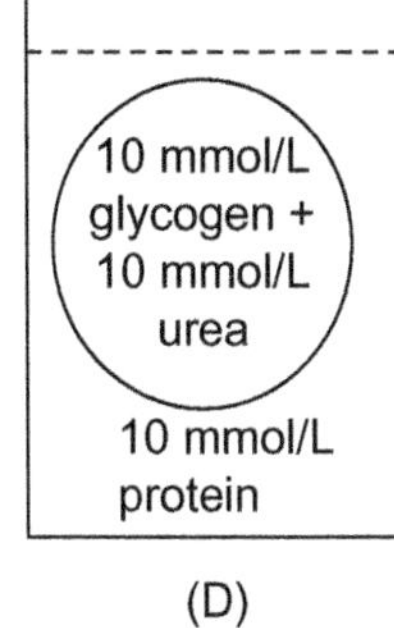

FIGURE 3.15 Iso-osmoticity versus isotonicity. (A) Iso-osmotic and isotonic, (B) initially iso-osmotic and hypotonic, (C) initially iso-osmotic and hypertonic, and (D) initially neither iso-osmotic nor isotonic but at equilibrium iso-osmotic and isotonic.

The distinction between osmotic pressure and tonicity is illustrated in the Figure 3.15, in which a hypothetical cell membrane is assumed to be permeable to a solvent, water, and urea, but impermeable to glycogen and a neutral protein. The solutes are assumed to be present at equal and low concentration (10 mmol/L) so that their solutions are iso-osmotic. The solutions inside and outside the cell are therefore initially iso-osmotic in examples A, B, and C.

In Figure 3.15A the solutes cannot pass through the cell membrane; therefore, the external solution is always isotonic as well as iso-osmotic with the internal solution. In Figure 3.15B, urea passes freely through the cell membrane into the cell; water also diffuses into the cell in an attempt to equalize the total concentration of solute molecules on both sides of the membrane. The external solution is therefore hypotonic with respect to the internal solution. Figure 3.15C is the reverse of Figure 3.15A. In C, both urea and water diffuse out of the cell so that the external solution is hypertonic relative to the internal solution. In both B and C, the external and internal solutions will cease to be iso-osmotic when some urea has diffused through the cell membrane. In Figure 3.15D, the total concentration of solute molecules inside the cell is initially twice that outside, so the solutions are not initially iso-osmotic. Urea diffuses out of the cell, and water diffuses in; therefore, the solutions are not initially isotonic. Eventually, urea and water distribute themselves so that their concentrations are equalized on both sides of the membrane. Consequently, at equilibrium, the external and internal solutions will be both iso-osmotic and isotonic.

Pharmaceutical preparations, which on administration come into contact with blood cells or other unprotected tissue cells, need to be made isotonic to prevent tissue damage or pain. Ophthalmic and otic preparations intended for installation into the eye or nose should be approximately isotonic to avoid irritation. Parenteral solutions for intravenous or intramuscular injection can cause tissue irritation, pain on injection, and electrolyte shifts if the solutions deviate from isotonicity with the blood. Solutions that are hypotonic with respect to blood and lacrimal secretions may be adjusted to isotonicity through the addition of suitable substances such as sodium chloride or dextrose. Hypertonic solutions cannot be adjusted; when given parenterally, they are usually administered slowly in small volumes or into a large vein such as the subclavian, where dilution and distribution occur rapidly.

The effects of hypotonic and hypertonic solutions on living cells are a function of (1) the volume of the solution added, (2) the concentration of the solute, and (3) the nature of the solute. While both hypertonic and hypotonic solutions may cause pain and damage to cells, the effects of hypotonic solutions are more easily seen because they result in the lysis of the cell. The process is irreversible. Hypertonic solutions result in crenation or shrinking of the cells, which is often reversible, but those processes can only be viewed with a suitable microscope.

3.6.4 Van't Hoff Equation for Osmotic Pressure

The osmotic pressure caused by nondissociating solute in a solution is given by

$$\pi V = nRT \tag{3.14}$$

where π is the osmotic pressure, V is the volume of the solution in liters, n is the number of moles of the solute, R the gas constant equal to 0.082 liter atm/mol deg, and T is the absolute temperature. Since osmotic pressure is a colligative property, there is a correction in the preceding equation for calculating the osmotic pressure of solutions containing electrolytes, i.e., dissociating solutes. Van't Hoff introduced a correction factor, i, which approaches a number equal to the number of ions, ν, produced by a solute upon complete dissociation. The ratio i/ν is called osmotic coefficient, Φ, which has been used in the following equation applicable for calculating osmotic pressure of a solution containing electrolytes:

$$\pi V = \Phi nRT \tag{3.15}$$

Calculating the activity coefficient is not easy; therefore, a concept of "dissociation factor" is used. This is a good approximation for "osmotic coefficient" and could be readily and easily calculated as follows:

Nonelectrolytes: 1
Substances dissociating into 2 ions: 1.8
Substances dissociating into 3 ions: 2.6
Substances dissociating into 4 ions: 3.4
Substances dissociating into 5 ions: 4.2
Tip: Contribution of 0.8 by each additional ion

The concept of dissociation factor is based on assuming 80% dissociation if no % dissociation is given, as shown in the following example.

Calculate the dissociation factor for zinc sulfate: $ZnSO_4$, if it is 40% ionized in weak solutions:

If we have 100 particles of $ZnSO_4$
40 Zn ions
40 SO_4 ions
60 $ZnSO_4$

---

140 Total particles = 1.4 times as many particles as there were before dissociation; thus, the dissociation factor is 1.4.

Example:

One gram of sucrose, molecular weight 342 g/mole, is dissolved in 100 mL of solution at 25°C. What is the osmotic pressure of the solution?

Solution:

The moles of sucrose = 1.0/342 = 0.0029 moles. $\pi = 0.71$ atm.

3.7. OSMOLARITY AND OSMOLALITY

Osmotic pressure is expressed as osmolarity or osmolality. You may conceptualize these terms by comparing them with molarity and molality, respectively. Osmolarity is the mass of a solute which produces the osmotic pressure equal to that produced by 1 mole of an ideal un-ionized (i.e., nonelectrolyte) when dissolved in sufficient quantity of solvent (e.g., water) to produce 1 L (i.e., 1000 cm^3) of solution. Osmolality differs from osmolarity in the sense that the amount of solvent is always 1 kg instead of a quantity sufficient to produce 1 L of solution.

To make an osmotically, i.e., physiologically stable, solution for *in vivo* use, you need 0.155 M NaCl, or 0.1033 M $CaCl_2$ or 0.31 M sucrose. Not one of these compounds is able to freely pass through the RBC plasma membrane. Here, NaCl, $CaCl_2$, and sucrose are all equivalent osmotically because each of them would have the same osmotic pressure since each solution contains approximately the same number of dissolved particles. Sucrose, a nondissociating substance, has 0.31 moles of particles in a 0.31 M solution. Since $CaCl_2$ dissociates into three separate ions (1 Ca^{2+} and 2 Cl^-), there are 0.31 moles of particles in a 0.103 M solution (3*0.1033 or ~0.31 moles of particles). Thus, the important concept is the total concentration of dissolved solute particles, which is expressed by osmolarity. The unit of osmolarity (osmole/L) indicates the number of moles of dissolved particles per liter. Thus, in the preceding example, 0.155 M NaCl is a 0.31 osM solution (0.155 M Na^+ + 0.155 M Cl^-). One liter of water weighs differently at different temperatures; e.g., at 25°C, 1 L of water weighs 997 g. Therefore, osmolality is generally greater than osmolarity and expressed by osmolality = (1000/997) × osmolarity at 25°C.

The mass of a solvent remains the same regardless of any changes in pressure or temperature; therefore, osmolality is the common method of measurement in osmometry and is used to determine medical conditions such as diabetes, shock, and dehydration, whereas osmolarity is used for the detection of the concentration of dissolved particles in urine.

Example:

A 0.9% (w/w) solution of sodium chloride has an osmotic coefficient 0.928. What is its osmolality?

Solution:

Osmolality is the number of moles of total ions in 1 kg of solvent. Therefore,

$$Osmolality = \#\ of\ ions\ x\ \#\ of\ moles\ of\ solutes\ \text{in}\ 1\ kg\ of\ solvent\ x\ osmotic\ coefficent$$

$$0.9\%\ \frac{w}{w}\ solution\ of\ Nacl$$

$$= \frac{9\ g\ of\ NaCl}{1\ kg\ of\ solvent}$$

$$= \frac{9\ g\ NaCl}{58.5\ g\ NaCl\ per\ mole} = 0.154\ mole\ NaCl$$

Therefore,

$$Osmolality = 2 \times 0.154 \times 0.928 = 0.286\ \frac{osmol}{kg}\ or\ 286\ mosmol/kg$$

3.7.1 Adjusting Tonicity

Due to the presence of numerous salts and osmotic ingredients, body fluids such as blood and lachrymal fluid exert a certain osmotic pressure. As a result, the tonicity or osmotic pressure of pharmaceutical solutions that are meant to be applied to delicate membranes of the body should be adjusted so that they are isotonic with body fluids. Isotonic solutions cause no swelling or contraction of the tissues with which they come in contact, and produce no discomfort when instilled in the eye, nasal tract, blood, or other body tissues. Isotonic sodium chloride is a familiar example of such a preparation, and consists of 0.9 g NaCl per 100 mL of water.

The tonicity of a hypotonic pharmaceutical solution can be adjusted by adding a sufficient amount of sodium chloride, which would increase the tonicity of the solution to isotonic levels. The amount of sodium chloride to be added can be measured by the cryoscopic method or the sodium chloride equivalent method. In the opposite case of hypertonic solution, isotonicity may by achieved by adding water calculated by the White–Vincent method or Sprowl method.

3.7.2 Adjusting Tonicity of Hypotonic Drug Solution

In the cryoscopic method, the freezing point depression is calculated for a drug concentration using the $\Delta T_f^{1\%}$ values available in the reference books [9,10]. For the remaining freezing point depression, the required NaCl is calculated using L_{iso} equal to 3.4 or ΔT_f of 1% solution equal to 0.58.

3.7.3 L_{iso} Values

The freezing point of human blood and lachrymal fluid is $-0.52°C$. Therefore, any drug solution having a freezing point depression, ΔT_f, equal to $-0.52°C$ would be isotonic. We therefore know that the freezing point depression, $\Delta T_f = K_f m = i\, K_f M = L_{iso}\, M$, so 0.9% NaCl is isotonic and equal to 0.154 M.

$$L_{iso} = \frac{\Delta T_f}{M} = \frac{0.52}{0.154} = 3.4 \qquad (3.16)$$

Therefore, L_{iso} is the decrease in freezing point brought about by a drug solution whose concentration is 1 M. It depends on the nature of ions (see Table 3.3).

Example:

How much NaCl is required to render 150 mL of a 1.1% solution of apomorphine hydrochloride isotonic with blood serum?

Solution:

In this problem, first you should calculate the amount that 100 mL of a 1.1% solution of apomorphine hydrochloride will decrease the freezing point. You will find the $\Delta T_f^{1\%}$ value for apomorphine hydrochloride equal to 0.08. Therefore, the decrease in freezing point by 1.1% solution $= 0.08 \times 1.1 = 0.088°$.

Therefore, you need to add NaCl to decrease the freezing point by (0.52 − 0.088) 0.43°, which can be calculated as follows.

Since a 0.52° decrease in freezing point happens due to 0.9% NaCl, a 0.43° decrease in freezing point would happen because $(0.9/0.52) \times 0.43 = 0.74\%$ NaCl. Therefore, the amount of sodium chloride required to make 150 mL 1.1% apomorphine solution isotonic $= 0.74/100 \times 150 = 1.11$ g. So, you would have to dissolve 1.65 g of apomorphine hydrochloride and 1.11 g of NaCl in sufficient water to make 150 mL, which will be isotonic with blood serum.

TABLE 3.3 L_{iso} Values for Various Types of Electrolytes*

Electrolytes	L_{iso}	Examples
Nonelectrolytes	1.9	Sucrose, dextrose
Weak electrolytes	2.0	Cocaine, ephedrine, atropine
Di-divalent electrolytes	2.0	Zinc sulfate
Uni-univalent electrolytes	3.4	Sodium chloride, oxycodone hydrochloride
Uni-divalent electrolytes	4.3	Sodium sulfate, ephedrine sulfate, atropine sulfate
Di-univalent electrolytes	4.8	Calcium chloride, zinc chloride
Uni-trivalent electrolytes	5.2	Sodium citrate
Tri-univalent electrolytes	6.0	Ferric chloride
Tetraborate electrolytes	7.6	Sodium borate

**Tabulated on the basis of various editions of the Merck Index, literature, and online searches.*

Sodium chloride equivalent method: In this method, the quantity of drug is multiplied by a factor, E, whose product is equal to the quantity of NaCl having similar osmotic pressure as that of the drug. This quantity is subtracted from the quantity of NaCl isotonic with blood (i.e., 0.9%) to obtain the quantity of NaCl required to be added to the drug solution to make it isotonic.

If the NaCl equivalent, E, is not available in any reference book, it can be calculated for 1 g of such drug as follows.

Here, the concept is that 1 g of drug and its equivalent amount of NaCl, E, will decrease the freezing point by the same amount. Therefore,

$\Delta T_f^{1\%} = L_{iso} \times 1\ g/M_w = 3.4 \times E/58.5$,

where 3.4 is L_{iso}value for sodium chloride.

Therefore, $E = 17 \times \dfrac{L_{iso}}{M_w}$

Example:

A solution contains 1.2 g apomorphine hydrochloride in a volume of 150 mL. What quantity of sodium chloride must be added to make the solution isotonic?

Solution:

The amount of apomorphine hydrochloride required for preparing 150 mL solution containing 1.2 % apomorphine hydrochloride = 1.2 mL/100 mL × 150 g = 1.8 g. The E value for apomorphine hydrochloride is 0.14. So, 1.8 g of apomorphine hydrochloride = 1.8 g × 0.14 = 0.252 g of NaCl.

To make a 150 mL solution isotonic, you need [0.9 g/100 mL × 150 mL = 1.35 g] 1.35 g NaCl, but here you already have 0.252 g. Therefore, you need to add 1.35 g − 0.252 g = 1.098 g NaCl and 1.8 g apomorphine hydrochloride in sufficient water to make 150 mL.

3.7.4 Adjusting Tonicity of Hypertonic Drug Solution

The White–Vincent method involves adding water to drugs to make an isotonic solution, followed by the addition of an isotonic or isotonic-buffered diluting vehicle to bring the solution to the final volume.

Example:

Make the following solution isotonic with respect to plasma.

Dibucaine hydrochloride: 0.08 g
Sodium borate: 0.40 g
Sterilized isotonic solution q.s.: 150.0 mL

Solution:

First, find E values from a reference book [9]; they are 0.13 and 0.42 for dibucaine hydrochloride and sodium borate, respectively:

$$\text{NaCl equivalents} = (0.08\text{ g} \times 0.13) + (0.40\text{ g} \times 0.42) = 0.178\text{ g NaCl}$$

Because 0.9 g NaCl is isotonic in 100 mL solution, 0.178 g would be isotonic in (100 mL/0.9 g) × 0.178 g = 19.78 mL. Therefore, 0.08 g dibucaine hydrochloride and 0.40 g of sodium borate will be dissolved in sterilized water sufficient to make 19.78 mL, to which sufficient diluting isotonic solution will be added to make 150 mL.

The Sprowls method uses the V value, which gives volumes in milliliters for 0.3 g of a drug whose solution will be isotonic. Sufficient diluting isotonic solution can be added to obtain the desired volume.

The preceding problem can be solved using this method as follows.

The V values for dibucaine hydrochloride and sodium borate are 4.3 mL and 14 mL, respectively. This means that for 0.3 g of dibucaine hydrochloride, you need 4.3 mL water. Hence, for 0.08 g dibucaine hydrochloride, you will need (4.3 mL/0.3 g) × 0.08 g = 1.15 mL. Likewise, for 0.3 g of sodium borate, you need 14 mL water. Hence, for 0.30 g sodium borate, you will need (14 mL/0.3 g) × 0.40 g = 18.67 mL. Thus, the total amount of water required = 1.15 mL + 18.67 mL = 19.82 mL. Therefore, 0.08 g dibucaine hydrochloride and 0.40 g of sodium borate will be dissolved in sterilized water sufficient to make 19.82 mL, to which sufficient diluting isotonic solution will be added to make 150 mL.

For a list of constants used for adjusting tonicity of drug solutions, see Table 3.4.

TABLE 3.4 List of Constants Used for Adjusting Tonicity of Drug Solutions

Drugs	E value	V value	$\Delta T_f^{1\%}$
Apomorphine hydrochloride	0.14	4.7	0.08
Atropine sulfate	0.13	4.3	0.07
Boric acid	0.52	16.7	0.29
Calcium lactate	0.23	7.7	0.14
Dextrose monohydrate	0.16	5.3	0.09
Dibucaine hydrochloride	0.13	4.3	0.08
Ephedrine hydrochloride	0.30	10.0	0.18
Ephedrine sulfate	0.23	7.7	0.14
Homatropine hydrobromide	0.17	5.7	0.10
Lactose	0.17	5.7	0.10
Morphine hydrochloride	0.15	5.0	0.09
Morphine sulfate	0.14	4.8	0.08
Phenylephrine hydrochloride	0.32	9.7	0.18
Pilocarpine nitrate	0.23	7.7	0.14
Sucrose	0.08	2.7	0.05
Tetracaine hydrochloride	0.18	6.0	0.11
Urea	0.59	19.7	0.35

E value = 1 g of drug would have osmotic pressure equal to E g of NaCl.
v value = 0.3 g of drug when dissolved in V mL of water would be isotonic.
$\Delta T_f^{1\%}$ = Decrease in freezing point of water by 1% solution of the drug.
Tabulated on the basis of various editions of Merck Index, literature, and online searches.

3.7.5 Clinical Significance of Osmosis

Existence of equal osmotic pressure inside and outside of living cells is required for their viability and maintenance of homeostasis. The osmotic imbalances can lead to many pathological conditions such as diarrhea. Oral rehydration therapy (i.e., administration of a mixture of glucose and salts in a physiological amount) is required to replenish and stop the water loss during diarrhea. *E. coli* and other diarrhea-causing microorganisms either increase the secretion of Cl- ions into the intestinal lumen or decrease the absorption of Na^+ ions onto the blood. Consequently, the ionic concentration in intestine becomes more than in blood, which creates an osmotic gradient in favor of intestine. Hence, there is net flow of water from systemic circulation to intestine.

Fortunately, in addition to absorption by intestinal villus cells, Na^+ ions are also actively transported from intestine to blood via transporters that are not impaired in diarrhea. However, these transporters require the presence of glucose molecules to transport Na^+ ions. Therefore, oral rehydration therapy (ORT) includes a mixture of glucose and other electrolytes that do not do anything about the severity of diarrhea but replace the lost fluids, thereby minimizing the risk of dehydration.

A higher concentration of glucose would not speed up the activity of the co-transport system; rather, an osmotic pressure would be built up, which would induce the flow of water from systemic circulation to the intestinal lumen. However, substituting glucose in ORT with starch is a better choice, because it releases hundreds of glucose molecules on being broken down by the normal, gradual digestive process, and they are immediately taken up by the co-transport systems and removed from the intestinal lumen. The presence of starch does not cause any generation of osmotic gradients because osmotic pressure is a colligative property. A similar useful effect can also be obtained by using proteins instead of starch because there is a co-transport system for amino acids, too. This forms the basis of food-based ORT, which can be prepared at home from inexpensive materials.

3.8. SOLUBILITY AND SOLUTIONS OF NONELECTROLYTES

Nonelectrolytes are substances that do not yield ions when dissolved in water.

Example: Solution of glucose in water
Electrolytes are substances that form ions in solution and conduct electric current.
Examples: Hydrochloric acid, sodium chloride, etc.
A true solution is a mixture of two or more components that form a homogeneous molecular dispersion. Particle size of the dispersed phase is less than 1.0 μm.
A coarse dispersion represents a system in which the diameter of the dispersed particles is larger than 0.5 μm.
Examples: Emulsions, suspensions
In the case of a colloidal dispersion, the particle size of the dispersed medium is in between true solutions and coarse dispersions.
Examples: Colloidal silver sols and polymeric solutions
A solution consists of two substances: a solute and a solvent. A substance that is dissolved is generally referred to as the solute, and the substance in which it is dissolved is called the solvent.
Example: Sodium chloride solution in water
Sodium chloride is the solute, and water is the solvent.

3.8.1 Saturated Solution

A solution that contains as much solute as the solvent can hold in the presence of dissolving substance (solute) at a stated temperature is called a saturated solution. Any solution that contains less than this amount is called unsaturated, and if it contains more than the amount, it is called a supersaturated solution.

Solubility is the extent to which the solute dissolves in a saturated solution at a specified temperature.

The United States Pharmacopoeia (USP) describes solubility in descriptive terms rather than exact solubility (see Table 3.5).

3.8.2 Concentration Expressions

The concentration of a solution can be expressed in a variety of ways:

Molarity (M, C): Gram molecular weights (moles) of solute in 1 L of solution.
Normality (N): Gram equivalent weights of solute in 1 L of solution.
Molality (m): Gram molecular weights (moles) of solute in 1000 g of solvent.
Mole fraction (X, N): Ratio of the moles of the solute to the total moles of all constituents (solute + solvent) in the solution.
Percent by weight (% w/w): Grams of solute in 100 g of solution.
Percent by volume (% v/v): Milliliters of solute in 100 mL of solution.

TABLE 3.5 Descriptive solubility terms

Descriptive Terms	Parts of Solvent per One Part of Solute
Very soluble	Less than 1
Freely soluble	1–10
Soluble	10–30
Sparingly soluble	30–100
Slightly soluble	100–1,000
Very slightly soluble	1,000–10,000
Practically insoluble	More than 10,000

Example:

A solution of sodium chloride is prepared by dissolving 317.1 g of sodium chloride in enough water to make 1,000 mL solution at 25°C. The density of the solution is 1.198 g/cc. The molecular weight of sodium chloride is 58.45.

Calculate the (1) molarity, (2) molality, (3) mole fraction of sodium chloride and water, and (4) percentage by weight of sodium chloride:

1. Molarity

$$Moles\ of\ NaCl = \frac{gNaCl}{mol\ wt\ NaCl} = \frac{317.1}{58.45} = 5.43$$

$$Molarity = \frac{moles\ of\ NaCl}{kg\ of\ solvent} = \frac{5.43}{1} = 5.43\ M$$

2. Molality

$$\text{weight of solution (g)} = \text{Vol} \times \text{density} = 1000 \times 1.198 = 1198\ \text{g}$$

$$\text{weight of solvent (g)} = \text{weight solution} - \text{weight solute} = 1198 - 317.1 = 880.9\ \text{g} = 0.8809\ \text{kg}$$

$$\text{Molarity} = \frac{\text{Moles of NaCl}}{\text{kg of solvent}} = \frac{5.43}{0.8809} = 6.16\ \text{m}$$

3. Mole fraction of sodium chloride and water

$$\text{Moles of water} = \frac{880.9}{18.02} = 48.88$$

$$\text{Moles fraction of NaCl} = \frac{\text{Moles of NaCl}}{\text{Moles of NaCl} + \text{Moles of water}} = \frac{5.43}{5.43 + 48.88} = 0.0999$$

$$\text{Moles fraction of water} = \frac{\text{Moles of water}}{\text{Moles of NaCl} + \text{Moles of water}} = \frac{48.88}{5.43 + 48.88} = 0.9001$$

4. Percent by weight

$$= \frac{\text{Gm of NaCl}}{\text{Gm of Solution}} \times 100$$

$$= \frac{317.1}{1198} \times 100 = 26.47\%\ w/w$$

NB: Equivalent weight

$$= \frac{\text{atomic weight}}{\text{Number of equivalents per atomic weight (Valence)}}$$

Example:

Magnesium has a valence of 2, and its atomic weight is 24.

$$\text{Therefore, the equivalent weight} = \frac{24}{2} = 12\ \text{g/equivalent}$$

$$\text{Equivalent weight (g/Eq)} = \frac{\text{molecular weight (g/mole)}}{\text{equivalent/mole}}$$

$$\text{Equivalent weight of NaCl} = \frac{58.5\ \text{g/mole}}{1\ \text{equivalent/mole}} = 58.5\ \text{g/equivalent}$$

3.8.3 Ideal and Real Solutions

An ideal solution is defined as that solution in which there is no change in the properties of the components other than dilution when they are mixed to form the solution. There is no absorption or evolution of heat during the solution process. The final volume of the solution also shows an additive property of the individual components. Ideality in gas implies the complete absence of attractive forces, whereas ideality in solution denotes complete uniformity of attractive forces. Furthermore, ideal solutions must strictly obey Raoult's law of vapor pressure throughout the complete range of temperature.

Raoult's law states that in an ideal solution, the partial vapor pressure of a component of a solution is equal to the vapor pressure of the pure constituent multiplied by its mole fraction in the solution.

If a solution of two volatile and miscible liquids is represented by A and B, then the partial vapor pressures of the two substituents above the solution are as follows:

$$P_A = P_A^{\circ} X_A$$

$$P_B = P_B^{\circ} X_B$$

where P_A and P_B are the partial vapor pressures of the constituents over the solution; X_A and X_B are the mole fractions of A and B in the solution, respectively; and P_A° and P_B° are the vapor pressures of the pure A and pure B, respectively. The total vapor pressure can be expressed graphically as shown in Figure 3.16.

Example:

What is the partial vapor pressure of ethylene chloride and benzene in solution at a mole fraction of benzene of 0.7. The vapor pressures of pure benzene and pure ethylene chloride are 268 mm and 236 mm at 50°C, respectively. Calculate the total pressure at this temperature.

Let B represent benzene, and let A represent ethylene chloride.

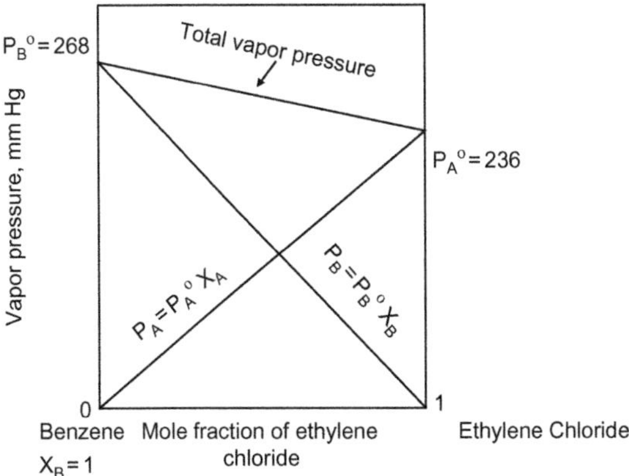

FIGURE 3.16 Vapor pressure-composition curve for an ideal binary system.

$$P_B = 268 \times 0.7 = 187.6 \text{ mm}$$
$$X_A = 1 - X_B = 1 - 0.7 = 0.3$$
$$P_A = 235 \times 0.3 = 70.5 \text{ mm}$$
$$\text{Total Pressure} = P = P_A + P_B$$
$$P = 187.6 + 70.5 = 258.1 \text{ mm.}$$

3.8.4 Real Solutions

In a real solution, complete uniformity of attractive forces does not exist, and it does not obey Raoult's law throughout the entire range of composition. Two types of deviation are generally recognized:

- Negative deviation
- Positive deviation

3.8.4.1 Negative Deviation

When the force of attraction between unlike molecules (adhesive force) exceeds the force of attraction between like molecules (cohesive force), the total vapor pressure of the system is less than that expected from Raoult's law, as shown in Figure 3.17.

Examples:

Chloroform and acetone which manifest greater adhesive forces via the formation of hydrogen bond as shown below:

Cl_3C——H------ O=C(CH_3)$_2$
Chloroform Acetone

3.8.4.2 Positive Deviation

When the adhesive forces are less than the cohesive forces, a positive deviation from Raoult's law is generally noticed. The total vapor pressure of the system is higher than that expected from Raoult's law, as shown in Figure 3.18.

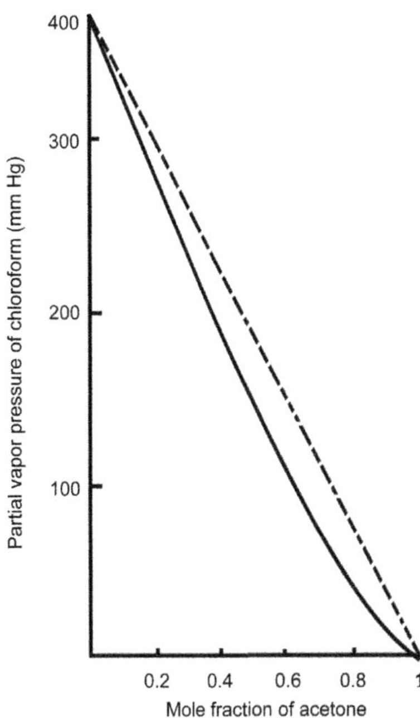

FIGURE 3.17 Decrease in partial vapor pressure of chloroform with increase in mole fraction of acetone. Key (----) vapor pressure calculated by using Raoult's law; (___) experimental data (*Adapted from [11]*).

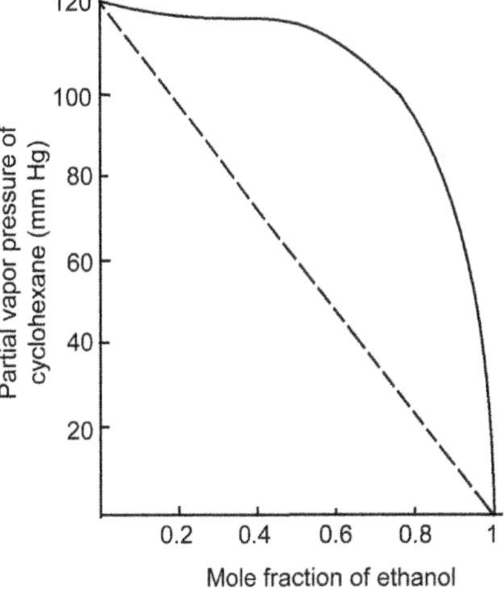

FIGURE 3.18 Increase in partial vapor pressure of cyclohexane with increase in mole fraction of ethanol. Key (----) vapor pressure calculated by using Raoult's law; (___) experimental data (*Adapted from [11]*).

Examples:

Cyclohexane and ethanol
Benzene and ethyl alcohol
Carbon disulfide and acetone

3.9. SPECTROSCOPY

The word *spectroscopy* is derived from *spectrum*, which means a blend of different colors formed when light

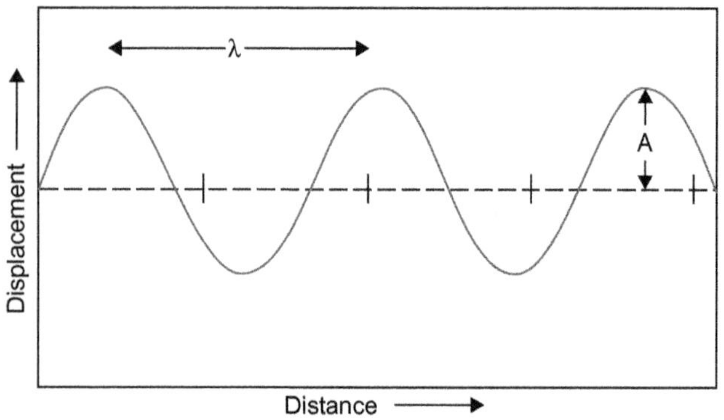

FIGURE 3.19 Diagrammatic representation of a wave.

(visible electromagnetic radiation, or EMR) passes through matter such as a prism, due to a difference in wavelength, and *skopin*, which means examination or evaluation. Thus, spectroscopy is the branch of science that deals with the interaction between EMR and matter.

EMR is the energy emitted in the form of photons by matter possessing either kinetic or potential energy or both. EMR has dual characteristics of both waves and particles. An EMR wave form consists of mutually perpendicular oscillating electric and magnetic fields and travels at the speed of light, *c*, which is given by

$$c = n\lambda \tag{3.17}$$

where *n* is frequency, which is the number of peaks passing a given point in 1 second; and λ is a wavelength of the radiation, which is the distance between two successive peaks, as shown in Figure 3.19.

Electromagnetic radiation is absorbed or emitted when the molecule atom or ion of the sample moves from a lower to higher or from a higher to lower energy state, resulting in changes in rotational, vibrational, and/or electronic energies that are measured by spectroscopic methods. Absorption spectroscopy, such as UV-visible and infrared spectroscopy, measures the absorption; whereas emission spectroscopy, such as fluorescence spectroscopy, measures the emission of radiation.

The full EMR spectrum is continuous, and each region merges partially into the neighboring regions. However, for convenience of reference, the Joint Committee on Nomenclature in Applied Spectroscopy has assigned wavelengths for various spectral regions, as shown in Table 3.6.

TABLE 3.6 Spectral Regions and their Wavelength

Spectral Regions	Wavelength (nm)
Gamma rays	0.2–10
Far ultraviolet	10–200
Near ultraviolet	200–380
Visible	380–780
Near infrared	780–3,000
Middle infrared	3,000–30,000
Far infrared	30,000–300,000
Microwave	300,000–1,000,000,000
Radiowave	1,000,000,000 <

3.9.1 UV-Visible Spectroscopy

The wavelength range of UV and visible radiation are in the range of 200–380 nm and 380–780 nm, respectively, which are expressed in nanometers or in angstroms; but their absorption is expressed in terms of wave number (cm^{-1}), which is the inverse of wavelength. Radiation in this region is of sufficient energy to cause electronic transition of outer valence electrons.

Electronic transitions are associated with vibrational as well as rotational transitions. A compound appears colored if it selectively absorbs light in the visible region. The main function of absorbed energy is to raise the molecule from ground energy state (E_0) to a higher excited energy state (E_1), the difference of which is given by

$$\Delta E = E_1 - E_0 = hn = h\frac{c}{\lambda} \tag{3.18}$$

where *h* is Plank's constant, *n* is the frequency of radiation absorbed, *c* is the velocity of light, and λ is the wavelength of radiation absorbed.

ΔE depends on bond strength, i.e., how tightly the electrons are held in the bonds, and accordingly, absorption will occur in the UV or visible range. For example, if the electrons of a molecule are held by sigma bonds (e.g., in saturated compounds), no visible range of radiation will be absorbed because the energy requirement for transitioning such electrons to the next higher energy level is so high that it cannot be provided by absorbing radiation in the visible range. The absorption of radiation in the UV region may provide energy sufficient for exciting sigma bond-held electrons, and hence such compounds appear colorless. Some sigma bond-held electrons, such as those found in alkanes, require such a large amount of energy for their excitation that only absorption of gamma radiation can provide sufficient excitation energy; hence, they are used as solvents in UV-visible spectroscopy. On the other hand, electrons held by π bonds or nonbonding electrons (located principally in the atomic orbital of N, O, S and halogens [X] as a lone pair of electrons) can be excited by the absorption of UV radiation. Thus, the energy requirement for such transitions can be represented by

$$n \rightarrow \pi^* < \pi \rightarrow \pi^* < n \rightarrow \sigma^* < \sigma \rightarrow \sigma^* \tag{3.19}$$

where the $n \rightarrow \pi^*$ transition requires the lowest energy, and $\sigma \rightarrow \sigma^*$ requires the highest amount of energy, as shown in Figure 3.20.

3.9.2 Correlation of Molecular Structure and Spectra Conjugation

Conjugation of unsaturated groups in a molecule increases the absorption intensity in comparison to the $n \rightarrow \pi^*$ transition occurring in an isolated group in a molecule. Consequently, the wavelength of maximum absorption shifts to a longer wavelength (i.e., bathochromic or red shift). Some examples are provided in Figure 3.21.

A similar effect happens when a group containing n electrons is conjugated with a group containing π electrons, as shown in the following, where oxygen contains n and the methylene group contains π electrons:

$CH_3C(=O)CH_3$ λmax = 290 nm $CH_3C(=O)CH_3{=}CH_2$ λmax = 325 nm

Aromatic systems that also contain π electrons strongly absorb UV radiation where hypsochromic or blue shift (i.e., a shift toward a lower wavelength) occurs, as shown in the following, where the order of electronegativity is C < S < N < O:

λmax = 254 nm λmax = 250 nm λmax = 232 nm λmax = 217 nm λmax = 210 nm

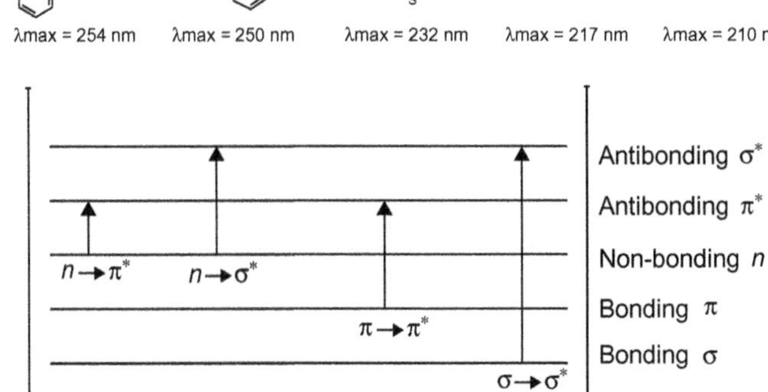

FIGURE 3.20 Energy levels of electronic transitions.

Thus, it appears that as the length of a conjugated system in a molecule increases, the λ max moves toward the visible region. Moreover, the absorption of radiation of a particular wavelength is characteristic of a group of atoms rather than the electrons themselves. Two types of groups—chromophores and auxochromes—can influence absorption of energy required for transition of electrons.

3.9.2.1 Chromophores

The term *chromophore* literally means "color-bearing," which is a functional group not conjugated with any other group and has a characteristic UV or visible absorption spectrum. Table 3.7 shows some typical chromophores.

TABLE 3.7 Some Important Chromophores and their Characteristic Absorption Bands

Chromophores	Formula	Wavelength (nm)
Nitrile	–CN	<180
Nitro	$-NO_2$	210
Nitrite	–O–NO	225
Nitrate	$-O-NO_2$	270
Azo	–N=N–	>290
Nitroso	–N=O	300
Ethene	–C=C–	190
Thiol	–SH	195
Benzene	Ph–H	184
CONJUGATED CHROMOPHORES		
Nitroethene	$C=C-NO_2$	230
Enamine	C=C–CN	220
Phenol	ArOH	280

λmax = 180–200 nm
Absorption intensity = 10,000

λmax = 217 nm
Absorption intensity = 21,000

λmax = 258 nm
Absorption intensity = 36,000

λmax = 250 nm
Absorption intensity = 1259

λmax = 290 nm
Absorption intensity = 3162

λmax = 360 nm
Absorption intensity = 12,589

FIGURE 3.21 The effect of increasing conjugation on spectral properties.

The conjugation of chromophores leads to absorption at longer wavelengths with an increase in absorptivity.

3.9.2.2 *Auxochromes*

Auxochromes do not absorb significantly on their own but rather increase the absorption of a chromophore to which it is attached. Their effect is related to polarity. For example, auxochromes such as CH_3-, CH_3CH_2-, and Cl^- have very little effect usually in the range of 5–10 nm, whereas $-NH_2$ and $-NO_2$ completely alter the spectra of chromophores; e.g., benzene does not display color because it does not have a chromophore, but nitrobenzene is pale yellow color because of the presence of a chromophore nitro group. Para-hydroxynitrobenzene exhibits a deep yellow color where an auxochrome (–OH) is conjugated with the chromophore $-NO_2$. Similar behavior occurs in azo benzene (red color), but para-hydroxy azobenzene is a dark red color.

3.9.3 Visible Spectra

Generally, a compound absorbs in the visible range if it contains at least five conjugated chromophoric and auxochromic groups; e.g., methylene blue absorbs at 660 nm, and its chemical structure is shown in Figure 3.22.

3.9.4 The Beer–Lambert Law

The Beer–Lambert law states that the concentration of a substance in solution is directly proportional to the "absorbance," A, of the solution, which can be written mathematically as

$$A = k \times c \times l \tag{3.20}$$

where c and l are concentration of the solution and length of sample cuvette, respectively; and k is a constant that is called the molar absorption coefficient if c and l are expressed as moles per liter and cm, respectively, or the specific absorption coefficient if c and l are g per liter and cm, respectively.

The law is true only for monochromatic light, which is light of a single wavelength or narrow band of wavelengths, and provided that the physical or chemical state of the substance does not change with concentration.

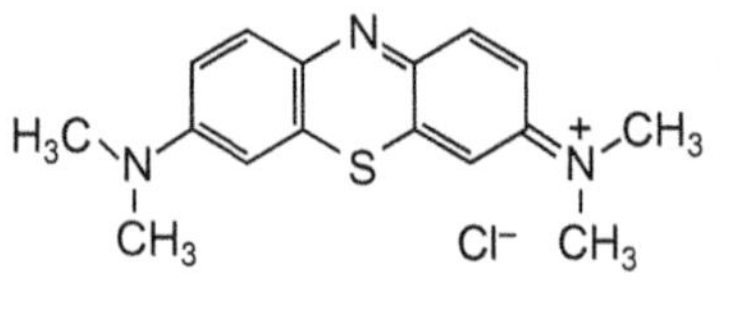

FIGURE 3.22 Methylene blue bearing conjugated chromophores and auxochromes.

When monochromatic radiation passes through a homogeneous solution in a cell, the intensity of the emitted radiation depends on l and c of the solution. Io is the intensity of the incident radiation, and I is the intensity of the transmitted radiation. The ratio I/Io is called transmittance, which is sometimes expressed as a percentage and referred to as %transmittance, $\%T$. Figure 3.23 schematically represents such phenomena.

Absorbance is equal to the inverse of T or $\%T$, which is expressed by Eq. 3.21:

$$A = log\left(\frac{I_0}{I}\right) = log\left(\frac{1}{T}\right) = log\left(\frac{1}{\%T}\right) = log\left(\frac{100}{T}\right) = kcl \tag{3.21}$$

According to the Beer–Lambert law, A is proportional to c, which means A doubles with twice an increase in c. Therefore, in all quantitative UV-visible spectroscopy, A is used instead of T.

3.9.5 Applications of Absorption Spectroscopy (UV, Visible)

3.9.5.1 *Detection of Impurity Present in a Compound*

UV absorption spectroscopy is one of the best methods for determination of impurities in organic molecules. Additional peaks can be observed due to impurities in the sample, and they can be compared with that of standard raw material. Impurities can also be detected by measuring the absorbance at specific wavelength; e.g., benzene appears as a common impurity in cyclohexane and can be detected by its absorption at 255 nm because cyclohexane absorbs at 200 nm.

3.9.5.2 *Quantitative Analysis*

UV-visible absorption spectroscopy can be used for the quantitative determination of compounds by applying the Beer–Lambert law.

3.9.5.3 *Qualitative Analysis*

UV-visible spectroscopy can be used for identification by comparing the absorption spectrum with the spectra of known compounds; e.g., aromatic compounds and aromatic olefins are generally characterized by using UV-visible spectroscopy.

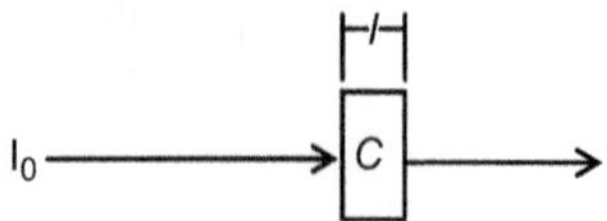

FIGURE 3.23 Diagrammatic representation of the change in intensity of radiation passing through a sample cuvette.

3.9.5.4 *Determination of Dissociation Constants of Acids and Bases*

To determine the dissociation constants of acids and bases, the Henderson-Hasselbalch (H-H) equation (see Chapter 4 for details about this equation) can be used, e.g. Eq. 3.22 is the H-H equation for an acid where $[A^-]$ and [HA] indicates concentrations of the ionized and unionized form of acid, respectively:

$$pH = pK_a + log\frac{[A^-]}{[\mathrm{HA}]} \tag{3.22}$$

pK_α of an acid can be calculated from Eq. 3.22 if the ratio $[A^-]/[HA]$ is known at different pH, which can be easily determined spectrophotometrically. A plot of pH vs log $[A^-]/[HA]$ will result in a straight line. The y intercept of this plot will provide the pKa value.

3.9.5.5 *Quantitative Analysis of Pharmaceutical Substances*

Many drugs can be assayed by making a suitable solution of the drug in a solvent and measuring the absorbance at a specific wavelength; e.g., diazepam tablets can be analyzed by making the solution in acidic methanol and measuring the absorbance at 284 nm.

3.9.5.6 *Quantification of Nucleic Acid Samples*

The polymeric nucleic acid absorbs at 260 nm, which can be used for their quantification. For example, it has been generally observed that an absorbance of 1.0 equals 50, 40, and 33 μg/mL for DNA, RNA, and short oligonucleotides, respectively.

3.9.5.7 *Detection of Impurity in Nucleic Acid Samples*

There is a probability of the presence of proteins/peptides in nucleic acid samples, which can be easily determined by using their absorbance at 280 nm because nucleic acid absorb at 260 nm. It has been found that pure DNA samples have a ratio of absorbance at 260 nm and 280 nm equal to 1.8. A ratio less than 1.8 indicates contamination of DNA samples with proteins and/or peptides. Similarly, the ratio is equal to 2 for a pure RNA sample.

3.9.5.8 *Quantification of Protein and Peptide Solutions*

Generally, proteins with no prosthetic group absorb at 280 nm, which is mainly contributed by tryptophan and tyrosine amino acid residues. Tryptophan and tyrosine have molar absorptivity of about 5,700 and 1,300 $M^{-1}\ cm^{-1}$ at 280 nm, respectively. Therefore, the molar absorptivity of a protein can be estimated by using Eq. 3.23 because no other amino acid residues contribute to the absorbance at 280 nm:

$$\text{The absorbance of } 1\frac{mg}{mL} \text{ protein solution in a sample cuvette of } 1\ cm = \frac{(5700 \times \#of\ Trp + 1300 \times \#of\ Tyr)}{M} \tag{3.23}$$

where M is molecular weight of the protein. It has been found that an absorbance of 1.0 at 280 nm indicates 1 mg/mL for protein but 0.33 mg/mL for a peptide sample solution.

3.9.6 Infrared Spectroscopy

A molecule is always vibrating as its bonds stretch, contract, or bend with respect to one another. Absorption of radiation in the infrared (IR) region causes changes in vibrational pattern of a molecule. This vibration is recorded in infrared spectroscopy, which is a plot of frequency of radiation absorbed in terms of wavenumber versus absorbance.

An infrared spectrum is a characteristic property of a drug molecule (see Figure 3.24), which can be used for both establishing the identity of a compound and revealing the structure of a new compound. An IR spectrum from 1,450 to 600 cm^{-1} is called the fingerprint region, which can be used for identification of a compound due to its uniqueness. The rest of the region from 4,000 to 1,450 cm^{-1} is due to various types of molecular vibration, and hence appropriately called the group frequency region.

The IR spectrum provides information about the functional groups present in a compound. This information, in turn, can be used for elucidating its structure in conjunction with other analytical techniques. A particular functional group absorbs radiation of certain frequencies that are almost the same irrespective of in which compound they are present. For example, the −OH group of alcohols absorb strongly at 3,200–3,600 cm^{-1}; but the OH group of carboxylic acid absorbs strongly at

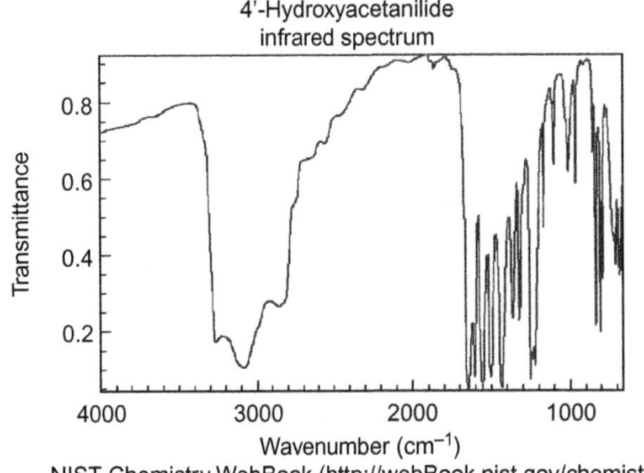

FIGURE 3.24 The IR spectrum of solid-state acetaminophen powder.

2,500–3,000, whose peak shape is broad due to involvement with making hydrogen bonds; the CO group of ketone absorb strongly at 1,710 cm^{-1}; and the CH_3 group absorb strongly at 1,450 and 1,375 cm^{-1}.

3.9.6.1 *Applications*

IR spectroscopy has been applied in pharmacy to solve many problems, such as investigating identity, purity, and crystalline structure of a drug and their interaction with excipients either as a stand-alone method or in combination with other analytical methods. Following are some of the important applications of IR spectroscopy in pharmacy:

- *Verification of drug identity:* IR spectroscopy was first introduced to identify drugs in USP XVI. The current USP 35 NF 30 lists 1,321 monographs that use the IR spectrum to identify drugs, which is based on a comparison of the IR spectrum of a drug with that of a reference standard. However, precautions should be taken because sometimes two drugs might have exactly identical overlapping spectra, such as in the case of the homologues of the long chain fatty acids and esters and drugs exhibiting polymorphism or pseudopolymorphism.
- *Testing purity of a drug:* The manufacturing process of a drug may introduce tiny amounts of some unwanted materials that might cause some adverse reactions or modify therapeutic outcomes which could be identified by IR spectroscopy. For example, the presence of dichloroacetic acid in chloramphenicol is detected by the appearance of a band at 1,745 cm^{-1} in the IR spectrum of chloramphenicol. Therefore, the peak at 1,745 cm^{-1} is defined as an analytical band of impurity.
- *Investigation of drug structure:* At one time there were three proposed structural formulas for penicillin. This issue was resolved by the presence of a strong band at 1,780 cm^{-1}, indicating a CO group related with the presence of a cyclic β-lactam ring. Therefore, the structural formula containing the β-lactam ring was accepted as the correct formula for penicillin.
- *Elucidation of crystalline structures:* IR spectroscopy has been reported to have an advantage over X-ray powder diffraction for obtaining information about conformational characteristics of polymorphs of a drug containing types of H-bonds that affect vibrations of OH, NH, or C = O groups. For example, α and β forms of chloramphenicol palmitate are characterized by peaks at 858 and 843 cm^{-1}, respectively; forms I, II, IV, and the solvates of indomethacin by means of their markedly different IR spectra at 1,700 cm^{-1}; forms I and II of rotenone in 800–850 cm^{-1}; a quantitative analysis of a mixture of acetylsalicylic acid (aspirin) and salicylic acid by bands at 920 and 760 cm^{-1}, respectively, etc.
- *Investigation of drug-excipient interaction:* The interaction of a drug with excipients involving complexation, hydrogen bonding, etc., modifies its physicochemical properties, resulting in changes in pharmacological actions and pharmacokinetic behaviors. Interactions are identified by the appearance of a new IR absorption peak indicating formation of a new complex compound, disappearance of a peak, shifting of a characteristic peak, broadening of a peak, or alteration in intensity of a particular peak.

3.9.7 Fluorescence Spectroscopy

In UV-visible spectroscopy, the absorption of electromagnetic radiation in the UV and visible region leads to transition of a molecule from the ground state to the excited state. Because the excited state possesses higher energy than the ground state, ultimately these excited electrons come back to the ground state by emitting absorbed energy as well as losing it in some other way. The emission of absorbed energy is broadly termed luminescence.

The electrons at the ground state (which contains the lowest energy) are paired in such a way that their spin is antiparallel to each other, which cancels the energy associated with both paired electrons, resulting in zero energy for the ground state. This is termed a singlet state of electrons. However, excited electrons can orient either parallel (triplet state, S = 1) or antiparallel (singlet state, S = 0). When electrons return to the ground state by emitting energy from the triplet state, the phenomenon is termed phosphorescence. Fluorescence is the phenomenon that occurs when excited electrons come back to the ground state from the singlet state. Phosphorescence has a long lifetime (10^{-2} to 100 sec), and its rate is slow. In contrast, fluorescence has a short lifetime (10^{-8} sec), and emission of energy is fast enough to be comparable with other processes such as collisional deactivation and intersystem crossing. The overall energy balance for the fluorescence process can be written as

$$E_{fluor} = E_{abs} - E_{vib} - E_{solv.relax.} \tag{3.24}$$

where E_{fluor} is the energy of the emitted radiation, E_{abs} is the energy of the radiation absorbed by the molecule during excitation, and E_{vib} is the energy lost by the molecule during vibrational relaxation. The term $E_{solv.relax.}$ indicates the energy lost to the solvent cage where the excited electrons reorient themselves or relax to the ground state. As is obvious from Eq. 3.24, the energy of fluorescence is always less than the energy absorbed during excitation. Therefore, the wavelength of emitted radiation during fluorescence is always greater than that of the absorbed radiation.

3.9.7.1 *Applications*

All the applications of fluorescence spectroscopy are based on comparisons of wavelengths of radiation required for the excitation of an electron and wavelengths of radiation emitted during the relaxation of the excited electron to the ground state. The difference between excitation and emission wavelengths is much less in comparison to wavelengths of incident and transmitted radiation involved in UV-visible spectroscopy. Thus, fluorescence intensity is measured above a low background, where a very low absorbance is measured by comparing two very large signals that are slightly different. In contrast, in UV-visible spectroscopy, a very high absorbance is measured by comparing one similarly high signal with another very low signal. Therefore, fluorescence spectroscopy is a very sensitive technique, up to 1,000 times more sensitive than UV-visible spectrophotometry. Moreover, recent advances in instrumentation have made it possible to detect fluorescence of even a single molecule.

Not all drugs are suitable for investigation by fluorescence spectrometry because they have to absorb radiation of a particular wavelength to get their electrons excited and must come back to ground state by emitting radiation of different wavelengths. Generally, the molecules capable of displaying fluorescence or phosphorescence contain a rigid conjugated structure, e.g., aromatic hydrocarbons, rhodamines, coumarins, oxines, polyenes, etc. Many drugs (e.g., morphine, riboflavin, bumetanide, chlorophyllin copper complex sodium, copovidone, digoxin, ergotamine, estradiol, fluorescein sodium, hydroxyprogesterone, quinine sulfate, stanozolol, thiamine hydrochloride, triamterene, etc.), some natural amino acids and cofactors (e.g., tyrosine, tryptophan, nicotinamide adenine dinucleotide, flavin adenine dinucleotide, etc.,) fluoresce and hence can be investigated using fluorometry for qualitative and quantitative characterization.

Manipulation of biopolymers such as nucleic acid and proteins and the imaging of biological membranes and living organisms are emerging areas utilizing extensively fluorescence-based detection and analysis. Since amino acids such as tyrosine and tryptophan fluoresce, fluorometry can differentiate proteins and peptides from biological matrices; this is not possible with UV-visible spectrometry due to an overlap of absorbance by proteins and peptides around 190 nm with other substances present in the cellular matrices. The recent development of dyes and fluorophores for biological applications is further expanding the applications of fluorescence spectroscopy.

3.9.8 Nuclear Magnetic Resonance Spectroscopy

The nuclei of certain atoms spin just like electrons do. Hydrogen is one such atom whose nucleus contains only one proton. Since a circulating charge creates a magnetic field along the axis of spin, a hydrogen atom or a proton placed in an external magnetic field would orient either parallel or antiparallel to the magnetic moment of it. A parallel arrangement or alignment along with the external magnetic field is more stable; therefore, energy must be absorbed by the proton to change its alignment against the field. Consequently, if a magnetic field is continuously changed over a proton placed in a constant radiation energy, at a certain magnetic field strength value, the energy required to flip the orientation of the proton matches with the applied radiation energy when energy is absorbed, which will appear as a peak on a plot between magnetic field versus absorption of energy.

3.9.8.1 *Nuclear Magnetic Resonance (NMR) Spectrum*

Different protons exist in different environments and thereby possess different magnetic field strengths. This would require different external magnetic fields to flip over their alignment, provided the applied radiation energy is constant. Therefore, a plot of magnetic field and energy absorbed would have various peaks corresponding to various protons present in the sample, which would differ in intensity as well as their location. Such a plot is called the NMR spectrum.

Thus, while one is interpreting an NMR spectrum, attention is focused on the following aspects:

Number of Peaks: This provides information about the number of different kinds of protons in the sample molecule because protons with the same environment absorb at the same applied magnetic field. For example, CH_3-CH_2-Cl would have two NMR peaks, but $CH_3-CH-Cl-CH_3$ (isopropyl chloride) would have three peaks because CH_3- in isopropyl chloride is not equivalent to CH_3- in the other molecule, since they are surrounded by different neighboring groups.

Locations of Peaks: This provides information about the electronic environment of each peak, i.e., whether the protons representing a peak are aromatic, aliphatic, primary, secondary, tertiary, benzylic, vinylic, acetylenic, or adjacent to halogen or to other atoms or groups.

In addition to protons, an atom/molecule also contains electrons, in which spinning can also generate a magnetic field in an NMR experiment called the secondary or induced magnetic field. The induced magnetic field either can oppose or reinforce the applied magnetic field depending on the relative location of protons. As a result, the field experienced by protons is diminished or reinforced, and the protons are called either shielded or deshielded, respectively, from the influence of the externally applied magnetic field.

Obviously, shielding means that a greater external magnetic field strength is required to change the orientation of the spinning proton, which results in an upfield shift in the NMR absorption peak. In contrast, deshielding causes a downfield shift of the NMR absorption peak. Benzene causes deshielding of aromatic protons, but acetylene causes shielding of acetylenic protons. Such up- or downfield shifts in NMR peaks due to electrons are called chemical shifts (see Table 3.8), in which the units are parts per million (ppm) of the total applied external magnetic field. The reference point for measuring chemical shifts is not a single proton but the compound tetramethylsilane, $(CH_3)_4Si$, where silicone is a very low electronegative compound. Therefore, the shielding of protons in silane is greater than in most of the other molecules. Consequently, the NMR signals from most of the other organic molecules appear downfield in comparison to those from silane.

There are two commonly used scales for measuring chemical shift values: δ (delta) and τ (tau). The position of tetramethylsilane in the δ scale is taken as 0.0 ppm, whereas most other chemicals have chemical shift values of 0–10 ppm. In the τ scale, the position of tetramethylsilane is taken as 10.0 ppm. Thus, the two scales are related by the equation $\tau = 10 - \delta$. The electron-withdrawing groups such as halogens cause deshielding by lowering the electron density in the vicinity of the proton.

Intensities of Peaks: This provides information about the number of protons in each kind; this number is proportional to the area under the peak. This intensity is due to the absorption of a quantum of energy required by a proton for flipping over in a magnetic field. Since the field strength is the same, the greater absorption of energy could be due only to the proportionally greater number of protons.

Splitting of a Peak: A chemical shift is caused by shielding and/or deshielding effects of electrons, but the splitting of a peak appearing at a particular position is due to the effect of neighboring protons, which is called spin-spin coupling. For example, the NMR spectrum of dichloroethane (see Figure 3.25) shows two peaks: one is a doublet and another is a quartet. The doublet is due to coupling of three CH_3- protons with a single CH– proton which spin align either along or opposite to the external applied magnetic field. On the contrary, the quartet is due to coupling of a single –CH– proton with three CH_3- protons, which can spin four different ways, as shown in Figure 3.26. It should be noted that peak intensity, i.e., the area under the peak, is proportional to the number of electrons represented by them; and the separation between two peaks, termed a coupling constant, is the same in both doublet and quartet peaks.

TABLE 3.8 Characteristic Proton NMR Chemical Shifts

Type of Proton	Type of Compound	Chemical Shift Range (ppm, δ)
RCH_3	1° aliphatic	0.9
R_2CH_2	2° aliphatic	1.3
R_3CH	3° aliphatic	1.5
C=C–H	vinylic	4.6–5.9
C=C–H	vinylic, conjugated	5.5–7.5
C≡C–H	acetylenic	2–3
Ar–H	aromatic	6–8.5
Ar–C–H	benzylic	2.2–3
C=C–CH_3	allelic	1.7
HC–F	fluorides	4–4.5
HC–Cl	chlorides	3–4
HC–Br	bromides	2.5–4
HC–I	iodides	2–4
HC–OH	alcohols	3.4–4
HC–OR	ethers	3.3–4
RCOO–CH	esters	3.7–4.1
HC–COOR	esters	2–2.2
HC–COOH	acids	2–2.6
HC–C=O	carbonyl compounds	2–2.7
RCHO	aldehydic	9–10
ROH	hydroxylic	2–4
ArOH	phenolic	4–12
C=C–OH	enolic	15–17
RCOOH	carboxylic	10.0–13.2
RNH_2	amino	1–5

3.9.8.2 Applications

NMR has been widely used for the analysis of body fluids to assess drug toxicity and therapeutic effects. Although it has intrinsically low sensitivity, it is a nondestructive technique, allows the simultaneous detection of many compounds usually present in samples of drug metabolites, and generally does not require sample preparations, or if any, they are minimal. Following are some of specific applications of nuclear magnetic resonance:

- *Anticancer drugs:* Tumors have numerous metabolic pathways that are altered in comparison to healthy normal tissue, which can be detected by HR NMR spectroscopy. Thus, changes in the spectral patterns of samples with respect to the control are used to diagnose or predict the progression of malignant diseases. A number of spectroscopic markers such as choline-containing compounds have been proposed to assess proliferative rates in the spectra of tumors. Fatty acid synthase (FAS) is overexpressed in tumors, which need *de novo* synthesis of fatty acids to accelerate membrane production for highly proliferative cancerous cells. Therefore, the treatment targets inhibiting FAS activity, which results in a decrease of phosphatidylcholine and its precursor phosphocholine levels that can be measured by NMR spectroscopy.

- *Drugs for infectious diseases:* The ability of NMR spectroscopy to detect metabolic changes in cells has been exploited to obtain information about the mechanism of action of antimicrobial agents. For example, it has been reported that 8-azaxanthine inhibits *Aspergillus nidulans* hyphal growth by *in vivo* inactivation of urate oxidase by using a mutant strain *A. nidulansuaZ14* mutant and comparative NMR metabolomics data.
- *Antidiabetic drugs:* Rosiglitazone is an antidiabetic drug that works by enhancing insulin sensitivity. In a small clinical study, NMR was used to obtain biomarkers in plasma and urine, indicating treatment outcomes of rosiglitazone. The multivariate analysis of NMR data showed that the rosiglitazone treatment led to a reduction in urine hippurate and aromatic amino acids, as well as an increase in plasma branched-chain amino acids, alanine, and glutamine/glutamate, which were linked to an increase in hepatic insulin sensitivity in diabetic patients.
- *Drug-induced toxicity:* The ability of NMR spectroscopy to provide information on metabolite changes has been used for figuring out drug-induced toxicities. Cyclosporine is an immunosuppressant drug widely used in organ transplants to reduce the activity of the patient's immune system and, thereby, the risk of organ rejection. However, its clinical use is limited by its nephrotoxicity, which is enhanced when combined with the immunosuppressive inhibitor sirolimus. The NMR spectroscopy analysis of urine metabolites after 6 days of cyclosporine treatment showed changes of 2-oxoglutarate, citrate, and succinate concentrations, together with increased urine isoprostane concentrations, that were indicative of oxidative stress. After 28 days of treatment, increased lactate and glucose concentrations in urine and decreased concentrations of Krebs cycle intermediates were detected, indicating proximal tubular damage. Thus, the urine NMR metabolic patterns indicated that cyclosporine and/or sirolimus induced damage of the renal tubular system, which is reported to be more sensitive than currently used clinical kidney function markers such as creatinine concentrations in serum.

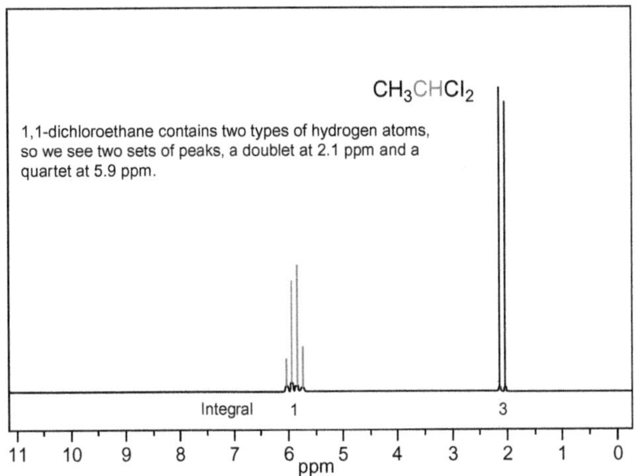

FIGURE 3.25 Splitting of a peak in the NMR spectrum of dichloroethane.

3.9.9 Mass Spectroscopy

Mass spectroscopy is an analytical technique used to separate electrically charged particles on the basis of their masses. It involves bombardment of the sample

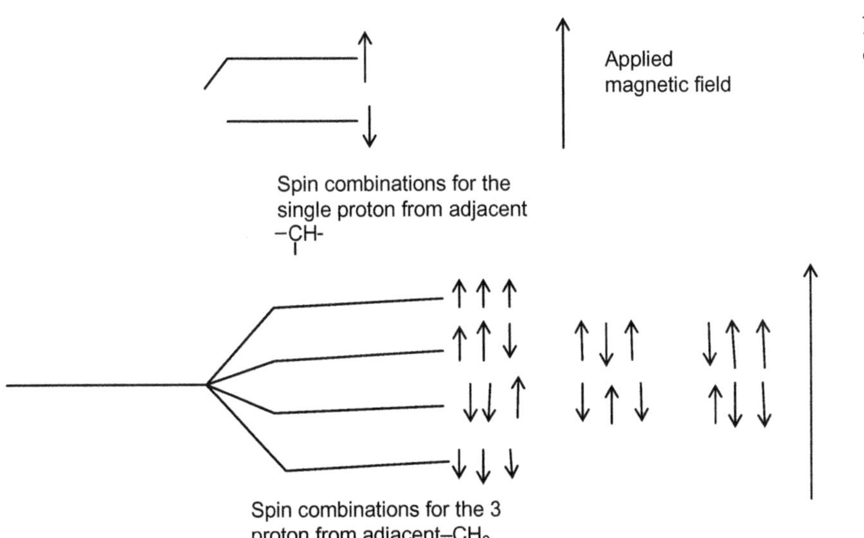

FIGURE 3.26 Spin-spin coupling in dichloroethane.

molecules with a beam of extremely energetic electrons. Consequently, molecules become charged and fragmented, some of which are positively charged ions. Each ion has a particular value for ratio of mass and charge (m/z ratio). Since the value of charge is generally 1; the m/z ratio is simply the mass of the ion. A mass spectrum is the plot of signals representing m/z ratios of all the ions produced due to fragmentation and their intensities, indicating relative abundance. Figure 3.27 shows the structure of acetaminophen, and Figure 3.28 shows its mass spectrum ($C_8H_9NO_2$; Mol. wt 151.16), where the prominent signals are numbered and their m/z ratios are shown in parentheses. Signal # 1 at 151 is called the molecular ion or parent ion and is generally represented by M^+. A molecular ion is produced when high-energy electrons bombarding on the sample (here e.g., acetaminophen) knock off one electron; hence, M^+ represent the molecular weight of the sample.

The molecular ions are highly unstable; therefore, some of them would further fragment into smaller pieces whose relative intensities or abundances are controlled by their relative stability. The tallest signal in the spectrum (signal # 2 in Figure 3.28) is called the base peak, whose intensity is arbitrarily assigned a height of 100 and the rest of the peak heights are assigned relative to it. The signal # 2 (Mol. Wt. 109) is due to knocking off CH_3CO- moiety (Mol. Wt. 43) from acetaminophen. Signal # 4 is representing CH_3CO- moiety because it corresponds to Mol. Wt. of 43. The appearance of tiny peaks 1 or 2 m/z ratios more or less of a significant peak is due to isotopes.

3.9.9.1 *Applications*

Mass spectra are useful in proving the identity of a compound as well as helping in establishing the structure of a new compound. Generally, we accept two compounds as the same if their physicochemical properties are same. Because a single mass spectrum provides the relative abundances of a number of fragments that are involved in many of the physicochemical properties, if the mass spectrum of an unknown compound is identical with the mass spectrum of a previously reported compound, the two compounds are the same without any doubt. Moreover, mass spectrum provides an exact molecular weight of a compound and also its molecular formula, which can be of immense help in establishing the structure of the new compound or at least confirming the presence of certain structural units.

Mass spectrometry-based techniques using electrospray and matrix-assisted laser desorption ionization have found use in the area of nucleic acid; for example, they include sequencing techniques for oligonucleotides, approaches to mixture analysis, microscale sample handling, and targeted DNA assays. Mass spectrometry coupled with liquid chromatography is of immense help in unraveling column-outlet multicompound bands, where it is universally applicable yet has excellent sensitivity. Tandem mass spectrometry has been used in studies with S-(N-methylcarbamoyl)glutathione, a metabolite of the antineoplastic agent N-methylformamide for characterizing derivatized glutathione conjugates.

3.10. CONCLUSIONS

This chapter discussed some of the physical properties of drug molecules that are of immense importance during the development of safe, effective, and reliable dosage forms. Some of the surface properties, such as surface tension, interfacial tension, and adsorption, and electrical properties play a very important role in various aspects of pharmaceutics and their application in dosage form design. The flow properties of different fluids encountered in pharmacy practice and their applications are discussed in the rheology section. Different colligative properties and their application in various aspects of pharmacy are also discussed. Some of the spectroscopic techniques and their basic principles and applications in evaluating quality products

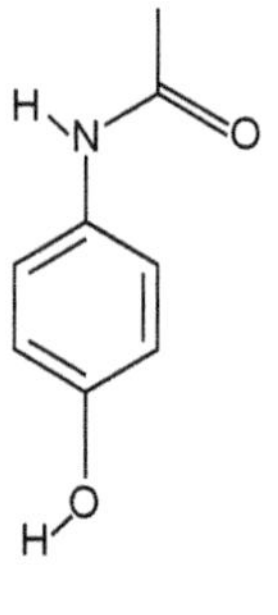

FIGURE 3.27 Structure of acetaminophen.

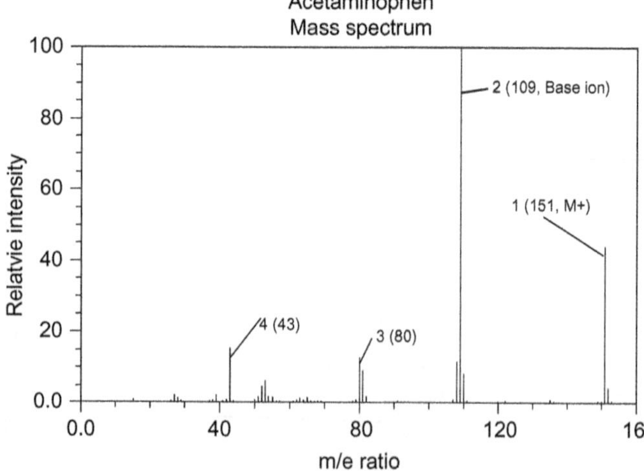

FIGURE 3.28 Mass spectrum of acetaminophen. Retrieved from http://webbook.nist.gov/cgi/cbook.cgi?ID=C103902&Units=SI&Mask=200#Mass-Spec

are critically evaluated. The concepts developed in this chapter would be useful in the overall quality assessment of the drugs and dosage forms influencing their therapeutic outcomes.

CASE STUDIES

Case 3.1

A patient suffering with osteoarthritis was administered a full course (one injection containing 20 mg of sodium hyaluronate in 2 mL phosphate buffered saline for 5 weeks) of Hyalgan® (sodium hyaluronate injection) intra-articularly in the knee joint, but the symptoms did not improve significantly. What option or options would you suggest?

Approach: One reason for pain in osteoarthritis is the decrease in lubrication between two bony joint surfaces provided by synovial fluid. Therefore, sodium hyaluronate is injected into the joint. Because it is antithixotropic in nature, the sodium hyaluronate supplements the loss in viscoelastic property of the synovial fluid. The viscoelasticity of sodium hyaluronate is mainly dependent on the molecular weight of hyaluronic acid used. The different brands of sodium hyaluronate vary in the molecular weight of hyaluronic acid used, as shown in Table 3.9.

Thus, the next logical viable option could be using Orthovisc or Euflexxa. Synvisc should be tried last because it consists of the highest-molecular-weight hyaluronic acid. Here, you should note that although a higher apparent viscosity is expected with an increasing molecular weight of hyaluronic acid, which could be expected to provide better cushioning and lubrication to joints, there could be limit because activity provided by hyaluronic acid is not only mechanical, but also could be biological. In fact, the lubricating and cushioning activity provided by synovial fluid is highly complex.

Case 3.2

You are the drug information pharmacist in your state, and a few pharmacy interns are working under your supervision. You receive a phone call from the local hospital emergency center regarding a case of acetaminophen poisoning. The patient has ingested 20 Tylenol caplets. What information do you need to collect to provide a better understanding of the dose of activated charcoal needed for this patient?

Approach: You have to look for a source for any review or meta-analysis on activated charcoal (AC) in acute poisoning. For one excellent source, see the review article in reference [7].

Understand the time of ingestion, time of treatment with other decontamination modalities before activated charcoal administration, and what type of activated charcoal to use. AC is produced by heating sawdust or coconut shells at 600°C–900°C followed by activation using a stream of hot air and a vacuum to create a more adsorptive surface area in them by degassing the surfaces. The typical surface area of AC is 800–1,200 m^2/g. A 50 g dose of AC has an adsorptive surface area equivalent to the surface area of seven football fields. Super-activated charcoal may have a surface area of 2,800–3,500 m^2/g. Activated charcoal acts as an adsorbent because of its higher surfaces by weak intermolecular (Van der Waals) forces. The usual dose to be administered is a 10:1 ratio (Dose of AC: Weight of drug ingested). For 1 g of drug, you need 10 grams of AC. In this case, 20 Tylenol caplets contain 10 g of active drug. Therefore, you need at least 100 g of AC for this patient.

Case 3.3

A study reported in the *British Journal of Dermatology* [8] suggests that ointment is evenly spread on the skin as compared to creams and solutions. Ointment showed an even spread to the applied areas. Cream, low-viscosity cream, and solution showed poor spreading, resulting in an uneven distribution of dose (lower dose in the periphery). Can you explain the reasons?

Approach: In this study, human volunteers applied four formulations (0.1 g each) to abdominal skin. In order to answer this question regarding spreading, you have to know the composition and surfactants used in each formulation. Creams and solutions have some disadvantages because rapid evaporation (alcohol/water),

TABLE 3.9 Commercially Hyaluronans [6]

Brand Name	Generic Name	Manufacturer	Mol. Wt. (K Da)
Hyalgan	Sodium hyaluronate	Sanofi-aventis	500–730
Supartz	Sodium hyaluronate	Smith & Nephew	620–1170
Synvisc	Hylan G-F 20	Genzyme Corporation	80% Hylan A (6,000) + Hylan B (>6,000)
Orthovisc	High-molecular-weight hyaluronan	DePuy Mitek	1000–2900
Euflexxa	Sodium hyaluronate	Ferring Pharmaceutical	2400–3600

which is measured as cooling, of formulation influences spreading, resulting in an uneven distribution of drug on the applied surface. Ointments, on the other hand, distribute and spread well to the applied area. The presence of surfactants also helps in spreading because they reduce the contact angle. Therefore, patients should be advised to apply creams and solutions to multiple sites and to spread them quickly.

Case 3.4

A community pharmacist engaged in compounding is preparing some Nystatin popsicles using the same recipe for drug, water, coloring agent, flavoring agent, and sugar as a sweetener as used previously. To his utter surprise, when he opens the freezer, he finds the batch he made last night has not solidified. Rechecking the calculation also reveals that all the weights of materials and volumes of solvents used were correct. Can you establish a cause of this problem?

Approach: The first issue you have to think about is why the solution is not freezing. Since the solvent is water, it should freeze at 0 degrees or less than that temperature. Checking the freezer to see whether it's in workable condition is the next issue. From the colligative properties, you know that the presence of salt decreases the freezing point of water. Because the pharmacist used the right amount and previously had success in making Nystatin popsicles, it could be some extra salt that might be causing this problem. That can be easily tested by using the organoleptic method. In this case, possibly the pharmacist added crystalline salt instead of crystalline sugar, which is stored in identical plastic containers. You must read labels carefully before selecting an active or inactive pharmaceutical ingredient.

Case 3.5

A 20% salicylic acid ointment was prepared for a patient to use as a wart treatment. After one week of treatment, the patient did not see a keratolytic effect of this particular batch of ointment. The patient reported this failure to the pharmacist who compounded the prescription. How should the pharmacist respond to this situation?

Approach: The first and foremost thing the pharmacist should do is report the complaint in the pharmacy's book. If possible, the pharmacist may request some of the prepared ointment from the patient. The lot number of the salicylic acid used and the ointment base should be retrieved from the batch and preparation records. If the pharmacy has a spectrophotometer, the concentration of salicylic acid in the used ointment should be measured at that time. If the pharmacy has an infrared spectrometer, the pharmacist should get an IR spectrum of the salicylic acid used in the preparation. This IR spectrum should be compared to the library data that already exists for salicylic acid. If the spectra are different, then the salicylic acid used in the preparation is not really salicylic acid. Therefore, the patient was not getting any keratolytic effect with its use.

Case 3.6

A higher frequency of occurrence of necrotizing enterocolitis (NEC) has been observed in premature infants in intensive care units fed enterally undiluted calcium lactate than those fed no calcium lactate or calcium lactate diluted with water or formula. Can you figure out why?

Approach: The tonicities of oral medications such as calcium lactate commonly used to feed premature infants kept in intensive care are very high, and this may lead to necrotizing enterocolitis if administered undiluted. Furthermore, orally administered calcium lactate or gluconate can have many additives, e.g., ethyl alcohol, sorbitol, and propylene glycol, in a significantly greater amount than generally found in parenterals, leading to unusually higher osmolalities in oral medications. The high osmolalities of orally fed nutritional supplements are the reason for the development of NEC in the premature infants. Therefore, extreme precaution should be taken while feeding premature babies in intensive care units.

References

[1] Holmes HN. Laboratory manual of colloid chemistry. New York: Wiley; 1922. p. 52.

[2] Attwood D, Udeala OK. The surface activity of some antihistamines at the air-solution interface. J Pharm Pharmacol 1975;27(10):754–8.

[3] Fukahoria S, Fujiwaraa T, Itob R, Funamizu N. pH-dependent adsorption of sulfa drugs on high silica zeolite: modeling and kinetic study. Desalination 2011;275(1–3):237–42.

[4] Rangel-Yagui CO, Pessoa Jr A, Costa Tavares L. Micellar solubilization of drugs. J Pharm Pharmaceut Sci 2005;8(2):147–63.

[5] Plasma viscosity and blood viscoelasticity. <http://www.vilastic.com/tech10.html> [accessed 05.06.2013].

[6] Vitanzo PC, Sennett BJ. Hyaluronans: is clinical effectiveness dependent on molecular weight? Am J Orthoped 2006:421–8.

[7] Olson KR. Activated charcoal for acute poisoning: one toxicologist's journey. J Med Toxicol 2010;6(2):190–8 [June].

[8] Ivens UI, et al. Ointment is evenly spread on the skin, in contrast to creams and solutions. Br J Derm 2001;145:264–7.

[9] The Merck Index, 13th Edition, Merck & Co., Inc., Whitehouse Station, NJ, 2001, pp. MISC 32-MISC42.

[10] Hammarlund ER. Sodium chloride equivalents, cryoscopic properties, and hemolytic effects of certain medicinals in aqueous solution IV: Supplemental values. J. Pharm., Sci. 1981;70:1161–3.

[11] Liron Z, Srebrenik S, Martin A, Cohen S. Theoretical derivation of solute-solvent interaction parameter in binary solution: case of the deviation from Raoult's law. J. Pharm. Sci. 1986;75:463–8.

CHAPTER

4

Equilibrium Processes in Pharmaceutics

Sunil S. Jambhekar

LECOM Bradenton, School of Pharmacy, Bradenton, FL, USA

CHAPTER OBJECTIVES

- Define and exemplify equilibrium processes applicable in pharmacy.
- Identify and define various physicochemical properties of drugs determined under equilibrium conditions.
- Explain the dependency of physicochemical properties on the equilibrium process.
- Define the "Rule of Five" and discuss its role in drug development.
- Define polar surface area and illustrate its role in predicting oral absorption of drugs.
- Discuss the importance of physicochemical properties of drugs in the drug discovery process, drug dissolution, drug absorption, and the bioavailability of drugs.
- Discuss the role of the gastrointestinal tract and biological membranes, diffusion and passive diffusion, and the pH-partition theory in drug absorption
- Apply the Henderson–Hasselbalch equation to predict drug absorption.
- Illustrate the interplay among partition coefficient, lipophilicity, and permeability of a drug.
- Explain the concept of drug dissolution, importance of drug dissolution, and various theories used to describe drug dissolution.
- Examine the factors affecting dissolution and solubility.
- Evaluate the biopharmaceutical classification of drugs on the basis of their solubility.

Keywords

- Convective absorption
- Diffusion
- Dissolution
- Drug dissolution and distribution
- Equilibrium
- Gastrointestinal physiology
- Henderson–Hasselbalch equation
- Ionization
- pH-Partition hypothesis
- Polar surface area
- Rule of Five
- Surface activity
- Viscosity

4.1. INTRODUCTION

The term *equilibrium* has been defined many ways in dictionaries. The definitions that closely apply to many processes, encountered in pharmaceutics, are as follows:

> A condition, at which, all acting influences are canceled by others, resulting in a stable, balanced, or unchanged system.
>
> The state of a chemical reaction in which its forward and reverse reactions occur at equal rate so that the concentration of the reactants and products remain unchanged with time.
>
> The state of a reversible chemical reaction in which the forward and reverse reactions occur at equal rates so that there are no further changes in the concentrations of the reactants and products.

The equilibrium process or condition is quite common in the life sciences, and pharmaceutics and biopharmaceutics, of course, are no exceptions. Following are a few examples of equilibrium processes that play

Pharmaceutics. DOI: http://dx.doi.org/10.1016/B978-0-12-386890-9.00004-2

an important role in pharmaceutics: ionization of weak acids and bases; partition coefficient and lipid solubility of a drug; equilibrium or saturation solubility; diffusion, in general and, passive diffusion, in particular. It is important to note that some of these properties are very much interrelated; for example, the ionization of weak acids and bases and solubility, solubility and drug dissolution, and lipophilicity and membrane permeation. There are other physicochemical properties that also play an equally important role in pharmaceutics and biopharmaceutics and that depend on the equilibrium processes mentioned earlier. They include drug dissolution, passive diffusion, drug absorption, drug distribution, etc.

Physicochemical properties of drugs depend on the equilibrium processes and play an important role in influencing the *in vivo* performance of a drug in a particular dosage form, as well as in the early stages of the drug discovery process. In the former, it is often reflected in the rate and extent of drug absorption following the administration of a dosage form, and, in the latter, it is frequently reflected in the extended time line and higher cost in developing new therapeutic agents or active pharmaceutical ingredients. It is becoming increasingly evident that drug discovery and development involves much more than finding the compound with optimum biological activity.

In an effort to reduce delays and attrition rate, most pharmaceutical companies are now evaluating their lead compounds for drug-like properties, many of which depend on equilibrium processes. Early assessment of a lead compound with respect to physicochemical properties provides the opportunities for early optimization of the therapeutic agent. These physicochemical properties also play an important role in the selection of the drug delivery system or dosage form. This chapter discusses the important physicochemical properties of a drug that depend on the equilibrium processes in the discipline of pharmaceutics and biopharmaceutics. The processes are ionization of weak acids and bases, partition coefficient, equilibrium solubility, drug dissolution, and passive diffusion.

The importance of physicochemical properties of drugs in the early drug development and discovery process has been recognized for long time. Moreover, these physicochemical properties have always been taken into consideration by pharmaceutical scientists in the optimization of formulation aspects of drug discovery and formulation processes. The publication of the so-called Rule of Five [1,2], combined with a combinatorial approach to discovering new chemical entities and the emergence of the Biopharmaceutics Classification System (BCS) [3] for drugs, however, has attracted widespread interest and recognition in deeper understanding of physicochemical properties of drugs in regard to their applications in the drug discovery and formulation processes and, hence, elevated their significance to a higher level. Early estimation of these properties enables scientists in the drug discovery process to separate out poor drug candidates from the desirable ones before these candidates go into clinical trials. Furthermore, the Rule of Five has allowed scientists to establish the connection between poor intestinal absorption and the drug molecule possessing any two of the following physicochemical properties of a drug: molecular weight greater than 750 Daltons, number of hydrogen bond donors greater than 5, number of hydrogen bond acceptors greater than 10, and calculated log P (partition coefficient) greater than 5. These properties are considered to contribute to the poor drug absorption due to poor intestinal permeability.

The guidelines, promoting the Rule of Five, have proven to be very useful for approximate predictions of intestinal drug absorption. Furthermore, since lipid solubility has played a critical role in the drug absorption process, measurement of lipid solubility has become a guiding principle in the early drug discovery and development process. And, because the lipid-solubility of a drug molecule is the sum of the individual partition coefficients for each of its functional groups, the prediction of lipid solubility (c log P) can be estimated.

Stewart et al. [2] examined the relationship between molecular surface properties of drugs with their biological performance and reported it to be revealing. Most notably, the relationship demonstrated a strong correlation between the polar surface area (PSA) of a drug molecule and drug transport from human intestine and across the drug membrane. The polar surface area is defined as the sum of the Van der Waals surface areas for the polar atoms, oxygens, nitrogens, and attached hydrogen atom (or the number of H-bond donors and H-bond acceptors). (See http://www.molinspiration.com for calculating the PSA.) The PSA is a major determinant for oral absorption and brain penetration of drugs that are transported by the transcellular route (movement across cell membranes). For this reason, this property should be recognized and considered important in the early drug discovery process of drug screening. Another related parameter, dynamic PSA (PSAd), has emerged [4] as a parameter of significance for its utility in predicting membrane permeability of a compound and its oral absorption in humans. Dynamic PSAd values obtained from the interpolation of the sigmoidal plot for 20 selected compounds suggest that when the PSAd is greater than 140 $Å^2$, absorption of a compound is incomplete (<10%), and when the PSAd value is less than 60 $Å^2$, drug absorption will be greater than or in excess of

90%. Amidon and his co-workers [3,5,6] contributed significantly in their seminal work by developing a Biopharmaceutics Classification System (BCS), which is based on physicochemical properties such as equilibrium solubility and partition coefficient, among others.

A consideration of these physicochemical properties is fundamental to discussing several important aspects of the overall effects they exert on drug absorption. For a given chemical entity (drug), there often will be a difference in physiological availability and, presumably, in clinical responses, primarily because of the fundamental requirement that drug molecules must pass through various biological membranes and interact with intercellular and intracellular fluids before reaching the elusive region termed the "site of action." Under these conditions, the physicochemical properties of the drug must contribute favorably to facilitate absorption and distribution processes to augment the drug concentration at various active sites. Equally important is the fact that these biopharmaceutical properties of a drug must ensure a specific orientation on the receptor surface so that a sequence of events is initiated that leads to the observed pharmacological effects. Drug molecules that are deficient in the required biopharmaceutical properties may display generally marginal pharmacological action or may even be totally ineffective.

Before these physicochemical properties are discussed in detail, however, it is important to understand gastrointestinal physiology, the biological membrane, the absorption process, and how orally administered drugs reach the general circulation and elicit their pharmacological effects.

Biopharmaceutics may be defined as the study of the influence of formulation factors on the therapeutic activity of a drug from a drug product or a dosage form. It involves the study of the relationship between some of the physicochemical properties of a drug and the biological effects observed following the administration of a drug via various dosage forms or drug delivery systems. Almost any formulation alteration in a dosage form or a drug delivery system is likely to influence drug absorption rate in the body. The formulation factors include the chemical nature of the drug (e.g., ester, salts, and complexes), the particle size and surface area of the drug, the type of dosage form (e.g., solution, suspension, capsule, and tablet), and the excipients and processes employed in the manufacturing of the dosage form or drug delivery system.

Drugs are frequently administered to human subjects via oral route. This route, compared to an intravenous as well as any other extravascular routes, is much more complex with respect to the physiological conditions existing at the absorption site. Additionally, complexity in drug absorption arises due to different environments the drug molecules encounter in the gastrointestinal tract as well as the nature of the membrane the drug molecules have to cross prior to reaching the general circulation. Therefore, it is prudent to review gastrointestinal physiology prior to discussing important physicochemical properties of drugs and the role they play in influencing the action and performance of a drug administered via dosage form.

4.2. GASTROINTESTINAL PHYSIOLOGY

Figure 4.1 provides a schematic representation of the gastrointestinal tract and illustrates some of the problems encountered by drug molecules at the site following their administration via an oral dosage form [7]. The stomach may be divided into two main parts: the body of the stomach and the pylorus. Histologically, these parts represent two main areas: the pepsin- and HCl-secreting area and the mucus-secreting area, respectively, of the gastric mucosa [8]. The pH range of the stomach contents, in humans, usually varies from 1 to 3.5; the most commonly

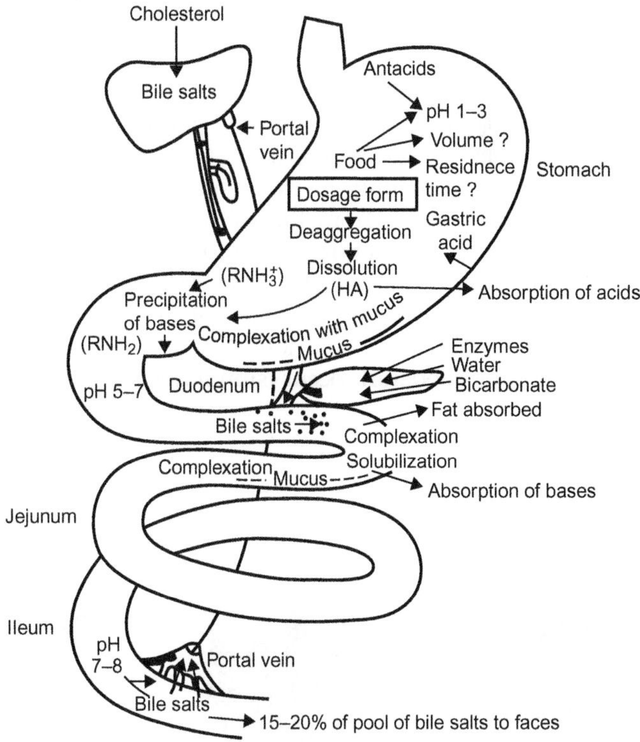

FIGURE 4.1 Processes occurring along with drug absorption when drug molecules travel down the gastrointestinal tract and the factors that affect to drug absorption [7]. *(From Florence AT, Attwood D.* Physiochemical Principles of Pharmacy, *5th ed. New York: Pharmaceutical Press, 2011, with permission.)*

reported range is 1 to 2.5. There is also the existence of a diurnal cycle of gastric acidity in humans. The stomach contents during nighttime are generally more acidic with approximate pH of 1.3; conversely, during the daytime, due to food consumption, the pH of stomach content is less acidic. The recovery of stomach acidity, however, occurs quite rapidly. Proteins, present in the membrane, being amphoteric in nature, provide excellent buffer effects and, as digestion of food occurs, the liberation of amino acids is accompanied by enormous increase in the neutralizing capacity.

The small intestine is divided anatomically into three sections: the duodenum, the jejunum, and the ileum. Each area of the small intestine contributes in the digestion and absorption of food. Compared to the stomach, the surface area available for absorption increases many folds in the intestinal lining, and the surfaces of theses folds possess villi and microvilli (Figure 4.2). Unlike the stomach contents, duodenal contents in humans exhibit a pH range of 5 to 7, with a gradual decrease in acidity along the length of the gastrointestinal tract, with the ultimate pH being 7 to 8 in the lower ileum. The volume of the fluid that enters the upper intestine is estimated to be approximately 8 liters; nearly 7 liters of this arises from digestive juices and fluids, and the remaining 1 liter is generated due to oral intake. Over the entire length of the large and small intestine and the stomach is the brush border, which consists of a uniform coating (thickness, 3 mm) of mucopolysaccharide. This coating layer serves as a mechanical barrier to bacteria or food particles.

Drug molecules, released from the dosage form, face a rapidly changing environment with respect to pH when they travel from the stomach, through the pylorus, into the duodenum. In addition to pH differences, digestive fluid secreted into the small bowel contains many enzymes not present in the gastric fluids. It is important to note that digestion and absorption of foodstuff occur simultaneously in the small intestine. Intestinal digestion is the terminal phase of preparing foodstuff for absorption and consists of two processes: completion of the hydrolysis of large molecules to smaller ones, which can be absorbed, and bringing the finished product of hydrolysis into an aqueous solution or emulsion.

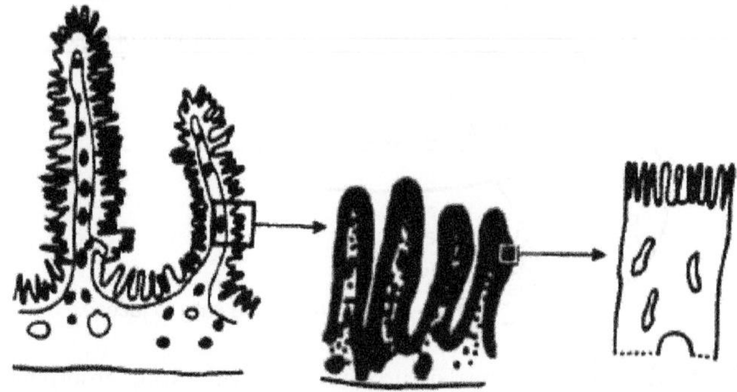

FIGURE 4.2 The epithelium of the small intestine at different levels of magnification. From left to right: the intestinal villi and microvilli that constitute the brush border.

Drug absorption, following the administration by an extravascular route, whether from the gastrointestinal tract or from other sites, requires the passage of the drug in a molecular form across the barrier membrane. Most drugs are presented to the body as solid or semi-solid dosage forms. Therefore, drug particles must first be released from these dosage forms, which is followed by their dissolution in the aqueous fluid prior to their passage, through the biological membrane, into the general circulation. These drug particles will dissolve rapidly if they possess the desirable physicochemical properties. The available drug molecules will travel from a region of high concentration to a region of low concentration, across the membrane, into the blood or general circulation (Figure 4.3). Therefore, knowledge of biological membrane structure and its general properties is imperative in understanding absorption processes and the role of the physicochemical properties of drug substances.

4.2.1 Biological Membrane

The gastrointestinal membrane is viewed as a bimolecular lipoid layer that is covered on each side by protein with the lipid molecule oriented perpendicular to the cell surface (Figure 4.4). Since the lipid layer is interrupted by small water-filled pores with a radius of approximately 4 Å, a molecule with a radius of 4 Å or less may pass through these water-filled pores. Membranes, therefore, provide a specialized transport system and assist the passage of water-soluble material and ions through the lipid interior, a process sometimes termed "convective absorption." The rate of transfer of small molecules through the membrane pore is influenced by the relative sizes of the holes as well as by the interaction between permeating molecules and the membrane. The occurrence of the passage of drug molecules through the membrane is

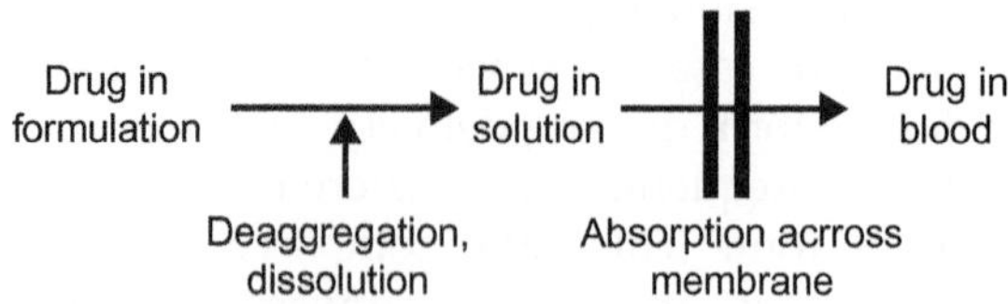

FIGURE 4.3 Sequence of events in drug absorption from formulations of solid dosage forms.

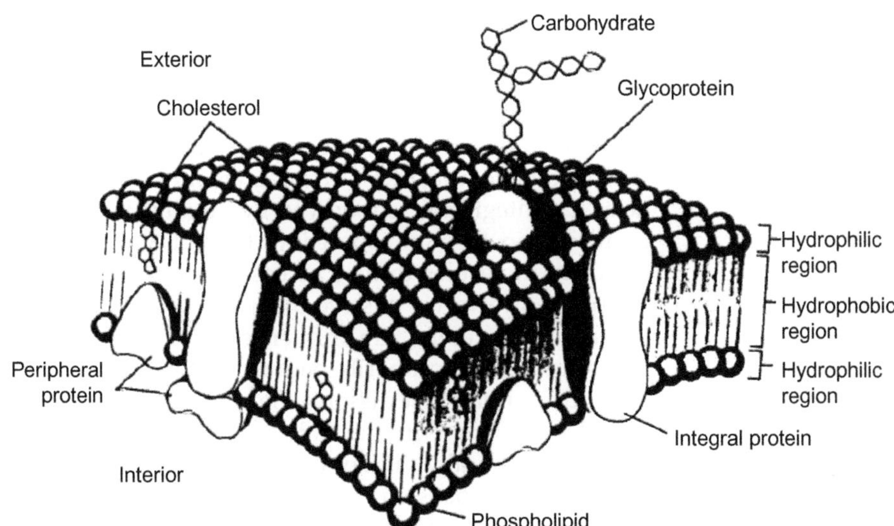

FIGURE 4.4 Basic structure of an animal cell membrane. *(From Smith C, Marks A, Lieberman M, eds.* Basic Medical Biochemistry. *Baltimore: Lippincott, Williams and Wilkins, 2004:159–163, with permission.)*

referred to as the transfer of drug molecules from the solution in the aqueous luminal phase to the lipophilic membrane, which is then followed by the transfer to the aqueous phase on the other side of the membrane.

Biological membranes are composed of small amphipathic molecules, phospholipids, and cholesterol. The protein layer associated with membranes is hydrophilic in nature. This constitutes the striking difference between biological membranes and polymeric membranes. Biological membranes, owing to their composition, have a hydrophilic exterior and a hydrophobic interior. Cholesterol is a major component of most mammalian biological membranes, and its removal will render the membrane highly permeable. The presence of a cholesterol complex with phospholipids, therefore, reduces the membrane permeability to water, cations, glycerides, and glucose. The shape of the cholesterol molecule allows it to fit closely with the hydrocarbon chains of unsaturated fatty acids in the bilayer. It is the presence of cholesterol that is attributed to the rigidity manifested by the biological membranes. Another important feature of the biological membrane is its ability to adapt to a changed environment. The details of membrane structure are still widely debated, and Figure 4.4 illustrates a more recent model of the membrane structure.

In addition to physicochemical properties, other physiological factors may affect the rate and extent of drugs from the gastrointestinal region. These factors are as follows: properties of epithelial cells, segmental activity of the bowel, degree of vascularity, effective absorbing surface area per unit length of gut, surface and interfacial tensions of the gastrointestinal fluids, electrolyte content and their concentration in luminal fluid, enzymatic activity in the luminal contents, and gastric emptying time of the drug from stomach.

4.2.2 Mechanisms of Drug Absorption

The passage of drug molecules is viewed as the movement of drug molecules across a series of membranes and spaces (Figure 4.5), which, collectively, serve as a macroscopic membrane. The cells and interstitial spaces that exist between the gastric lumen and the capillary blood or the structure between sinusoidal space and the bile canaliculi are examples. The drug transfer, therefore, may be impeded by each membrane and the space to a different degree; this process of drug transfer, therefore, may become a rate-limiting step to the overall process of drug passage from the site of administration to the general circulation in the body. This complexity of a membrane structure makes quantitative prediction of drug transport a challenging task. A qualitative description of the processes of drug transport across functional membranes follows.

4.2.3 The pH-Partition Hypothesis on Drug Absorption

Physiological factors often play an important and influential role in the drug absorption process. Additionally, drug absorption is influenced by many physicochemical properties of the drug itself. Shore, Brodie, Hogben, Schanker, Tocco, and others [8–14] reported from their research that passive diffusion is responsible for absorption of most drugs, and drugs are preferentially absorbed in an un-ionized form across lipid membrane from the gastrointestinal tract. Therefore, the dissociation constant, lipid solubility, and pH of the fluid at the absorption site determine the extent of drug absorption from a solution. This interrelationship among these parameters is referred to as the pH-partition theory. This theory, therefore, has

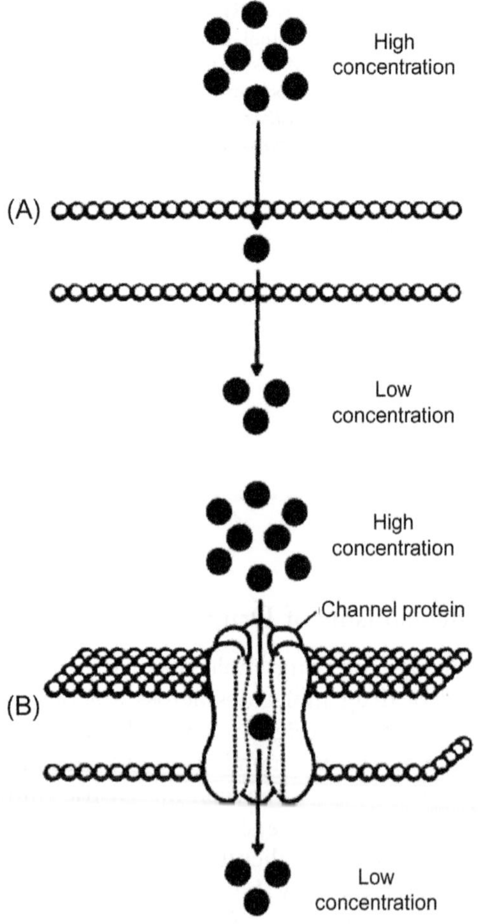

FIGURE 4.5 (A) Simple diffusion ; (B) Membrane channels. *(From Smith C, Marks A, Lieberman M, eds.* Basic Medical Biochemistry. *Baltimore: Lippincott, Williams and Wilkins, 2004:159–163, with permission.)*

been viewed as a guide for the understanding of drug absorption and drug transfer from the gastrointestinal tract and drug transport across the biological membrane. The highlights of this theory are as follows:

- The gastrointestinal and other biological membranes act as lipid barriers.
- The un-ionized form of the acidic or basic drug is preferentially absorbed.
- Most drugs are absorbed by passive diffusion.
- The rate of drug absorption and amount of drug absorbed are related to its oil–water partition coefficient (i.e., the more lipophilic the drug, the faster is its absorption).
- Weak acidic and neutral drugs may be absorbed from the stomach, but basic drugs are not.

Before we discuss the role of various physicochemical factors that influence drug absorption, let us examine the fate of a drug following its administration. When a drug is administered intravenously, it is immediately available to body fluids for distribution and to the site of action and, hence, its effects are observed quickly. However, when it is administered via oral route through solid dosage forms, additional barriers come into the picture. A solid dosage form such as a tablet must first disintegrate into smaller particles. Disintegration is followed by dissolution of drug particles and their transport into the gut and, thereafter, drug molecules diffuse across gut lumen and into the blood stream via passive diffusion. All extravascular routes, therefore, can influence the overall performance of a drug, primarily because of the requirement that a drug must first dissolve and become available in a molecular form in the solution. When a drug is administered orally via dosage form such as a tablet, a capsule, or suspension, the rate of absorption across the biological membrane frequently is controlled by the slowest step as illustrated here:

$$\text{Dosage form} \xrightarrow{\text{dissolution}} \text{Drug in solution} \xrightarrow{\text{absorption}} \text{Drug in general circulation}$$

The slowest or rate-limiting step in many instances is the drug dissolution. And, if drug dissolution is the slowest step, any factors that affect the rate of dissolution will also influence the rate of drug transfer from the absorption site. This, in turn, affects the onset as well as duration of action. A number of factors can influence the dissolution rate of drug from solid dosage forms and, therefore, the therapeutic activity of a drug. These factors include solubility of the drug, particle size and surface area of drug particles, crystalline and salt form of the drug, and the rate of disintegration.

4.3. IONIZATION

Most therapeutic agents exist as either weakly acidic or basic in nature. For a compound containing acidic or basic functional groups, solubility at a given pH is dictated by the compound's dissociation constant (pK_a). The ionized state of a compound exhibits greater aqueous solubility than the un-ionized or the neutral states. Therefore, solubility of a weakly acidic or basic drug depends on the pH of the solution. Many weakly acidic and basic drugs, therefore, are subjected to ionization in the gastrointestinal tract; therefore, solubility, dissolution, and absorption of a weak acidic or basic drug are very much influenced by the pH of the surrounding fluid.

Solubility, dissolution, and absorption of a weakly basic drug can be altered by changes in the gastric pH (co-administration of antacids). While a weakly basic compound might fully dissolve in the acidic environment of the stomach and result in high exposure levels under such conditions, co-administration of drugs that raise the pH can lead to greatly decreased solubility and lower exposure. Ionization of a drug can also alter the stability and permeability. For compounds containing both acidic and basic functional groups, the formation of zwitterions may lead to lowest solubility at an isoelectric point.

If a compound is ionizable, a salt can be formed, which may exhibit greater solubility and therefore faster dissolution. The greater solubility presents an advantage in the formulation of dosage forms such as an injectable solution and oral solution. The faster dissolution, on the other hand, is an advantage for the formulation development of a solid dosage form such as a tablet or capsule and liquid dosage form such as suspension.

4.3.1 Ionization of Weakly Acidic and Basic Drugs

The fraction of a drug that exists in its un-ionized form in a solution is a function of both the dissociation constant of the drug and the pH of the solution. The dissociation constant, for both weak acids and bases, is expressed as the pK_a (the negative logarithm of a dissociation constant, K_a). The Henderson–Hasselbalch equation for the ionization of a weak acid, HA, is derived from the following equation:

$$\mathbf{HA + H_2O \rightarrow A^- + H_3O^+} \tag{4.1}$$

We may express the equilibrium constant as

$$K_a = \frac{[_aH_3O^+][_aA^-]}{[_aHA]} \tag{4.2}$$

where K_a is the dissociation constant under the equilibrium condition and the subscript a is the activity coefficient. Assuming the activity coefficients approach unity in dilute solutions, the activity coefficients may be replaced by concentration terms, and Eq. 4.2 becomes

$$K_a = \frac{[H_3O^+][A^-]}{[HA]} \tag{4.3}$$

The negative logarithm of K_a is referred to as the pK_a. Thus,

$$pK_a = -\log K_a \tag{4.4}$$

Taking the logarithm of the expression for the dissociation constant of a weak acid in Eq. 4.4 yields

$$-\log K_a = -\log [H_3O] - \log [A^-] + \log [HA] \tag{4.5}$$

where A^- is the ionized form of a weak acid, and HA is the un-ionized form.

$$pH - pK_a = \log \frac{[\text{Ionized}]}{[\text{Un-ionized}]} \tag{4.6}$$

Defining α as the fraction of ionized species and 1 − α as the fraction remaining as the un-ionized form, we can write Equation 4.6 as

$$pH - pK_a = \log \frac{\alpha}{1-\alpha} \tag{4.7}$$

or

$$\frac{\alpha}{1-\alpha} = \text{antilog}\,(pH - pK_a) \tag{4.8}$$

Equation 4.8 permits determination of the fraction or percentage of the absorbable and nonabsorbable forms of a weak acid if the pH of the solution at the site of administration is known. Analogously, the dissociation or basicity constant for a weak base is derived as follows:

$$B + H_2O \leftrightarrow BH^+ + OH^- \tag{4.9}$$

The dissociation constant, K_b, is derived as follows:

$$K_b = \frac{[_aOH^-][_aBH^+]}{[_aB]} = \frac{[OH^-][BH^+]}{[B]} \tag{4.10}$$

and

$$pK_b = -\log K_b \tag{4.11}$$

The pK_a and pK_b values provide a convenient means of comparing the strength of weak acids and bases. The lower the pK_a, the stronger the acid; and the lower the pK_b, the stronger the base. The values for pK_a and pK_b of conjugate acid-base pairs are linked by the expression

$$pK_a + pK_b = pK_w \tag{4.12}$$

where pK_w is the negative logarithm of dissociation constant of water. Taking the logarithm of Equation 4.10 and rearranging yields

$$-\log K_b = -\log [OH^-] - \log [BH^+] + \log [B] \tag{4.13}$$

Although the dissociation constant of a weak base, under equilibrium condition, is described by the term K_b, it is conventionally expressed in terms of K_a because of the relationship expressed in Equation 4.12.

Equation 4.13 can then be written as

$$pH = pK_w - pK_b - \log \frac{[BH^+]}{[B]} \tag{4.14}$$

Because $pK_w - pK_b = pK_a$, Equation 4.14 takes the following form for a weak base (where BH^+ is the ionized form, and B is the un-ionized form):

$$pK_a - pH = \log \frac{[\text{Ionized}]}{[\text{Un-ionized}]} \tag{4.15}$$

Again, assuming that α is the fraction of ionized species and that 1 − α is the fraction of un-ionized species, Equation 4.15 becomes

$$pK_a - pH = \log\frac{\alpha}{1-\alpha} \quad (4.16)$$

or

$$\frac{\alpha}{1-\alpha} = \text{antilog}\,(pK_a - pH) \quad (4.17)$$

From Equation 4.17, one can readily calculate the fraction or percentage of absorbable and nonabsorbable form of a weak basic drug if the pH of the solution at the site of drug absorption is known. Figure 4.6 shows the pK_a values of several drugs and the relative acid or base strength of these compounds.

The relationship between pH and pK_a and the degree of ionization are provided by Eqs. 4.8 and 4.17 for weak acids and weak bases, respectively. Accordingly, most weak acidic drugs are predominantly present in an un-ionized form at lower pH of the gastric fluid and, therefore, may be absorbed from the stomach as well as from the upper part (duodenum) of the intestine. On the other hand, some very weakly acidic drugs, such as phenytoin and many barbiturates, whose pK_a values are greater than 8.0, essentially remain in an un-ionized form at all pH values. Therefore, for very weak acidic drugs, passage is faster and independent of pH. This, of course, assumes that the un-ionized species are adequately lipophilic or nonpolar. Furthermore, it is important to recognize that the fraction available in an un-ionized form changes dramatically only for weak acids whose pK_a values are between 3 and 7. Therefore, for the weak acids, a change in the rate of transport with pH is expected, as shown in Figure 4.7 [15]. Although the transport of weak acids with pK_a values less than 3.0 should theoretically depend on pH, the fraction available in an un-ionized form is so low that transport across the gut membrane may be slow even under the most acidic conditions.

Most weak bases, on the other hand, are poorly absorbed, if at all, in the stomach because they exist largely in the ionized form at pH 1–2. Codeine, a weak base with a pK_a of approximately 8, will have about 1 in every 1 million molecules in its un-ionized form at gastric pH 1.0. Weakly basic drugs with a pK_a value of less than 4, such as dapsone, diazepam, and chlordiazepoxide, remain essentially un-ionized through the intestine. Strong bases, which are those with pK_a values between 5 and 11, show pH-dependent absorption. Stronger bases, such as guanethidine ($pK_a > 11$) are ionized throughout the gastrointestinal tract and tend to be poorly absorbed.

Data provided in Tables 4.1 and 4.2 illustrate the importance of dissociation of drugs in the drug

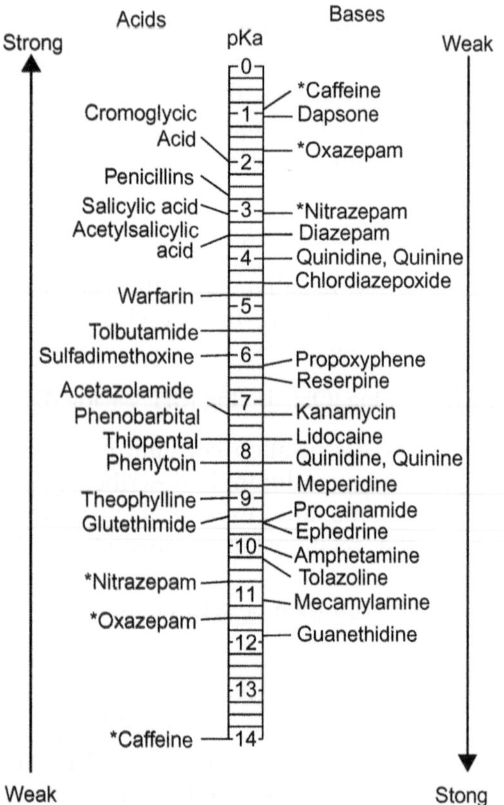

FIGURE 4.6 The pK_a values of certain acidic and basic drugs. Drugs denoted with an asterisk are amphoteric [15]. *(From Rowland M, Tozer T.* Clinical Pharmacokinetics: Concepts and Application, *2nd ed. Philadelphia: Lea and Febiger, 1989, with permission.)*

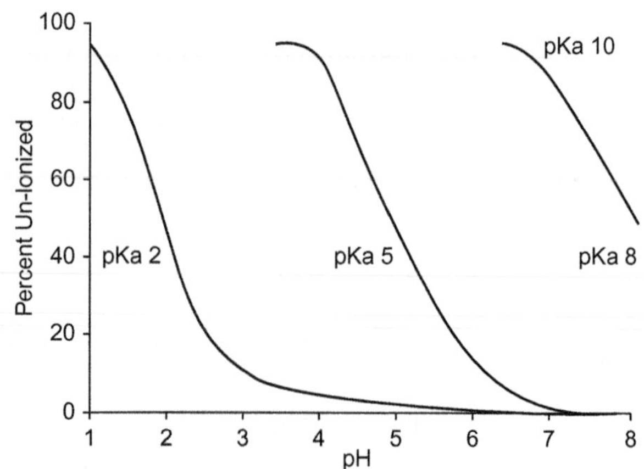

FIGURE 4.7 For very weak acids, pK_a values greater than 8.0 are predominantly un-ionized at all pH values between 1.0 and 8.0. Profound changes in the un-ionized fraction occur with pH for an acid with a pK_a value that lies within the range of 2.0 to 8.0. Although the fraction un-ionized of even strong acids increases with hydrogen ion concentration, the absolute value remains low at most pH values shown [15]. *(From Rowland M, Tozer T.* Clinical Pharmacokinetics: Concepts and Application, *2nd ed. Philadelphia: Lea and Febiger, 1989, with permission.)*

TABLE 4.1 Comparison of Gastric Absorption of Acids and Bases at pH 1 and 8 in the Rat [8,16]

	pK_a	% Absorbed at pH 1	% Absorbed at pH 8
ACIDS			
5-Sulfosalicylic acid	<2.0	0	0
5-Nitrosalicylic acid	2.3	52	16
Salicylic acid	3.0	61	13
Thiopental	7.6	46	34
BASES			
Aniline	4.6	6	56
p-Toluidine	5.3	0	47
Quinine	8.4	0	18
Dextromethorphan	9.2	0	16

TABLE 4.2 Comparison of Intestinal Absorption of Acids and Bases at pH 1 and 8 in the Rat at Several pH Values [8,16]

		% Absorbed from Rat Intestine			
	pK_a	pH 4	pH 5	pH 7	pH 8
ACIDS					
5-Sulfosalicylic acid	2.3	40	27	0	0
Salicylic acid	3.0	64	35	30	10
Acetylsalicylic acid	3.5	41	27	–	–
Benzoic acid	4.2	62	36	35	5
BASES					
Aniline	4.6	40	48	58	61
Aminopyrine	5.0	21	35	48	52
p-Toluidine	5.3	30	42	65	64
Quinine	8.4	9	11	41	54

absorption process reported in the result of studies in which pH at the absorption site is changed. Table 4.2 clearly shows the decreased absorption of a weak acid at pH 8.0 compared to pH 1.0 [15]. On the other hand, an increase to pH 8.0 promotes the absorption of a weak base, with practically nothing absorbed at pH 1.0. The data in Table 4.2 also enable a comparison of intestinal absorption of acidic and basic drugs from buffered solutions ranging from pH 4.0 to 8.0 [17]. These results concur with the pH-partition hypothesis.

The pH-partition theory provides a basic concept and framework necessary to understand why drug absorption occurs. At times, this theory arguably is an

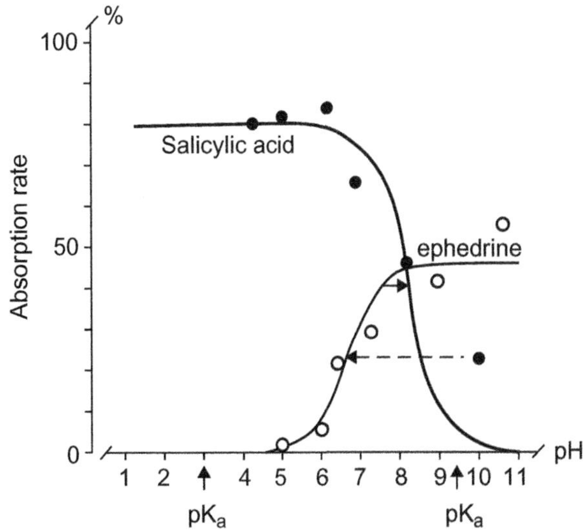

FIGURE 4.8 Relationship between absorption rates of salicylic acid and ephedrine and bulk phase pH in the rat small intestine *in vivo*. Dashed lines represent curves predicted by the pH-partition theory in the absence of an unstirred layer [18]. *(From Winne D. The influence of unstirred layers on intestinal absorption in intestinal permeation. In: Kramer M, Lauterbach F, eds.* Workshop Conference Hoechest, *vol 4. Amsterdam: Excerpta Medica, 1977:58–64, with permission.)*

oversimplification of a more complex drug absorption process. For example, experimentally observed pH-absorption curves are less steep (Figure 4.8) than that is expected theoretically and are shifted to higher pH values for bases and lower pH values for acids. Several investigators have attributed this experimentally observed deviation to a number of factors, such as limited absorption of ionized species of drugs, the presence of an unstirred diffusion layer adjacent to the cell membrane, and a difference between lumenal pH and cell membrane surface pH.

4.4. PARTITION COEFFICIENT: LIPOPHILICITY

The lipophilicity property has received considerable additional attention and importance since the emergence and acceptance of the Biopharmaceutics Classification System [3] for drugs and recognition of the importance of the Rule of Five [1] in the early drug discovery process. This is also the most important physicochemical property of a drug in a molecular structure/biological activity relationship. This physicochemical property affects the solubility and permeability of a drug, which, in turn, will influence other properties of the drug such as dissolution, absorption, distribution, metabolism, elimination, and protein binding. The partitioning of a compound between two completely immiscible phases depends on the availability of a drug in un-ionized form. Therefore, ionization of a compound plays an important role in determining the lipophilicity and permeability of a compound.

Following oral administration, some drugs may be poorly absorbed even though they are available predominantly in the un-ionized form in the gastrointestinal tract. This is attributed to the low or poor lipid solubility of the un-ionized species of the drug molecules. A physicochemical property, partition coefficient (*P*), provides a guide to lipid solubility or lipophilic nature of a drug. This property of a drug, therefore, influences the transport and absorption processes of the drug, and it is one of the most widely used properties in quantitative structure–activity relationships.

The movement of drug molecules from one liquid phase to another liquid phase is called partitioning. It is a commonly observed equilibrium process phenomenon in many pharmaceutical processes. In the body, for example, drugs partition themselves between the aqueous phase and lipophilic membrane. Preservative in an emulsion dosage form partitions between the water and oil phases; partitioning of antibiotics from body fluids to microorganisms is common; and drugs and excipients used in injectable dosage form can partition into the plastic and rubber stoppers of containers. It is therefore important that this process and property are well understood.

If two immiscible liquid phases are placed adjacent to each other, with one containing a solute soluble to some degree in both phases, the solute molecules will begin to migrate from back and forth from an aqueous or lower phase to the oil or upper phase (Eqs. 4.21 and 4.21a); eventually reaching a condition when the rates of transfer of drug molecules become equal. When the rates of transfer are equal, we have attained the equilibrium condition. Under such a condition, there is no further change in the concentration of a solute in each phase. At equilibrium, the chemical potential of the solute (free energy of the solute in solvent) in one phase is equal to its chemical potential in the other phase. If we consider an aqueous (w) and an organic (o) phase, we write according to theory

$$\mu_w^\ominus + RT \ln a_w = \mu_o^\ominus + RT \ln a_o \tag{4.18}$$

where *a* represents the activity coefficient of a solute (the effect of solute concentration on intersolute interactions). Rearranging Equation 4.18 yields

$$\frac{\mu_w^\ominus - \mu_0^\ominus}{RT} = \ln \frac{a_w}{a_o} \tag{4.19}$$

The term on the left side of Equation 4.19 is a constant at a given temperature and pressure. Therefore,

$$\frac{a_w}{a_o} = \text{constant or } \frac{a_o}{a_w} = \text{constant} \tag{4.20}$$

These constants are the partition (*P*) or distribution coefficients (*D*). Because most drugs are ionic, their partition coefficients are pH-dependent and usually reported at pH 7.4 and are therefore appropriately called distribution coefficients. If the solute under consideration forms an ideal solution in either phases or in solvent, the activity coefficient can be replaced by the concentration term, and Equation 4.20 becomes

$$P = \frac{C_o}{C_w} \tag{4.21}$$

or

$$\log P = \log \frac{C_o}{C_w} \tag{4.21a}$$

Equations 4.21 and 4.21a are conventionally used to calculate the partition coefficient and log of partition coefficient, respectively, of a drug. In both equations, C_o, the concentration of drug in the organic or oil phase, is divided by the concentration in the aqueous phase once the equilibrium is attained. The greater the value of *P* or *log of P*, the higher the lipid solubility of the solute. Please note, according to the Rule of Five [1], a *log of P* value for a compound should ideally be less than 5. *Log of P* is an operational definition of lipophilicity or hydrophobic bonding and, like the partition coefficient (P) value, plays an important role in the transfer of a drug through the lipophilic membrane. There are number of methods available for determination of partition coefficient experimentally. By far, the most commonly used method to measure lipophilicity is the shake-flask method to determine the octanol/water partition coefficient.

It has been demonstrated for several systems that the partition coefficient can be approximated by the solubility of the solute in the organic phase divided by the solubility in the aqueous phase. Therefore, the partition coefficient is a measure of the relative affinities of the solute for an aqueous or nonaqueous or oil phase. Octanol is often used as the nonaqueous or organic phase in experiments to measure the partition coefficient of drugs. The polarity of octanol suggests that water is solubilized to some extent in the octanol phase, and thus, partitioning is bit more complex than with an anhydrous solvent. Its usefulness, however, stems from the fact that biological membranes are also not simple anhydrous phases. While octanol is favored, other alcohols have also been used to determine the partition coefficient. One example is isobutanol.

The effect of lipid solubility and, therefore, the partition coefficient on the absorption of a series of barbituric acid derivatives is shown in Table 4.3. The term

TABLE 4.3 Comparison of Barbiturate Absorption in Rat Colon and Partition Coefficient (Chloroform/Water) of Undissociated Drug [8,16]

Barbiturate	Partition Coefficient	% Absorbed
Barbital	0.7	12
Aprobarbital	4.9	17
Phenobarbital	4.8	20
Allylbarbital	10.5	23
Butethal	11.7	24
Cyclobarbital	13.9	24
Pentobarbital	28.0	30
Secobarbital	50.7	40
Hexethal	>100	44

partition coefficient is more commonly expressed exponentially as log *P*. Tables 4.4 and 4.5 provide the partition coefficient values for various analogues of tetracycline and for different drugs, respectively.

Data provided in Table 4.4 illustrates the inverse correlation between the lipid solubility of four tetracyclines and mean antibiotic plasma concentration and with renal excretion. Only the more lipophilic minocycline and doxycycline pass through the blood brain and blood ocular barriers in measurable concentrations. It must be clearly understood that even though drugs with greater lipophilicity and, therefore, partition coefficient are better absorbed, it is imperative that drugs possess some degree of aqueous solubility because the availability of the drug molecule in a solution form is a prerequisite for drug absorption and the biological fluids at the site of absorption are aqueous in nature. Therefore, from a practical viewpoint, drugs must manifest a proper balance between hydrophilicity and lipophilicity. This factor is always taken into account and plays a critical role when a chemical modification is being considered for the purpose of improving the efficacy of a therapeutic agent.

Several drugs are good examples of polar or hydrophilic molecules that are poorly absorbed following oral administration and, therefore, must be administered parenterally. They include gentamicin, ceftrixine (ceftriaxone and cefotaxime), and streptokinase. In general, lipid-soluble drugs with favorable partition coefficients are well absorbed following oral administration. Frequently, the selection of a compound with a higher partition coefficient from a series of research compounds provides improved pharmacological activity. The researchers may occasionally consider a modification of the chemical structure of an existing compound to improve drug absorption. Chlortetracycline, which differs from tetracycline by the substitution of a chlorine at C-7; the substitution of an n-hexyl (Hexethal) for a phenyl ring in phenobarbital; or the replacement of the 2-carbonyl of pentobarbital with a 2-thio group (thiopental) are examples of enhanced lipophilicity (Figure 4.9).

It is important to recognize that there is risk of compromising the efficacy and safety profile of a drug even with a minor chemical modification in a drug molecule. This is due to alteration in the lipophilicity and other physicochemical properties of drugs. For this reason, medicinal chemists in a drug discovery group prefer the development of a lipid-soluble prodrug of a drug with poor oral absorption characteristics.

TABLE 4.4 Partition Coefficients of Four Analogues of Tetracycline [7]

Analogues of Tetracycline	Partition Coefficient*	Partition Coefficient**
Minocycline	30.0	1.1
Doxycycline	0.48	0.60
Tetracycline	0.09	0.036
Oxytetracycline	0.007	0.025

**Measured by using chloroform/water system*
***Measured by using octanol/water system*
Adapted from Florence AT, Attwood D. Physiochemical Principles of Pharmacy, 5th ed. New York: Pharmaceutical Press, 2011, with permission.

TABLE 4.5 Log of *P* Values for Representative Drugs*

Drug	Log *P*
Acetylsalicylic acid (Aspirin)	1.19
Amiodarone	6.7
Benzocaine	1.89
Caffeine	0.01
Chlorpromazine	5.30
Ciprofloxacin	− 1.12
Indomethacin	3.1
Lidocaine	2.26
Methadone	3.9
Phenytoin	2.50
Prednisone	1.46

**Modified from reference [7].*
Adapted from Florence AT, Attwood D. Physiochemical Principles of Pharmacy, 5th ed. New York: Pharmaceutical Press, 2011, with permission.

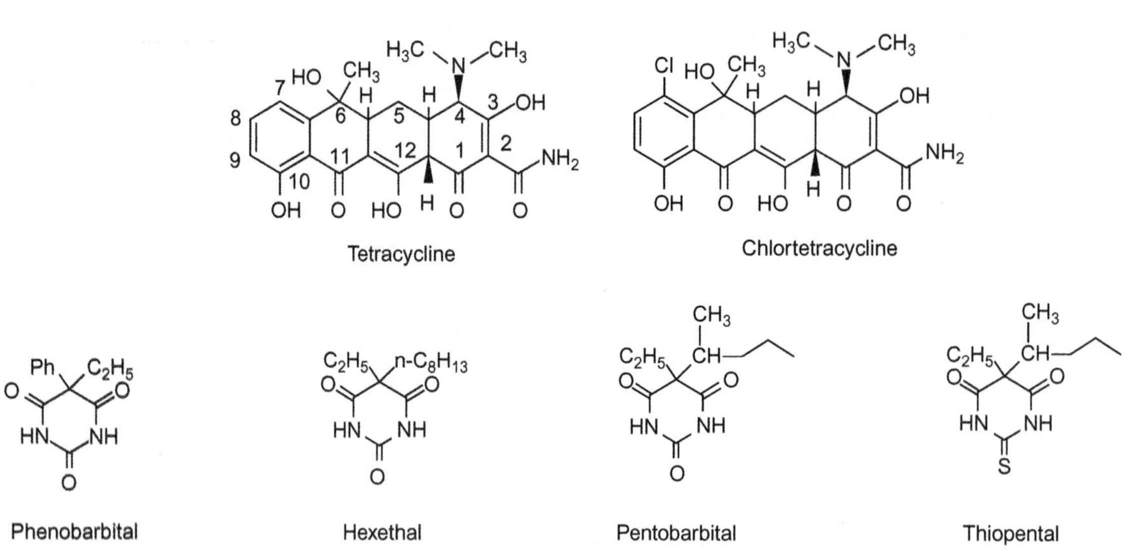

Tetracycline Chlortetracycline

Phenobarbital Hexethal Pentobarbital Thiopental

FIGURE 4.9 Drug pairs in which chemical modification enhances lipophilicity.

4.5. EQUILIBRIUM SOLUBILITY

The aqueous solubility of a drug substance is a fundamental physicochemical property and should be evaluated early in the discovery stage. Inadequate solubility can affect the results in the early screening process, may preclude the development of certain dosage forms, and may influence the drug dissolution and, therefore, the rate and extent of drug absorption. Solubility depends on the solvation energy of the solute in a solvent overcoming both the crystal lattice energy of the solid and the energy to create space in the solvent for the solute.

Equilibrium or saturated solubility can be defined as the maximum amount of solute that is present in a solution form per unit volume of a solvent at a constant temperature and pressure. It can also be defined as the maximum amount of solute present in solution per unit volume of a solvent when the rate of transfer of a solute from solid into solution is the same as the rate of transfer of solute molecules from the solution on to the powder particles. The attainment of equal transfer rates indicates that equilibrium condition is reached and, therefore, there will be no change in the concentration of solute in a solvent.

4.5.1 Expressions of Solubility

The solubility of a solute in a solvent can be expressed quantitatively in several ways. They include grams/liter, moles/liter, molal concentration, etc. Other less specific and less common forms of reporting solubility include parts per parts of solvent (for example, parts per million, ppm).

Many pharmacopoeia and other chemical and pharmaceutical compendia frequently use this form and also the expressions *insoluble, very highly soluble,* and *soluble.* These terms are imprecise and often not very helpful; however, they provide general guidance about the solubility of a drug. For quantitative work, specific concentration terms must be used.

Most substances have at least some degree of solubility in water, and while they may appear to be "insoluble" by a qualitative test, their solubility can be measured and quoted precisely. In aqueous media at pH 10, chlorpromazine base has a solubility of 8×10^{-6} mol/L; that is, it is very slightly soluble, but it might be considered to be "insoluble" if judged visually by the lack of disappearance of solid placed in a test tube of water.

There are many reasons why it is important to understand the way in which drugs dissolve in solution and the factors that maintain solubility or cause drugs to come out of solution, that is, to precipitate. These include the facts that

- Many drugs are formulated as solutions or are added in powder or solution form to liquids such as infusion fluids in which they must remain in solution for a given period.
- In whatever way drugs are presented to the body, they must usually be in a molecularly dispersed form (that is, in solution) before they can be absorbed across biological membranes.
- Drugs of low aqueous solubility (e.g., Taxol) frequently present problems in relation to their formulation and bioavailability.
- Patients are frequently advised to take poorly soluble drugs with plenty of water or fluids.

- For injectable solutions, high solubility of a drug under conditions close to the physiological pH of 7.4 is essential. For small-volume injectables such as intramuscular and subcutaneous, the solubility should be as high as possible to accommodate the dose to be administered in 0.5–2 mL for subcutaneous or up to 5 mL for intramuscular administration. The solubility requirement for intravenous injections is less stringent because volumes up to 20 mL can be administered. With lower solubility drugs, one has to resort to infusions of volumes of up to 1000 mL.
- Injectable solutions of drugs require particularly high chemical stability. Ideally, a drug substance must withstand heat sterilization in solution and subsequent storage for up to five years. For those drug substances lacking such optimum stability it is possible to circumvent heat stress by sterile filtration. Naturally, for injectables, solid-state drug properties are of minor importance as long as they do not hamper processing or the dissolution of a lyophilizate.
- For solid oral dosage forms (tablets and capsules) the most critical step, after swallowing a tablet or capsule (i.e., unit dose), is the release of the drug substance. Solubility, and therefore dissolution, can control or limit this important process. Therefore, a solubility that is reasonably high in relation to the drug dose is desirable.

Knowledge and understanding of the equilibrium solubility of a drug, therefore, are absolutely essential and play a critical role in the drug discovery process, drug formulation process, selection of a dosage form for a drug, drug dissolution in the gastrointestinal tract, and drug absorption. Tables 4.6 and 4.7 provide the equilibrium solubility of some commonly used drugs in water as well as other solvents.

TABLE 4.6 Solubility Comparison of Selected Drugs

Name of Drug	Solubility in Water (mg/mL)	Solubility in Alcohol (mg/mL)
Acetaminophen	Slightly soluble	100 mg/mL
Alprazolam	Insoluble	Soluble
Chlorpropamide	2 mg/mL	Soluble
Methocarbamol	25 mg/mL	Soluble
Terfenadine	0.01 mg/mL	38 mg/mL

TABLE 4.7 Aqueous Solubility of Tetracycline and Erythromycin salts*

Name of Drug	Solubility in Water (mg/mL)
Tetracycline	1.70
Tetracycline HCl	10.90
Tetracycline Phosphate	15.90
Erythromycin	2.10
Erythromycin Estolate	0.16
Erythromycin Stearate	0.33
Erythromycin Lactobionate	20.0

**Modified from reference [7].*
Adapted from Florence AT, Attwood D. Physiochemical Principles of Pharmacy, 5th ed. New York: Pharmaceutical Press, 2011, with permission.

4.5.2 Factors that Affect Solubility

A number of factors influence the solubility of a drug. They include temperature, molecule shape and substituent groups, pH of the aqueous solution, and solvent system.

4.5.2.1 Temperature

In general, the higher the temperature, the greater the solubility of a drug. This is particularly true if the drug possesses a high heat of solution, a property of a solid. If the heat of solution is very low or almost zero, the temperature may not have any effect on the solubility of that solute. In other words, increasing the temperature will not alter the solubility of that compound. And, if the solute exhibits negative heat of solution, increasing the temperature will result in a decrease in the solubility of that drug. Based on the influence of temperature on the solubility of a solute, solids have been classified as endothermic and exothermic. Endothermic solutes will absorb heat from the surrounding during the formation of a solution, and exothermic solutes will liberate heat during the formation of a solution. The magnitude of the influence of temperature on the solubility, however, depends on the intrinsic solubility of a solute as well as the availability of the solute in a salt form or weak acid or weak base form. If the intrinsic solubility of a solute is very low and the solute is either a weak acid or base, the temperature will exert greater influence on the solubility. Salts of weakly acidic or basic drugs are generally more soluble than the corresponding weakly acidic and basic drugs and, therefore, their solubility is less influenced by the temperature.

4.5.2.2 Shape and Substituent Groups

Interactions between nonpolar groups and water are important in determining its influence on the solubility. The straight chain carbon compounds exhibit

TABLE 4.8 Correlation between Melting Points of Sulfonamide Derivatives and Aqueous Solubility [7]

Compound	Melting Point (°C)	Solubility (g/Liter)
Sulfadiazine	253	0.077
Sulfamerazine	236	0.200
Sulfapyridine	192	0.285
Sulfathiazole	174	0.588

Reproduced from Florence AT, Attwood D. Physiochemical Principles of Pharmacy, 5th ed. New York: Pharmaceutical Press, 2011, with permission.

TABLE 4.9 Substituent Group Classification [7]

Substituent	Classification
$-CH_3$	Hydrophobic
$-CH_2-$	Hydrophobic
–Cl, –Br, –F	Hydrophobic
$-N(CH_3)_2$	Hydrophobic
$-SCH_3$	Hydrophobic
$-OCH_2CH_3$	Hydrophobic
$-OCH_3$	Slightly hydrophilic
$-NO_2$	Slightly hydrophilic
–CHO	Hydrophilic
–COOH	Slightly hydrophilic
–COO	Very hydrophilic
$-NH_2$	Hydrophilic
$-NH_3$	Very hydrophilic
–OH	Very hydrophilic

Reproduced from Florence AT, Attwood D. Physiochemical Principles of Pharmacy, 5th ed. New York: Pharmaceutical Press, 2011, with permission.

solubility that is related to the length of the carbon chain. As the carbon chain gets longer, the solubility will decrease as a consequence of the molecule becoming larger, with an increase in the molecular weight. These molecules exhibit a more compact molecular arrangement. Chain branching of hydrophobic groups makes a molecule less compact and, as a result, it exhibits greater solubility. The melting point of solids is an indicator of the solubility of a compound (Table 4.8). The melting point of a compound reflects the strength of interactions between the molecules in the solid state.

The influence of substituent groups on the solubility of molecules in water can be due to the molecular cohesion or to the effect of the substituent on its interaction with water molecules. It is not easy to predict the effect a particular substituent will have on crystal properties; however, as a guide to the solvent

TABLE 4.10 The Effect of Substituents on Solubility of Acetanilide Derivatives in Water [7]

Derivative	Substitutents	Solubility (mg/liter)
Acetanilide	H	6.38
	Methyl	1.05
	Ethoxyl	0.93
	Hydroxyl	0.93
	Nitro	15.98
	Aceto	9.87

Reproduced from Florence AT, Attwood D. Physiochemical Principles of Pharmacy, 5th ed. New York: Pharmaceutical Press, 2011, with permission.

interactions, substituents can be classified as either hydrophobic or hydrophilic, depending on their polarity (Table 4.9). The position of the substituent on the molecule can influence its effect, however. This can be seen in the aqueous solubilities of *o*-, *m*-, and *p*-dihydroxybenzenes; as expected, all are much greater than that of benzene, but they are not the same, being 4, 9, and 0.6 mol/L, respectively. The relative low solubility of *para* compound is due to its greater stability of its crystalline state. The melting points of the derivatives indicate that this is so, as they are 105°C, 111°C, and 170°C, respectively. In the case of the *ortho* derivative, the possibility of intramolecular hydrogen bonding in aqueous solution, decreasing the ability of the OH group to interact with water, may explain why its solubility is lower than that of its *meta* analogue.

Information in Table 4.9 best illustrates the influence of substituents on solubility by considering the solubility of a series of substituted acetanilides for which data are provided in Table 4.10. The strong hydrophilic characteristics of polar groups capable of hydrogen bonding with water molecules are evident. The presence of hydroxyl groups can therefore markedly change the solubility characteristics of a compound; phenol, for example, is 100 times more soluble in water than is benzene. In the case of phenol, which has considerable hydrogen-bonding capability, the solute-solvent interaction outweighs other factors in the solution process. But, as we have discovered, the position of any substituent on the parent molecule will affect its contribution to solubility.

4.6. THE EFFECT OF PH

pH of a solvent is one of the primary influences on the solubility of drugs because the great majority of drugs are either weak acidic or weak basic in nature and contain ionizable groups.

The solubility of weak acids and bases clearly depends on the pH of the surrounding solution as well as the dissociate constant (pK_a) of the drug. This, therefore, contributes to the differences in the dissolution rate of drugs in different regions of the gastrointestinal tract. The solubility of weak acid is obtained by

$$C_s = [HA] + [A^-] \tag{4.22}$$

where [HA] is the intrinsic solubility of the un-ionized species of the acid (i.e., C_o) and $[A^-]$ is the concentration of its anion, which can be expressed in terms of its dissociation constant, K_a, and intrinsic solubility, C_o; that is,

$$C_s = C_o + \frac{K_a C_o}{[H^+]} \tag{4.23}$$

It is ostensible from Eq. 4.23 that at a higher hydrogen ion concentration of solution (i.e., the lower the pH of the solution), weak acidic drugs will display lower solubility. Therefore, weakly acidic drugs, such as non-steroidal anti-inflammatory agents, barbituric acid derivatives, aspirin, and phenytoin, are less soluble in acidic solution than in alkaline solution; the available predominant undissociated species of drugs, being in unhydrated form, are unable to interact with water molecules to the same extent as the ionized form, which are readily hydrated. It is also obvious from Eq. 4.23 that the knowledge of the dissociation constant (pK_a) of a drug as well as the intrinsic solubility (C_o) is essential to calculate the solubility of a weak acidic drug at a particular pH.

Analogously, the solubility of a weak base is obtained by

$$C_s = C_o + \frac{C_o[H^+]}{K_a} \tag{4.24}$$

Contrary to Eq. 4.23, Eq. 4.24 suggests that the higher the hydrogen ion concentration of solution (i.e., the lower the pH of the solution), the greater the solubility of a drug. Therefore, weakly basic drugs, such as tetracycline, erythromycin, and ciprofloxacin, are more soluble when the hydrogen concentration of the solution is high (i.e., solution of low pH). Analogues to the weak acidic drugs, the predominant dissociated species of the drug, being in hydrated form, can interact with water molecules much readily compared to the un-ionized form, which is not readily hydrated. Equation 4.24 also suggests that solubility of weakly basic drugs at any pH can be calculated if the dissociation constant (pK_a) and the intrinsic solubility (C_o) of the drug are known. Both equations (Eqs. 4.23 and 4.24), therefore, permit the determination of the pH required to keep the weakly acidic and basic drugs, respectively, in solution form or the pH above or below which the drug will precipitate out from the solution form. This information is very practical and useful in a practice setup because many drugs, particularly oral solution and injectable solutions, prior to their use, are stored in different types of glass and plastic containers. During the storage period, some of the additives present in the glass and plastic may leach into the solution and alter the pH of the solution. The change in the pH may cause precipitation or separation of a drug from solution.

4.7. USE OF CO-SOLVENTS

The technique of using a co-solvent is considered when drug solubility in a single solvent is limited and, therefore, preparation of oral solution or injectable solution in a single solvent is not possible or perhaps when the chemical stability of a drug is compromised by the use of a single solvent. Many pharmaceutical dosage forms are complex systems. Water-miscible solvents commonly used in liquid dosage forms include glycerol, propylene glycol, ethyl alcohol, and polyethylene glycols. The addition of another component complicates the system, so one needs to exercise prudence in balancing between the improvement of solubility and other potential adverse effects, such as lesser stability of a drug. The technique of using co-solvent is vital in the formulation of liquid oral solutions and injectable solutions.

Solubility of phenobarbital in glycerol-water, ethanol-water, and ethanol-glycerol mixtures has been reported in the literature. Phenobarbital dissolves up to 0.12% w/v in water at 25°C. Glycerol, even when used in high concentrations, does not significantly increase the solubility of phenobarbital. Ethanol, on the other hand, is a much more efficient co-solvent than glycerol, as it is less polar. Solubility is at a maximum at 90% ethanol in ethanol-water mixtures, and at 80% ethanol in ethanol-glycerol mixtures. It is naïve to assume that the drug dissolves in "pockets" of the co-solvent (for example, ethanol in ethanol-water mixtures), although obviously the affinity of co-solvent for the solute is of importance.

Additives will influence solute-solvent interfacial energies or dissociation of electrolytes through changes in the dielectric constant. A reduction in ionization through a decrease in the dielectric constant will favor decreased solubility, but this effect may be counterbalanced by the greater affinity of the undissociated species in the presence of the co-solvent (Table 4.11).

We have now addressed four physicochemical properties, mentioned in the introduction, which work on the principles of the equilibrium condition and which play vitally important roles in influencing a drug's

TABLE 4.11 Solubility of Phenobarbital and Sodium Phenobarbital in Various Solvents

Solvent	Free Acid (mg/mL)	Sodium Salt (g/mL)
Water	1.0	1.00
Alcohol	125	0.100
Chloroform	25	Practically Insoluble
Ether	76.92	Practically Insoluble

availability from the dosage form. Also mentioned in the introduction is the role of another physicochemical property, drug dissolution, which depends on the equilibrium property and plays an equally important role in influencing the drug's availability from solid dosage forms. It is, therefore, important to discuss this property to some extent in the following section.

4.8. DRUG DISSOLUTION AND DISSOLUTION PROCESS

When a drug is administered orally via tablet, capsule, or suspension, the rate of absorption often is dictated by the ability of drug particles to dissolve in the surrounding fluid at the absorption site. If the drug particles dissolve slowly, it may take a longer time for the drug to reach the general circulation and elicit its effects. For this reason, the dissolution rate often results in being rate limiting (slowest), as presented in the following sequence:

$$\text{Solid drug} \xrightarrow[\text{Step I}]{\text{Dissolution}} \text{Drug in solution} \xrightarrow[\text{Step II}]{\text{Absorption}} \text{Drug in systemic circulation}$$

If the dissolution of the drug (Step I) is slow, or dictates the rate of absorption, then dissolution is the rate-determining step in passage of the drug to the general circulation. Under such conditions, factors controlling dissolution, such as solubility, ionization, or surface area of a drug particle, will then dictate and influence the overall dissolution process. Figure 4.10 depicts the absorption of aspirin from solution and from two different types of tablets. It is clear from Figure 4.10 that aspirin absorption is much more rapid from solution than from tablet formulations. This rapid absorption of aspirin suggests that the rate of absorption is dissolution rate limited. The drug is available in a molecular form in the solution dosage form.

A general and mathematical relationship describing the dissolution of a drug was first reported by

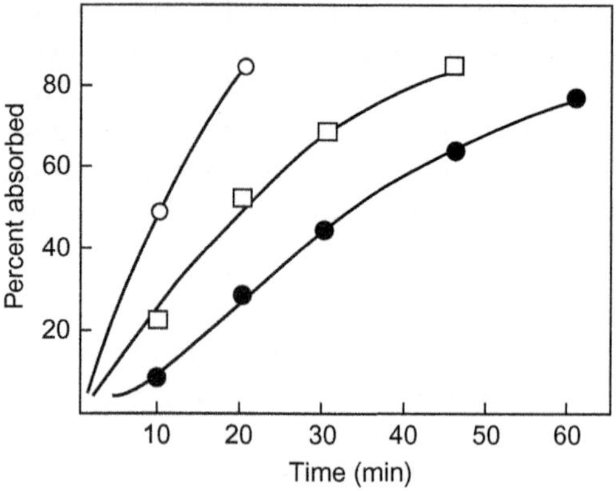

FIGURE 4.10 Absorption of aspirin after oral administration of a 650 mg dose in solution (O), in buffered tablets (□), or in regular tablets (●) [19]. *(From Levy G, Leonard JR, Procknal JA. Development of* in vitro *dissolution tests which correlate quantitatively with dissolution rate limited absorption.* J Pharm Sci, *1965;54:1319–25, with permission.)*

Noyes and Whitney [20,21]. The equation derived by those authors is

$$\frac{dc}{dt} = KS(C_s - C_t) \tag{4.25}$$

where dc/dt is the dissolution rate, K is a constant, S is the surface area of the drug or solute undergoing dissolution, C_s is the equilibrium solubility of the drug in the surrounding solvent or dissolution fluid, and C is the concentration of the drug in the solvent or dissolution fluid at time t.

The constant K in Eq. 4.25 has been shown to be equal to D/h, where D is the coefficient of the dissolving material or the drug, and h is the thickness of the diffusion layer surrounding the dissolving solid drug particles. This diffusion layer is a thin, stationary film of a solution saturated [7] with drug, and it is adjacent to the surface of a solid particle (Figure 4.11); in essence, this simply means that the drug concentration in the diffusion layer corresponds to C_s, the equilibrium solubility of the drug. The term $(C_s - C_t)$ in Eq. 4.25 represents the concentration gradient for the drug between the diffusion layer and the bulk solution. If a sink condition exists and dissolution is the rate-limiting step in the absorption process, the term C_t in Eq. 4.25 is negligible compared to C_s. Under this condition, Eq. 4.25 collapses to

$$\frac{dc}{dt} = \frac{DSC_s}{h} \tag{4.26}$$

Equation 4.26 describes a diffusion-controlled dissolution process [7]. It is presumed that when solid drug particles are introduced to fluids at the absorption sites, the drug instantly saturates the diffusion layer (Figure 4.11); subsequently, drug molecules begin to diffuse from the diffusion layer into the bulk solution,

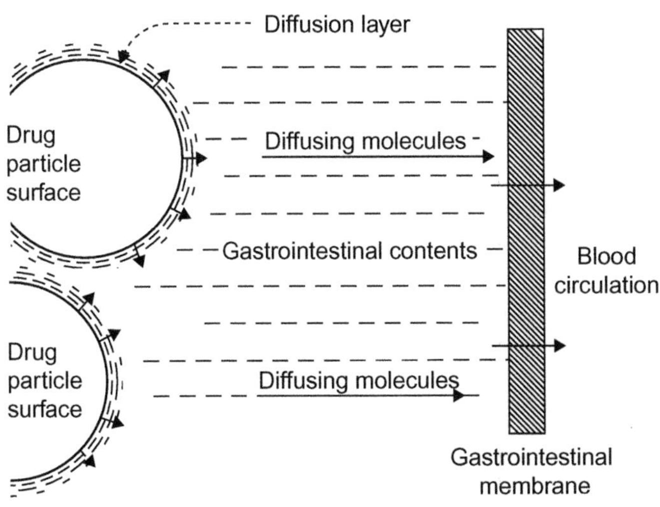

FIGURE 4.11 Dissolution from a solid surface. *Reproduced with permission from, Physiochemical Principles of Pharmacy (5e), (Florence and Atwood [7]), Pharmaceutical Press, 2011.*

TABLE 4.12 The Effect of Changing Parameters from the Dissolution Equation on the Rate of Solution [7]

Equation Parameter	Comments	Effect on Rate of Solution
D (diffusion coefficient of drug)	May be decreased in the presence of substances that increase viscosity of the medium	(−)
A (area exposed to solvent)	Increased by micronization and in "amorphous drugs"	(+)
h (thickness of diffusion layer)	Decreased by increased agitation in gut or flask	(+)
C_S (solubility in diffusion layer)	That of weak electrolytes altered by change in pH, by use of appropriate drug salt or buffer ingredients	(−) (+)
C (concentration in bulk)	Decreased by intake of fluid in stomach, by removal of drug by partition or absorption	(+)

Reproduced from Florence AT, Attwood D. Physiochemical Principles of Pharmacy, 5th ed. New York: Pharmaceutical Press, 2011, with permission.

which is instantly replaced in the diffusion layer by molecules from the solid crystal or particle. This is a continuous process and, although the process is an oversimplification of the dynamics of the dissolution process, Eq. 4.26 is qualitatively very useful in understanding the effects of some important factors on the dissolution and, therefore, the absorption rate of drugs. When dissolution is the rate-limiting factor in absorption, then bioavailability of a drug is adversely affected. These factors are listed in Table 4.12.

A closer examination of Noyes–Whitney equations (Eqs. 4.25 and 4.26) clearly signifies that equilibrium solubility (C_s) is one of the major factors determining the rate of dissolution. Other important factors that influence drug dissolution include the characteristics of solvents and the surface area of powder particles. The former includes the characteristics of a solvent such as pH, which affects the solubility of a drug and also affects its dissolution rate. Similarly, the use of a different salt or other physicochemical form of a drug, which exhibits solubility that is different from the parent drug, also generally affects the dissolution rate. The latter, on the other hand, includes the surface area of the drug particles that is exposed to the dissolution fluid. In the discussion to follow, some of the more important factors affecting dissolution and, therefore, absorption are presented in greater detail.

In the drug dissolution process, according to the Noyes–Whitney equations (Eqs. 4.25 and 4.26), the drug dissolution rate is directly proportional to the drug solubility. Therefore, drugs that exhibit high solubility generally do not present bioavailability problems. The solubility of a drug, in turn, can be altered by the salt formation as well as incorporation of a solubilizing agent in the dissolution medium or in the formulation of a dosage form. Other factors that influence drug solubility include the hydrous versus anhydrous forms of a drug, amorphous versus crystalline nature of the drug, and availability of the drug in different polymorphic forms.

A factor that plays a pivotal role in the drug dissolution process is the surface area (S) of the powder exposed to the surrounding dissolution fluid. A drug dissolves more rapidly when its surface area is increased. This is usually accomplished by reducing the particle size by employing techniques such micronization and coprecipitation. Many poorly soluble drugs are marketed in micronization or microcrystal form. Particle size reduction generally results in more rapid and complete absorption. Drugs such as spironolactone, digoxin, micronized glyburide, and griseofulvin are good examples. Generally, the smaller the powder particle size and, therefore, greater the number of particles, the larger is the total surface area exposed compared to larger but fewer particles of an identical total mass. It is implicitly assumed in this example that the powder particles are capable of being completely surrounded by the dissolution fluid. Under this condition, drug dissolution will be faster from smaller particles due to greater available surface area.

The relationship of particle size–surface area–dissolution rate is not so straightforward, in particular, for problematic hydrophobic drugs. Reduction in the particle size alone of hydrophobic drugs may not always translate into enhanced drug dissolution due to inadequate effective surface area available. It is the effective surface area that is critical in the drug dissolution process. Because of high interfacial tension, hydrophobic drugs display a lower effective surface area and slower dissolution. The effective surface area of hydrophobic drugs may be increased by incorporation of a small amount of wetting or surface active agent to the formulation or in the dissolution fluid. These agents will lower the surface tension between the powder particle and surrounding liquid as well as increase the fluid penetration of the powder particles and reduce aggregation of the suspended particles.

Other equations are also employed to describe drug dissolution under specific conditions. The Hixson and Crowell [22,23] cube-root equation for dissolution kinetics is based on the assumptions that dissolution takes place normal to the surface of the solute, there is no stagnation, agitation is identical on all exposed surfaces, and the solute particle retains its geometric shape. By appropriate substitution, the general form of the cube-root equation expresses the factors related to the solid in terms of weight; this is advantageous, as the surface is constantly changing and is difficult to experimentally evaluate.

Although the general form is cumbersome, it may be greatly simplified by imposing certain restrictions. If the concentration change is negligible [i.e., $(C_s - C)$ is almost constant], dw/dt, the amount dissolved per unit time, is proportional to the surface. This special case is expressed by the equation

$$\frac{dW}{dt} = 3KS = 3KaW^{2/3} \tag{4.27}$$

where $a = \alpha_{sv}/\rho^{2/3}$. The integrated form of this equation is

$$Kt = W_0^{1/3} - W^{1/3} \tag{4.28}$$

where W_o is the initial weight, W the weight of the solid at the time t, and K is the rate constant for a given set of conditions. A plot of $W_0^{1/3} - W^{1/3}$ against time is linear, with a slope of rate constant K.

As dissolution is a surface phenomenon, a given weight of smaller particles of a substance dissolves in a shorter time than larger particles of the same weight by virtue of the greater surface area exposed to the dissolving medium. For example, 1 g of powdered alum dissolves faster than 1 g of lump alum in a given amount of water; however, the dissolution rate is not changed by further reduction of particle size. It should be stressed that the dissolution rate is expressed in terms of the amount of solute dissolved per unit surface, e.g., g hr^{-1} cm^{-2}.

If absorption of a dissolved substance from the gastrointestinal tract is rapid, and dissolution is the rate-limiting step in drug availability, the drug is absorbed and removed from the gastrointestinal tract as fast as it dissolves. Consequently, there is no change in concentration in the gastrointestinal lumen. Thus, the effect of various factors on the *in vitro* dissolution rate determined with negligible concentration change may be extrapolated to a similar effect of these factors on *in vivo* dissolution rate.

4.9. FACTORS INFLUENCING THE DISSOLUTION RATE

4.9.1 Unreacting Additives

When neutral electrolytes and nonionic organic compounds are additives in the solvent phase, the dissolution rate of the solid is linearly dependent on the solubility of the solid in the solvent system. The dissolution rate of benzoic acid in aqueous solutions of sodium chloride or sodium sulfate decreases as its solubility decreases. The ion-dipole interaction competitively binds the water so that it is not as available for hydrogen bonding with the benzoic acid. Dextrose also decreases the solubility and dissolution rate.

In examining the dissolution rates and solubility of 55 compounds, it has been found that the ratio of rate to solubility ranged from 1.5 to 3. Thus, the dissolution rate of a new chemical entity or derivative may be roughly estimated by a consideration of its solubility.

As dissolution proceeds, the concentration of a solute in solution is increased, and the concentration gradient is decreased. This results in a slowing of the dissolution rate. Constituents of the gastrointestinal tract and excipients in solid dosage forms may absorb a drug. If an additive adsorbs the dissolved solute, the concentration gradient $(C_s - C)$ remains large, and the dissolution rate remains rapid.

4.9.2 Viscosity

In most dissolution processes applicable in pharmacy, the reaction at the interface of the solid and the solvent occurs much faster than the rate of transport or diffusion of the reactants from the interface to the bulk solution. An increase in viscosity therefore decreases the dissolution rate of a diffusion-controlled process. Numerous equations have been proposed that show the dissolution rate to be a function of the viscosity raised to a power where the exponent ranged from -0.25 to -0.8.

4.9.3 Surface Activity

In highly irregular particles with pores and crevices, the total surface area of the powder particles may be incompletely exposed to the solvent, due to occlusion by air. In the presence of surface-active agents, the surface tension between the powder particle and liquid medium is lowered, and the entire surface is wetted. This increase of surface contact between the solid and solvent, i.e., effective surface, increases the apparent dissolution rate.

Surface-active agents in low concentrations, i.e., below the critical micelle concentration, do not markedly affect dissolution rate. It has been postulated that a slight increase in rate at low concentrations can be attributed to the orientation of the dissolved solute between ionized surfactant molecules and the reduction of their repulsive force. When used in high concentrations, surface-active agents tend to increase the dissolution rate. This is probably a consequence of the greater total solubility resulting from the incorporation of the dissolved solute in a micellar structure.

4.9.4 Temperature

In general, solids dissolve faster if the system is warmed. If a substance absorbs heat in the dissolution process, its solubility is increased by an increase in temperature. The increase in solubility provides an increased concentration gradient that results in an increased dissolution rate. The increase in temperature increases kinetic motion and diffusion of the solute through the diffusion layer into the bulk solution, which increases the dissolution area. A flow pattern in which the velocity is variable and the path is curved is known as curvilinear flow. In the region of curvilinear flow for each 10° C rise in temperature, the dissolution rate increases approximately 1.3 times.

4.9.5 Agitation

As most dissolution procedures in pharmacy are accomplished by stirring, this discussion is limited to rotational agitation. The intensity of agitation is one of the most important factors in determining the dissolution rate of a solid. Generally, higher stirring rates yield faster dissolution rates because the thickness of the diffusion layer is inversely proportional to the agitation. This has been expressed in the empirically developed relationship

$$K = aN^b \tag{4.29}$$

where N is the agitation in terms of revolutions per minutes, K represents the dissolution rate, and a and b are constants. For a diffusion-controlled process, $b \to 1$. If the dissolution is controlled by an interfacial reaction, the agitation does not influence the dissolution rate and $b \to 0$.

When a stirrer is operated in a liquid so that the only friction is from the walls and bottom of the container and the viscosity of the fluid, the type of agitation is known as free rotational agitation. In free rotational agitation, the flow of fluid may be one of three types.

At very low rotations per minute (rpm), the flow is passive. The solids do not move, and the dissolution rate depends on the manner in which the solid is scattered on the bottom of the container. The solid and solution are not transported to the top of the system, and the system has layers of different concentrations. Dissolution does not occur where the particles touch one another in the pile at the center of the tank bottom. At very high rpm, the flow is turbulent. The centrifugal force of the rotating fluid tends to force the particles outward and upward. The cube-root equation does not apply to turbulent or passive flow.

Between these two extremes of flow is the useful curvilinear type of flow. In the curvilinear region, the dissolution rate is nearly linearly proportional to the rpm. In curvilinear flow, the particles move to the center and pile up, and then they move around circularly to the center. The cube-root equation applies to curvilinear flow.

4.9.6 Dissolution in a Reactive Medium

The discussion has been concerned with dissolution of a solid in a nonreactive medium. This is applicable to the preparation of solutions and the dissolution of drugs that do not undergo chemical reaction in body fluids. With these slightly soluble nonreacting drugs, e.g., chloramphenicol and griseofulvin, an increase in specific surface of the administered solid is a practical means of decreasing the time required for the drug to dissolve and to speed up onset of therapeutic activity. Because physiological conditions are not neutral, acidic and basic drugs react to the various pHs of the gastrointestinal tract with marked changes in solubilities and dissolution rates.

The dissolution rate in a reactive medium is decreased as the viscosity is increased. The dissolution rate is slowed by the addition of other solutes that compete for the solvent molecules and effectively decrease the solubility of the drug. Conversely, if the solubility of the drug in the diffusion layer is increased, the dissolution rate of the drug is increased. The solubility of acidic and basic drugs may be increased by modifying the pH of the diffusion layer.

The dissolution of a solid acidic drug may be increased by increasing the pH of the diffusion layer. In the administration of oral dosage forms, antacids may be administered to raise the pH of the stomach. This method has its limitations and is impractical because of the massive dose of antacid required.

Certainly, it is an uninspiring method if one is attempting to formulate a product as a single tablet or capsule.

A second method for increasing the dissolution rate of a solid acid is to mix the acid with a solid basic substance, e.g., sodium bicarbonate or sodium citrate. This mixture provides an increased pH of the immediate environment of the acid. There is an optimum ratio of the two constituents, depending on the fraction of the total surface of each and the strength of the acid. The maximum dissolution rate of the mixture for a given surface is not as great as the dissolution rate of the true salt.

4.10. PASSIVE DIFFUSION

Strictly speaking, diffusion is the tendency of gas molecules or liquid molecules or dissolved solute molecules to distribute uniformly over the space available at a constant temperature. It is a spontaneous process by which molecules move from the region of high concentration to the region of low concentration and, therefore, as long as the concentration gradient is maintained, molecules will continue to move in this manner. Diffusion is the result of random molecular motion, and the concentration gradient is the driving force. In 1855, Fick, quantitatively, described diffusion of molecules. It is described as Fick's first law of diffusion. It is expressed, mathematically, as

$$J = -D \times \frac{dC}{dX} \tag{4.30}$$

where J is the flux, D is the diffusion coefficient, and dC/dX is the concentration gradient in the direction of X (distance in the direction). The negative sign indicates that the direction of molecular movement is opposite to the increase in the concentration.

The drug transfer process is often viewed as the movement of a drug molecule across a series of membranes and spaces (Figure 4.5), which, collectively, serve as a macroscopic membrane. The cells and interstitial spaces lying between the gastric lumen and the capillary blood or structure between the sinusoidal space and the bile canaliculi are examples. Each of the cellular membranes and spaces may impede drug transport to varying degrees; therefore, any one of them can be a rate-limiting step to the overall process of drug transport. This complexity of structure makes quantitative prediction of drug transport difficult. A qualitative description of the processes of drug transport across functional membranes follows.

Passive diffusion is a natural tendency of drug molecules to move from the region of high concentration to the region of low concentration. The transfer of most drugs across a biological membrane occurs by passive diffusion. This movement of drug molecules is attributed to the kinetic energy of the molecules. The rate of diffusion, therefore, depends on the magnitude of the concentration gradient across the biological membrane and can be represented by

$$-\frac{dC}{dt} = K \cdot dC = K(C_{abs} - C_b) \tag{4.31}$$

where $-dC/dt$ is the rate of diffusion across a membrane; K is a complex proportionality constant that comprises the area of membrane (A), the thickness of the membrane (h), the partition coefficient (P) of the drug molecule between the lipophilic membrane and the aqueous phase on each side of the membrane, and the diffusion coefficient (D) of the drug; C_{abs} is the drug concentration at the absorption site; and C_b is the drug concentration in the blood.

The gastrointestinal absorption is the transfer of drug molecules from an aqueous solution of the gastrointestinal tract or from the lumen of the gut wall, followed by the penetration of the epithelial membrane by a drug molecule to the capillaries of the systemic circulation. Upon its entrance in the blood, the drug distributes itself rapidly in the blood. And, owing to the volume differences at absorption (GI tract) and distribution (blood) sites, the drug concentration in blood (C_b) will be much lower than the concentration at the absorption site (C_{abs}). This continuous transfer of drug maintains the sink condition and the concentration gradient throughout the absorption process—that is, ($C_{abs} - C_b$). Consequently, the concentration gradient is approximately equal to C_{abs}, so Equation 4.31 reduces to

$$-\frac{dC}{dt} = K \cdot C_1 \tag{4.32}$$

Because drug absorption by passive diffusion is a first-order process, the rate of absorption (dC/dt in Eq. 4.32) is directly proportional to the concentration at the absorption site (C_1 in Eq. 4.32). This suggests that the greater the concentration of drug at the absorption site, the faster the rate of absorption (Figure 4.12). It is, however, important to note that the percentage of dose absorbed at any time remains unaffected.

A major source of variation in absorption is the membrane permeability, which depends on the lipophilicity of the drug molecule. As discussed earlier, it is often characterized by its partition between octanol and water. The lipid solubility of a drug, therefore, is a very important physicochemical property governing the rate of transfer through a variety of biological membrane barriers. Figure 4.13 illustrates the role of partition coefficients in the drug absorption process from the colon, and that a good correlation exists between the percentage of drug absorption and the partition coefficient of an un-ionized drug.

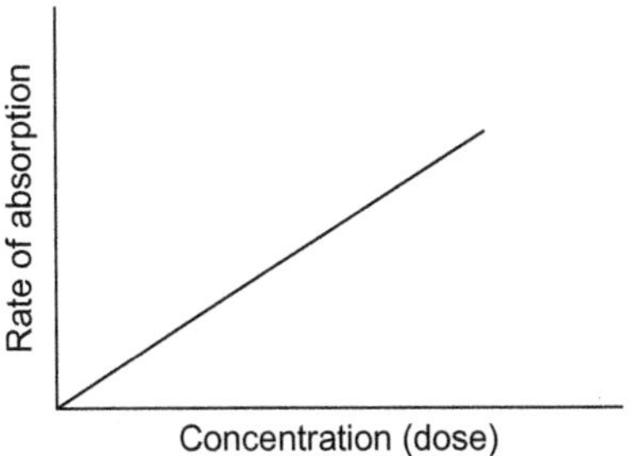

FIGURE 4.12 Effect of drug concentration on the rate of absorption when passive diffusion is operative.

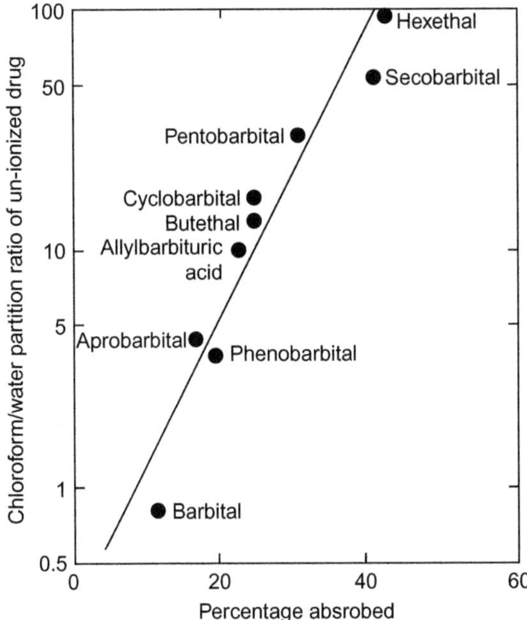

FIGURE 4.13 Comparison between colonic absorption of barbiturates in the rat and lipid-to-water partition coefficient of the un-ionized form of the barbiturates [9]. *(From Schanker LS. Absorption of drugs from the colon.* J Pharmacol Exp Ther *1959;126:283–94; with permission.)*

4.11. BIOPHARMACEUTICS CLASSIFICATION SYSTEM (BCS)

As mentioned in the introduction of the chapter, Amidon and co-workers [3,5,6] in their seminal work created the Biopharmaceutics Classification System (BCS). It was reported [24–27] that factors that affect the rate and extent of drug absorption from the gastrointestinal (GI) tract include physiochemical factors (e.g., p*K*a, solubility, stability, diffusivity, lipophilicity, polar-nonpolar surface area, presence of hydrogen-bonding functionalities, particle size, and crystal form), physiological factors (e.g., GI pH, GI blood flow, gastric emptying, small intestinal transit time, colonic transit time, and absorption mechanisms) and factors related to the dosage form (e.g., tablet, capsule, solution, suspension, emulsion, and gel).

Though all factors stated here contribute to drug absorption, the fundamental events that control oral drug absorption are the permeability of the drug through the GI membrane and the solubility/dissolution of the drug dose in the GI milieu. These key parameters are characterized in the Biopharmaceutics Classification System [24] by three dimensionless numbers: absorption number (A_n), dissolution number (D_n), and dose number (D_o). These numbers take into account both physiochemical and physiological parameters fundamental to the oral absorption process [5]. Based on their solubility and intestinal membrane permeability characteristics, drug substances have been classified into one of four categories according to the BCS.

4.11.1 Class I Drugs: High Solubility and High Permeability

Class I drugs provide both rapid dissolution and high membrane permeation. This class includes small molecule hydrophilic drugs that are not ionized in the gastrointestinal tract. Examples include acetaminophen, valproic acid, ketoprofen, dysopyramide, verapamil, and metoprolol. Class I drugs are well absorbed and are affected by a limited set of interactions that alter drug absorption. Since gastric emptying will frequently control the rate of absorption for this class of drugs, interactions that delay gastric emptying will delay drug absorption. This can be important for class I analgesic drugs where a rapid rate of absorption and quick rise in the plasma level to within the therapeutic range is needed to alleviate pain quickly.

4.11.2 Class II Drugs: Low Solubility and High Permeability

Dissolution appears to be a rate-limiting step from the immediate-release formulations of problematic or poorly water-soluble drugs. If such a drug requires a high dose for the therapeutic effects, then it will have a much greater impact on drug absorption. For example, the antifungal drug griseofulvin and the cardiac glycoside drug digoxin are both poorly water-soluble and possess similar dissolution profiles that limit the rate of drug absorption. However, the extent of griseofulvin absorption is incomplete for a typical dose of 500 mg, whereas a normal 0.25 mg oral dose of digoxin usually provides a fairly complete absorption.

For class II drugs, therefore, any interactions that enhance drug solubility and dissolution rate in the gastrointestinal tract will exert a positive effect on the gastrointestinal absorption. Furthermore, the absorption of this class of drugs often increases in proportion to the fat content of the co-administered meal. This is attributed to the increased gastrointestinal fluid volume as a result of the co-administered meal, stimulated gastrointestinal secretions, and biliary solubilization effects that increase the dissolution rate. Additionally, increased gastric residence time due to the calorie density permits greater time for drug dissolution.

4.11.3 Class III Drugs: High Solubility and Low Permeability

For drugs that belong to class III and are administered via immediate release formulations, the intestinal membrane permeation rate is often the rate-limiting step in drug absorption. Many drugs in this class also exhibit region-dependent absorption with better absorption in the upper small intestine. Therefore, any interactions that compromise upper intestinal absorption may result in a significant decrease in oral bioavailability. Consequently, these drugs show a sharp decrease in absorption with a co-administered meal that is independent of fat content. Meals tend to decrease the absorption of some drugs in this category as a result of a simple physical barrier that compromises the availability of drug molecules to the upper intestinal membrane.

4.11.4 Class IV Drugs: Low Solubility and Low Permeability

Poor aqueous solubility does not always translate into high lipophilicity and, therefore, high membrane permeation for a drug. Drugs that belong to class IV possess both low solubility and low permeability, both of which hinder good drug absorption. Drugs in this class, however, may still be administered orally if the resultant plasma concentrations are sufficient to produce the desired therapeutic effect, and the drugs do not exhibit a narrow therapeutic index.

The BCS has been recognized as the one of the most significant prognostic tools created to facilitate oral drug product development in recent years; the validity and broad applicability of the BCS have been the subject of extensive research and discussion [28–31]; it has been adopted by the U.S. Food and Drug Administration (FDA), the European Medicines Agency (EMEA), and the World Health Organization (WHO) for setting bioavailability/bioequivalence (BA/BE) standards for immediate-release (IR) oral drug product approval; and the BCS principles are extensively used by the pharmaceutical industry throughout drug discovery and development.

Up to now, the FDA has implemented the BCS system to allow waiver of *in vivo* BA/BE testing of IR solid dosage forms for class I, high-solubility, high-permeability drugs. As for class III (high-solubility, low-permeability) drugs, as long as the drug product does not contain agents and/or excipients that may modify intestinal membrane permeability, *in vitro* dissolution tests can ensure BE. The absorption of a class III is likely limited by its permeability and less dependent upon its formulation, and its bioavailability may be determined by an *in vivo* pattern. If the *in vitro* dissolution of a class III drug product is rapid under all physiological pH conditions, its *in vivo* behavior will essentially be similar to that of an oral solution (i.e., controlled by gastric emptying), and as long as the drug product does not contain permeability modifying agents (this potential effect is largely mitigated by the large gastric dilution), an *in vitro* dissolution test can ensure BE. Hence, biowaivers for BCS class III drugs are scientifically justified and have been recommended [32–34].

4.12. CONCLUSIONS

From the information presented in this chapter, it is clear that a number of important physicochemical properties of a drug, which play an important and influential role in the drug discovery process, drug dissolution process, and drug absorption process, are measured under equilibrium conditions. They include equilibrium solubility, partition coefficient, ionization, and diffusion, particularly passive diffusion. With the acceptance of the Rule of Five and an emergence of the Biopharmaceutics Classification System of drugs, these properties have attained greater importance in the early drug discovery process. A number of other properties such as powder particle size and pH of the gastrointestinal fluid are discussed here because they play an equally important role in drug dissolution and absorption processes. The importance of these properties and other factors such as pH of the dissolution fluid, solubility of a drug in the diffusion layer, and composition of the fluid is evident when one examines the drug absorption process, Noyes–Whitney equation, biological membrane, and gastrointestinal physiology.

CASE STUDIES

Case 4.1

An oil-in-water (o/w) emulsion uses both methyl paraben and propyl paraben as preservatives.

Recently, a compound pharmacist found out that he did not have methyl paraben; instead, he used butyl paraben and propyl paraben as preservatives for this emulsion. To his surprise, he found his emulsion showed some growth after a few days. Explain the possible cause of this problem, accounting for the antimicrobial mechanism of parabens.

Approach: Parabens are esters of (4-hydroxybenzoic acid) used as preservatives in liquid dosage forms. Preservation of an emulsion is an important issue because in this system there are two immiscible phases. Some of the parabens are more water soluble than others. As the chain length of the paraben increases, its aqueous solubility decreases and oil solubility increases. They can partition more to the oil phase than to the water phase. Due to the solubility and partition effects in the oil phase, and the interaction with emulsifiers, they may not attain an effective concentration in the aqueous phase. Since bacterial contamination happens in the aqueous phase, one may expect instability in the emulsion. In this case, both propyl and butyl parabens are more hydrophobic, and one expects more partition of both of these preservatives to the oil phase, causing even a further decrease of the effective antibacterial concentration in the aqueous phase and causing an instability in this (o/w) emulsion.

The alternative way to avoid this problem is to use different preservatives or switch over to a methyl and propyl paraben combination.

Case 4.2

A 65-year-old HIV+ male patient is taking Atripla® (a combination of three medicines: efavirenz, tenofovir, and emtricitabine). A Foley catheter was inserted into his urinary bladder to help him pass urine. When he was also administered acyclovir (which has two pKas, 2.27 and 9.25), a white cloudy precipitate was observed in the catheter, indicating some sort of crystallization of acyclovir. This was further confirmed by the appearance of needle-like structures in the urine samples. What is your advice to this patient to overcome this problem of crystalluria?

Approach: Atripla® is a non-nucleoside reverse transcriptase inhibitor. Therefore, according to FDA guidelines, it is combined with a nucleoside reverse transcriptase inhibitor such as acyclovir. Obviously, the idea is that these two different mechanisms would inhibit reverse transcriptase in viruses more efficiently. The two pKas of acyclovir, an amphipathic drug, suggest its minimum solubility of 2.5 mg/mL at physiologic pH [35]. Generally, acyclovir intravenous infusion contains 50 mg of acyclovir per mL. Therefore, to prevent formation of crystals in urine, both the infusion rate of acyclovir and the water intake should be manipulated. The former should be decreased, whereas the latter should be increased.

References

[1] Lipinsky CA, Lombordo F, Dominy W, et al. Experimental and computational approaches to estimate solubility and permeability in drug discovery and development settings. Adv Drug Deliv Rev 1997;23:3–25.

[2] Stewart B, Wang Y, Surendran N. Ex. *In vivo* approaches to predicting oral pharmacokinetics in humans. 6th ed. Ann Repts Med Chem Trauma, Academic Press 2000;35:299–307.

[3] Amidon G, Lenncranas H, Shah V, et al. A theoretical basis for a biopharmaceutics drug classification: the correlation of *in vitro* drug product and *in vivo* bioavailability. Pharm Res 1995;12:413–20.

[4] Ertl P, Rohde B, Selzer P. Fast calculation of molecular polar surface area as a sum of fragment-based contributions and its application to the prediction of drug transport properties. J Med Chem 2000;43:3714–7.

[5] Martinez MN, Amidon GL. A mechanistic approach to understanding the factors affecting drug absorption: a review of fundamentals. J Clin Pharmacol 2002;42:620–43.

[6] Lennernas H. Human intestinal permeability. J Pharm Sci 1998;87:402–10.

[7] Florence AT, Attwood D. Physiochemical principles of pharmacy. 5th ed. London and Chicago: Pharmaceutical Press; 2011.

[8] Schanker LS. Absorption of drugs from the rat colon. J Pharmacol Exp Ther 1959;126:283–94.

[9] Shore PA, Brodie BB, Hogben CAM. The gastric secretion of drugs: a pH partition hypothesis. J Pharmacol Exp Ther 1957;119:361–9.

[10] Hogben CAM, Tocco DJ, Brodie BB, et al. On the mechanism of intestinal absorption of drugs. J Pharmacol Exp Therap 1959;125:275–82.

[11] Schanker LS. On the mechanism of absorption of drugs from the gastrointestinal tract. J Med Pharm Chem 1960;2:343–59.

[12] Schanker LS. Mechanism of drug absorption and distribution. Annu Rev Pharmacol 1961;1:29–44.

[13] Schanker LS. Passage of drugs across the gastrointestinal epithelium in drugs and membrane. In: Hogben CAM, editor. Proceedings of the first international pharmacology meeting, vol. 4. New York: The Macmillan Company; 1963.

[14] Schanker LS. Physiological transport of drug. In: Harper NJ, Simons AB, editors. Advances in drug research. London: Academic Press; 1966. p. 71–106.

[15] Rowland M, Tozer T. Clinical pharmacokinetics: concepts and application. 2nd ed. Philadelphia: Lea and Febiger; 1989.

[16] Gibaldi M. Biopharmaceutics and clinical pharmacokinetics. 4th ed. Philadelphia: Lea and Febiger; 1991.

[17] Schanker LS. Absorption of drugs from the rat small intestine. J Pharmacol Exp Ther 1958;128:81–7.

[18] Winne D. The influence of unstirred layers on intestinal absorption in intestinal permeation. In: Kramer M, Lauterbach F, editors. Workshop conference hoechest, vol 4. Amsterdam: Excerpta Medica; 1977. p. 58–64.

[19] Levy G, Leonard JR, Procknal JA. Development of *in vitro* dissolution tests which correlate quantitatively with dissolution rate limited absorption. J Pharm Sci 1965;54:1319–25.

[20] Noyes NA, Whitney WJ. The rate of solution of solid substances in their own solution. J Am Chem Soc 1897;19:930–42.

[21] Noyes NA, Whitney WJ. Ueber Die Auslosungsgesch Wingdigkeit Von Festen Stossen In Ihern Eigenen Losungen. Z Physik Chem 1897;23:689–92.

[22] Hixson A, Crowell J. Dependence of reaction velocity upon surface and agitation I: theoretical consideration. Ind Eng Chem 1931;23:923–31.

[23] Hixson A, Crowell J. Dependence of reaction velocity upon surface and agitation II: theoretical consideration. Ind Eng Chem 1931;23:1002–9.

[24] Dahan A, Miller J, Amidon G. Prediction of solubility and permeability membership: Provisional BCS Classification of the world's oral drugs. AAPS J 2009;3(4):740–6.

[25] Dahan A, Amidon G. Gastrointestinal dissolution and absorption of class II drugs. In: Van de Waterbeemdand H, Testa B, editors. Drug bioavailability: estimation of solubility, permeability, absorption, and bioavailability. Weinheim: Wiley-VCH; 2008, p. 33–51.

[26] Sun D, Yu L, Hussain M, Wall D, Smith R, Amidon G. *In vitro* testing of drug absorption for drug 'developability' assessment: forming an interface between *in vitro* preclinical data and clinical outcome. Curr Opin Drug Discov Develop 2004;7:75–85.

[27] Dahan A, Amidon GL. Small intestinal efflux mediated by MRP2 and BCRP shifts sulfasalazine intestinal permeability from high to low, enabling its colonic targeting. Am J Phys Gastro Liver Physiol 2009;297:G371–7.

[28] Polli J, Abrahamsson B, Yu L, Amidon G, Baldoni J, Cook J, et al. Summary of workshop report: bioequivalence, biopharmaceutics classification system, and beyond. AAPS J 2008;10:373–9.

[29] Thiel-Demby VE, Humphreys JE, St. John Williams LA, Ellens HM, Shah N, Ayrton AD, et al. Biopharmaceutics classification system: validation and learning of an *in vitro* permeability assay. Mol Pharm 2009;6:11–8.

[30] Yang Y, Faustino PJ, Volpe DA, Ellison CD, Lyon RC, Yu LX. Biopharmaceutics classification of selected beta blockers; solubility and permeability class membership. Mol Pharm 2007;4:608–14.

[31] Blume HH, Schug BS. The biopharmaceutics classification system (BCS): class III drugs—better candidate for BA/BE waiver? Eur J Pharm Sci 1999;9:117.

[32] Cheng CL, Yu XL, Lee HL, Yang CY, Lu CS, Chou CH. Biowaiver extension potential to BCS class III high solubility low permeability drugs: bridging evidence for metformin immediate release tablet. Eur J Pharm Sci 2004;22:297.

[33] Jantratid E, Prakongpan S, Amidon GL, Dressman J. Feasibility of biowaiver extension to biopharmaceutics classification system class III drug products: cimetidine. Clin Pharmacokinet 2006;45:385–99.

[34] Stavchansky S. Scientific perspective on extending the provision for waivers of *in vivo* bioavailability and bioequivalence studies for drug products containing high solubility–low permeability drugs (BCS Class 3). AAPS J 2008;10:300–5.

[35] DrugPoints® System. 2012, Thomson Reuters. STAT! Ref Online Electronic Medical Library. Available from: http://online.statref.com.cuhsl.creighton.edu/Document.aspx?fxId=6&docId=599.

Suggested Readings

Avdeef A. *Absorption and Drug Development: Solubility, Permeability, and Charge State*. New York: Wiley-Interscience, 2003.

Florence, Alexander and Attwood, David. *Physiochemical Principles of Pharmacy*, 5th ed., London: Pharmaceutical Press, 2011.

Ganellin C, Roberts S. eds. *Medicinal Chemistry: The Role of Organic Chemistry in Drug Research*, 2nd ed. New York: Academic Press, 1993.

Gibaldi M. *Biopharmaceutics and Clinical Pharmacokinetics*, 4th ed. Philadelphia: Lea and Febiger, 1991.

Grant, David and Higuchi, T. *Solubility Behavior of Organic Compounds; Techniques of Chemistry*, Vol. 21. New York: Wiley Interscience, 1990.

Horter D, Dressman JB. Influence of physiochemical properties on dissolution of drugs in the gastrointestinal tract. *Adv Drug Deliv Rev* 2001;46:75–87.

Jambhekar, Sunil. In *Foye's Principles of Medicinal Chemistry*, 7th ed., Williams and Lemke (Ed.), Baltimore: Wolters Kluwer/Lippincott, Williams and Wilkins, 2012.

Pandit, Nita K. *Introduction to Pharmaceutical Sciences*. Baltimore: Lippincott, Williams, and Wilkins. 2007.

Rowland M, Tozer T. *Clinical Pharmacokinetics: Concepts and Application*, 3rd ed. Philadelphia: Lea and Febiger, 1994.

Sinko, Patrick, (Ed.), *Martin's Physical Pharmacy and Pharmaceutical Sciences*, 6th ed., Baltimore: Lippincott, Williams and Wilkins, 2006.

Taylor J, Kennewell P. *Modern Medicinal Chemistry: Ellis Horwood Series in Pharmaceutical Technology*. New York: Ellis Horwood, 1993.

Wermuth C, Koga N, Konig H, et al. *Medicinal Chemistry for the 21st Century*. Boston: Blackwell Scientific Publications, 1992.

CHAPTER

5

Kinetic Processes in Pharmaceutics

Ramprakash Govindarajan

Research and Development, GlaxoSmithKline, Research Triangle Park, North Carolina, USA

CHAPTER OBJECTIVES

- Understand the fundamental principles of kinetic processes in pharmaceutics.
- Recognize various kinetic processes in pharmacy.
- Apply the principles of chemical kinetics to drug stability.
- Understand the various factors that can affect drug stability.
- Understand the shelf-life of a drug and its determination.
- Appreciate the kinetics involved in the process of drug diffusion.
- Understand the kinetics involved in the process of drug dissolution.
- Understand the kinetics of drug release from a dosage form or drug delivery system.

Keywords

- Chemical kinetics
- Diffusion
- Dissolution
- Drug product stability
- Drug release
- Mass transport
- Pharmaceutics
- Reaction order
- Stability testing

5.1. INTRODUCTION

Pharmaceutics involves the study of physical, chemical, biological, and technological processes, which influence the pharmacological response of a biologically active molecule upon administration to humans or animals. The knowledge of these processes is applied in the development of safe, effective, commercially manufacturable, and patient-acceptable medicinal products that provide the desired therapeutic benefits. Each subdiscipline of pharmaceutics therefore requires the understanding of various processes and the interplay between them.

As in all other disciplines, the ability to accelerate certain processes and to slow down others can be used to maximize desirable occurrences and effects. Very often, this ability to change the rates of processes, relative to each other, enables us to utilize windows of opportunity to 'make things happen'.

5.2. THERMODYNAMICS VS. KINETICS

The laws of thermodynamics dictate whether a process will occur spontaneously and define the position of chemical, thermal, and mechanical equilibria. All systems spontaneously move toward lower free energy (chemical potentials) and higher entropy. These laws therefore form the basis of the *driving force* for processes to occur. The rates of these processes, however, will be influenced by several environmental factors. In pharmaceutics, the resulting time course of various processes and their interplay can have a major influence on the quality and performance of medicinal products. For example, the equilibrium solubility of an active pharmaceutical ingredient (API) under a given set of *in vivo* conditions is a thermodynamic property. However, when a tablet is administered, the *rates* of tablet disintegration and drug dissolution will dictate the concentration of dissolved drug near the sites of absorption. The time course of this *in vivo* dissolution will affect *rates* of absorption and hence the plasma levels of the drug. Similarly, when an extended release

Pharmaceutics. DOI: http://dx.doi.org/10.1016/B978-0-12-386890-9.00005-4

dosage form is designed to provide therapeutic levels of a drug over a prolonged period, the *rates* of drug release from the dosage form will dictate the pharmacokinetics of the drug. In the case of molecules that have an absorption window in the gastrointestinal tract, the *rates* of transit of gastrointestinal contents and the *rates* of drug dissolution will both influence the drug concentrations available within the absorption window, and hence the bioavailability. While a degradation process in a drug product may be thermodynamically favored, the *rates* of these physical/chemical processes can be controlled, for example, by providing protective packaging or storage at lower temperatures, thereby allowing for reasonably long shelf-lives. Thus, an understanding and control, if possible, of physical, chemical, and biological processes is critical for ensuring that a pharmaceutical product consistently exhibits the desired level of stability and *in vivo* performance.

This chapter provides an overview of physical and chemical rate processes, an understanding of which is important for both pharmaceutical scientists as well as practicing pharmacists. The chapter is divided into sections dealing with kinetics of chemical changes and physical mass transport processes (diffusion and dissolution). Transport processes in biological systems are discussed in Chapter 13.

The objective of this chapter is to introduce students of pharmacy to the fundamental principles of kinetic processes relevant to pharmaceutics. While this chapter intends to provide an overview of the key concepts, readers are encouraged to refer to additional texts, found in the reference list, for more detailed discussion of these topics [1–4].

5.3. CHEMICAL REACTION KINETICS AND DRUG STABILITY

One of the major challenges for a pharmaceutical scientist is to provide the required dose of the active ingredient in a dosage form that retains the chemical integrity of the drug molecule under the defined conditions of storage over the claimed shelf-life. Drug molecules can undergo various chemical degradation processes including hydrolysis, oxidation, isomerization, polymerization, and photochemical decomposition, resulting in a decrease in potency of the active ingredient. These processes can occur after synthesis, during storage prior to drug product manufacture, and over the shelf-life of the manufactured drug product, resulting in generation and growth of unwanted degradation products in the drug substance or the drug product.

Therefore, there is a need to understand these processes mechanistically and kinetically to develop stable pharmaceutical products, prescribe suitable storage conditions, and establish expiration dates. This section deals with the fundamental concepts of chemical kinetics, stability testing of pharmaceuticals, and prediction of the shelf-life of drug products.

5.3.1 Fundamental Principles and Terminology

5.3.1.1 Process Rates and Orders

The rate or speed of a process (a physical or chemical change) can be defined by the rate at which the concentration of a species undergoing the change decreases or the concentration of the resulting species increases with time.

Let us consider a reaction in which reactants A and B react to form products X and Y:

$$mA + nB \rightarrow pX + qY \tag{5.1}$$

The rate of progress of the reaction at time t can be measured in terms of changes in the concentrations of the reactants or the products:

$$\text{Rate} = -\frac{1}{m}\frac{d[A]}{dt} = -\frac{1}{n}\frac{d[B]}{dt} = \frac{1}{p}\frac{d[X]}{dt} = \frac{1}{q}\frac{d[Y]}{dt} \tag{5.2}$$

The *rate equation* relating the reaction speed with the concentration of the reactants can be expressed as follows:

$$Rate = k[A]^{\alpha}[B]^{\beta} \tag{5.3}$$

It is important to note that α and β are *not always* the stoichiometric numbers m and n in Eq. 5.1, but have to be obtained from rate experiments and hence are empirical. When the reaction rate follows the concentration dependence as defined in Eq. 5.3, it is of the order α with respect to A and order β with respect to B (partial orders). The overall reaction order is the sum of the exponents in the rate equation, i.e., $(\alpha + \beta)$, and k is the rate constant. *Reaction order is defined based on the rate equation obeyed and hence is a kinetic property of the process.*

5.3.1.2 Order vs. Molecularity

Molecularity refers to the number of molecules participating in a given step of a reaction and hence is related to the mechanism of the reaction. For a single-step (elementary) reaction, the molecularity and order are the same. In other words, the partial orders are the same as the stoichiometry values in a balanced chemical equation. This statement also applies to an elementary step of a complex, multistep process. For example, an elementary bimolecular reaction exhibits second-order kinetics, and the observed rate depends on the concentrations of both the reacting species.

For a complex multistep reaction, each elementary reaction has an order (molecularity). However, the overall rate equation might be much more complicated than Eq. 5.3. The equation might include concentration terms of intermediates, products and catalysts, and fractional exponential terms. Thus, molecularity and order of a chemical process may be different. For example, while a reaction may exhibit zero-order or fractional-order kinetics, it is not conceivable for a reaction to have zero or fractional molecularity.

5.3.1.3 *Classifying Reactions: Order and Pseudo-Order*

Let us first deal with the simplest form of rate equations before addressing reaction kinetics in complicated pharmaceutical systems. Consider a bimolecular reaction, alkaline hydrolysis of ethyl acetate in a dilute aqueous solution:

$$CH_3COOC_2H_5 + OH^- \rightarrow CH_3COO^- + C_2H_5OH \quad (5.4)$$

The rate equation can be expressed as follows, where the rate of disappearance of ethyl acetate from solution at any given time t is directly proportional to the concentrations of ethyl acetate and hydroxide ions:

$$\text{Rate} = -\frac{d[CH_3COOC_2H_5]}{dt} = k_2[CH_3COOC_2H_5]^1[OH^-]^1 \quad (5.5)$$

Equation 5.5 represents a second-order rate expression, and k_2 is the second-order rate constant.

If the same reaction were to be carried out in a buffered system, where the concentration of hydroxide ions is maintained constant, then the equation can be rewritten as follows:

$$\text{Rate} = -\frac{d[CH_3COOC_2H_5]}{dt} = k_1'[CH_3COOC_2H_5]^1$$

$$k_1' = k_2[OH^-]^1 \quad (5.6)$$

The overall reaction appears to follow first-order kinetics, and the rate of disappearance of ethyl acetate exhibits dependence only on the concentration of ethyl acetate. This is referred to as a *pseudo first-order reaction* and k_1' is the pseudo first-order rate constant.

Consider a suspension formulation of a poorly soluble ester drug RCOOR′ in a vehicle buffered at an alkaline pH that promotes hydrolysis of the ester:

$$RCOOR'_{solution} + OH^- \longrightarrow RCOO^- + R'OH \quad (5.7)$$

In such cases, due to presence of undissolved excess ester in the system, the ester concentration in solution would remain constant (and equal to its solubility in the vehicle) as long as there is excess solid present. If OH^- catalyzed hydrolysis is the sole reaction pathway, then the rate equation can be expressed as follows:

$$\text{Rate} = -\frac{d[RCOOR']}{dt} = k_0' \quad (5.8)$$

$$k_0' = k_1'[RCCOOR']^1 = k_2[OH^-]^1[RCOOR']^1 \quad (5.9)$$

The reaction rate therefore appears to be independent of the concentrations of the reactants and is constant. The constant k_0' is called the pseudo zero-order rate constant and is related to the second-order and pseudo first-order rate constants as expressed in Eq. 5.9. This kinetic behavior would continue as long as there is excess undissolved ester replenishing the solution and maintaining a constant reactant concentration. Once the entire excess solid disappears, the solution concentration of the ester begins to decrease, and the reaction will exhibit first-order kinetics with respect to the ester.

5.3.1.4 *Half-Life and Shelf-Life*

The half-life of a reaction ($t_{0.5}$) is defined as the time required to decrease the reactant concentration to 50% of the initial concentration. It can be expressed as a function of the rate constants.

For pharmaceutical products, shelf-life is defined as the time duration after manufacture until which the critical quality attributes of the product are within acceptable limits, i.e., the time duration between the dates of manufacture and expiry of the product. Solely in terms of the content of the API, it is the time until which the concentration of the API is above defined minimum acceptable levels (say 90% or 95% of the label claim). It is important to note that changes in product attributes other than API content (for example, changes in drug release behavior or physical properties of the dosage unit) may influence the determination of shelf-lives.

An understanding of the kinetics and mechanisms of these deterioration processes is necessary to stabilize the formulation as well as predict the shelf-life of drug products.

5.3.2 Zero-Order Reactions

As mentioned earlier, a zero-order reaction proceeds at a constant rate and hence appears to be independent of the concentration of the reactant in the system. If a represents concentration of the reactant after time t and a_0 is the initial concentration of the reactant at time zero, the rate of reaction can be expressed as follows. Unless otherwise specified, similar concentration symbols will be used in subsequent sections on chemical kinetics:

$$\text{Rate} = -\frac{da}{dt} = k_0 \tag{5.10}$$

The integrated form can be written as follows:

$$a = a_0 - k_0 t \tag{5.11}$$

A zero-order reaction can occur if the reaction rate, for example, is limited by the concentration of a catalyst. In such cases, k_0 may be proportional to the catalyst concentration or, for example, the intensity of light in a photochemical process. This highlights the fact that the observed order often cannot be deduced from a balanced chemical equation. The constant k_0 has the units of [concentration × time^{-1}].

From Eq. 5.11, the half-life, i.e., the time at which $[a = \{^1/_2\}\, a_0]$, can be expressed as follows:

$$t_{0.5} = \frac{a_0 - 0.5a_0}{k_0} = \frac{a_0}{2k_0} \tag{5.12}$$

The half-life for a zero-order reaction therefore is dependent on the initial concentration of the reactant.

As an example, let us consider the hydrolysis of acetylsalicylic acid (ASA 180.2 g/mole) in an aqueous solution to yield salicylic acid (138.1 g/mole):

ASA + H_2O ⟶ Salicylic acid + Acetic acid (5.13)

Maulding and coworkers monitored the extent of hydrolysis of ASA in a powder mixture with microcrystalline cellulose, starch, lactose, stearic acid, and magnesium trisilicate, with varying amounts of added water, when stored at 40°C [5]. In Figure 5.1, the reaction progress is depicted in terms of the formation of salicylic acid, in mixtures initially containing 400 mg of aspirin. As seen in the figure, in the time period over which the reaction was monitored, the amount of salicylic acid formed increased linearly with time, suggesting a constant reaction rate and no dependence on the overall reactant concentration in the system.

For any given system, the excess solid ASA maintains a constant reactant concentration in solution. Therefore, although the reaction is first order with respect to ASA, it exhibits zero-order kinetics.

It can also be inferred from the figure that the overall reaction rate exhibits a dependence on the concentration of water. This is reasonable if one considers the role of water as a reactant as well as a solvent (a higher amount of water resulting in a higher fraction of the total ASA in solution). However, it is important to note that in complex heterogeneous pharmaceutical systems, reaction rates can be affected by a multitude of interrelated factors. The amount of water can influence other rate-determining factors such as concentrations of products formed and the concentrations and catalytic activity of other components of the system.

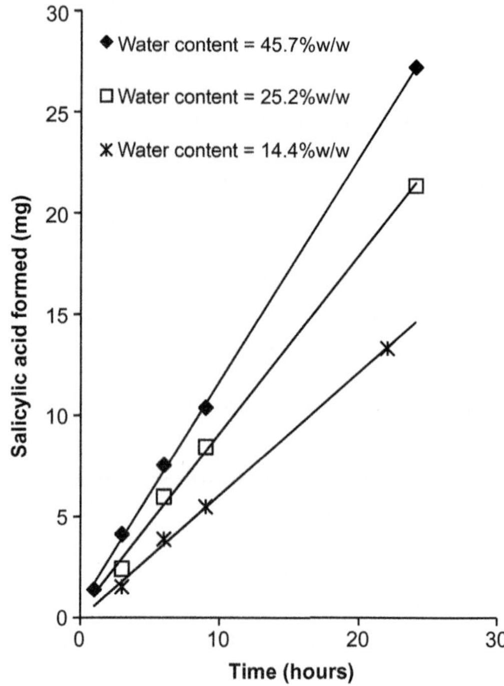

FIGURE 5.1 Formation of salicylic acid at 40°C, in powder mixtures initially containing 400 mg of ASA, with varying amounts of added water. The reaction exhibits pseudo zero-order kinetics as seen by a constant rate of formation of salicylic acid. Note that the reaction rates (slope of the lines) increase with an increase in the water concentrations in the system. *(Plots reconstructed from data in reference [5])*

5.3.3 First-Order Reactions

Using the same symbols as in Eq. 5.10, the rate equation for a first-order reaction can be written as follows:

$$\text{Rate} = -\frac{da}{dt} = k_1 a \tag{5.14}$$

The integrated forms of the rate equation can be obtained as follows

$$\int_{a_0}^{a} \frac{da}{a} = -\int_0^t k_1 dt \tag{5.15}$$

$$\ln a - \ln a_0 = -k_1 t \tag{5.16}$$

$$a = a_0 . e^{-k_1 t} \tag{5.17}$$

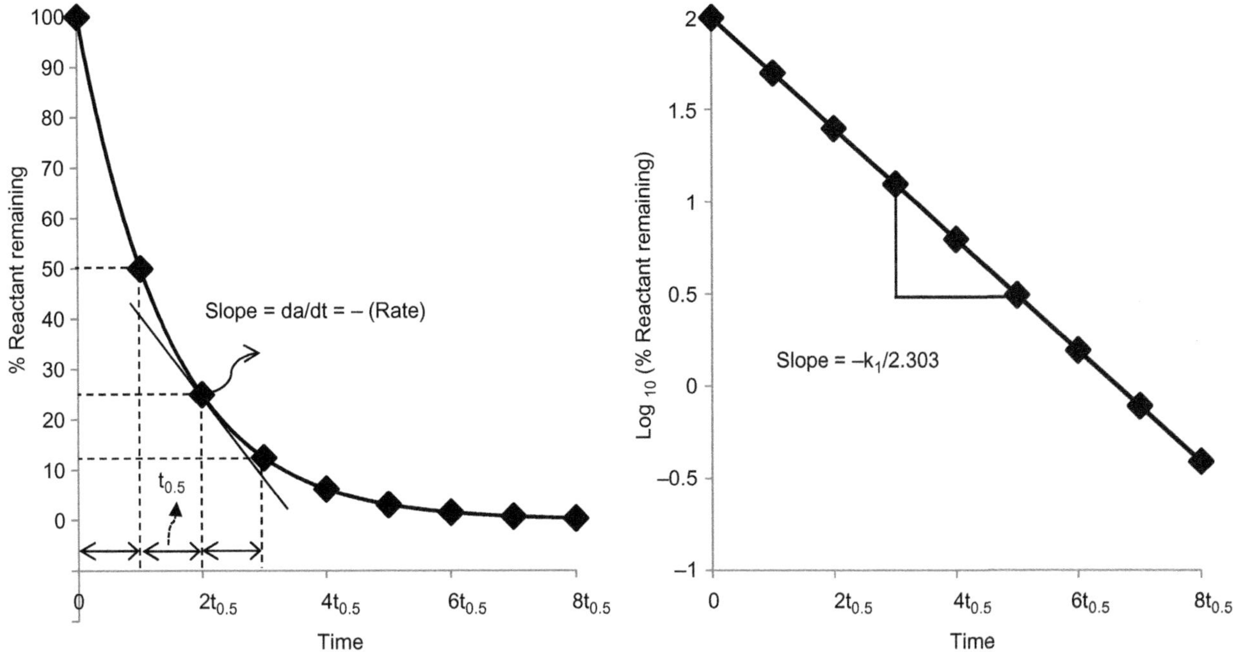

FIGURE 5.2 First-order reaction progress. The time-axis has been scaled as multiples of the half-life ($t_{0.5}$).

Rearranging and converting logarithms to the base 10, we can obtain

$$\log\left[\frac{a}{a_0}\right] = \frac{-k_1 t}{2.303} \tag{5.18}$$

A first-order reaction therefore implies an exponential decrease in the concentration of the reactant and hence an exponential decrease in the reaction rate as seen in Eqs. 5.14–5.17. The unit of the first-order rate constant k_1 is time^{-1}.

Mathematically, the half-life for the reaction can be obtained by substituting a with 0.5 a_0 in Eq. 5.18:

$$t_{0.5} = \frac{2.303}{k_1}\log\left[\frac{a_0}{0.5a_0}\right] = \frac{0.693}{k_1} \tag{5.19}$$

Therefore, the half-life of a first-order reaction is independent of the initial concentration of the reactant. Figure 5.2 represents a first-order decrease of reactant as the reaction progresses. As seen in the figure in each subsequent half-life, the reactant content is reduced by half. A semi-log plot of the same data yields a straight line with a slope of [$-k_1/2.303$].

Oberholtzer and Brenner investigated the solution stability of cefoxitin sodium at various solution pH values [6]. As seen in Figure 5.3, cefoxitin sodium underwent rapid hydrolytic degradation in solution. The in Figure 5.3 yielded first-order constants of 3.42E-03, 2.46E-03, and 7.83E-03 hour^{-1} at 25°C and a cefoxitin half-life of 212, 288, and 89 hours at pH values of 3.0, 7.0, and 9.0, respectively. The shelf-life (the time over which >90% of the original content of the drug is intact) can be calculated for a first-order reaction as follows:

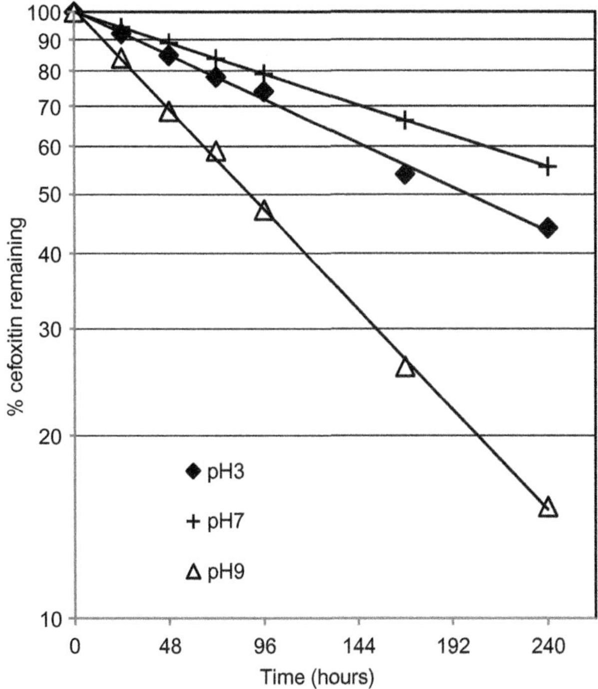

FIGURE 5.3 Observed first-order degradation plots for cefoxitin sodium at different solution pH values at 25°C. The drug was found to undergo hydrolysis of the beta-lactam ring in solution. The degradation rates exhibited dependence on the solution pH. *(Adapted from reference [6])*

$$t_{0.9} = \frac{2.303}{k_1} \log\left[\frac{a_0}{0.9a_0}\right] = \frac{0.105}{k_1} \tag{5.20}$$

The calculated shelf-lives for these solutions were 40, 49, and 14 hours at pH 3.0, 7.0, and 9.0, respectively. These short half-lives preclude the formulation of aqueous parenteral solution formulations for cefoxitin. These studies revealed the need for the drug to be provided as a sterile solid for reconstitution prior to parenteral administration.

5.3.4 Second-Order Reactions

For a bimolecular process, where two reactant molecules collide during the reaction to finally yield the products, it is reasonable to assume that the rate of product formation would depend on the rates of collisions and hence the concentrations of both reactants. For a second-order reaction of the type $A + B = X$, the rate equation can be written as follows:

$$\text{Rate} = -\frac{da}{dt} = -\frac{db}{dt} = k_2\, a\, b \tag{5.21}$$

Let us consider a simple case in which the initial molar concentrations of both the reactants is the same; i.e., $a_0 = b_0$ and A and B react with a 1:1 stoichiometry, then at any given time t, $a = b$.

$$\text{Rate} = -\frac{da}{dt} = -\frac{db}{dt} = k_2\, a^2 \tag{5.22}$$

$$-\int_{a_0}^{a} \frac{da}{a^2} = \int_0^t k_2 dt \tag{5.23}$$

$$\left(\frac{1}{a}\right) - \left(\frac{1}{a_0}\right) = k_2 t \tag{5.24}$$

$$\left(\frac{a_0 - a}{a\, a_0}\right) = k_2 t \tag{5.25}$$

Therefore, a plot of the LHS term in Eq. 5.25 versus time should yield a straight line with the value of the slope equal to the second-order rate constant. As seen from the equation, the units of k_2 are concentration^{-1}time^{-1}. For this simple case in which $a_0 = b_0$, the half-life of the reaction can be expressed as follows by modifying Eq. 5.25:

$$t_{0.5} = \left(\frac{a_0 - 0.5a_0}{0.5k_2\, a_0^2}\right) = \left(\frac{1}{k_2\, a_0}\right) \tag{5.26}$$

The half-life of the second-order reaction therefore is inversely proportional to the initial concentration of the reactant.

Let us once again consider the saponification of ethyl acetate in Eqs. 5.4–5.6. A reaction mixture containing equimolar concentrations (0.064 M) of ethyl acetate and sodium hydroxide was monitored for the loss of ethyl acetate, by measuring the acetic acid formed [7]. The progress of the reaction and

Time (min.)	Millimolar ethyl acetate remaining, (a)	Millimolar ethyl acetate reacted, (a_0-a)	$\left(\frac{a_0 - a}{a\, a_0}\right)$
0	a_0 = 64	0	0.000
5	40.9	23.1	0.009
15	24.5	39.5	0.025
25	17.3	46.7	0.042
35	13.7	50.3	0.057
55	9.3	54.7	0.092

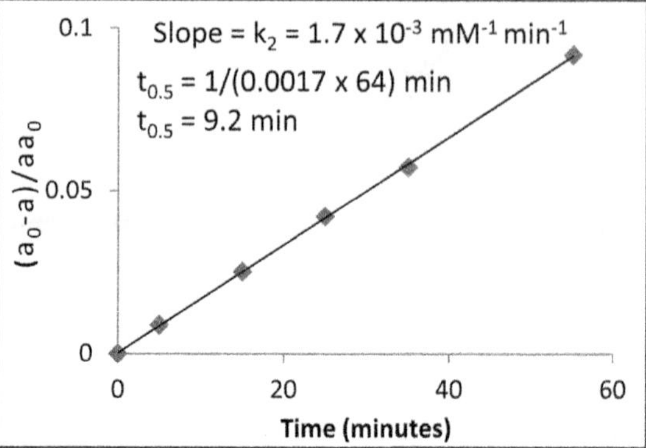

FIGURE 5.4 Second-order reaction: saponification of ethyl acetate in a solution containing equal concentrations (64 mM) of ethyl acetate and sodium hydroxide. *(Data adapted from reference [7].)*

calculation of k_2 and $t_{0.5}$ using the expression in Eq. 5.25 are shown in Figure 5.4.

For a second-order reaction ($A + B \rightarrow X$) in which the initial concentrations of the reactants are not equal ($a_0 \neq b_0$), the rate equation can be expressed as follows, where 'x' is the concentration of A and B that has reacted at time t:

$$\text{Rate} = -\frac{da}{dt} = -\frac{db}{dt} = \frac{dx}{dt} = k_2(a_0 - x)(b_0 - x) \tag{5.27}$$

Integrating the rate equation and appropriate substitution yields

$$\left(\frac{2.303}{a_0 - b_0}\right) \log \frac{a \cdot b_0}{b \cdot a_0} = k_2 t \tag{5.28}$$

As seen from Eq. 5.28 again, the units for k_2 are [concentration^{-1} time^{-1}]. When the initial concentrations of the reactants are different ($a_0 \neq b_0$), it is not possible to define a single $t_{0.5}$.

5.3.5 Determination of Reaction Order

For simpler systems, the easiest method of determining the order of a reaction would be to obtain experimental data on the progress of a reaction under the defined conditions. This data can be *substituted* into rate equations to calculate k values at each time point; for example, Eqs. 5.11, 5.16, and 5.25. The rate equation, which yields a consistent calculated value for k, represents the reaction order.

The reaction orders can also be determined *graphically* by plotting the experimental data in the form of the rate equations (Eqs. 5.11, 5.16, and 5.25) and determining the equation that provides the best fit.

The *isolation method* can also be employed, say for a reaction, which follows the rate equation:

$$\text{Rate} = k[A]^{\alpha}[B]^{\beta} \quad (5.29)$$

As a first step, the reaction can be carried out with a large excess of A, say a concentration A′ such that $k[A]^{\alpha}$ remains fairly constant as the reaction proceeds and B disappears. The reaction therefore exhibits pseudo β-order and the equation can be written as follows:

$$\text{Rate} = k'[B]^{\beta}, \text{ where } k' = k(A')^{\alpha} = \text{constant} \quad (5.30)$$

By following the disappearance of B, one can experimentally determine the value of β and k'.

In the second step, by holding the concentration of B at a large excess, similarly, one can infer the value of α. Thus, the partial orders and the overall reaction order can be obtained. Alternately, in the second step, the reaction could be repeated, still with a large excess of A, but at a different concentration, say A″. The rate equation can be similarly written as follows:

$$\text{Rate} = k''[B]^{\beta}, \text{where } k'' = k(A'')^{\alpha} = \text{constant} \quad (5.31)$$

The value of α can be determined from the following relationship:

$$\log\frac{k'}{k''} = \alpha \log\frac{A'}{A''} \quad (5.32)$$

From our earlier discussions on reaction half-lives, it can be inferred that the $t_{0.5}$ of a reaction can be related to the initial concentration of the reactant, depending on the reaction order (n). In general, if the initial concentrations of reactants (a_0, b_0, c_0...) can be expressed as a_0 ($a_0 = b_0 = c_0$...), the dependence of the half-life on initial reactant concentration can be expressed as follows:

$$t_{0.5} \propto \left(\frac{1}{a_0^{n-1}}\right) \quad (5.33)$$

If the same reaction is carried out at two *different* initial concentrations (a_0' and a_0'') and the corresponding half-lives are determined to be $t_{0.5}'$ and $t_{0.5}''$, the order of the reaction n can be determined from the following relationship:

$$n = 1 + \frac{\log(t'_{0.5}/t''_{0.5})}{\log(a''_0/a'_0)} \quad (5.34)$$

5.3.6 Complex Reactions

Very often in pharmaceutical systems, it is not possible to express the kinetics of drug degradation as simple zero-, first-, or second-order reactions. Drugs may react in reversible reactions, multiple pathways, or in sequential reaction steps. The rate equations need modifications to describe these complex reaction pathways.

5.3.6.1 *Reversible Reactions*

In reversible processes, one has to account for the rates of forward and reverse reactions. Let us consider a simple reversible reaction with first-order forward and reverse reactions:

$$\mathbf{A} \underset{k_r}{\overset{k_f}{\rightleftharpoons}} \mathbf{B} \quad (5.35)$$

$$\text{Rate of forward reaction} = k_f a \quad (5.36)$$

$$\text{Rate of reverse reaction} = k_r b \quad (5.37)$$

At equilibrium, the rates of forward and reverse reactions are the same i.e. $k_f\, a_{eq} = k_r\, b_{eq}$, where a_{eq} and b_{eq} are the equilibrium concentrations of A and B.

When equilibrium is attained, the concentrations of A and B (a_{eq} and b_{eq}) are constant and the equilibrium constant K_{eq} can be expressed as follows:

$$K_{eq} = \frac{b_{eq}}{a_{eq}} = \frac{k_f}{k_r} \quad (5.38)$$

The overall rate of reaction, i.e., the approach to equilibrium from a system starting from A, can be expressed as follows:

$$\text{Rate} = -\frac{da}{dt} = k_f a - k_r b \quad (5.39)$$

Since b can be expressed as $(a_0 - a)$, the rate can be expressed as follows:

$$\text{Rate} = -\frac{da}{dt} = (k_f + k_r)a - k_r a_0 \quad (5.40)$$

The integral form of the rate equation can be written as follows:

$$\log(a - a_{eq}) = \log(a_0 - a_{eq}) - t\left[\frac{k_f + k_r}{2.303}\right] \quad (5.41)$$

Observe that when the experimental conditions favor the forward reaction much more, and the equilibrium is shifted far to the right, and a_{eq} and k_r approach zero, K_{eq} would approach infinity and Eq. 5.41 would be similar to the first-order rate equation, Eq. 5.18.

Konishi and coworkers [8] studied the equilibrium between Triazolam (B) and its hydrolysis product (A) in aqueous solution, at several solution pH values. The reaction represents a dehydration-hydrolysis equilibrium, with Triazolam being the dehydration product of the forward reaction (Figure 5.5). The left

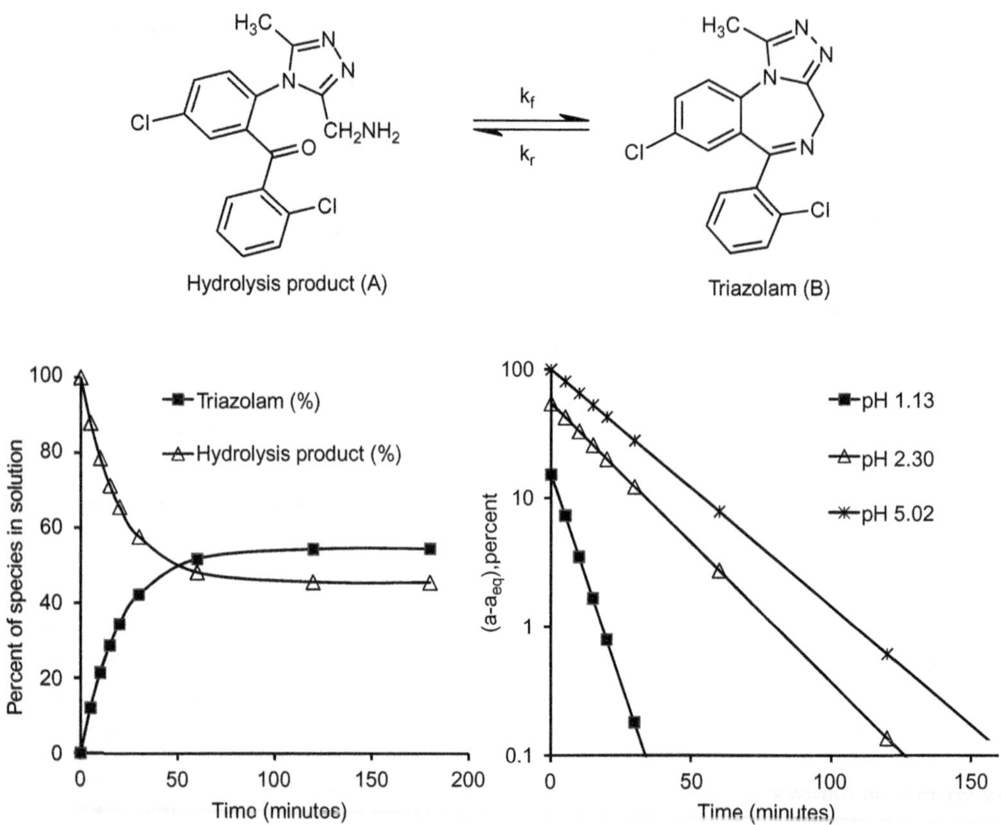

FIGURE 5.5 Hydrolysis-dehydration equilibrium of Triazolam (B) in solution. Left panel: the attainment of equilibrium starting from 100% hydrolysis product (A) at pH 2.3, ionic strength 0.5 M, and a temperature of 37°C. Right panel: semi-log plots of (a-a$_{eq}$) versus time at different pH values. Additional description is included in the text. *(Graphs plotted using data obtained from reference [8].)*

panel in the figure represents the change in concentrations of the two species, starting with 100% A in a solution at pH 2.30, ionic strength 0.5 M, and 37°C. This plot, when followed to equilibrium, enables determination of the equilibrium concentrations of the hydrolysis product and Triazolam (a_{eq} and b_{eq}, respectively) and the equilibrium constant K_{eq} using Eq. 5.38. As seen from Eq. 5.41 and the right panel of Figure 5.5, a semi-log plot of $(a - a_{eq})$ versus time yields a straight line with a slope equal to $(k_f + k_r)/2.303$. Here, a and a_{eq} refer to the concentration of the hydrolysis product, at time t and at equilibrium. The slope of the line represents the speed of attainment of equilibrium (i.e., $a - a_{eq} = 0$). From the slope and the equilibrium constant, the individual rate constants k_f and k_r were computed using Eqs. 5.38 and 5.41.

The right panel in Figure 5.5 also reveals the pH dependence of this equilibrium. The Y-intercepts of the lines are equal to $a_0 - a_{eq} = b_{eq}$, i.e., the equilibrium amount of B under the defined conditions. As seen in the figure, the equilibrium fractions of Triazolam at pH 1.13, 2.30, and 5.02 were approximately 15%, 55%, and 100%, respectively. Therefore, Triazolam solutions, when maintained at pH values >5, would exhibit minimal formation of the hydrolysis product.

5.3.6.2 *Consecutive Reactions*

The product of one reaction can further react, leading to a series of consecutive reactions. For example, ethyl eicosapentaenoate (EPA ethyl ester), an omega-3 polyunsaturated fatty acid ester derived from fish oil, undergoes autoxidation. Teraoka et al. studied autoxidation kinetics of EPA ethyl ester, which followed consecutive reaction kinetics with an initial induction period (see Eq. 5.42) [9].

$$\left[\text{EPA} \xrightarrow{R_i} \text{EPA}^*\right] \xrightarrow{k'} \text{Peroxide} \xrightarrow{k''} \text{Secondary products} \tag{5.42}$$

The oxidation reaction starts after the concentration of initiator radicals reaches a minimum concentration and the induction time required to attain this state EPA* is t_0. R_i represents the rate of generation of initiator radicals. The first-order rate constants of (i) formation of peroxide from the activated EPA* and (ii) conversion of the peroxide to secondary oxidation products (aldehydes and acids) are referred to as k' and k'', respectively.

The first-order rate equation for the conversion of EPA to peroxide can be represented as in Eq. 5.43

where $[EPA]_0$ represents the initial concentration of EPA. Note the similarity with the first-order rate equation, Eq. 5.17, with the addition of the induction period t_0, which precedes the formation of peroxide:

$$[EPA] = [EPA]_0 e^{-k'(t-t_0)} \quad (5.43)$$

The rate of change of peroxide concentration (rate of formation − rate of consumption) can be expressed as follows:

$$\begin{aligned}\frac{d[\text{Peroxide}]}{dt} &= k'[EPA] - k''[\text{Peroxide}] \\ &= k'[EPA]_0 e^{-k'(t-t_0)} - k''[\text{Peroxide}]\end{aligned} \quad (5.44)$$

which upon integration yields

$$[\text{Peroxide}] = \frac{k'[EPA]_0}{k''-k'}\left[e^{-k'(t-t_0)} - e^{-k''(t-t_0)}\right] \quad (5.45)$$

The concentration of products of secondary oxidation can be expressed as follows:

$$[\text{Secondary products}] = [EPA]_0 - [EPA] - [\text{Peroxide}] \quad (5.46)$$

From Eqs. 5.43, 5.45, and 5.46, we can write

$$\begin{aligned}&[\text{Secondary products}] \\ &= [EPA]_0\left[1 + \frac{1}{k''-k'}\left(k'e^{-k''(t-t_0)} - k''e^{-k'(t-t_0)}\right)\right]\end{aligned} \quad (5.47)$$

If the mechanism does not involve a lag time (induction time), the term $t - t_0$ can be replaced by t.

5.3.6.3 *Parallel Reactions*

Several drugs degrade simultaneously by multiple pathways, the predominant pathway being dependent on the conditions. These pathways could include different chemical transformations or different catalytic pathways for the same transformation.

For a molecule A, which degrades by parallel pathways as shown below and where both pathways exhibit first-order kinetics, the rate equations can be expressed as follows:

$$A \xrightarrow{k_b} B, \quad A \xrightarrow{k_c} C \quad (5.48)$$

$$\text{Rate of loss of A} = -\frac{da}{dt} = k_b a + k_c a = (k_b + k_c)a = (k_{obs})a \quad (5.49)$$

In Eq. 5.49, k_b and k_c are the first-order rate constants for formation of B and C, respectively, and k_{obs} is the observed first-order rate constant for loss of A. When the reaction is monitored by following the appearance of B and C, the following relationships can be used to determine the rate constants of the individual reactions:

$$\frac{k_b}{k_c} = \frac{b}{c}; \quad k_{obs} = k_b\left(1 + \frac{c}{b}\right) = k_c\left(1 + \frac{b}{c}\right) \quad (5.50)$$

Bundgaard and Hansen studied the kinetics of degradation of pilocarpine, which underwent simultaneous epimerization and hydrolysis to yield isopilocarpine and pilocarpic acid, respectively, as shown in Eq. 5.51. While the epimerization was determined to be a reversible reaction, the hydrolysis reactions of both epimers under the conditions of the experiment were irreversible. In addition, there was no interconversion between hydrolysis products C and D [10].

Pilocarpine (A) ⇌ (k_1, k_2) Isopilocarpine (B); Pilocarpine (A) → (k_3) Pilocarpic acid (C); Isopilocarpine (B) → (k_4) Isopilocarpic acid (D) (5.51)

Let us first consider the parallel reactions (epimerization and hydrolysis) leading to loss of pilocarpine in solution. The overall loss of pilocarpine (A) as well as the individual parallel reactions followed pseudo first-order kinetics. The observed rate of loss of A can be expressed as a sum of the rates of the two parallel reactions:

$$\text{Rate} = -\left[\frac{da}{dt}\right]_{epimerization} - \left[\frac{da}{dt}\right]_{hydrolysis} \quad (5.52)$$

From Eqs. 5.51 and 5.52, the overall observed rate of loss of pilocarpine can also be expressed as follows:

$$\text{Rate of loss of A} = (k_1a - k_2b) + k_3a \quad (5.53)$$

Here, a and b refer to the concentrations of pilocarpine (A) and isopilocarpine (B, epimerization product), respectively. From the first-order loss of pilocarpine in a solution containing 1 mg/mL of pilocarpine HCl in a 0.1 M carbonate buffer (pH 10.9) at 37°C, the authors determined the overall first-order degradation rate constant, $k_{obs} = 0.047\ min^{-1}$. At the end of the reaction, it was determined that 86% of the pilocarpine had degraded to pilocarpic acid (C), and the remaining was accounted for by isopilocarpic acid (D). Therefore, the value of k_3 was determined as $0.86 \times (k_{obs}) = 0.040\ min^{-1}$.

The reader would appreciate that the irreversible hydrolysis of isopilocarpine to yield isopilocarpic acid would consume the product of the reversible epimerization reaction (decrease the value of b and hence the value of k_2b in Eq. 5.53). This would drive the forward reaction, i.e., epimerization to maintain the equilibrium. An apparent first-order rate constant for loss of pilocarpine via the epimerization route was determined as $k_{epimerization} = k_{obs} - k_3 = 0.007\ min^{-1}$.

For drugs with multiple degradation pathways, the relative proportions of each degradation product would therefore be a function of the rate constants associated with each pathway. The reaction conditions (i.e., formulation composition, packaging, and storage conditions) will influence the relative rates of these parallel pathways. Often it might be necessary to perform a "balancing act" to minimize overall degradation. In such cases, a thorough understanding of the mechanism and kinetics of all the pathways is valuable.

5.3.7 Enzyme Catalysis

Enzymes are proteins that catalyze several biochemical reactions. The interaction between an enzyme (E) and a substrate (S) yields an enzyme-substrate complex, which then results in formation of the product (P), as shown here:

$$E + S \underset{k_2}{\overset{k_1}{\rightleftharpoons}} E \cdot S \xrightarrow{k_3} E + P \quad (5.54)$$

The total initial enzyme concentration $[E_0]$ can be expressed as follows:

$$[E_0] = [E] + [E \cdot S] \quad (5.55)$$

Based on the preceding scheme, we can express the rate of formation of E·S and the rate of product formation as follows:

$$\frac{d[E \cdot S]}{dt} = k_1[E][S] - k_2[E \cdot S] - k_3[E \cdot S] \quad (5.56)$$

$$\frac{d[E \cdot S]}{dt} = k_1[E][S] - (k_2 + k_3)\,[E \cdot S] \quad (5.57)$$

$$\frac{d[P]}{dt} = k_3[E \cdot S] \quad (5.58)$$

During the course of the reaction, if we can assume that the rate of formation of E·S is the same as the rate of breakdown of E·S to product, then the concentration of E·S remains fairly constant (a steady-state approximation):

$$\text{At steady state,} \frac{d[E \cdot S]}{dt} = 0 \quad (5.59)$$

Therefore, from Eqs. 5.57 and 5.59, the steady-state concentration of the complex can be expressed as follows:

$$[E \cdot S]_{ss} = \frac{k_1[E][S]}{k_2 + k_3} \quad (5.60)$$

Since no enzyme is consumed in the reaction

$$\text{at steady state, } [E_0] - [E \cdot S]_{SS} = [E] \quad (5.61)$$

From equations Eqs. 5.60 and 5.61

$$[E \cdot S]_{SS} = \frac{k_1[S]([E_0] - [E \cdot S]_{SS})}{k_2 + k_3} \quad (5.62)$$

Therefore,

$$[E \cdot S]_{SS} = \frac{k_1[S][E_0] - k_1[S][E \cdot S]_{SS}}{k_2 + k_3} \quad (5.63)$$

$$(k_2 + k_3)[E \cdot S]_{SS} = k_1[S][E_0] - k_1[S][E \cdot S]_{SS} \quad (5.64)$$

$$(k_2 + k_3 + k_1[S])[E \cdot S]_{SS} = k_1[S][E_0] \quad (5.65)$$

K_m, the Michaelis–Menton constant, is defined as $K_m = (k_2 + k_3)/k_1$. In other words, it is the tendency of the E·S complex to yield product or dissociate back to the substrate, relative to the tendency to form the complex.

Therefore,

$$[E \cdot S]_{SS} = \frac{k_1[S][E_0]}{k_2 + k_3 + k_1[S]} = \frac{[S][E_0]}{K_m + [S]} \quad (5.66)$$

Under steady-state conditions, the overall velocity of the reaction is the rate of formation of product:

$$V = \frac{dP}{dt} = k_3[E \cdot S]_{SS} = \frac{k_3[S][E_0]}{K_m + [S]} \tag{5.67}$$

When the substrate concentration is very large, then all the enzyme is saturated with the substrate, i.e., $[E_0] = [E \cdot S]$, and the reaction proceeds at maximum velocity V_{max}:

$$\text{Therefore, maximum velocity} = V_{max} = k_3[E \cdot S] = k_3[E_0] \tag{5.68}$$

Therefore, the velocity equation (Eq. 5.67) can be written in terms of the Michaelis–Menton equation:

$$V = \frac{k_3[S][E_0]}{K_m + [S]} = \frac{V_{max}[S]}{K_m + [S]} \tag{5.69}$$

From the Michaelis–Menton equation, at very high concentration of substrate, i.e., when $[S] >> K_m$, the velocity approaches V_{max} and is independent of substrate concentration. On the other hand, when the substrate concentration is low, i.e., $[S] << K_m$, then the velocity is directly proportional to the substrate concentration.

By rearranging the Michaelis–Menton equation, we obtain the Lineweaver–Burke equation, which can be graphically used to obtain the values of K_m and V_{max} from V versus [S] data:

$$\frac{1}{V} = \frac{1}{V_{max}} + \frac{K_m}{V_{max}[S]} \tag{5.70}$$

5.3.8 Reaction Kinetics in the Solid State

The chemical reaction kinetics described in earlier sections were derived from kinetic behavior in homogeneous liquid and gaseous systems. When a reaction occurs in a solid state, the reaction sites are not homogeneously distributed in the solid mass. In a crystalline solid, for example, the reaction occurs or is initiated at higher energy sites such as crystal defects on surfaces and edges of the particle. The direct application of kinetic equations developed for homogeneous systems, for processes occurring in nonhomogeneous systems, is therefore limited. The kinetic treatment of chemical reactions of pure solids, for example, can be based on (i) contracting geometries of reactant phases, (ii) nucleation and growth of the product phase, or (iii) liquid decomposition product layers. Interested readers are directed to literature that discusses solid-state reaction kinetics in greater detail [11,12].

5.3.8.1 *Prout–Tompkins Model*

In this chapter, we look at one specific kinetic model that describes chemical reactions in the solid state.

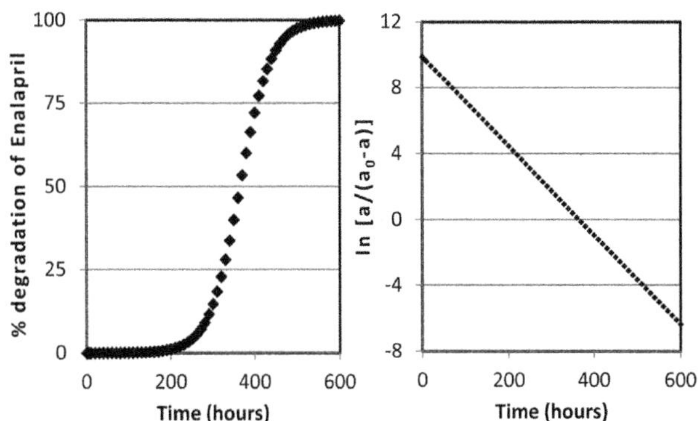

FIGURE 5.6 Solid-state decomposition kinetics of enalapril at 80°C and 0% RH. Additional details are provided in the text. *(The plots have been constructed using data reported in reference [13].)*

Mechanistically, this model is based on initiation and propagation of reactions from active nuclei in the solid, and the reaction rate is assumed to be proportional to the number of nuclei. The model includes an induction time required for generation of an appropriate density of active nuclei and is mathematically expressed in Eq. 5.71:

$$\ln\left[\frac{a}{(a_0 - a)}\right] = kt + c \tag{5.71}$$

In Eq. 5.71, a_0 represents the initial amount of reactant, a is the amount remaining at time t, k is the reaction rate constant, and c is a term that accounts for the induction time. Stanisz studied the solid-state decomposition of enalapril, an inhibitor of angiotensin-converting enzyme [13]. The progress of the degradation reaction plotted as % decomposition versus time reveals a sigmoidal relationship with induction, acceleration, and decay periods (Figure 5.6, left panel). A log-linear relationship, as expressed in the Prout–Tompkins equation, Eq. 5.71 was obtained (Figure 5.6, right panel) when $\log_e[a/(a_0 - a)]$ was plotted as a function of time. This suggested that the reaction followed a solid-state nucleation and propagation mechanism.

Pharmaceutical formulations are highly complicated multicomponent systems with several factors influencing the mechanisms and kinetics of drug degradation. We address some of the key factors in subsequent sections.

5.3.9 Factors Affecting Reaction Kinetics

5.3.9.1 *Temperature*

The shelf-life of pharmaceutical products is defined under specified packaging configurations and conditions of storage (temperature and humidity). Often, higher temperatures are utilized to accelerate decomposition reactions in order to study the degradation behavior of drug substances and drug products. An increase in temperature by 10°C near room temperature is known to cause a two- to four-fold increase in reaction rate for many reactions. An increase in temperature causes an increase in the velocities of molecules and hence the rates of collisions between them. These collisions between reacting molecules can be considered as a prerequisite for bimolecular reactions. However, not all collisions will result in the conversion of reactants to products. The molecules possess a distribution of velocities and hence a distribution of energy levels. The energy of activation, E_a, is a measure of the minimum energy required for the colliding molecules to overcome repulsive forces, interact, form high-energy intermediates, and yield reaction products. The *Arrhenius equation*, which describes the relationship between temperature and reaction rate, can be written as follows:

$$k = Ae^{-E_a/RT} \tag{5.72}$$

$$\log k = \log A - \frac{E_a}{2.303\ RT} \tag{5.73}$$

In the Arrhenius equation, R is the universal gas constant (1.987 cal K^{-1} $mole^{-1}$), T is the absolute temperature, E_a is the activation energy, and the term A is referred to as the frequency factor. This factor is a measure of the number of collisions that occur, satisfying conditions, such as molecular orientation. The term $e^{(-Ea/RT)}$ is a measure of the fraction of molecules that possess energies greater than or equal to E_a at temperature T. With an increase in temperature, the fraction of molecules that possess adequate energy increases. This leads to an increase in the reaction rate.

According to the transition state theory, reactant molecules must first achieve an activated higher energy state before the formation of products. This requires the formation of transition states, involving bond formation and cleavage, which lead to generation of product molecules. The energy difference between the reactants and this high-energy state is the *energy of activation* required for the forward reaction (Figure 5.7). The reaction scheme is shown in Eq. 5.74, where K* is the equilibrium constant for the formation of the complex and k′ is the rate constant for its breakdown.

$$\underset{\text{Reactants}}{A + B} \underset{}{\overset{K^*}{\rightleftharpoons}} \underset{\text{Activated complex}}{[A \cdots B]} \xrightarrow{k'} \text{Products} \tag{5.74}$$

$$\text{Reaction Rate} = k'[A \cdots B] = K^*k'[A][B] = k[A][B] \tag{5.75}$$

In Eq. 5.75, *k*, the rate constant of the overall reaction, is numerically equal to the product of the equilibrium constant for formation of the activated complex and the first-order rate constant for decomposition of the activated complex to the product phase.

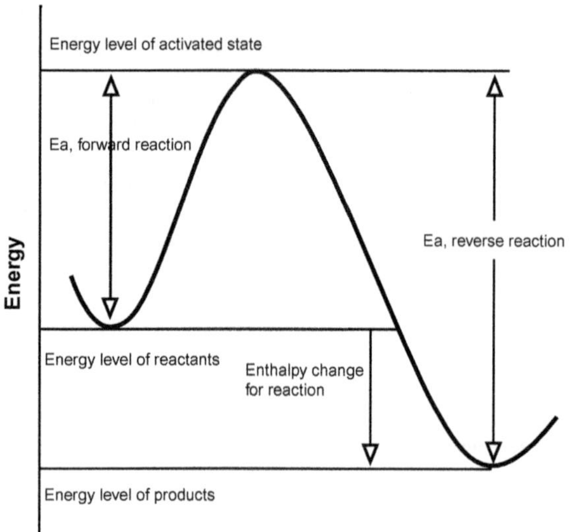

FIGURE 5.7 Energy relationship between reactants, products, and activated state.

Based on thermodynamic considerations, the equilibrium constant K* can be expressed as

$$K^* = e^{-\Delta G^*/RT} = e^{-[\Delta H^* - T\Delta S^*]/RT} = e^{-[\Delta H^*/RT]}e^{[\Delta S^*/R]} \tag{5.76}$$

$$k = k'K^* = k'e^{[\Delta S^*/R]} \cdot e^{-[\Delta H^*/RT]} \tag{5.77}$$

In the preceding equations, ΔG*, ΔH*, and ΔS* represent the free energy, enthalpy, and entropy change associated with formation of the activated complex.

A comparison between Eq. 5.77 and the Arrhenius equation, Eq. 5.72, reveals the similarity between the activation energy E_a and ΔH*, which is also seen in Figure 5.7. The comparison also suggests a parallel between the entropy change involved with the formation of the activated complex and the Arrhenius frequency factor A. The higher the entropy change associated with the formation of the activated complex, the greater is the probability of formation of the complex, i.e., higher is the frequency factor.

$$A = k'e^{[\Delta S^*/R]} \tag{5.78}$$

Catalysis, as seen before for enzymatic reactions, refers to a phenomenon in which a molecule, the catalyst, interacts with a reactant to reduce the activation energy for the reaction that is catalyzed. Consequently, at a given temperature, the fraction of reactant molecules that are energetic enough to cross the energy barrier is higher, in the presence of a catalyst. Hence, the reaction rate is faster. The net concentration of the catalyst does not change during the reaction, since it itself does not undergo any change in the process.

As a representative example, let us consider the effect of temperature on OH^- catalyzed degradation of

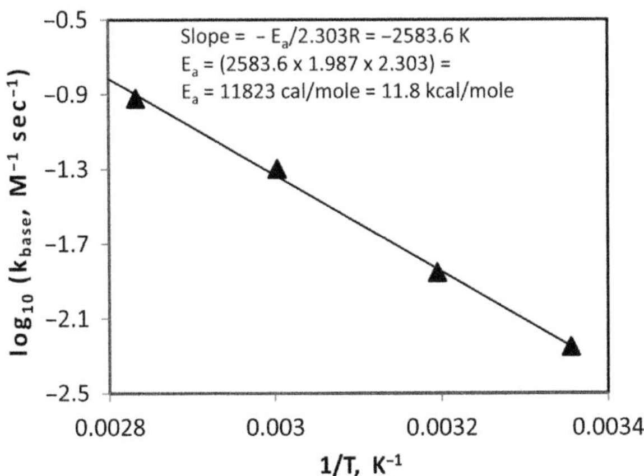

FIGURE 5.8 Arrhenius plot of log of specific base-catalyzed degradation rate constant of moexipril versus reciprocal of absolute temperature. A temperature range of 25°C–80°C is plotted. The calculation of the activation energy E_a for this catalyzed pathway is shown in the figure. *(Graph plotted using data adapted from reference [14].)*

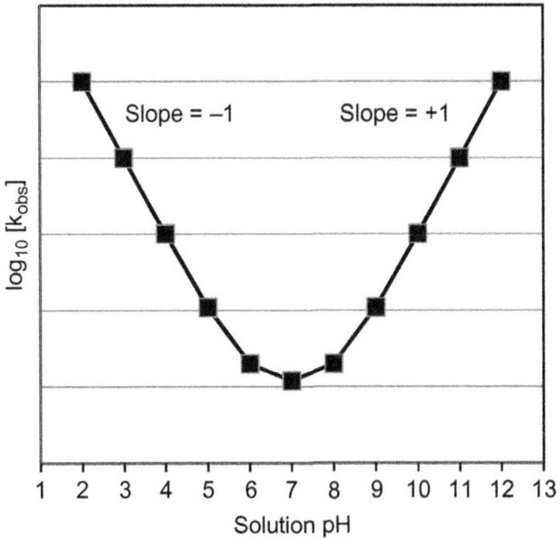

FIGURE 5.9 pH-rate profile for a hypothetical reaction with equal specific acid- and base-catalyzed rate constants (k_{acid} and k_{base}), with a minimum reaction rate at pH = 7. Since both the specific acid- and base-catalyzed pathways are of partial first order with respect to the catalysts (H^+ and OH^- ions), the slopes of the arms of the U-shaped profile are −1 and +1. The ratio of the catalyzed rate constants (k_{acid} or k_{base}) to the uncatalyzed or solvent-catalyzed rate constant (k') in this hypothetical case was 10^6.

moexipril, an inhibitor of angiotensin-converting enzyme [14]. A plot of the logarithm of the second-order rate constant, k_{base}, as a function of the reciprocal of absolute temperature, is shown in Figure 5.8. The straight-line relationship obtained is described in Eq. 5.73. The calculation of energy of activation from the slope of the line is presented in Figure 5.8.

5.3.9.2 Solution pH

The influence of solution pH on chemical reactivity in liquid formulations has been extensively studied. In particular, the rates of hydrolytic reactions can exhibit a dependence on solution pH, due to catalytic effects of H^+ or OH^- ions and various buffer species in solution. The effect of solution pH on reaction kinetics can be complicated and influenced by several factors. In the following paragraphs, we attempt to understand these effects in a stepwise fashion.

The terms *specific acid-catalysis* and *base-catalysis* describe the catalytic effect of hydrogen (or hydronium) ions and hydroxide ions in solution. We saw an example of this in the alkaline hydrolysis of ethyl acetate, Eqs. 5.4–5.6. When the reaction is catalyzed by the acidic or basic components of buffers used in the formulations, it is termed as *general acid-catalysis* or *base-catalysis*.

5.3.9.3 Specific Acid- and Base-Catalysis

Let us first consider the kinetics of specific acid- and base-catalyzed degradation of a compound E. In dilute aqueous solution, if the degradation proceeds along solvent-catalyzed (or uncatalyzed) as well as specific acid- and base-catalyzed pathways, the observed pseudo first-order rate constant, k_{obs}, can be expressed as a sum of three rate constants, as shown in Eq. 5.80:

$$\text{Rate} = -\frac{d[E]}{dt} = k_{obs}[E] \quad (5.79)$$

$$k_{obs} = k' + k_{acid}[H^+] + k_{base}[OH^-] \quad (5.80)$$

Equation 5.80 reveals that the specific acid- and base-catalyzed reactions are second-order processes, which will appear first order at constant H^+ or OH^- concentrations. The rates of these catalyzed pathways will depend on the concentration of the respective catalysts, i.e., H^+ or OH^- ions, and hence the solution pH. The terms k_{acid} and k_{base} are the second-order specific acid- and base-catalyzed rate constants. The term k' describes the rate constant associated with the solvent (water)-catalyzed process. It also represents a pseudo first-order process because the term includes the concentration of water, which is constant and in large excess.

Figure 5.9 is a plot of $\log_{10}$ (k_{obs}) versus solution pH, in a hypothetical situation, in which the specific acid- and base-catalyzed rate constants k_{base} and k_{acid} are of equal magnitude. The minimum value of the observed rate constant is therefore at pH 7. If the reaction represented degradation of a drug in solution, the pH of maximum stability would therefore be 7. Since the partial order of the catalyzed pathways with respect to

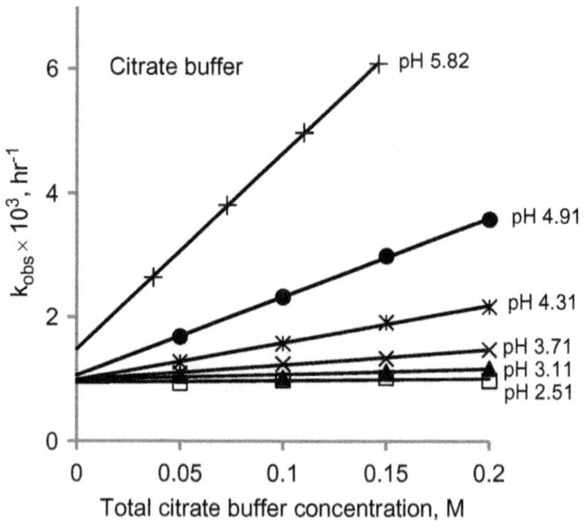

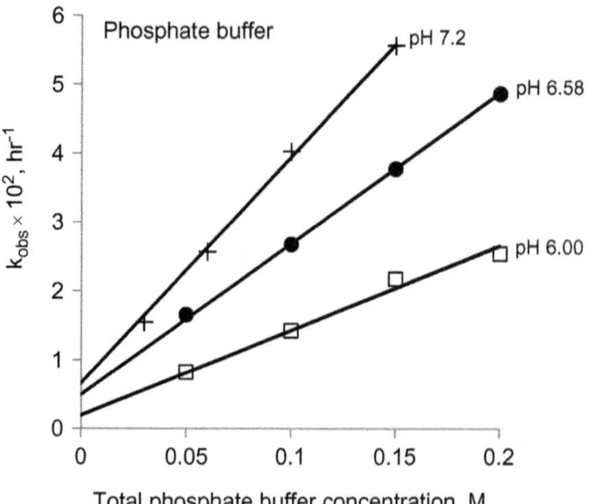

FIGURE 5.10 Effect of buffer concentrations and solution pH on the pseudo first-order rate constant (k_{obs}) of degradation of cefadroxil at 35°C and an ionic strength of 0.5. The left panel depicts the effects of a citrate buffer in an acidic pH range, and the right panel depicts the influence of a phosphate buffer in a higher pH range. *(Graphs were plotted based on data obtained from reference [15].)*

the catalysts (H^+ and OH^-) is one (Eq. 5.80), the two arms of the profile will have slopes of -1 and $+1$, respectively.

When the catalytic effects of H^+ and OH^- are not of equal magnitude (i.e., $k_{acid} \neq k_{base}$), the pH of maximum stability will shift. For example, the pH rate profile for the hydrolysis of atropine at 30°C revealed maximum stability at pH 3.7 due to $k_{base} > k_{acid}$[3].

The shape of the pH-rate constant profile will depend on the magnitude of k' relative to k_{base} and k_{acid}. For example, the ratio of the catalyzed rate constants (k_{acid} or k_{base}) to the solvent-catalyzed rate constant (k') in the hypothetical case in Figure 5.9 was 10^6. This reveals a very narrow pH range of maximum stability due to relatively high catalytic rates for both the specific acid- and base-catalyzed pathways. If this ratio of catalyzed to uncatalyzed rate constants were lower in magnitude, the base of the pH-rate curve would be "flatter," resulting in a broader pH range over which the reaction rates would be low.

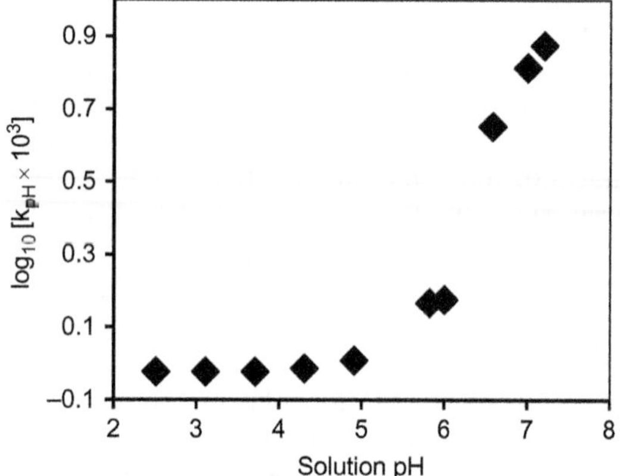

FIGURE 5.11 Buffer-independent, pseudo first-order rate constants for degradation of cefadroxil at 35°C and an ionic strength of 0.5, plotted as a function of solution pH. These rate constants were obtained by extrapolation of the "rate constants vs. buffer concentration" plots in Figure 5.10 to zero buffer concentration. *(Graphs were plotted based on data obtained from reference [15].)*

5.3.9.4 General Acid- and Base-Catalysis

The solution pH of pharmaceutical formulations therefore is frequently adjusted with buffers to achieve minimum degradation rates and hence maximum stability. The choice of buffer can be critical because, in addition to specific acid- and base-catalysis, the reaction can be catalyzed by the buffer species utilized to maintain the desired solution pH, i.e., general acid-base catalysis. For example, if a buffer system comprising a weak acid HX and its conjugate base X^- is utilized to control the solution pH, Eq. 5.80 can be further written as follows, where k_{HX} and k_{X^-} are the general acid- and base-catalyzed rate constants:

$$k_{obs} = k' + k_{acid}[H^+] + k_{base}[OH^-] + k_{HX}[HX] + k_{X^-}[X^-] \tag{5.81}$$

Let us consider the pH dependence of degradation of cefadroxil, a cephalosporin antibiotic, in buffered aqueous solutions [15]. Each of the plots in Figure 5.10 represents the effect of total buffer molarity on the observed rate constant of cefadroxil degradation at a given solution pH. The *buffer-independent rate constants* at each pH value were obtained by extrapolation of this straight-line relationship to zero buffer concentration and are expressed as k_{pH} in Figure 5.11. These k_{pH} values, when plotted as a function of solution pH, yield the buffer-independent pH-rate constant profiles as shown in Figure 5.11 for cefadroxil. Such plots reveal the influence of pH on reaction rates in the absence of general catalysis by buffer species.

$$k_{pH} = k' + k_{acid}[H^+] + k_{base}[OH^-] \quad (5.82)$$

In the left panel of Figure 5.10, at low pH values (2.51 and 3.11), the citrate buffer molarity from 0.05 M to 0.2 M had only a small effect on reaction rate. The influence of citrate buffer concentration on reaction rate (i.e., the slope of the line) increased with an increase in solution pH, between pH 3.71 and 5.82. The slope of these lines is the catalytic rate constant for the overall buffer-catalyzed degradation. If we represent this constant as k_{cit}, Eq. 5.82 can be rewritten as follows:

$$k_{obs} = k' + k_{acid}[H^+] + k_{base}[OH^-] + k_{cit}[\text{total citrate}] \quad (5.83)$$

Citric acid is a triprotic acid with p*Ka* values of 3.1, 4.7, and 5.4. In the pH range studied, the total citrate buffer concentration can be expressed as a sum of the concentrations of the un-ionized acid and all the ionized species:

$$[\text{Total citrate}] = [H_3Cit] + [H_2Cit^-] + [HCit^{2-}] + [Cit^{3-}] \quad (5.84)$$

The buffer catalysis can therefore be expressed as a sum of the contributions from each buffer species:

$$k_{obs} = k' + k_{acid}[H^+] + k_{base}[OH^-] + k_{H_3Cit}[H_3Cit] + k_{H_2Cit^-}[H_2Cit^-] + k_{HCit^{2-}}[HCit^{2-}] + k_{Cit^{3-}}[Cit^{3-}] \quad (5.85)$$

Based on the p*Ka* values of citric acid, the solution pH and the total concentration of citrate, the concentrations of the individual buffer species can be calculated. Using the k_{cit} values determined from the slopes in Figure 5.10, and the distribution of the different citrate species, the authors determined the values of the second-order catalytic rate constants for each of the buffer species [15]:

$$k_{H_3Cit} = 9.7 \times 10^{-5}\ M^{-1}\ h^{-1}$$
$$k_{H_2Cit^-} = 1.85 \times 10^{-3}\ M^{-1}\ h^{-1}$$
$$k_{H_2Cit^{2-}} = 1.86 \times 10^{-2}\ M^{-1}\ h^{-1}$$
$$k_{Cit^{3-}} = 9.47 \times 10^{-2}\ M^{-1}\ h^{-1}$$

With an increase in solution pH, the degree of ionization of citric acid increases. The extent of ionization also progressively increases the catalytic rate constants of the citrate ions. Therefore, a change in solution pH could affect reaction rates by influencing the rates of specific acid- and base-catalyzed pathways as well as by influencing the rates of general acid/base catalysis.

The phosphate buffer in the pH range plotted in Figure 5.10 exists predominantly as $H_2PO_4^-$ and HPO_4^{2-}. A similar treatment of the phosphate buffered solutions yields Eq. 5.86:

$$k_{obs} = k' + k_{acid}[H^+] + k_{base}[OH^-] + k_{H_2PO_4^-}[H_2PO_4^-] + k_{HPO_4^{2-}}[HPO_4^{2-}] \quad (5.86)$$

The authors also determined the following values [15].

$$k_{H_2PO_4^-} = 6.8 \times 10^{-2}\ M^{-1}\ h^{-1}$$
$$k_{HPO_4^{2-}} = 0.378\ M^{-1}\ h^{-1}$$

5.3.9.5 *Ionization States of the Degradant*

Solution pH can also affect the ionization states of the drug undergoing degradation. The rate constants of uncatalyzed and specific- and general-, acid- and base-catalyzed reactions of the drug molecule in different states of ionization can be different. Cefadroxil is an amphoteric molecule with three p*Ka* values and can exist as a cation, a zwitterion, an anion, and a di-anion. The entire solution pH-reaction rate profile for cefadroxil can therefore be more complicated than the simplistic treatment discussed in the previous section [15].

Let us consider a simpler example of ciclosidomine (p*Ka* 4.6), depicted as D, which undergoes specific- and general-, acid- and base-catalyzed degradation in solution. The ionization equilibrium and the concentration of ionized (DH^+) and un-ionized (D) species can be expressed as follows:

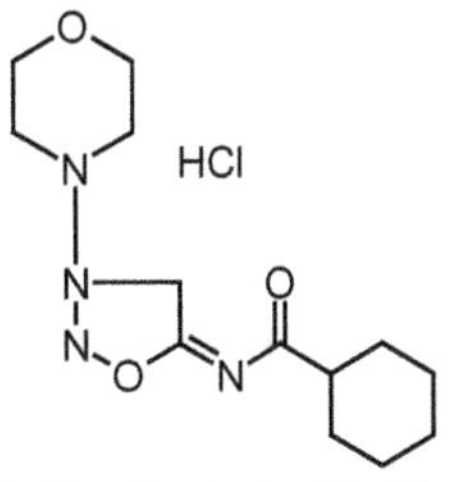

HCl

$$DH^+ \underset{}{\overset{K_a}{\rightleftharpoons}} D + H^+ \quad (5.87)$$

Ciclosidomine hydrochloride (D. HCl)

$$K_a = \frac{[D][H^+]}{[DH^+]} \quad (5.88)$$

$$[D]_{total} = [D] + [DH^+] \quad (5.89)$$

$$[D] = [D]_{total}\left(\frac{K_a}{K_a + [H^+]}\right) \quad (5.90)$$

$$[DH^+] = [D]_{total}\left(\frac{[H^+]}{K_a + [H^+]}\right) \quad (5.91)$$

Using the relationships in Eqs. 5.90 and 5.91, we can write an expression for the observed degradation rate constant, k_{obs}, in terms of k_D and k_{DH+}, the apparent first-order rate constants for overall degradation of the un-ionized and the ionized species, respectively:

$$k_{obs} = k_{DH^+}\frac{[DH^+]}{[D]_{Total}} + k_D\frac{[D]}{[D]_{Total}}$$

$$k_{obs} = \frac{k_{DH^+}[H^+]}{K_a + [H^+]} + \frac{k_D K_a}{K_a + [H^+]} = \frac{k_{DH^+}[H^+] + k_D K_a}{K_a + [H^+]} \quad (5.92)$$

If each species degrades by uncatalyzed and specific- and general-, acid- and base-catalysis, we can write the following expressions in which the rate constants with * correspond to the protonated species and the rate constants with the # correspond to the deprotonated form:

$$k_{DH^+} = k'^{*} + k^{*}_{acid}[H^+] + k^{*}_{base}[OH^-] + k^{*}_{HX}[HX] + k^{*}_{X^-}[X^-] \quad (5.93)$$

$$k_D = k'^{\#} + k^{\#}_{acid}[H^+] + k^{\#}_{base}[OH^-] + k^{\#}_{HX}[HX] + k^{\#}_{X^-}[X^-] \quad (5.94)$$

These expressions for k_{DH+} and k_D can be substituted in Eq. 5.92 to obtain the kinetic equation describing the sum of all pathways for both the un-ionized and the ionized forms of ciclosidomine.

It is also important to note that not all the terms in Eqs. 5.93 and 5.94 may be relevant. For example, concentrations of the protonated form of a weak base might be negligible in a pH range where significant specific base catalysis occurs, and hence, the corresponding term may be neglected (k^*_{base} $[OH^-]$, in the preceding example). Similarly, if the buffers used in the system have been shown not to exhibit any general catalysis, all the buffer terms can be removed from the equation.

Adjustment of solution pH, the choice of buffer and buffer concentration can therefore be critical in maintaining the chemical stability of a liquid formulation over shelf-life. A thorough understanding of all potential reaction pathways is therefore a prerequisite for formulation of a stable solution.

In the case of solid dosage forms as well, the use of acidic or basic excipients has been reported to control the microenvironment around the drug particles, thereby conferring enhanced chemical stability. It is suggested that the mechanism of action of these pH modifiers in the "near dry" solid state is based on their ability to influence the pH of the sorbed water on the solid surface, thereby providing an environment conducive to chemical stability [16,17].

5.3.9.6 Ionic Strength

Electrolytes are often added to solution formulations, for example, as buffers to adjust solution pH or as salts to adjust tonicity. In addition to these additives, ionizable drugs can contribute to the ionic strength of the formulation. The ionic strength of a solution, μ, can be expressed as follows, where m is the molar concentration and z is the charge of each ionic species:

$$\mu = 0.5\,\Sigma(mz^2) = 0.5(m_A z_A^2 + m_B z_B^2 \ldots\ldots) \quad (5.95)$$

The influence of ionic strength on the rate constants of interacting ionic species can be expressed by the Brønsted–Bjerrum equation:

$$\log k = \log k_0 + A\ Z_1 Z_2 \sqrt{\mu} \quad (5.96)$$

Z_1 and Z_2 are the charges on the two interacting ions, k is the rate constant at the ionic strength of μ, and k_0 is the rate constant at zero ionic strength, i.e., in an infinitely dilute solution. A in this equation is a constant that depends on the dielectric constant, density, and temperature of the solution and for dilute aqueous solutions at 298 K is equal to 1.018. Although this relationship is strictly obeyed up to an ionic strength of only ~0.01, a linear relationship between log k and $\mu^{0.5}$ is often seen in solutions of higher ionic strengths. Figure 5.12 depicts such a linear relationship up to an ionic strength of ~0.19 [18].

Based on a modified Debye–Huckel equation, a modified Brønsted–Bjerrum equation can be written and is preferable for higher ionic strengths of up to 0.1:

$$\log k = \log k_0 + A\ Z_1 Z_2 \left(\frac{\sqrt{\mu}}{1 + \sqrt{\mu}}\right) \quad (5.97)$$

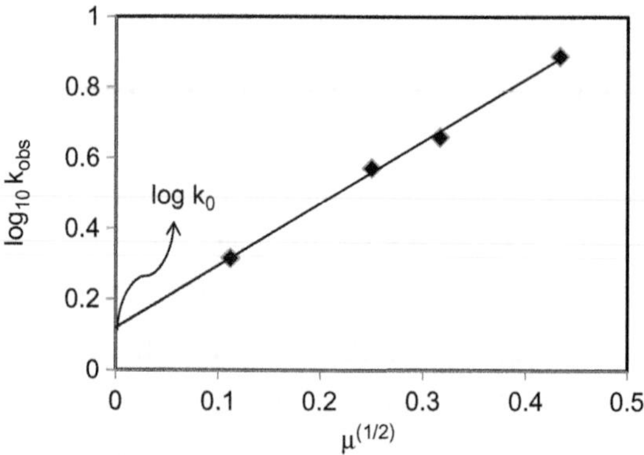

FIGURE 5.12 The effect of ionic strength on the rate constant of dismutation of a semiquinone free radical of chlorpromazine, in an HCl-KCl buffer at 25°C and a pH of 1.96. The straight-line relationship between the logarithm of the observed second-order rate constant (liter mole^{-1} sec^{-1}) and the square root of the ionic strength yields a Y intercept, which is the rate constant at zero ionic strength. The ionic strength range of the data points is from 0.013 to 0.19. *(Graph plotted with data reported in reference [18].)*

The ionic strength also influences the dissociation constants of ionizable drugs in solution due to its effect on ionic activity coefficients. At ionic strengths of up to 0.3 M, the influence of ionic strength on dissociation constants can be expressed as follows:

$$pK' = pK + \left(\frac{0.51(2Z-1)\sqrt{\mu}}{1+\sqrt{\mu}}\right) \quad (5.98)$$

In Eq. 5.98, K′ is the apparent dissociation constant at an ionic strength of μ, the term K is the thermodynamic dissociation constant at zero ionic strength, and Z is the charge on the conjugate acid.

If the ionized and un-ionized forms of a drug molecule exhibit different chemical reactivity, the ionic strength could also alter the rates of chemical reactions by altering the degree of ionization.

The kinetic salt effect in pharmaceutical systems has been discussed in detail elsewhere [19].

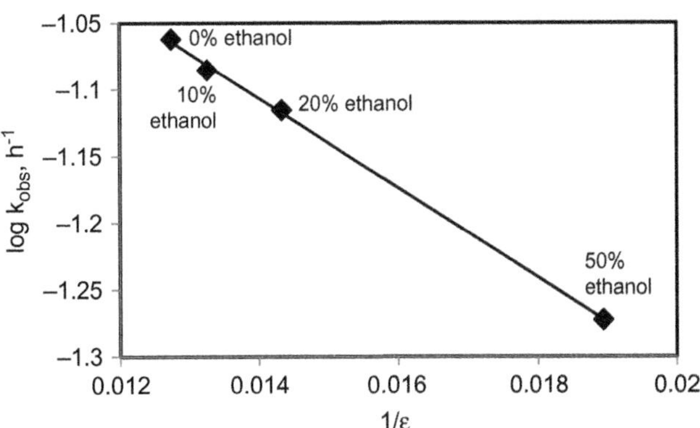

FIGURE 5.13 Effect of dielectric constant of solvent on the observed first-order rate constant of degradation of ampicillin in 0.08 N HCl. The dielectric constant was altered by addition of ethanol (0% to 50% ethanol, dielectric constant of 78.5 to 52.8). The measured pH was in the range of 1.2–1.25. *(Graph was plotted using data obtained from reference [20].)*

5.3.9.7 Dielectric Constant

Nonaqueous co-solvents are often used to enhance the solubility of drugs and prepare solution formulations. While the presence of the drug in solution itself may be detrimental to chemical stability, the solvent used may influence the dielectric constant of the system and hence the chemical reactivity.

The ability of a medium to facilitate interaction of reactants and to make the formation of transition states energetically favored will enhance the rates of reaction. For example, solvents having a high dielectric constant will favor reactions that involve formation of a polar transition state from neutral molecules. Reactions between oppositely charged ions, on the other hand, are accelerated in solvents of lower dielectric constants. The effect of dielectric constant on the rate of reaction can be expressed by the following equation [20]:

$$\log k_{obs} = \log k_0 - \frac{1}{\varepsilon}\left(\frac{N Z_A Z_B e^2}{2.303 R T d_{AB}}\right) \quad (5.99)$$

The term k_0 represents the rate constant in a medium with infinite dielectric constant, k_{obs} is the observed rate constant in a medium of dielectric constant ε, N is Avogadro's number, Z_A and Z_B are the charges of two interacting ions, e is the unit of electrical charge, and d_{AB} is the distance between the ions in the activated complex.

The degradation of ampicillin in 0.08 N HCl was evaluated as a function of alcohol concentration in solution (Figure 5.13). A plot of log k_{obs} versus 1/ε revealed a linear relationship in agreement with Eq. 5.99. The reaction rate decreased with an increase in the alcohol fraction, i.e., a decrease in the dielectric constant. The mechanism of degradation under acidic conditions is thought to involve an interaction of the ampicillin cation with a hydrated proton to form a dication activated complex. The interaction of these ions with like charge to form a higher-charged complex is favored by media of higher dielectric constant. Therefore, the reaction rate increases with a decrease in the fraction of ethanol [20].

5.3.9.8 Oxidizing Agents

For drugs susceptible to oxidation, availability of oxygen from the atmosphere can be detrimental to stability. In addition, oxygen dissolved either in liquid formulations or in the adsorbed water layers in solid formulations can promote oxidative degradation. Protective packaging, and removal of oxygen from the headspace in the packed product, can be employed to stabilize formulations against oxidation. Film-coating polymers with reduced oxygen permeability, for example, can be used to minimize oxygen penetration into tablet cores during storage.

Oxidation reactions can proceed by uncatalyzed auto-oxidation with molecular oxygen or by a chain process, which includes initiation, propagation, and termination steps involving free radicals. The chain processes can be initiated via free radicals generated by the action of light, heat, or transition metal impurities. Antioxidant strategies include (i) initiation inhibitors such as chelating agents (for example, EDTA and citric acid) to sequester metal ion initiators; (ii) protection against a part of the UV-visible spectrum by using colored glass containers; (iii) chain-breakers such as butylated hydroxy toluene and alpha-tocopherol, which react with the free radicals and form less-reactive free radicals; and (iv) reducing agents or oxygen scavengers such as sodium metabisulfite and ascorbic acid [21].

5.3.9.9 *Light*

Photo-labile compounds when exposed to light absorb certain frequencies and sufficient energy to get activated. This might lead to a photochemical reaction. Photochemical oxidation and reduction reactions are common. The reaction mechanisms are often multistep and complex. Protection of photo-labile drugs from light may be required during processing or compounding of the drug substance into the drug product and during storage of the drug product over its shelf-life.

5.3.9.10 *Water*

While water is present in large excess in aqueous liquid formulations, solid dosage forms have the advantage of having lower water content and hence may be comparatively less susceptible to degradation reactions mediated by water.

The humidity of the immediate surroundings and the affinity of the solid phase for water influence the water content in the solid formulation. Presence of hygroscopic materials and amorphous phases may result in a large uptake of water from the surroundings into the solid dosage forms. Water, when present, either adsorbed on the solid surface or absorbed into amorphous regions in the solid, can influence chemical reactivity as a reactant or a reaction product, or as a medium for the reaction to occur. Water can also plasticize amorphous regions in solid formulations, thus increasing the mobility of the molecules and their reactivity. When sufficient water is adsorbed on the surface to cause surface dissolution of the solid, the reactivity in this solution phase will be influenced by all the factors described earlier for solution systems. This might also provide avenues for stabilization of drugs, for example, by using acidic or basic excipients to control the chemical environment in these water layers.

For solid formulations, which need protection from water, drug product manufacturing operations that avoid the use of water are preferred. These formulations may also need special protective coatings and packaging materials and use of a desiccant in the packed product to act as water scavenger during shelf-life storage.

5.3.10 Stability Evaluation and Assignment of Shelf-Life

Each marketed pharmaceutical product must be assigned a shelf-life, over which it will retain its identity, safety, and efficacy by staying within established physical chemical, microbiological, therapeutic, and toxicological specifications. Stability studies are carried out on the drug product during development stages to understand storage-induced changes in any critical product attributes. When carried out under normal storage conditions, these studies can often take a long time to provide meaningful and useful data to guide development. Therefore, in order to speed up the process of identifying the right formulation and optimizing key product properties, accelerated stability studies are carried out. These studies subject the drug product to exaggerated environmental conditions to accelerate the rates of chemical degradation and physical changes. Data from accelerated and long-term stability studies are used together to understand the nature and extent of changes in the product over time. During the product development phase, these data aid in making appropriate changes to the formulation to enhance it stability. Stability studies on the final product at the commercial manufacturing scale, in the final container-closure system, guide the assignment of storage conditions and expiration dates (shelf-lives) for the marketed product.

Stress testing of a drug substance or drug product is often carried out under harsher conditions (for example, 50°C–60°C and 75% RH) than for accelerated testing (40°C/75% RH). This is done in most cases to identify degradation products and pathways, characterize the stability of the drug substance, and validate the analytical methods for their ability to be "stability indicating."

Accelerated stability studies are carried out at a series of higher-temperature conditions. As discussed earlier, the reaction order can be determined by plotting the data obtained, according to equations for each reaction order, and determining the order that provides the best fit. The values of the rate constant for that reaction order can then be determined for all the temperatures. A plot of log k versus 1/T would reveal an Arrhenius relationship with a slope of $[-E_a/2.303\ R]$, enabling the calculation of the energy of activation:

$$\log k = \log A - \frac{E_a}{2.303\ RT} \tag{5.100}$$

This straight-line relationship can also be used to determine the value of the rate constant at room temperature or any desired temperature of storage. By subtracting the Arrhenius equations at temperatures T_1 and T_2, we can obtain the following equations, if the value of frequency factor A is the same at T_1 and T_2:

$$\log \frac{k_2}{k_1} = \frac{E_a(T_2 - T_1)}{2.303\ R\ T_2 T_1} \tag{5.101}$$

If the energy of activation is known and the rate constant at any one temperature is known, the value of rate constant at another desired temperature can be determined.

If the reaction is of the first order, the time required for 10% loss of potency can be expressed as follows:

$$t_{0.9} = \frac{2.303}{k_1} \log \left[\frac{a_0}{0.9 a_0} \right] = \frac{0.105}{k_1} \tag{5.102}$$

Substituting for k in Eq. 5.100, we obtain, for a first order reaction:

$$\log t_{0.9} = \log 0.105 - \log A + \frac{E_a}{2.303\,RT} \qquad (5.103)$$

$$\log\frac{(t_{0.9})_1}{(t_{0.9})_2} = \frac{E_a(T_2 - T_1)}{2.303\,R\,T_2T_1} \qquad (5.104)$$

Therefore, if we define the shelf-life as time for 10% loss of potency, the shelf-life at any chosen temperature can be calculated from the knowledge of the activation energy and the value of $t_{0.9}$ at another temperature.

Figure 5.14 depicts plots of log k and log $t_{0.9}$ for the degradation of thiamine HCl in a multivitamin preparation as a function if 1/T [22]. The energy of activation was calculated from the slope of the log k versus 1/T plot, and was determined to be 25.8 kcal/mole. The time required for 10% of the thiamine HCl to degrade increased with decreasing temperature. Equation 5.103 can be utilized to calculate the shelf-life at the desired storage temperature.

Accelerated stability testing is meaningful only if the degradation is a thermal phenomenon. For example, if the rate of decomposition of the drug is determined by light-catalyzed reactions, extrapolation of data from higher temperatures may not accurately predict shelf-life under room temperature conditions. In addition, accelerated stability conditions may have limited utility for formulations that exhibit physical transitions such as melting, vaporization and glass transitions, crystallization of amorphous forms, and polymorphic transformations at higher temperatures—for example, melting of cream and ointment formulations. In such cases, there might be a discontinuity in the Arrhenius relationship of reaction rate with temperature.

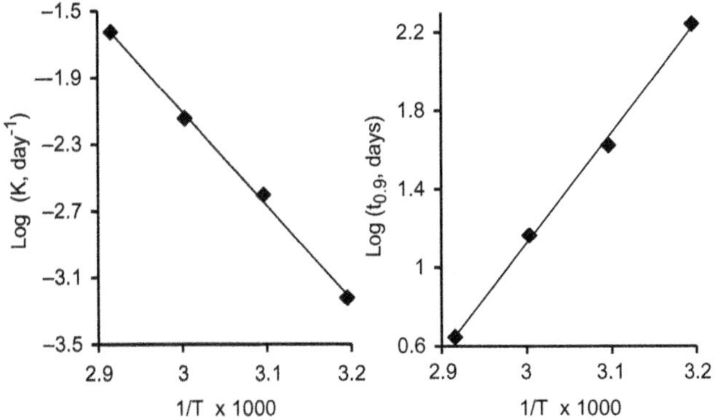

FIGURE 5.14 Left panel: Arrhenius plot of log (first-order degradation rate constant) of thiamine HCl in a multivitamin preparation versus 1/T (temperature range = 40°C–70°C). Right panel: Plot of log $t_{0.9}$ versus 1/T. *(Graphs plotted based on data obtained from reference [22].)*

Increased temperature can also decrease the solubility of volatile reactive species like oxygen. On the other hand, in suspension formulations, higher temperature storage can result in increased concentrations of the drug in the continuous phase. Higher temperatures can also affect solution pH and the relatively humidity in the headspace of sealed drug product containers. All these factors can influence reaction rates significantly and result in non-Arrhenius behavior [23]. Data from higher temperature storage should therefore be treated carefully with a thorough understanding of any additional factors that might influence reaction rates.

5.4. DIFFUSION

In the preceding sections, we discussed chemical-change processes, focusing mostly on chemical degradation in pharmaceuticals. We classified these chemical changes in terms of their progress as a function of time and looked at factors that could be altered to either speed up these changes (accelerated stability studies) or minimize the extent of their occurrence (stabilization of drug products against decomposition). In this and the next section, we focus on physical mass transport processes relevant in pharmaceutics.

Diffusion is the mass transport of individual molecules of a substance. This transport is a result of random motions of the molecules and is related to a *driving force*—for example, a chemical or electrical potential difference, pressure, temperature differences. The driving force determines the direction of mass transport.

Examples of diffusion processes relevant to pharmaceutics include (i) transport of drug out of controlled-release formulations, (ii) transport of drug molecules across biological barriers in the body during absorption and disposition processes, and (iii) diffusion of reactive gaseous molecules such as oxygen and water vapor into and out of pharmaceutical drug product containers. The objective of this section is to introduce the fundamental concepts of these transport processes. Applications of these concepts are also included in other chapters. Applications of these concepts, and discussions on diffusion in biological systems and membrane transport, are included in other chapters.

5.4.1 Fick's First Law of Diffusion

Fick's first law of diffusion describes the relationship between the amount of mass transfer occurring and the driving force responsible for the transfer.

Flux (J), is the amount of material moving across unit cross-sectional area of a barrier (which poses a resistance to the movement) in unit time. For a membrane with surface area = S, the flux can be mathematically expressed in terms of the mass transfer rate as follows:

$$\text{Flux} = J = \frac{1}{S}\frac{dM}{dt} \tag{5.105}$$

The units of flux are $gcm^{-2}sec^{-1}$. Flux is proportional to the driving force, which is responsible for the movement of material, i.e., the concentration gradient across the membrane. The expression of Fick's first law of diffusion is given in Eq. 5.106:.

$$\text{Flux} = J = -D\frac{dC}{dx} \tag{5.106}$$

D is the *diffusion coefficient or diffusivity* of the material undergoing transport (the diffusant). D is *not* a constant of proportionality, and changes depending on the properties and composition of the diffusion medium, temperature, pressure, and the nature and concentration of the diffusant. The units of D are cm^2/sec. The negative sign in the expression signifies that the movement of material is in a direction that is opposite to the direction of the concentration gradient. In other words, the movement of material is from a high er to lower concentration.

5.4.2 Fick's Second Law of Diffusion

Fick's second law of diffusion deals with changes in concentration of the diffusant, in a given region of the barrier, as a function of time. Let us consider a particular volume unit of the barrier. The change in concentration of the diffusant in that region with time is related to the movement of material into and out of the region, i.e., the change in flux of the material as a function of distance, along the direction of diffusion. Since both concentration and flux are functions of time as well as distance, we can express this relationship as follows:

$$\frac{\partial C}{\partial t} = -\frac{\partial J}{\partial x} \tag{5.107}$$

Differentiating the first law equation with respect to *x* (distance), we obtain

$$-\frac{\partial J}{\partial X} = D\frac{\partial[\partial C/\partial x]}{\partial x} = D\frac{\partial^2 C}{\partial x^2} \tag{5.108}$$

From Eqs. 5.107 and 5.108, we obtain the expression for Fick's second law of diffusion:

$$\frac{\partial C}{\partial t} = D\frac{\partial^2 C}{\partial x^2} \tag{5.109}$$

Fick's second law states that in a given region, the change in concentration as a function of time is directly proportional to the change in the concentration gradient as a function of distance.

Equation 5.109 represents diffusion only in one direction, say along the x-axis. The change in concentration of the diffusing agent in all three dimensions can be expressed as follows:

$$\frac{\partial C}{\partial t} = D\left(\frac{\partial^2 C}{\partial x^2} + \frac{\partial^2 C}{\partial y^2} + \frac{\partial^2 C}{\partial z^2}\right) \tag{5.110}$$

5.4.3 Diffusion across a Thin Membrane

Let us consider a thin membrane separating a donor compartment with a higher concentration of the diffusant (C_d) and a receptor compartment from which the solution is removed and replenished constantly with fresh solvent, to keep the concentrations of the diffusant low (C_r) and maintain sink conditions (Figure 5.15). After this system has been allowed to equilibrate for a while, the concentrations in the two compartments will become fairly constant. Under these conditions, the concentration of diffusant in a given location in the film will be constant, i.e., the rate of change of concentration a fixed location in the film (dC/dt) will be zero. By Fick's second law of diffusion

$$\frac{dC}{dt} = D\frac{d^2C}{dx^2} = 0 \tag{5.111}$$

This implies that under these conditions, the change in concentration gradient as a function of distance in the film is zero. The concentration gradient is constant, and the concentration of the diffusant (C) has a linear

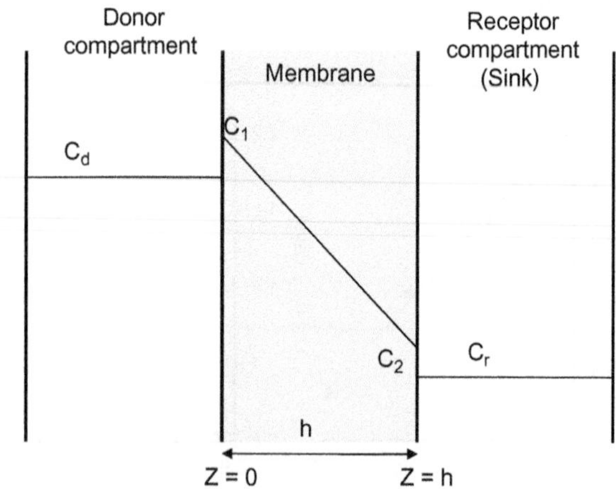

FIGURE 5.15 Diffusion across a thin membrane. The membrane of thickness *h* separates a donor compartment with a higher diffusant concentration of C_d and a receptor compartment with a lower diffusant concentration of C_r. The concentrations in the film at the donor end and the receptor end are C_1 and C_2, respectively.

relationship with the distance into the film (x). The concentrations may not be strictly constant but will only vary slightly with time giving rise to a "quasi-stationary state." Under these conditions of constant concentration gradient across the film thickness, dC/dx, the concentration gradient can be approximated as $[C_2 - C_1/h]$, where C_2 and C_1 represent the concentration of the diffusant molecule *in the membrane* at the receptor side and the donor side, respectively. Therefore, the first law of diffusion can be written as follows:

$$\text{Flux} = J = -D\frac{dC}{dx} = -D\frac{(C_2 - C_1)}{h} = D\frac{(C_1 - C_2)}{h} \tag{5.112}$$

In addition to the assumption of quasi-stationary state described previously, this treatment also ignores the influence of the static aqueous layers on either side of the membrane (aqueous boundary layers) on the mass transport process.

The concentrations of the diffusant in the membrane edges cannot be easily determined. The concentrations C_1 and C_2 have been shown in Figure 5.15 as being higher than C_d and C_r. This is accounted for by the distribution coefficient K having a value greater than unity. If the value of K is known, the membrane concentrations can be expressed in terms of the solution concentrations in the donor and receptor compartments:

$$K = \frac{C_1}{C_d} = \frac{C_2}{C_r} \tag{5.113}$$

$$KC_d = C_1 \text{ and } KC_r = C2 \tag{5.114}$$

$$\text{Flux} = J = \frac{dM}{S\,dt} = \frac{DK}{h}(C_d - C_r) \tag{5.115}$$

$$\frac{dM}{dt} = \frac{D\,S\,K}{h}(C_d - C_r) = P\,S(C_d - C_r); \quad \text{where } P = \frac{D\,K}{h} \tag{5.116}$$

The term P is known as *permeability* or *the permeation coefficient* and has units of linear velocity. If the receptor compartment can be maintained as a perfect sink, $Cr \approx 0$ and the equation is simplified as follows:

$$\frac{dM}{dt} = \frac{D\,S\,K\,C_d}{h} = P(S\,C_d) \tag{5.117}$$

5.4.4 Multilayer Diffusion

In this chapter, we briefly touch on multilayer diffusion. The diffusing molecules often have to cross multiple layers—for example, water vapor diffusing through multiple layers of a packaging materials, and drug molecules diffusing through lipophilic and hydrophilic barriers after oral administration before getting into the systemic circulation. For a controlled-release oral formulation, where the drug molecule has to diffuse out though an insoluble polymer coat on a tablet to be available for absorption, the presence of a static, unstirred aqueous layer on the outer surface of the coat would represent a second barrier layer.

The permeability across each layer, P_i, can be represented as $P_i = D_iK_i/h_i$, where K_i is the partition coefficient of a barrier phase relative to the next layer; h_i is the thickness of the barrier layer; and D_i is the diffusivity of the system and depends on the diffusion layer, the diffusant, and the temperature.

The resistance of each layer to diffusion, R_i, is defined as the reciprocal of the permeability of that layer, and the total resistance of multiple layers is a sum of the resistance of each layer:

$$R_i = \frac{1}{P_i} = \frac{h_i}{D_iK_i} \tag{5.118}$$

For diffusion across n layers, the total resistance is expressed as the sum of the reciprocal of the permeability of each layer:

$$R_{multilayer} = \frac{h_1}{D_1K_1} + \frac{h_2}{D_2K_2} \cdots\cdots\cdots \frac{h_n}{D_nK_n} \tag{5.119}$$

Therefore, for a two-layer diffusion system, the overall permeability can be described by Eq. 5.120:

$$P = \frac{D_1K_1D_2K_2}{h_1D_2K_2 + h_2D_1K_1} \tag{5.120}$$

5.4.5 Vapor Diffusion

Gaseous molecules such as water vapor and oxygen can diffuse through walls of drug product containers, plastic films used for packaging, and through polymer film coatings intended for protection of the drug product. This can be detrimental to the stability of molecules that are susceptible to hydrolytic or oxidative degradation.

Let us consider a packed pharmaceutical product bottle containing tablets of an active ingredient susceptible to hydrolysis. The relative humidity in the immediate headspace of the tablets can influence the hydrolytic reaction rates. When the bottle is stored under given conditions of temperature and external humidity, the kinetics of change in the headspace humidity in the bottle will depend on the following:

- The *permeability* of the packaging configuration to water vapor
- The difference in the relative humidity between the headspace in the bottle and the outside (the driving force for diffusion)

- The contents of the container (product, desiccant etc.), their initial water contents, and their water uptake behavior as a function of relative humidity at the given temperature

Chen and Li developed a model accounting for the factors listed here to predict the water uptake by tablets packed in bottles and stored under different temperature and humidity conditions [24].

5.4.5.1 Water Vapor Transmission Rates

Water vapor transmission rates (WVTRs) can be defined as the mass of water vapor permeating through barrier films, plastic container walls, etc., under given conditions of temperature and for a given difference in the relative humidity (ΔRH) on either side of the barrier. It must be noted that relative humidity at a given temperature is a measure of the water activity in the atmosphere. ΔRH is a measure of the difference in water activity across the barrier and hence the driving force for water diffusion. When WVTR is determined for sealed high-density polyethylene (HDPE) bottles, it is usually expressed in units of milligrams of water per day [25].

The *permeability* of the bottle to water vapor can be expressed as follows:

$$P = \frac{WVTR}{\Delta RH} \tag{5.121}$$

WVTR can be expressed as the amount of water permeated into the bottle, *m*, over a time period *t*:

$$m = P\ t\ \Delta RH \tag{5.122}$$

Note the similarity in the permeability term for water vapor diffusion into induction-sealed HDPE bottles and diffusion of solutes through membranes, Eqs. 5.121, 5.122, and 5.116.

When the bottles are empty, any water diffusion from or into the bottles is added or removed from the headspace of the bottles. If V is the volume of the bottle, and if C_{sat} is the saturation water vapor concentration (mass per unit volume) at the temperature of the experiment, then VC_{sat} is the saturation amount of water vapor in the bottle at the given temperature (corresponding to 100% RH). At time *t*, with an additional water vapor quantity *m* permeated into the bottle, the relative humidity inside the bottle $RH_{int,t}$ can be expressed as follows:

$$RH_{int,\,t} = \left(\frac{m_0 + m}{VC_{sat}}\right)100 = RH_{int,\,0} + \left(\frac{m}{VC_{sat}}\right)100 \tag{5.123}$$

Here, m_0 and $RH_{int,\,0}$ represent the initial amount of water vapor and the initial relative humidity within the bottle.

The rate of change of internal RH at a given temperature is equal to the rate of water entry into the bottle, and hence, a differential form of Eq. 5.123 can be rewritten as follows. Here the subscripts 'ext' and 'int' refer to outside and inside the bottle respectively:

$$\frac{dRH_{int}}{dt} = P\Delta RH = P(RH_{ext} - RH_{int}) \tag{5.124}$$

$$\frac{dRH_{int}}{(RH_{ext} - RH_{int})} = P\ dt \tag{5.125}$$

The integral form of the equation can be written as:

$$\ln\frac{(RH_{ext} - RH_{int})_0}{(RH_{ext} - RH_{int})_t} = P\ t \tag{5.126}$$

$$(RH_{ext} - RH_{int})_t = (RH_{ext} - RH_{int})_0(e^{-P\,t}) \tag{5.127}$$

$$RH_{ext,\,t} - RH_{int,\,t} = (RH_{ext,\,0} - RH_{int,\,0})(e^{-P\,t}) \tag{5.128}$$

At constant external RH i.e., $RH_{ext,\,0} = RH_{ext,\,t}$, then

$$RH_{int,\,t} = RH_{ext}(1 - e^{-P\,t}) + RH_{int,\,0}(e^{-P\,t}) \tag{5.129}$$

These relationships were obtained for empty bottles, where all the water, which diffused into the bottle, contributed entirely to the vapor pressure and the relative humidity of the bottle contents. Presence of drug product or desiccants in the bottles will introduce additional materials. These will compete for binding with water. The affinity of water for these materials, and the distribution of water between them and the headspace in the bottle, will also influence the kinetics of RH change within the bottle.

The external relative humidity during shelf-life can therefore influence the headspace RH, even in sealed plastic bottles. Once the bottle is opened, the contents are exposed directly to the external RH. For water-sensitive products, desiccant pouches (containing silica gel, for example) are often added to the bottles to maintain lower RH of the headspace despite repeated opening and closing of the containers to withdraw the dosage units.

5.5. DISSOLUTION

The process by which molecules of a solid substance in contact with a liquid solvent leave the solid phase and form a one-phase, homogeneous, molecular mixture with the solvent is known as dissolution. In this section, we focus on the kinetics of dissolution of solid drug substances, or the mechanisms and kinetics of their release from formulated drug products. Related topics including dissolution testing of solid dosage forms and biopharmaceutics are discussed in other chapters.

5.5.1 Noyes–Whitney Equation

Availability of the drug in solution in most cases is a prerequisite for absorption, disposition, and pharmacological activity of the drug at the site of action. Therefore, dissolution of a drug after being administered as a solid is an important process influencing its activity.

The rate at which a solid dissolves when in contact with a solvent is expressed by the Noyes–Whitney equation:

$$\frac{dM}{dt} = \frac{DS}{h}(Cs - C) \tag{5.130}$$

where M is the mass of the solute that goes into solution in time t; dM/dt is the dissolution rate; S is the surface area of the solid available to interact with the solvent; D is the diffusion coefficient of the solute in the solvent and depends on the nature of the solute, the solvent composition, viscosity, and temperature; C_s is the saturation solubility of the solute in the given solvent at the temperature of the experiment; and C is the concentration of the solute in bulk solution.

The surface of the solid exposed to an aqueous medium has an aqueous diffusion layer, which is a stagnant liquid film on the solid surface (Figure 5.16). Molecules of the solute dissolve in the liquid film and achieve a saturation concentration (C_s) at the interface of the solid and the liquid film. These molecules then diffuse through the liquid film toward the bulk solution, where the drug has a lower concentration. The driving force for this step is the concentration gradient across the diffusion layer. The thickness of this diffusion layer is written as h in Eq. 5.130. As we get beyond the static, unstirred diffusion layer, into the bulk solution phase, mixing of contents occurs and the solute concentrations are uniform. If the concentration of the solute in the bulk solution is significantly lower than the saturation solubility of the drug (say $C < 0.15\,C_s$, and $C_s - C \approx C_s$), then sink conditions apply. The Noyes–Whitney equation for sink conditions can be expressed as follows:

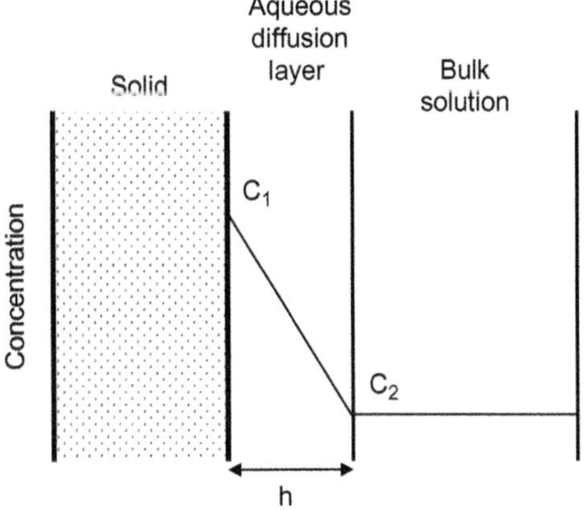

FIGURE 5.16 Schematic representation of the dissolution process. The concentration gradient across the stagnant liquid layer is shown.

$$\frac{dM}{dt} = \frac{DSC_s}{h} \tag{5.131}$$

It is easy to notice the similarity between the expressions for the rate of diffusion through a membrane (Fick's law) and the rate of dissolution from a solid (Noyes–Whitney equation) and the parallel between these processes.

5.5.1.1 *Surface Area (S)*

As seen from Eq. 5.130, the dissolution rate of a solid in contact with the solvent depends on the total surface available for interaction with the solvent and hence for diffusion of the drug across the stagnant solvent layer. As seen in Figure 5.17, when a solid formulation is ingested orally, it comes in contact with the gastrointestinal contents. Dosage forms designed for immediate release of the drug often break apart by *disintegration* of the tablet into smaller aggregates (granules) and then by *de-aggregation* to yield the individual particles. If the tablet does not disintegrate, *dissolution* and *erosion* would occur only on the tablet surface as the tablet geometry shrinks.

When disintegration occurs, an increase in effective surface area of the drug is achieved, resulting in an increase in the dissolution rate. For the same dose of a drug substance, a decrease in particle size distribution of the drug could result in a large increase in the overall drug surface area available upon tablet disintegration. Particle size reduction and increase in surface area are among the primary strategies for improving the dissolution rate of poorly soluble drugs.

5.5.1.2 *Solubility of the Drug (C_s)*

The dissolution rate of a solid drug substance, as seen from the Noyes–Whitney equation (Eq. 5.130), is directly influenced by the saturation solubility of the drug, C_s, which is the concentration of the drug achieved at the interface of the solid surface and the aqueous diffusion layer. Dissolution rate is directly proportional to the difference in the concentrations across this diffusion layer (concentration gradient, driving force, $C_s - C$).

The saturation solubility of a stable crystalline solid form of a drug at a given temperature in a specified solvent is a thermodynamic property of the drug. However, when a metastable solid form of the same compound possessing higher free energy (for example, the amorphous form of a drug) is used, concentrations higher than the thermodynamic solubility of the drug may be attained. This will provide a higher concentration gradient in the diffusion layer and hence faster

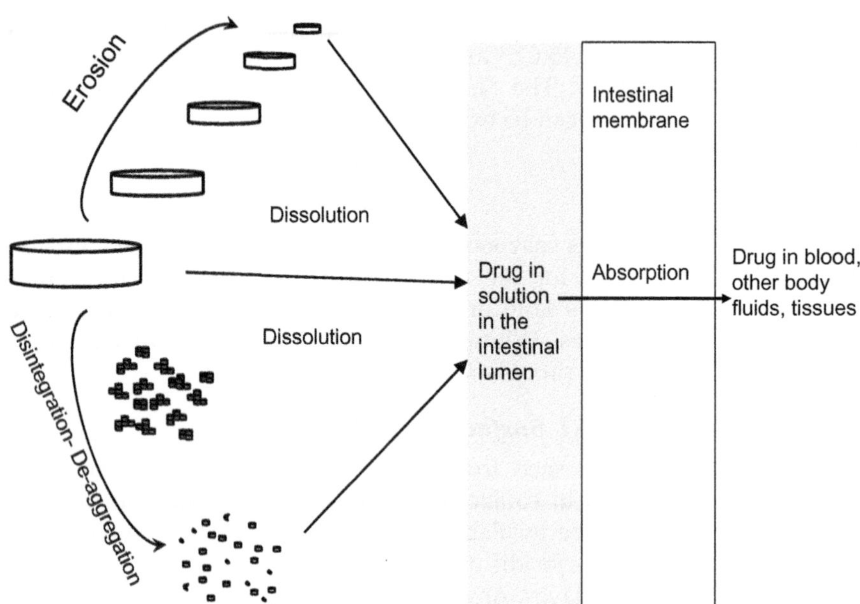

FIGURE 5.17 Schematic representation of the breakdown of tablet formulation on oral administration (by erosion or disintegration). Dissolution from all stages provides the drug in solution, which is available for absorption in the intestine.

rates of dissolution and faster availability of the dissolved drug at the site of absorption, *in vivo*. Supersaturation of the bulk solution phase is also a possibility while using metastable forms. If a supersaturated solution is available at an absorption site, and if absorption rates are faster than the rates of crystallization and precipitation of the stable solid, higher bioavailability of the drug may be achieved. Use of stabilized amorphous forms of drugs is a widely reported approach for improving the bioavailability of poorly water-soluble drugs [26].

The pH of the diffusion layer surrounding the drug particle can also influence the solubility of ionizable drugs in the diffusion layer and hence the concentration gradient across it. For example, use of salt forms of drugs can significantly increase dissolution rates compared to the free acid or base forms of the drugs [27,28]. During dissolution of sodium salicylate in acidic media (say 0.1 M HCl), the high concentration of the sodium salt close to the solid surface would buffer the diffusion layer to a pH higher than the pH of the bulk medium. This would result in a higher solubility of the acidic drug in the diffusion layer, a higher concentration gradient, and a higher dissolution rate. This buffering effect would not be seen with solid salicylic acid in 0.1 M HCl. Therefore, although the saturation solubility of both the free acid and the sodium salt in the bulk medium are the same, the sodium salt provides a higher dissolution rate [27].

5.5.1.3 *Diffusion Layer Thickness*

The term *h* in the Noyes–Whitney equation is the thickness of the diffusion layer, and it influences the diffusion path length and hence the rate of dissolution. In laboratory dissolution tests, the stirring speed and the hydrodynamics in the dissolution vessels can influence the diffusion layer thickness and hence the dissolution profiles. *In vivo*, the peristaltic movements of the gastrointestinal tract and the composition of the gastrointestinal contents can dictate the thickness of the diffusion layers around the exposed surfaces of the solid drug substance.

5.5.2 Intrinsic Dissolution Rates

During dissolution tests, the surface area changes as dissolution progresses, and this influences the dissolution rate. It is difficult to measure this change in surface area with reasonable accuracy. Therefore, for comparisons of dissolution rates of pure drug substances during screening of drug candidates and to assess the effect of different solid forms of a given active pharmaceutical ingredient, dissolution tests are often carried out under fixed conditions of temperature, medium composition, agitation, as well as surface area of the solid. The drug substance sample to be evaluated is compressed into a flat disc holder such that a fixed surface area is exposed during the test. The initial dissolution rates under these controlled conditions can therefore be normalized for surface area and compared across different samples. These normalized rates are called intrinsic dissolution rates and have units of mass per unit time per unit area:

$$\text{Intrinisic dissolution rate} = \frac{1}{S}\frac{dM}{dt} = \frac{DCs}{h} \qquad (5.132)$$

5.5.3 Hixson–Crowell Cube Root Law

If the dissolution of a solid phase—for example, a solid dosage form—proceeds such that its geometric shape stays the same while the dimensions shrink, then the Hixson–Crowell cube-root model can be used to describe the dissolution kinetics. This model can also be applied to dissolution of the drug from a particulate sample, where the particles are of uniform size and dissolution proceeds uniformly across the entire surface of all particles.

The dissolution kinetics from uniform *spherical* particles can be expressed in terms of the mass of total undissolved solid as follows:

$$\sqrt[3]{M} = \sqrt[3]{M_0} - \kappa t \quad (5.133)$$

$$\kappa = \frac{\sqrt[3]{M_0}}{d}\frac{2DC_S}{h\rho} \quad (5.134)$$

M is the mass of undissolved solid at time t, and M_0 is the initial amount of solid. D and C_s are the diffusion coefficient and saturation solubility of the solute in the medium, respectively. The thickness of the static diffusion layer around each particle is termed as h. The density and the particles is ρ, and the particle diameter at time t is d.

5.5.4 Drug Release Kinetics

So far, our discussions have focused on the dissolution of drug from the solid surface of the drug substance, which is made quickly available for dissolution either in a dissolution test or after oral administration. Frequently, formulations are designed to slow down the availability of drug for absorption, by prolonging the release of the drug from the dosage form. In these instances, the availability of the drug is not dictated by dissolution kinetics alone. The mechanism of retardation of drug release will dictate the availability of the drug at the site of absorption as a function of time. In the following sections, we look at the kinetics of key controlled-release approaches employed for oral drug delivery.

5.5.5 Matrix Systems

Matrix controlled-release systems refer to solid formulations where the drug is dispersed in a polymer matrix, which controls the release of the drug. The release of drug often occurs through a combination of several processes, including (i) penetration of medium into the matrix; (ii) dissolution of the drug and diffusion out of the matrix; (iii) erosion of the matrix material, exposing fresh surfaces for release of drug; and (iv) in some cases, drug dissolved in the polymer matrix partitioning into the surrounding media. The kinetics of release can therefore be complicated.

5.5.5.1 Inert/Insoluble Matrices

In these formulations, the drug is dispersed in a matrix of an inert polymer such as ethyl cellulose, methylmethacrylate, or polyvinyl acetate. The drug and any soluble components in the matrix dissolve initially from the surface of the tablet into the dissolution medium. This creates channels for deeper medium penetration, drug dissolution, and diffusion of the drug out of the system. The Higuchi model describes drug release behavior from such systems as follows:

$$Q = \sqrt{\left(\frac{D\varepsilon Cs}{\tau}\right)(2A - \varepsilon\, C_s)t} \quad (5.135)$$

Here, Q is the quantity of drug released from unit surface area of the matrix at time t, D is the diffusion coefficient of the drug in the release medium, ε is porosity of the matrix, τ is tortuosity of the matrix, C_s is saturation solubility of the drug in the release medium, and A is the initial quantity of drug per unit volume of the matrix. As evident from the equation, the total amount released is proportional to the square root of time.

An increased porosity of the matrix increases the volume of water influx, drug dissolution, and release. The tortuous nature of the channels and pores in the matrix through which the drug diffuses out is represented by the term τ. An increase in tortuosity, by increasing the diffusion path length for transport of the drug out of the matrix, causes a decrease in the rate of drug release. The tortuosity and porosity of the matrix can be influenced by the formulation composition. For example, the incorporation of soluble excipients that will dissolve in the invading fluids and leach out of the system will increase the effective porosity and decrease the tortuosity of the system, thereby increasing release rates.

5.5.5.2 Hydrophilic, Swellable Matrix Systems

Hydrophilic, swellable matrix systems represent one of the most common approaches employed to formulate sustained-release formulations. These matrices utilize hydrophilic polymers like polyethylene oxide and hydroxypropyl methylcellulose. Upon exposure to the dissolution medium, these polymers take up water and form a viscous gel layer, which controls drug release (Figure 5.18). Often, there is a fraction of the dose that dissolves in the medium as it fills the surface pores and diffuses out of the system before the gel layer is formed. This causes an initial burst-release effect. Once the polymer particles start hydrating, the mobility of the polymer chains increases, the polymer

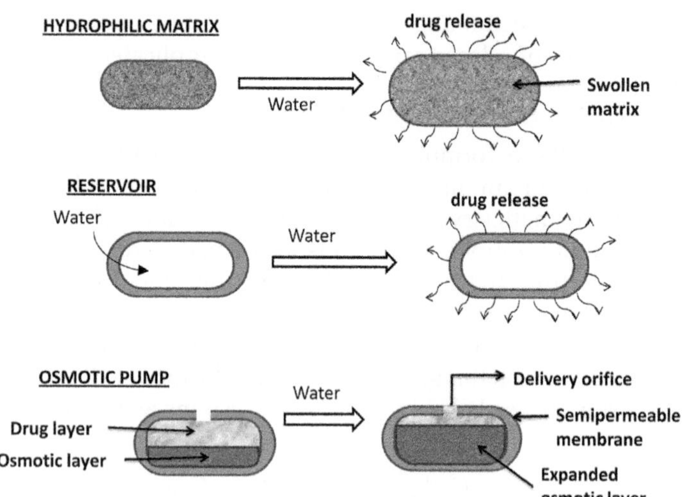

FIGURE 5.18 Schematic representation of three different oral controlled-release systems. The release mechanisms and drug release kinetics are described in the text.

chains relax, and there are structural changes in the porosity of the matrix. The drug substance dispersed in the matrix dissolves and diffuses out through the swollen polymer and the water-filled pores. Hydration and formation of the gel proceed toward the core of the tablet, and drug diffusion out of the matrix continues. In addition, depending on the composition of the core, the polymer chains on the surface continue to fully hydrate, disentangle, and relax, leading to erosion of the core and direct exposure of inner surfaces to the dissolution medium. Release from such systems is therefore by a combination of dissolution, diffusion, and erosion mechanisms.

The release rates from these systems can be modified by altering the viscosity grade and concentration of the polymer in the system. Lower viscosity grades and lower concentrations of the swellable polymers lead to faster influx of water and faster diffusional transport of the drug. It might also cause greater rates of polymer disentanglement and matrix erosion [3]. The matrix properties, release rates, and predominant mechanisms can be altered by careful choice of polymers and other excipients.

The power law equation by Korsmeyer et al. has been used frequently to describe the kinetics and to propose the mechanisms of release from swellable matrix systems. The logarithmic version of the equation is as follows [29]:

$$\log\left(\frac{M_t}{M_\infty}\right) = \log k = n \log t \tag{5.136}$$

The ratio M_t/M_∞ represents the fraction of drug-released at time t; k is a kinetic constant and depends on the nature of the system. The term n has been used to characterize the drug-release mechanisms from hydrophilic matrix systems as follows:

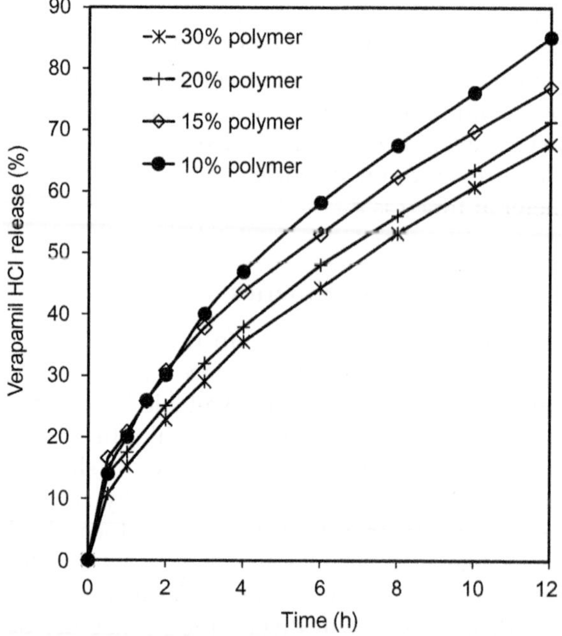

FIGURE 5.19 Release profiles for Verapamil HCl from hydrophilic matrix systems containing different levels of swellable polymer (hydroxypropyl methylcellulose K4M). The tablets also contained succinic acid, dibasic calcium phosphate, magnesium stearate, and talc. The dissolution study was carried out in 900 mL of simulated intestinal fluid, pH 7.5 at 37°C in a USP dissolution testing apparatus with paddles at 50 rpm.

$0.43 < n < 0.50$: Fickian diffusion (first-order release)
$0.50 < n < 0.89$: Anomalous release
$0.89 < n < 1.00$: Case II transport where the transport is entirely controlled by polymer chain relaxation (zero order)
$n > 1$: Super case II transport (unknown order)

Figure 5.19 depicts the effect of polymer (hydroxypropyl methylcellulose) concentration, in hydrophilic matrix tablets containing verapamil HCl, on the rate of drug release in simulated intestinal fluid. Increased polymer load caused a decrease in release rates in the dissolution test. When treated by the power law model, (Eq. 5.136) the exponent values (*n*) for all the release profiles were between 0.5 and 0.6, suggesting anomalous release.

5.5.6 Reservoir Systems

These systems have a drug-containing core, which is coated with a release-controlling polymer film. The film controls the rate of water entry into the core as well as diffusion of drug back out through the film (Figure 5.18). The release mechanism from these systems can be described by Fick's laws of diffusion. If the diffusional surface area is S, the diffusion coefficient of the drug is D, ΔC is the concentration gradient across the film, h is the film thickness, and K is the partition coefficient, then the rate of drug release can be written as follows:

$$\frac{dM}{dt} = \frac{S\,D\,K\Delta C}{h} \tag{5.137}$$

For a given formulation, S, D, K, and h are constant. If we can assume sink conditions, i.e., low concentrations in the external medium compared to the concentrations of the drug achieved inside the tablet, ΔC is maintained constant until most of the drug is depleted from the system. Therefore the drug release rate is expected to be constant (zero order). The release rates can be altered by altering the thickness of the release-controlling film (increased film thickness will proportionally decrease release rate) and/or its permeability.

5.5.7 Osmotic Pumps

Osmotic pumps are delivery systems that rely on entry of water into a tablet core through a semipermeable membrane. The water then aids in transport of the drug through predrilled apertures or through pores created by dissolution of soluble materials in the coating. Let us discuss the mechanism and release kinetics of one particular type: the push-pull osmotic pump (Figure 5.18).

The core of the push-pull system is a bilayer tablet, with one layer containing the drug and other excipients, which upon entry of water promote the formation of a homogeneous suspension of the drug. The other layer contains an osmotically active expandable pushing layer (Figure 5.18). The bilayer tablet is coated with a semipermeable membrane with an aperture drilled on the drug layer side.

When the tablet is exposed to the dissolution medium or gastrointestinal fluids, osmotic water uptake occurs in both layers of the tablet core. The drug layer is converted to a homogeneous drug suspension, while the osmotic push layer expands to pump out the drug suspension through the orifice. It is evident from the mechanism described that dissolution of the drug is not a prerequisite for release from this system, and hence, it is a big advantage, especially for poorly water-soluble drugs.

The kinetics of release is controlled by water entry into the tablet and can be described by the following equations [30]:

$$\frac{dM}{dt} = \left[\frac{dV}{dt}\right]_{total} C_{D,\ susp} \tag{5.138}$$

where dM/dt is the rate of release of the drug, dV/dt is the rate of total volume flow from the dosage form, and $C_{D,\ susp}$ is the concentration of the drug in the dispensed suspension. The volume changes in the two layers (osmotic layer, O; and drug layer, D) can be expressed as follows, and their sum equals the total volume flow out of the device:

$$O = \left[\frac{dV}{dt}\right]_O, \text{ and } D = \left[\frac{dV}{dt}\right]_D \tag{5.139}$$

$$O + D = \left[\frac{dV}{dt}\right]_{total} \tag{5.140}$$

The rates of volume flow for each compartment can be expressed in terms of the osmotic membrane permeability (k), thickness of the membrane (h), area of the osmotic compartment, (A_O), total area of the dosage form (A), imbibition pressure of the drug compartment (π_D), and imbibition pressure of the osmotic compartment, (π_O):

$$O = \frac{k}{h} A_O\, \pi_O \tag{5.141}$$

$$D = \frac{k}{h}[A - A_O].\ \pi_D \tag{5.142}$$

The concentration of the drug in the dispensed suspension $C_{D,\ susp}$ can be expressed in terms of the fraction of the drug layer that is drug substance (f_d) and the total solids concentration of the dispensed suspension (C_{solids}):

$$f_d C_{solids} = C_{D,susp} \tag{5.143}$$

The mass delivery rate for the drug is expressed as follows

$$\frac{dM}{dt} = (O + D) f_d C_{solids} \tag{5.144}$$

Zero-order release rates, independent of medium pH, have been achieved from such systems [30].

Although different mechanisms of drug release might provide sustained delivery of an administered dose of the drug over the same time duration, their release kinetics may be different. Therefore, the time course of availability of the drug for absorption might be different. These kinetic differences in drug release, when overlaid on in-vivo rate processes like gastric emptying and gastrointestinal transit, and absorption rate differences in different regions of the gastrointestinal tract, can result in major differences in the pharmacokinetics of the drug.

5.6. CONCLUSIONS

In the field of pharmaceutics, an understanding of various physical, chemical, and biological processes and their interrelationships is critical for development of pharmaceutical products. The study of factors that influence the rates of these critical processes, and strategies to control these rates to our advantage, very broadly defines the subject of this chapter.

Thermodynamics defines the stability of systems, the position of equilibria, and hence the direction of spontaneous processes. However, kinetic factors dictate the rates at which these processes will occur.

Chemical stability is a key requirement for pharmaceutical products, in order to maintain the safety, efficacy, and acceptability of drug products. Major chemical degradation processes in pharmaceuticals include hydrolysis, oxidation, isomerization, and photochemical reactions. Knowledge of the kinetics of these processes allows us to predict the rate and extent of these changes under given conditions. Knowledge of the mechanisms of change allows us to develop strategies for stabilization.

Kinetically, chemical reactions can be classified based on reaction order. Reaction order is the sum of the exponents of all the concentration terms in a reaction rate. Zero-order, first-order, and second-order reactions are most common. Pseudo orders are often encountered because one of the reactants is either in large excess (for example, water in dilute aqueous solutions) or if a reactant concentration does not change because of the reaction (for example, specific acid or base catalysis in buffered solutions). For pharmaceutical systems, reaction rates are influenced by various factors, the key ones being temperature, water content (relative humidity), solution pH, ionic strength, dielectric constant, oxygen, light, and presence impurities that can catalyze reactions. Knowledge of these factors also helps to develop stabilization strategies.

Accelerated stability testing involves evaluating stability of the drug substances or drug products under higher temperature and humidity conditions. Data generated at higher temperature as well as during longer-term shelf-life-storage allow for assignment of appropriate storage conditions and associated shelf-lives. Use of the Arrhenius equation helps to predict the reaction progress at lower temperatures based on higher temperature data and hence can help during pharmaceutical development. However, extrapolation to lower temperatures must be done carefully because complicated pharmaceutical systems can exhibit non-Arrhenius behavior due to a variety of reasons [23].

Physical mass transport processes are also very critical in pharmaceutics. Diffusion of a drug across biological membranes is vital for availability of the drug at the site of action. Diffusion of a drug through polymer membranes and out of prolonged release formulations controls the availability of the drug for absorption and hence influences the pharmacokinetics of the formulation. Diffusion of reactive gaseous molecules through protective pharmaceutical packaging can be detrimental to chemical stability.

Key physical rate processes discussed in this chapter include molecular diffusion, including water vapor diffusion into drug product bottles, dissolution of solid drug substances, and kinetics of drug release from selected controlled-release systems. Applications of these concepts are covered in other chapters.

CASE STUDIES

Case 5.1

The implantable Infusaid drug pump model 100 (Shiley Infusaid, Norwood, MA) underwent clinical trials as a drug delivery system in the treatment of osteomyelitis in your hospital. This study evaluated the stability of vancomycin (1 mg/mL) incubated at 37°C for 4 weeks in the pump. Both bioassay and high-pressure liquid chromatography data demonstrated a loss of at least 38% of activity over 4 weeks and colloidal precipitation of vancomycin in the pump at the end of the experiment [31].

As the lead pharmacist on your team, explain your recommendation to the company.

Approach: This study demonstrated that vancomycin activity is reduced when the drug is incubated for 4 weeks at 37°C using a stability-indicating HPLC method. The drug also forms colloidal aggregates in the Infusaid drug pump model 100. Recommendations are not to use vancomycin in this drug pump. Future work that needs to be performed on vancomycin solutions, stability, and the drug pump should consider testing solutions with a pH of <3.0 or a solution prepared with some other diluent. This study suggests that vancomycin is not stable enough for use in the Infusaid drug pump model 100 over a prolonged period of time.

Case 5.2

You are a third-year pharmacy student in a reputed school of pharmacy. You receive a call from a friend who is a final year chemistry student regarding an OTC medication. He usually stores all his medicine in a medicine cabinet in his apartment bathroom. Recently, while removing aspirin tablets from the bottle, he discovered something unusual. There are some white crystal-like materials on the tablet surface, and he also noticed the smell of vinegar from the bottle. He wants to know whether it is safe to use this medicine. If not, then why?

Approach: Aspirin, or acetylsalicylic acid, can undergo a hydrolytic degradation in the presence of moisture to form salicylic acid and acetic acid (see Figure 5.20). The vinegar smell is possibly coming from acetic acid. The white crystal-like material is possibly due to salicylic acid, one of the toxic degradation products of this drug. So the recommendation is not to take this medication any more. Doing so may cause gastric irritation and ulcer.

Case 5.3

Some heat-labile drugs are freeze dried, and some protein and other drug products are kept in the freezer to enhance shelf-life. Do you agree that these facts are always true? If not, then what are the possible factors that might affect stability at these low temperatures?

Approach: Low temperature, freeze concentration, and ice formation are the three chief stresses resulting during cooling and freezing. Because of the increase in solute concentrations, freeze concentration could also facilitate second-order reactions, crystallization of buffer or nonbuffer components, phase separation, and redistribution of solutes. An understanding of these stresses is critical to the determination of when, during freezing, a protein suffers degradation and therefore is important in the design of stabilizer systems [32].

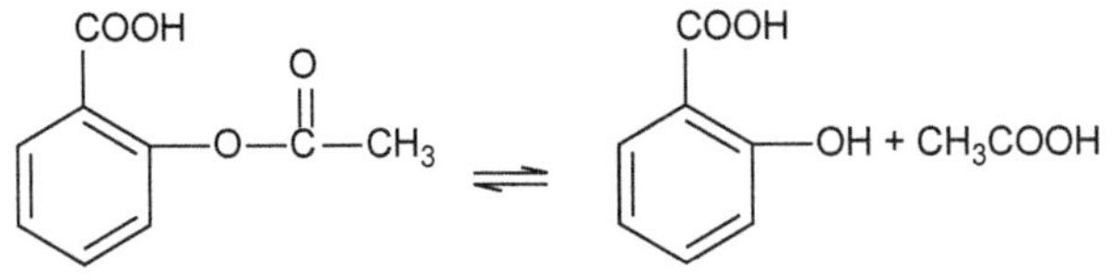

COOH, O, —O—C—CH_3 ⇌ COOH, —OH + CH_3COOH

Aspirin (acetylsalicylic acid) salicylic acid acetic acid

FIGURE 5.20 The degradation of acetylsalicylic acid into salicylic acid and acetic acid in presence of moisture.

References

[1] Florence AT, Attwood D, Attwood D. Physicochemical principles of pharmacy. London: Pharmaceutical Press; 2011.

[2] Sinko PJ, Allen Jr LV, Popovich NG, Ansel HC. Martin's physical pharmacy and pharmaceutical sciences. Lippincott Williams & Wilkins, Philadelphia, PA; 2006.

[3] Allen Jr Loyd V. Remington: the science and practice of pharmacy. 22nd ed. London: The Pharmaceutical Press; 2012.

[4] Carstensen JT, Rhodes CT. Drug stability: principles and practices. Marcel Dekker, New York; 1990.

[5] Maulding HV, Zoglio MA, Pigois FE, Wagner M. Pharmaceutical heterogeneous system. IV. A kinetic approach to the stability screening of solid dosage forms containing aspirin. J Pharm Sci 1969;58:1359–62.

[6] Oberholtzer ER, Brenner GS. Cefoxitin sodium: solution and solid-state chemical stability studies. J Pharm Sci 1979;68: 863–6.

[7] Mee AJ. Chemical kinetics. In: Speakman, JC, editor. Physical chemistry. London: Heinemann Educational Books, Ltd.; 1965. p. 566–589

[8] Konishi M, Hirai K, Mori Y. Kinetics and mechanism of the equilibrium reaction of triazolam in aqueous solution. J Pharm Sci 1982;71:1328–34.

[9] Teraoka R, Otsuka M, Matsuda Y. Chemical stability of ethyl icosapentate against autoxidation. II. Effect of photoirradiation on oxidation kinetics. Pharm Res 1994;11:1077–81.

[10] Bundgaard H, Hansen SH. Hydrolysis and epimerization kinetics of pilocarpine in basic aqueous solution as determined by HPLC. Int J Pharm 1982;10:281–9.

[11] Carstensen JT. Advanced pharmaceutical solids. Drugs and the Pharmaceutical Sciences, Vol 110. New York: Marcel Dekker; 2001.

[12] Khawam A, Flanagan DR. Solid-state kinetic models: basics and mathematical fundamentals. J Phys Chem B 2006;110: 17315–28.

[13] Stanisz B. Evaluation of stability of enalapril maleate in solid phase. J Pharm Biomed Analysis 2003;31:375–80.

[14] Gu L, Strickley RG. Diketopiperazine formation, hydrolysis, and epimerization of the new dipeptide angiotensin-converting enzyme inhibitor RS-10085. Pharm Res 1987;4:392–7.

[15] Tsuji A, Nakashima E, Deguchi Y, Nishide K, Shimizu T, Horiuchi S, et al. Degradation kinetics and mechanism of aminocephalosporins in aqueous solution: cefadroxil. J Pharm Sci 1981;70:1120–8.

[16] Serajuddin A, Thakur AB, Ghoshal RN, Fakes MG, Ranadive SA, Morris KR, et al. Selection of solid dosage form composition through drug-excipient compatibility testing. J Pharm Sci 1999;88:696–704.

[17] Badawy SIF, Hussain MA. Microenvironmental pH modulation in solid dosage forms. J Pharm Sci 2007;96:948–59.

[18] Felmeister A, Schaubman R, Howe H. Dismutation of a semiquinone free radical of chlorpromazine. J Pharm Sci 1965; 54:1589–93.

[19] Carstensen JT. Kinetic salt effect in pharmaceutical investigations. J Pharm Sci 1970;59:1140–3.

[20] Hou JP, Poole JW. Kinetics and mechanism of degradation of ampicillin in solution. J Pharm Sci 1969;58:447–54.

[21] Hovorka SW, Schöneich C. Oxidative degradation of pharmaceuticals: theory, mechanisms and inhibition. J Pharm Sci 2001;90:253–69.

[22] Garrett ER. Prediction of stability in pharmaceutical preparations. III. Comparison of vitamin stabilities in different multivitamin preparations. J Am Pharm Assoc 1956;45:470–3.

[23] Waterman KC, Adami RC. Accelerated aging: prediction of chemical stability of pharmaceuticals. Int J Pharm 2005;293: 101–25.

[24] Chen Y, Li Y. A new model for predicting moisture uptake by packaged solid pharmaceuticals. Int J Pharm 2003;255:217–25.

[25] Waterman KC, MacDonald BC. Package selection for moisture protection for solid, oral drug products. J Pharm Sci 2010; 99:4437–52.

[26] Serajuddin A. Solid dispersion of poorly water-soluble drugs: early promises, subsequent problems, and recent breakthroughs. J Pharm Sci 1999;88:1058–66.

[27] Serajuddin A, Jarowski CI. Effect of diffusion layer pH and solubility on the dissolution rate of pharmaceutical acids and their sodium salts. II: salicylic acid, theophylline, and benzoic acid. J Pharm Sci 1985;74:148–54.

[28] Serajuddin A, Jarowski CI. Effect of diffusion layer pH and solubility on the dissolution rate of pharmaceutical bases and their hydrochloride salts. I: Phenazopyridine. J Pharm Sci 1985;74: 142–7.

[29] Korsmeyer RW, Gurny R, Doelker E, Buri P, Peppas NA. Mechanisms of solute release from porous hydrophilic polymers. Int J Pharm 1983;15:25–35.

[30] Swanson DR, Barclay BL, Wong PS, Theeuwes F. Nifedipine gastrointestinal therapeutic system. Am J Med 1987;83:3–9.

[31] Greenberg, et al. Instability of vancomycin in Infusaid drug pump model 100. Antimicrob Agents Chemother 1987;31(4):610–1.

[32] Bhatnagar B, et al. Protein stability during freezing: separation of stresses and mechanisms of protein stabilization. Pharmaceutical development and technology. Pharm Dev Technol 2007;12 (5):505–23.

CHAPTER

6

Biopolymers

Somnath Singh and Justin Tolman
Department of Pharmacy Sciences, Creighton University, Omaha, NE, USA

CHAPTER OBJECTIVES

- Define and differentiate polymer, protein, and oligonucleotide.
- Discuss the structural properties that distinguish polymers from other molecules.
- Describe some polymers that are commonly used as excipients in the pharmaceutical industry, and their uses.
- Discuss the important physical properties of pharmaceutical polymers.
- Discuss briefly the properties of polymers in solution.
- Discuss briefly the solid-state properties of polymeric materials.
- Discuss pharmaceutical applications of polymers.

Keywords:

- Oligonucleotides
- Peptides
- Polymers
- Polymer properties
- Polymers as excipients
- Proteins

6.1. INTRODUCTION TO POLYMERS

Polymers are natural or synthetic compounds made up of numerous repeated monomer units. Chemical properties of a polymer depend on the monomer units and the way they have been arranged. Polymers can be either linear or branched. Branched polymers are then categorized as isotactic (similar side chains), atactic (random pattern of side chains), and syndiotactic (a regular pattern of alteration in side chains). Linear or branched chains can be covalently bonded together using cross-linking agents. Polymers with only one type of monomer unit are called homopolymers. Polymers with different monomer units are referred to as copolymers. Various copolymers can be prepared in which monomers may repeat in a specific regular pattern, termed alternating polymers, or arranged in no pattern at all, referred to as random copolymers, respectively (see Figure 6.1).

6.1.1 Properties of Polymers

6.1.1.1 Polydispersity

Almost all naturally and synthetically produced polymers exist as a mixture of molecules with varying molecular weights. This polydispersity can sometimes be reduced by purifying polymers or isolating polymer fractions. The average molecular weight (M_n) of a polymer containing n_1, n_2, $n_{3,\ldots}$ molecules with molecular weights M_1, M_2, $M_{3,\ldots}$ is calculated using the formula shown in Eq. 6.1:

$$M_n = \frac{n_1M_1 + n_2M_2 + n_3M_3 + \cdots}{n_1 + n_2 + n_3 + \cdots} = \frac{\Sigma n_iM_i}{\Sigma n_i} \qquad (6.1)$$

6.1.1.2 Solubility

After addition of polymer to a solvent, the polymer undergoes wetting and then swelling. Solvent takes a longer time to diffuse into high-molecular-weight polymers because more energy is required to break the intramolecular bonds, which are more prevalent than those in polymers of low molecular weight. If the solubility parameter of a polymer is the same as or close to the solubility parameter of the solvent, the solvent is considered a good solvent and can dissolve the polymer to yield a polymer solution. Water-soluble polymers increase the solution viscosity at low concentrations.

Pharmaceutics. DOI: http://dx.doi.org/10.1016/B978-0-12-386890-9.00006-6

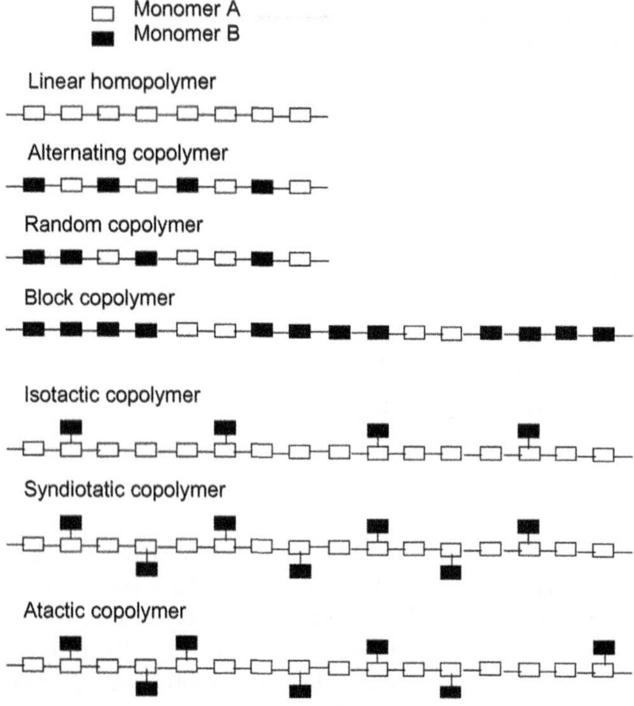

FIGURE 6.1 Various polymer structures attained due to alteration in polymerization pattern of two different monomers diagrammatically represented by □ and ■.

These water-soluble polymers have numerous pharmaceutical applications, including functioning as suspending agents in pharmaceutical suspensions by slowing the settling of solid insoluble particles in suspension. Some pharmaceutically utilized water-soluble polymers include hydroxyethyl cellulose, alginates, chitosan, etc. Hydrophilic polymers are a separate group of polymers that will absorb water and swell but do not completely dissolve. Some hydrophilic polymers are used pharmaceutically to control the release rate of drugs. Some polymers have a high melting point due to strong internal bonds. This high internal stability might cause the polymer to take a longer time to dissolve or not dissolve at all. Some poorly or insoluble polymers are also used in pharmaceutical preparations to form thin films, film-coating materials, surgical dressings, etc.

6.1.2 General Properties of Polymer Solutions

6.1.2.1 Viscosity

Polymers will increase the viscosity of solutions and suspensions. This increase in viscosity is one of the key properties for pharmaceutical polymer use. Numerous terms are used to describe the influence of polymers on solution viscosities. Note that η_0 is the viscosity of pure solvent and η is the viscosity of the polymer solution:

1. **Relative viscosity, η_r:** This is the viscosity of a polymer solution relative to the normal viscosity of the solvent as given in Eq. 6.2:

$$\eta_r = \frac{\eta}{\eta_0} \tag{6.2}$$

2. **Specific viscosity, η_{sp}:** Specific viscosity describes the difference of viscosities of a solvent and polymer solution relative to viscosity of the polymer solution and is shown in Eq. 6.3. It is the fractional increase in viscosity due to the addition of the polymer relative to the solvent viscosity:

$$\eta_{sp} = \frac{\eta - \eta_0}{\eta_0} = \eta_r - 1 \tag{6.3}$$

3. **Inherent viscosity, η_i:** The inherent viscosity is another way to describe the relative increase in viscosity due to the polymer in relation to the concentration of that polymer in the solution. It is calculated by taking the natural log of relative viscosity of a polymer solution divided by its concentration (c), as shown in Eq. 6.4:

$$\eta_i = \frac{\ln \eta_r}{c} \tag{6.4}$$

4. **Intrinsic viscosity[η]:** The intrinsic viscosity is not a true viscosity measurement but the inverse of molecular density; it describes the polymer's ability to increase the viscosity of a given solute. It is defined as the limit of the ratio of specific viscosity to polymer concentration (referred to as reduced viscosity) as polymer concentration approaches zero and is represented in Eq. 6.5:

$$[\eta] = \lim_{c \to 0} \frac{\eta_{sp}}{c} \tag{6.5}$$

The intrinsic viscosity of solutions of linear high-molecular-weight polymers is proportional to the molecular weight, M, of the polymer as given by the Mark–Houwink equation (Eq. 6.6):

$$[\eta] = KM^a \tag{6.6}$$

where a is a constant in the range 0–2 (most high-molecular-weight polymers have a value between 0.6 and 0.8), and K is a constant for a given polymer-solvent system.

6.1.2.2 Gelling

A concentrated polymer solution induces a highly viscous solution that is known as a gel. A gel contains a three-dimensional network of stable physical or chemical bonds characterized by high viscosity and rubber-like appearance. There are two main types of gels:

- **Type I:** Irreversible gel system made of covalent bonds
- **Type II:** Heat-reversible gels held together by weak hydrogen bonds

Polymer solutions can have a gel point that defines the state at which sufficient polymer bonding has occurred to create a coextensive polymer phase (i.e., the solution turns into a dense semisolid). Gel points can be temperature values, with some polymer solutions forming gels with a decrease in temperature, whereas others gel with an increase in temperature. Type I gels are more prevalent in pharmacy.

Some copolymers have differing solubility characteristics due to varied monomer units in the polymer. Copolymers can also form gels when dissolved in high concentration and can be referred to as heterogels. A common pharmaceutical example of a gel-forming block copolymer is polyoxyethylene–polyoxypropylene–polyoxyethylene, also known as Pluronic® or poloxamer; it can be found in a wide variety of pharmaceutical preparations.

6.1.2.3 *Crosslinking*

Crosslinking is the formation of covalent bonds between polymer chains to form networks of varying densities based on the degree of crosslinking. Water-soluble polymers can form gels when they are crosslinked. Several pharmaceutical polymers are crosslinked to affect solution or gel viscosities and drug release characteristics. One example is drug-containing hydrophilic contact lenses made from crosslinked poly(2-hydroxyethyl methacrylates). Other ophthalmologic solutions and gels are prepared with crosslinked polymers to increase the contact time of the drug with the cornea by increasing the viscosity of the formulation.

6.1.3 Application of Water-Soluble Polymers in Pharmacy and Medicine

Water-soluble or hydrophilic polymers are widely used in pharmaceutical preparations and drug products as suspending agents, surfactants, emulsifying agents, binding agents in tablets, thickening or viscosity-enhancing agents in liquid dosage forms, film-coating agents, etc. Some of the most common water-soluble polymers and their applications in pharmaceutical preparations can be found in Table 6.1. Other polymers that are not included in Table 6.1 have specific functions for uses such as coatings, enteric coatings, film formation, and hot melt extrusion.

6.1.4 Application of Water-Insoluble Polymers in Pharmacy and Medicine

Water-insoluble polymers are often used in pharmaceutical preparations in controlled drug release preparations and as membranes, containers, or tubing material. Permeability of drugs and its adsorption are two important parameters deciding the suitability of these polymers for use in pharmacy. Some drug

TABLE 6.1 Examples of Water-Soluble or Hydrophilic Polymers and Their Pharmaceutical Applications

Polymers	Description	Applications
Carboxymethylcellulose Sodium	This polymer is the sodium salt of substituted polycarboxymethyl cellulose. It is hygroscopic and soluble in water at all temperatures. Once hydrated or solubilized, it has acidic characteristics (p*K*a ~4.3).	It is used in oral and topical formulations as a coating agent, stabilizer, suspending agent, tablet binder, tablet disintegrant, and viscosity-increasing agent.
Carboxypolymethylene or Polyacrylic acid (Carbomer®, Carbopol®)	These high-molecular-weight polymers of acrylic acid that contain carboxylic acid groups (p*K*a ~6). These polymers form viscous gels in neutralized water due to repulsion between ionized functional groups.	They are used as controlled drug release agents, emulsifiers, emulsion stabilizers, viscosity enhancing agents, gelling agents, suspending agents, and tablet binders.
Methylcellulose	These methyl ether substituted long-chain cellulosic polymers are poorly soluble in cold water. Physical properties are influenced by the degree of substitution.	Low-viscosity grades are used as tablet binders, sustained release agents, emulsifiers, suspending agents, and thickeners. High-viscosity grades are used as tablet disintegrants and topical thickening agents.
Hydroxyethylcellulose (HEC)	HEC is a partially substituted poly(hydroxyethyl) ether of cellulose. This is soluble in both hot and cold water; it does not form gel.	It is used as a thickening agent in ophthalmic and topical preparations.

(*Continued*)

TABLE 6.1 (*Continued*)

Polymers	Description	Applications
Hypromellose (Hydroxypropylmethylcellulose, HPMC)	This is a partially substituted cellulose derivative of methoxy and hydroxyl propanoyl groups. The degree and composition of substitutions affect polymer properties. It forms a viscous colloidal solution.	Hypromellose is widely used in a wide variety of pharmaceutical preparations including oral, ophthalmic, otic, nasal, and topical preparations. It is used as a film-coating agent, tablet binder, controlled drug release modifier, dispersing and suspending agent, emulsifier and emulsion stabilizer, thickener, and gelling agent.
Povidone (polyvinylpyrrolidone, Kollidon®)	This is a variable-length linear polymer of 1-vinyl-2-pyrrolidone groups. The polymer viscosity is used to categorize molecular weight grades described by "K-values."	Povidone has a variety of uses but is principally used in oral dosage forms as a tablet binder and disintegrant. It can also be used as a suspending and viscosity-enhancing agent. Povidone also increases the solubility of numerous poorly soluble drugs.
Polyoxyethylene glycol (PEG, Macrogols)	PEG is a linear polymer of oxyethylene groups of varying lengths. Low-molecular-weight PEGs (PEG 200–700) are liquid at room temperature, whereas higher-molecular-weight PEGs are solid.	PEG is a widely used polymer in oral, rectal, topical ophthalmic/otic, and parenteral products. It is a solvent, diluent, viscosity-enhancing agent, suspending agent, ointment base, suppository base, tablet binder, plasticizer, lubricant, controlled drug release agent, etc.
Acacia (arabic gum)	This natural polymer is a complex and branched loose aggregate of cellulosic compounds and sugars that is soluble in water up to 30%. It is very viscous and has pH-dependent viscosity enhancement.	Acacia is principally used in topical formulations as a stabilizing, suspending, and viscosity-enhancing agent. It has also been used in controlled-release tablets.
Alginate Salts (Sodium salt, Potassium salt, Calcium salt, etc.)	These are salts of natural alginic acid polymer, which is a block mixture of polyuronic acids (D-mannuronic and L-glucoronic acid residues).	Alginate salts have a variety of pharmaceutical uses, such as tablet binder and disintegrant, suspending agent, viscosity-increasing agent, and sustained drug release agent.
Chitosan	This natural polymer is partially deacetylated and depolymerized from chitin. Polymer properties are based in part on the degree of acetylation. It is soluble at acidic pH values and gels at neutral pH values due to the presence of amine groups (p*K*a 5.5–6.5.)	Chitosan is used as a coating and film-forming agent, disintegrant, tablet binder, and viscosity-enhancing agent.
Pectin	Pectin is a high-molecular-weight complex polysaccharide obtained from the rind of citrus fruit. It consists of partially methoxylated polygalacturonic acid. Gelation is affected by the extent of esterification.	It is used as an adsorbent, thickening, emulsifying, gelling, and stabilizing agent.
Tragacanth (tragacanth gum)	This natural polymer composed of insoluble and soluble polysaccharides. It dissolves partially in water to produce highly viscous suspensions.	It is used topically as a suspending and viscosity-enhancing agent.

solutions that come in contact with insoluble polymers can be adsorbed onto the polymer surface depending on drug-polymer affinity. Some small molecule drugs as well as many biological medications (therapeutic proteins, peptides, antibodies, and oligonucleotides) will bind to insoluble polymers, especially in intravenous syringes, bags, and tubing. Some institutions will have special precautions and practices to avoid or minimize drug product binding to insoluble polymers that the drug product might come in contact with. In addition to surface adsorption, some small drug molecules can permeate into and possibly diffuse through insoluble polymers. The intercalation of small drug molecules into the insoluble plastics can affect polymer strength and integrity as well as interfere with the patient receiving the desired medication dose.

6.2. INTRODUCTION TO PEPTIDES AND PROTEINS

The tremendous advances in biotechnology and the sequencing of the human genome have made it possible to develop and produce an increasingly diverse number of therapeutically active proteins and peptides. Some examples of biotechnology-enabled pharmaceutical products include hemophiliac globulins, growth hormones, erythropoietin, colony-stimulating factors, interferon, natural proteins or "first-generation recombinant proteins," viral or bacterial proteins (as vaccines), monoclonal antibodies, and older products such as insulin and immunoglobulins. Despite this expansion in therapeutic proteins and peptides, they possess unique physical and chemical properties that present substantial difficulties in formulation and delivery.

Unlike conventional small-molecular-weight compounds, therapeutic proteins and peptides are biological macromolecules that are polypeptides and consist of polymerized amino acids. The linear polymers are composed of covalently linked amino acid monomers. Short peptide polymers are often referred to as polypeptides, whereas longer-chain-length molecules are considered proteins. Proteins and polymers are characterized by a regularly repeating backbone with distinctive functionalized amino acid side chains that interact with each other to promote the formation of a therapeutically essential three-dimensional conformational structure. This structure has four principal different levels of organization—namely, a primary structure, secondary structure, tertiary structure, and a quaternary structure—that determine the therapeutically active or functional three-dimensional structure.

6.2.1 Primary Structure

The primary structure of a protein consists of the protein's linear amino acid sequence. The primary structure is held in a fixed sequence by covalently linked amino acids through peptide (amide) bonds that provide flexibility and allow rotational movement. The primary structure also has definitive orientation due to carboxy-terminal and amino-terminal functional groups that make up the two ends of the amino acid chain. Ultimately, the structure and function of therapeutic proteins and peptides depend on the unique primary structure of a protein.

6.2.2 Secondary Structure

Secondary structures are composed of localized patterns of orientation due to hydrogen bonds between the amino acid backbone and side-chain amide and the carboxyl groups. Generally, the amino acid backbone N-H residues form hydrogen bonds with C = O bonds on a separate residue. Secondary structures are classified based on their localized geometries with common structures described as α helices and β pleated sheets. The α helix is a structurally ridged single-stranded right-handed spiral where hydrogen bonding occurs between amino acid residues that are spaced approximately four residues apart based on the primary structure sequence. Fibrous structural proteins, such as keratins, are mainly made up of α helical structures. The β pleated sheet is a weaker structural unit formed as a twisted and pleated sheet of amino acid strands. The hydrogen bonds might or might not form between residues that are in proximity to each other based on the primary structure sequence. Proteins can contain numerous secondary structural regions of both α helix and β pleated sheets in the same polypeptide chain. It is important to note that the hydrogen bonding potential in secondary structures depend on the relative orientation, spacing, and sequence of amino acids as well as the spatial proximity of amino acid residues based on the tertiary structures.

6.2.3 Tertiary Structure

The tertiary structure is the actual three-dimensional spatial structure of the protein. It is often composed of secondary structures packed into compact globular units known as domains. Domains then are the precisely folded, bent, and arranged secondary structures. Tertiary structures are principally folded and formed based on the properties of side chain functional groups. Domains form in part to minimize hydrophobic side-chain exposure to aqueous environments, promote hydrogen bonding, stabilize polar or ionized functional groups, form disulfide bonding, and ensure the protein is conformed in such a manner to be in an energy state minimum.

6.2.4 Quaternary Structure

Quaternary structures are composed of multiple separate polypeptide chains, known as subunits, arranged into complex three-dimensional structures. These subunits may be connected to each other through disulfide bonds and are stabilized by ionic bonds, hydrogen bonds, and Van der Waals interactions. While common for many biological proteins, not all therapeutic proteins exhibit quaternary structures. Figure 6.2 depicts the four different levels of protein structure [1].

6.2.5 Protein Stability

Many therapeutic proteins are chemically and structurally unstable and have the potential to lose their conformational stability and biological activity. Much of this instability is due to normal physiologic processes for protein digestion, cleavage, and processing throughout the body due to lowered pH

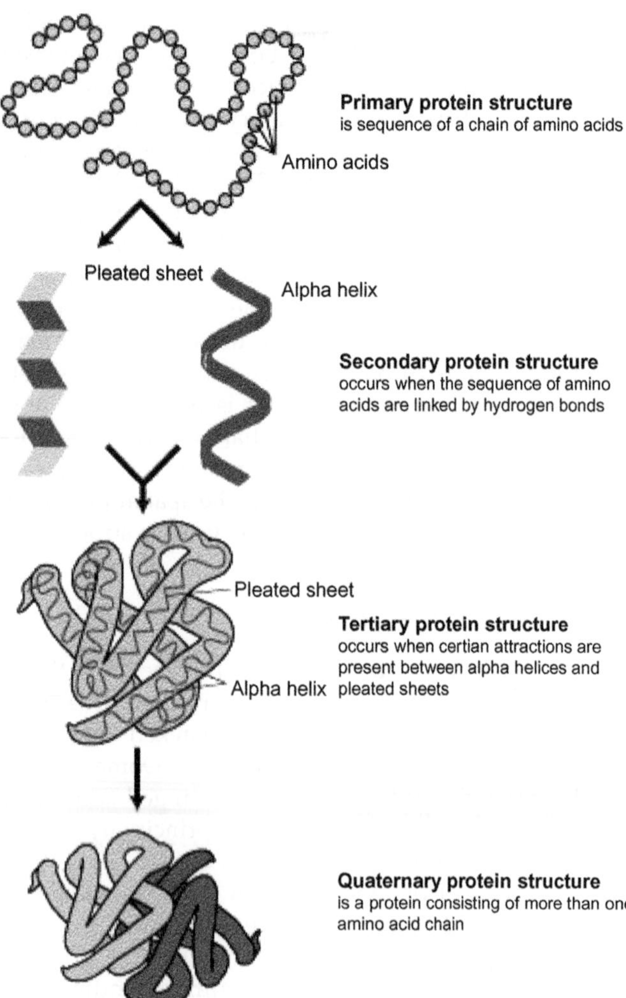

FIGURE 6.2 Primary, secondary, tertiary, and quaternary structure of proteins. *(Courtesy of the National Human Genome Institute)*

biological conditions, enzymatic cleavage and modifications, and antigen processing and preparation. Moreover, most proteins are impermeable across biological membranes and have short elimination half-lives in biological conditions. Therefore, the development of effective and efficient delivery systems and method for peptides and proteins is a substantial pharmaceutical challenge.

Protein and peptide delivery systems must be able to supply conformationally active molecules to the site of drug action. These systems should also include (i) the ability to control the release rate and/or location of drug release to ensure the therapeutic drug is maintained at the site of action for the intended duration of time, (ii) mechanisms to protect the stability and biological activity of the protein/peptide in the body, and (iii) mechanisms to maintain drug product stability during shipping and long-term storage. In-depth knowledge about protein structure, product stability, and handling requirements is then essential for the healthcare provider to educate and communicate appropriately to patients and other providers.

Protein stability refers to the maintenance of the primary, secondary, tertiary, and quaternary structures. Various interactions between charged groups, hydrophobic interactions, and hydrogen bonds help in increasing stability of the native protein structures. Peptidyl–prolyl isomerization, disulphide bridges methylation, phosphorylation, or glycosylation provides covalent contributions to protein stability. Noncovalent factors that contribute to protein stability are hydrophobic effects, hydrogen bonds, Van der Waals forces, aromatic interactions, and ion pairs/salt bridges. Hydrophobic polypeptide segments are buried in the interior of protein molecules, normally out of contact with water. If these interactions are not optimized, an increase in entropy can occur and may lead to disruption of protein stability.

Protein instability then results when the structure is disrupted by conversion of native protein (i.e., therapeutically active and folded) to non-native or denatured states (i.e., unfolded, cleaved, or inactivated proteins). Typically, these instabilities ultimately result in an alteration to pharmacologic effects or the complete loss of the protein's biological activity. Many therapeutic proteins have fragile three-dimensional structures and are susceptible to various degradation pathways. These pathways are referred to as physical and chemical instability. Physical instability refers to alteration in secondary or higher degrees of structures, whereas chemical instability refers to any changes leading to the formation of a new chemical entity such as formation or deletion of an amide bond between any two amino acids or alterations to the side chain functional groups.

6.2.6 Physical Instability

6.2.6.1 Aggregation

Aggregation is typically the reversible association of materials to form small, loose composite particles. For therapeutic proteins, this association can result in the loss of a protein's native structure due to disruption of tertiary or quaternary structural bonds or associations and potentially lead to irreversible protein instability. Aggregation can occur in the presence or absence of thermal, chemical, or physical stress. Aggregates can form due to the creation of non-native β sheet structures. Some factors that contribute to protein aggregation include elevated temperature, altered solution pH values, changes in salt concentration, and the presence of co-solutes including preservatives and surfactants.

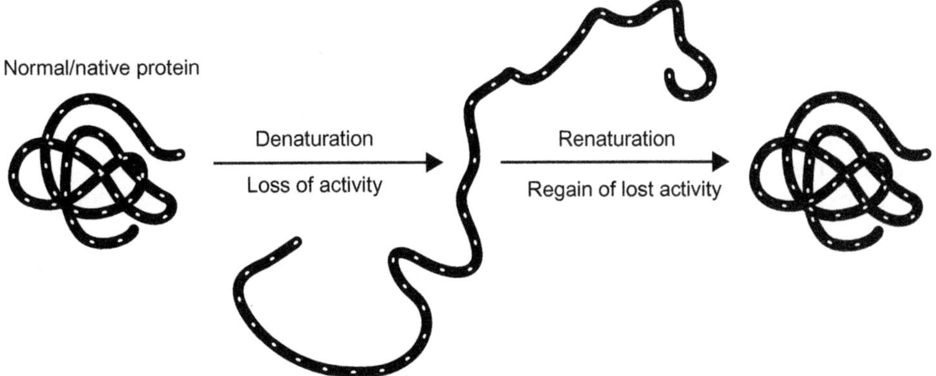

FIGURE 6.3 Schematic representation of normal and denatured protein [3].

6.2.6.2 Adsorption

Adsorption is the physical association of particles to an encountered surface. It is related to the adhesion of the proteins to various surfaces due to favorable interactions to coat or form a monolayer. Many therapeutic proteins have a high likelihood to adsorb onto the surfaces of water-insoluble polymers used in plastics related to drug delivery (e.g., syringe bodies, IV fluid bags, tubing, seals, plungers). Adsorption to these surfaces can alter the physicochemical properties of the protein to cause degradation. Protein adsorption to plastics can also lead to a reduction in drug dose and suboptimal pharmacologic responses. Although some adsorbed proteins can be disassociated, most are irreversibly adsorbed, unable to be recovered under normal clinical conditions.

6.2.6.3 Precipitation

Precipitation is similar to aggregation but occurs at a macroscopic level when irreversible particle flocculation occurs. Precipitated protein particles have lost important structural elements and are unable to be resuspended. Precipitation can be caused due to the presence of salts, addition of organic solvent or other additives, and change in pH of the protein solution. Insulin frosting is a type of protein precipitation, where finely divided insulin precipitation occurs on the walls of a container. This occurs due to denaturation of insulin at the air-water interface.

6.2.6.4 Denaturation

Denaturation is described as the disruption of the secondary and tertiary structure of proteins. It can occur due to various physical factors such as temperature, pH, and addition of organic solvents or other denaturants. Protein denaturation is often irreversible but might be reversible in specific circumstances. For example, elevated temperature can cause an increase in the energy of the system to promote bond rotation, which could lead to unfavorable interactions that could then disrupt protein structure and cause the unfolding of the protein. Sometimes, lowering the temperature can reverse the effect and allow the favorable interactions to reform to promote the proper folding of the therapeutic protein in a phenomenon called reversible denaturation. Figure 6.3 shows protein denaturation (http://www.bio.miami.edu). In cases of irreversible denaturation, the unfolding or misfolding occurs, but the process is not reversible; hence, the protein does not regain its native state [2].

6.2.7 Chemical Instability

6.2.7.1 Deamidation

In deamidation, hydrolysis of the side chain amide linkage in asparagine or glutamine residues occurs, resulting in the formation of free carboxylic acid. The rate of deamidation is affected by temperature, pH, ionic strength, and the presence of buffer ions in the solution. In a neutral pH solution, deamidation causes introduction of a negative charge and results in isomerization, which then affects the biochemical properties of peptides and proteins.

6.2.7.2 Racemization

Racemization of amino acids can occur in all amino acids except glycine because of a chiral center at the carbon bearing a side chain. Racemization generally occurs via the removal of α-methine hydrogen by base to form a carbanion ion. The rate of racemization is controlled by the stabilization of the carbanion ion, typically by the close association of electronegative functional groups or molecules. Racemization can result in formation of nonmetabolizable forms of amino acids or form peptide bonds that are accessible to proteolytic enzymes. Racemization of therapeutic proteins and peptides has the potential to disrupt protein structure and chemically stabilizing interactions.

6.2.7.3 *Oxidation*

The side chains of methionine, histidine, cysteine, tryptophan, and tyrosine residues in proteins are sites that are susceptible to oxidation. Methionine residues can be oxidized even by atmospheric oxygen. The thioether group of methionine is a weak nucleophile and is not protonated at a low pH, which can allow oxidation under acidic conditions. The rate of oxidative degradation will increase in the presence of visible light and is thought to be related to the formation of free radicals. The solution pH is also found to affect the rate of oxidation with slow histidine oxidation occurring at low pH values.

6.2.7.4 *Disulfide Exchange*

The interchanging of disulfide bonds in proteins can cause incorrect pairing and distort protein structure and loss of pharmacologic activity. Thiol ions cause a nucleophilic attack on the sulfur ion of the disulfide in neutral and alkaline conditions. Thiol scavengers such as p-mercuribenzoate and copper ions can be used to prevent disulfide exchange as they catalyze the oxidation of thiols in air.

6.2.7.5 *Hydrolysis*

Hydrolysis of amide bonds in the peptide backbone can occur under a variety of circumstances. Enzymatic cleavage, pH-dependent hydrolysis, and intramolecular catalysis at the N-terminal or C-terminal end at a residue adjacent to an aspartic acid residue via the ionized carboxyl group can all cause protein hydrolysis. Often, cleavage of peptide linkages and chemical hydrolysis can cause complete loss of pharmacologic activity and protein denaturation.

6.2.8 Protein and Peptide-Based Drugs

The number of marketed therapeutic proteins and peptides continues to expand. The clinical utility of these agents is also expanding to diverse groups of therapeutic applications such as replacing a deficient or an abnormal endogenous protein or peptide, providing some novel function or activity, augmenting an existing physiological pathway or process, binding with a molecule or receptor, delivering other compounds, eliciting an immune response for the purpose of vaccination, or diagnosis. Table 6.2 gives brief descriptions of select marketed drug products with clinically relevant approaches to the pharmaceutical principles of therapeutic proteins and peptides.

6.3. INTRODUCTION TO OLIGONUCLEOTIDES

Oligonucleotides are short linear nucleic acid polymers that typically have 50 or fewer nucleotide bases.

TABLE 6.2 Protein and Peptide-Based Drugs

Proteins/Peptides	Trade Name	Description
Insulin lispro	HumaLOG®	This is a rapid-acting insulin (onset, peak glycemic effect, and duration are 0.25–0.5, 0.5–2.5, and <5 hours, respectively).
Insulin regular	HumuLIN® R Novolin® R	This is a short-acting insulin (onset, peak glycemic effect, and duration are 0.5, 2.5–5, and 4–12 hours, respectively). HumuLIN R and Novolin R are obtained from *E. Coli* and *Saccharomyces cerevisiae*, respectively, using recombinant DNA technology.
Insulin NPH (isophane suspension)	(HumuLIN® N, NovoLIN® N)	This is an intermediate-acting insulin (onset, peak glycemic effect, and duration are 1–2, 4–12, and 14–24 hours, respectively).
Insulin NPH suspension and insulin regular solution	NovoLIN® 70/30	This is a combination of two types of insulin for which onset, peak glycemic effect, and duration are 0.5, 2–12, and 8–24 hours, respectively.
Insulin zinc	Lente®	Insulin zinc, like insulin NPH, is an intermediate-acting insulin that consists of a mixture of crystalline and amorphous insulin in a ratio of approximately 7:3.
Insulin glargine	Lantus®	This is a long-acting insulin (onset and duration are 3–4 and >24 hours, respectively) that does not have any pronounced peak glycemic effect.
Calcitonin	Fortical®, Miacalcin®	This is a peptide hormone that is used in osteoporosis. Salmon calcitonin (SCT) is more potent than human calcitonin (HCT) because it is not fibrillated in physiological solution. The p*K*a of SCT and HCT are 10.4 and 8.7, respectively; therefore, SCT remains charged at pH 7.4, which repels each other, thereby inhibiting fibrillation.
Erythropoietin	Procrit	It stimulates erythropoiesis and therefore is used in anemia due to some chronic diseases, renal failure, or chemotherapy.

(*Continued*)

TABLE 6.2 *(Continued)*

Proteins/Peptides	Trade Name	Description
Blood clotting factor VIII	Advate	It is used to treat Hemophilia A.
Blood clotting factor IX	BeneFIX®	This factor IX of recombinant DNA origin is used in the prevention and control of hemorrhagic episodes in patients with a deficiency of coagulation factor IX associated with hemophilia B (Christmas disease).
β-Gluco-cerebrosidase	Cerezyme	It hydrolyzes glucocerebroside to glucose and ceramide. Therefore, it is used in Gaucher's disease, in which the patient is genetically deficient of enzyme β-Gluco-cerebrosidase, resulting in an accumulation of the harmful fatty acid substance glucocerebroside in liver, spleen, lungs, and bone marrow.
Lactase	Lactaid	This is able to digest lactose; hence, it is used in gas, bloating, cramps, and diarrhea due to the patient's inability to digest lactose.
Interferon-α2b (IF Nα2b)	Intron A	It works as an immunoregulator although the exact mechanism is not known. It is used in hepatitis B and C, melanoma, Kaposi's sarcoma, follicular lymphoma, etc.
Peginterferon-α2b	Peg-Intron	This is IF Nα2b conjugated with polyethylene glycol to increase its half-life.
Growth hormone, somatotropin	Genotropin®, Nutropin®	This anabolic and anticatabolic effector is used in growth failure due to growth hormone deficiency or chronic renal insufficiency, Prader–Willi syndrome, Turner syndrome, and AIDS wasting (or cachexia) with antiviral therapy.
Lutropin-α	Luveris®	It is a recombinant human luteinizing hormone that increases estradiol secretion and therefore is used in treating infertility due to luteinizing hormone deficiency.
Botulinum toxin type A	Botox	This is a neurotoxin produced by *Clostridium botulinum*, which appears to affect only the presynaptic membrane of the neuromuscular junction in humans, where it prevents calcium-dependent release of acetylcholine and produces a state of denervation. Muscle inactivation persists until new fibrils grow from the nerve and form junction plates on new areas of the muscle-cell walls. This is used to treat cervical dystonia and minimize the appearance of glabellar lines.
L-Asparaginase	Elspar®	Asparaginase inhibits protein synthesis by hydrolyzing asparagine to aspartic acid and ammonia. It is used in acute lymphocytic leukemia, which requires exogenous asparagine for proliferation.
Bevacizumab	Avastin®	It is a recombinant, humanized monoclonal antibody that binds to all isoforms of vascular endothelial growth factor (VEGF), preventing its association with endothelial receptors, Flt-1, and KDR required for angiogenesis; therefore, it is used in the treatment of colorectal cancer and non-small-cell lung cancer.
Trastuzumab	Herceptin®	Trastuzumab is a monoclonal antibody that binds to the extracellular domain of the human epidermal growth factor receptor 2 protein (HER-2) and controls cancer cell growth. Therefore, it is used in the treatment of breast cancer, which overexpresses HER-2 receptors.
Denileukin diftitox	Ontak	It is a fusion protein (a combination of amino acid sequences from diphtheria toxin and interleukin-2) that directs the cytocidal action of diphtheria toxin to cells expressing the IL2 receptor. Therefore, it is used in the treatment of T-cell lymphoma, whose malignant cells overexpress the IL2 receptor.
Human papillomavirus (HPV) vaccine	Gardasil	It contains major capsid proteins from four HPV strains and is used as a vaccine for the prevention of HPV infection.
Hepatitis B surface antigen (HBsAg)	Engerix	This is derived from the hepatitis B surface antigen (HB_sAg) produced through recombinant DNA techniques from yeast cells and is used for immunization against infection caused by all known subtypes of the hepatitis B virus.
Pentagastrin	Gastrodiagnost	This synthetic pentapeptide simulates the action of natural gastrin. This is used as a diagnostic aid for evaluation of gastric acid secretory function.

Although only very few oligonucleotides have been approved as therapeutic agents, a great deal of research is being devoted to the development of these drug products. Oligonucleotides typically exert their pharmacologic activity as antisense oligonucleotides by interfering with normal DNA replication to silence a gene expression. As natural polymers, oligonucleotides present substantial barriers to drug product development, absorption, formulation, and delivery.

6.3.1 Antisense Oligonucleotides

Therapeutic oligonucleotides (oligo) typically have very specific nucleotide sequences that target specific sequences of DNA or RNA that are exposed during normal cellular processes. The therapeutic oligo is complementary to a chosen sequence with which it can bind with very high affinity. Antisense oligonucleotide containing complementary nucleotide sequences target mRNA or DNA but with modifications to promote cellular degradation of the complex into nucleotide residues (see Figure 6.4). The oligo-DNA/RNA hybrid duplex is then enzymatically degraded and results in inhibition of the expression of the chosen gene sequence.

6.3.2 Therapeutic Oligonucleotides

The drug delivery challenges for therapeutic oligonucleotides are substantial. They are not capable of permeating through biological membranes, are sensitive to widespread nuclease activity throughout the body, and are susceptible to chemical degradation and nonspecific adsorption to surfaces. Various chemical modifications and formulations have been investigated to overcome these barriers. Currently, only a few approved oligonucleotide-based drug products are available. However, future scientific advancements will likely lead to more marketed oligonucleotides. Examples of currently marketed products are described in the following sections.

6.3.2.1 *Pegaptanib Sodium (Macugen®)*

Pegaptanib is a modified oligonucleotide that is conjugated to PEG and is selective to inhibit vascular endothelial growth factor (VEGF). It is approved for the treatment of age-related macular degeneration as an intravitreal injection directly into the fluid of the eye. The invasive intraocular injection then bypasses biological membranes and eliminates the need for membrane permeation. Pegaptanib is available as a prefilled, single-dose, glass syringe with an attached needle that is all enclosed in a sterile foil pouch. The

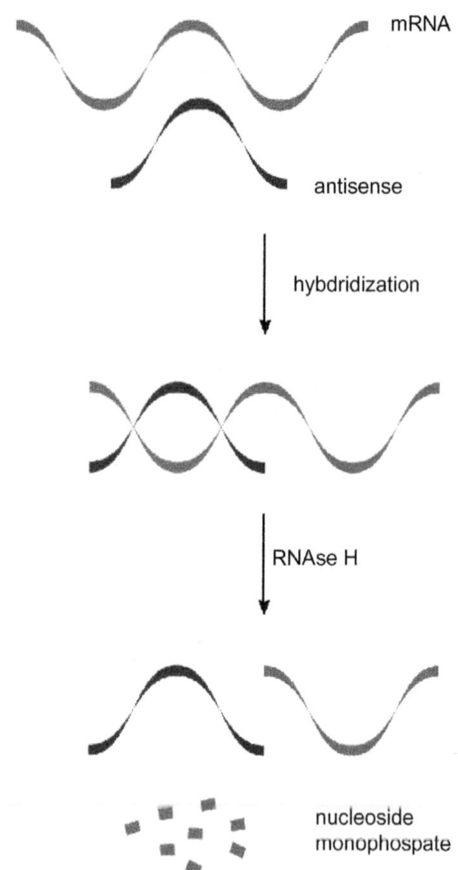

FIGURE 6.4 Diagrammatic representation of RNase-mediated destruction of mRNA bound to an antisense oligonucleotide. *(Modified and adapted from reference [4])*

drug solution is preservative-free and contains only sodium chloride and phosphate salts to ensure the solution is isotonic and has a neutral pH.

6.3.2.2 *Fomivirsen (Vitravene®)*

Fomivirsen is an antisense oligonucleotide that inhibits human cytomegalovirus (CMV) replication. It too is approved for injected into the vitreous fluid in the eye and is active against strains of CMV resistant to ganciclovir, foscarnet, and cidofovir. It is a sterile, preservative-free, buffered solution in a single-use glass vial. A sterile filter needle should be used to withdraw the solution and injected intravitreally using a new small gauge needle (30G).

6.3.2.3 *Mipomersen (Kynamro®)*

Mipomersen is an antisense oligonucleotide that inhibits the synthesis of apo B-100 involved in the production of low-density lipoprotein and very low-density lipoprotein associated with familial hypercholesterolemia. It is injected subcutaneously into the abdomen, thigh, or upper and outer part of the arm and is highly protein bound to blood plasma proteins. Mipomersen is available as a sterile, preservative-free, single-dose, prefilled glass syringe. The drug solution contains only pH adjustment ingredients.

6.4. CONCLUSIONS

The pharmaceutical utilization of polymers provides key functions in formulations and as pharmacologically active drugs. However, polymers are unlike many other active pharmaceutical ingredients and excipients in numerous ways. Many polymers used as pharmaceutical excipients have formulation-specific functions that are dependent on their chemical structure and molecular weight. Many polymers are used for the enhancement of viscosity, gelation, tablet binding of other ingredients, film formation, coatings, etc. Other polymers are therapeutically active proteins, peptides, and oligonucleotides. Scientific advances in pharmaceutical biotechnology will further expand the clinical utility and availability of these therapeutic biopolymers.

CASE STUDIES

Case 6.1

Lyophilization is generally used to provide long-term storage stability to protein and peptide pharmaceuticals. Explain how. What important considerations should you, as a pharmacist, provide to enhance stability during storage?

Approach: Lyophilized proteins exist in highly viscous amorphous glassy states with low molecular mobility and low reactivity and very stable under this condition. According to the "vitrification hypothesis," stability is highly dependent on storage temperature. If the same material is stored at a temperature higher than its glass transition temperature (Tg), the viscous glass will be transformed to a less viscous "rubbery" state with increased heat capacity, molecular mobility, and decreased stability. Crystallization of the glass-forming excipients can occur above the Tg value, further decreasing its stability. Excipients such as sugars are thought to hydrogen bond with the protein in the same manner as water, conserving its native structure by replacing water lost during drying and stabilizing the formulation during storage. Recent studies have shown that optimal stabilization is provided by glass-forming excipients that hydrogen bond to the protein molecule, thus preserving its native structure during lyophilization and storage. Storage temperature and moisture are the two important considerations you have to consider for stability. Moisture can act a plasticizer and affect Tg and thereby stability.

Case 6.2

As a manufacturing pharmacist, you are supposed to determine the drug load of a silicone rubber implantable delivery of a steroidal drug. You have no information available regarding how to proceed on this issue. What information will help you address this issue? Do you think this particular implant is a biodegradable or nonbiodegradable polymeric implant?

Approach: A silicone implant is not biodegradable. To determine the drug load, you have to use a food analytical method for the drug. You also need to know a good solvent system for dissolving the polymer and how to extract the drug from the polymeric solution. A good solvent is one for which the solubility parameter is close to that of the polymer. All this information can be obtained from the literature or a polymer handbook. In the case of silicone rubber, hexane is good solvent to dissolve the implant. You can find an assay method for the drug in the literature and use it to determine the concentration in the implant.

Case 6.3

The major component of hard gelatin and soft gel capsules is gelatin. Knowing some of the properties of polymer, explain why such differences occur between those two.

Also, one of your patients refuses to take such capsules because of his religious beliefs. What alternatives do you have for this patient?

Approach: The difference between hard and soft gel capsules is the amount of plasticizer used. The use of plasticizer in a polymer decreases the glass transition temperature (Tg) of a polymer. It can exist as a rubbery polymer at room temperature, but not as a glass. Glycerol or sorbitol is used as plasticizer for gelatin.

To provide other alternatives for your patient, you can do the following:

- Dispense the same drug in a different dosage form (suspension) if its physicochemical properties allow.
- Dispense capsules from which alternative sources besides animals are used to create the gelatin. Some hard shell capsules are made from materials other than gelatin. For alternatives to gelatin that will be of interest to those who, for religious, cultural, or other reasons, wish to avoid capsules manufactured from animal sources, consider offering Starch hydrolysate (Capill is the commercial product) or

Hydroxypropyl methyl cellulose (Vegicaps, or V-caps, is the commercial product in the market).

References

[1] Brooklyn College's three-dimensional structure of proteins. <http://academic.brooklyn.cuny.edu/biology/bio4fv/page/3d_prot.htm>, [retrieved on 18.05.2010].

[2] Lai MC, Topp EM. Solid-state chemical stability of proteins and peptides. J Pharm Sci 1999;88:489–500.

[3] Lehninger AL. Biochemistry: the molecular basis of cell structure and function. Worth Publishers; Richmond, UK.

[4] Oligonucleotides as drugs. <http://www.atdbio.com/content/13/Oligonucleotides-as-drugs>, [retrieved on 16.07.2012].

Suggested Readings

Yamamoto T, Nakatani M, Narukawa K, Obika S. Antisense drug discovery and development. *Future Med Chem*. 2011, 3:339–65.

Labarre DJ, Ponchel G, Vauthier C. *Biomedical and Pharmaceutical Polymers*. Pharmaceutical Press, London, UK; 2011.

Rowe RC, Sheskey PJ, Quinn ME, AP Association. *Handbook of Pharmaceutical Excipients*, 6th Edition. Pharmaceutical Press, London, UK; 2009.

Sinko PJ. *Colloidal Dispersions. Martin's Physical Pharmacy and Pharmaceutical Sciences: Physical Chemical and Biopharmaceutical Principles in the Pharmaceutical Sciences*. Lippincott Williams, New York, USA; 2006. p. 386–409.

PART II

PRACTICAL ASPECTS OF PHARMACEUTICS

CHAPTER

7

Drug, Dosage Form, and Drug Delivery Systems

Alekha K. Dash

Department of Pharmacy Sciences, School of Pharmacy and Health Professions, Creighton University, Omaha, NE, USA

CHAPTER OBJECTIVES

- Recognize the difference between drug, dosage forms, and drug delivery systems.
- Appreciate the need for various dosage forms and drug delivery systems.
- Identify the role of active and inactive materials in a dosage form.
- Recognize the importance of preformulation studies in dosage form design.
- Understand some of the important preformulation strategies commonly used in dosage form development.

Keywords

- Dosage form
- Dosage form design
- Excipients
- Pharmaceuticals ingredients
- Preformulation

7.1. INTRODUCTION

Drug substances are seldom administered alone; rather, they are administered either as dosage forms or drug delivery systems. Acetaminophen is the drug or, more precisely, the active pharmaceutical ingredient in a Tylenol tablet. Dosage form is a physical form of a pharmaceutical formulation containing the drug and some inactive ingredients necessary to make that particular physical form. In the preceding example of the Tylenol tablet, acetaminophen is the drug, and the tablet is the dosage form. Other dosage forms may include capsules, powders, emulsions, solutions, suspensions, syrups, lotions, elixirs, parenterals, suppositories, ointments, creams, pastes, etc. Drug delivery systems, on the other hand, are specialized dosage forms through which one can predict the release of the drug from such systems. The nicotine transdermal patch and Procardia XL are examples of drug delivery systems. Dosage forms as well as drug delivery systems contain various inactive ingredients besides the active drug. These inactive ingredients are also called pharmaceutical ingredients. They are incorporated into the dosage form to accomplish one or more of the functions outlined in Table 7.1.

Pharmaceutics is the science of dosage form design and belongs to a branch of pharmacy that deals with the general area of study concerned with the formulation, manufacture, stability, and effectiveness of various pharmaceutical dosage forms and drug delivery systems.

Various dosage forms need to do the following:

- Provide safe and convenient delivery of an accurate dosage of a drug
- Protect the drug from the destructive influences of atmospheric oxygen and humidity (for example, coated tablets, sealed ampoules)
- Protect tablets from the destructive influences of gastric acid during oral administration (for example, enteric coated tablets)
- Mask the unpleasant taste or odor of the drug substance (for example, flavored syrup, sugar-coated tablet or capsule)
- Administer a high dose of an insoluble drug in a liquid dosage form (for example, suspension)
- Provide clear liquid dosage forms for a drug substance (for example, syrups, solutions)
- Provide optimal drug action from topical administration sites (for example, ointments;

Pharmaceutics. DOI: http://dx.doi.org/10.1016/B978-0-12-386890-9.00007-8

TABLE 7.1 Functions of Pharmaceutical Ingredients

Functions to Be Accomplished	Pharmaceutical Ingredient	Examples
Solubilize	Surfactants	Tween 20
Suspend	Suspending agent	Methyl cellulose
Thicken	Thickening agent	Gum acacia
Dilute	Solvent	Water
Emulsify	Emulsifying agent	Tween 20, Span 80
Preserve	Preservatives	Methyl and propyl paraben
Color	Coloring agent	FD&C yellow color
Flavor	Flavoring agent	Peppermint oil
Disintegrate	Disintegrating agent	Starch
Bind	Binders	Starch

creams; transdermal patches; ophthalmic, otic, and nasal routes)

- Provide delivery of drugs by insertion into one of the body's orifices (for example, suppositories)
- Administer a drug directly into the body tissues (for example, parenterals)
- Provide optimal drug action through inhalation therapy (for example, aerosols)
- Provide time-controlled drug action (for example, controlled-release tablets, capsules, and suspensions)

7.2. PHARMACEUTICAL INGREDIENTS

Pharmaceutical ingredients generally establish the primary features of the dosage form and contribute to the physical form, texture, stability, taste, and overall appearance of the dosage form.

In the preparation of liquid dosage forms, the following pharmaceutical ingredients may be used:

- Solvents and co-solvents are used for the formulation of solutions.
- Preservatives are used to prevent microbial growth in solutions.
- Stabilizers are used to prevent drug decomposition.
- Flavoring agents are added to enhance palatability.
- Coloring agents are used to enhance product appeal.

In the preparation of tablet dosage forms, the following pharmaceutical ingredients are generally used:

- Diluents or fillers are used to increase the bulk of the formulation.
- Binders are used to adhere the powdered drug and pharmaceutical ingredients.
- Disintegrants are used to promote tablet disintegration (break-up) in the gastrointestinal tract.
- Lubricants are used to assist proper powder flow during tablet manufacturing.
- Coatings are applied to improve stability and enhance appearance.

In the preparation of semisolid dosage forms (ointments, creams), the major pharmaceutical ingredient used is the ointment base.

7.3. PREFORMULATION STUDIES

Preformulation is the process of optimizing a drug through the determination of its physical and chemical properties considered important in the formulation of a stable, effective, and safe dosage form. This also includes the determination of any possible interactions with various ingredients in the final formulation.

Pharmaceutical preformulation work is generally initiated when a compound shows sufficiently impressive results during biological screening. The preformulation flow sheet in Figure 7.1 illustrates the various steps involved in the preformulation process [1,2].

7.4. PHYSICAL DESCRIPTION

The majority of drug substances in use today occur as solids. However, they may be available as a liquid or even less frequently as a gas. This physical form plays an important role in detecting the ultimate dosage form. If the drug is available as a liquid, and the dosage form is requested as a solid, the preformulation scientist does not have enough options available to fulfill this request. In such instances, more preferred options are providing different salt forms of the product or even rethinking different dosage forms.

7.5. LIQUID DOSAGE FORMS

Examples of some liquid drugs and their clinical use in parentheses follow:

- Amyl nitrite (vasodilator)
- Nitroglycerin (anti-anginal)
- Ethchlorvynol (hypnotic)
- Clofibrate (antihyperlipidemic)
- Paraldehyde (sedative-hypnotic)
- Undecylenic acid (antifungal)

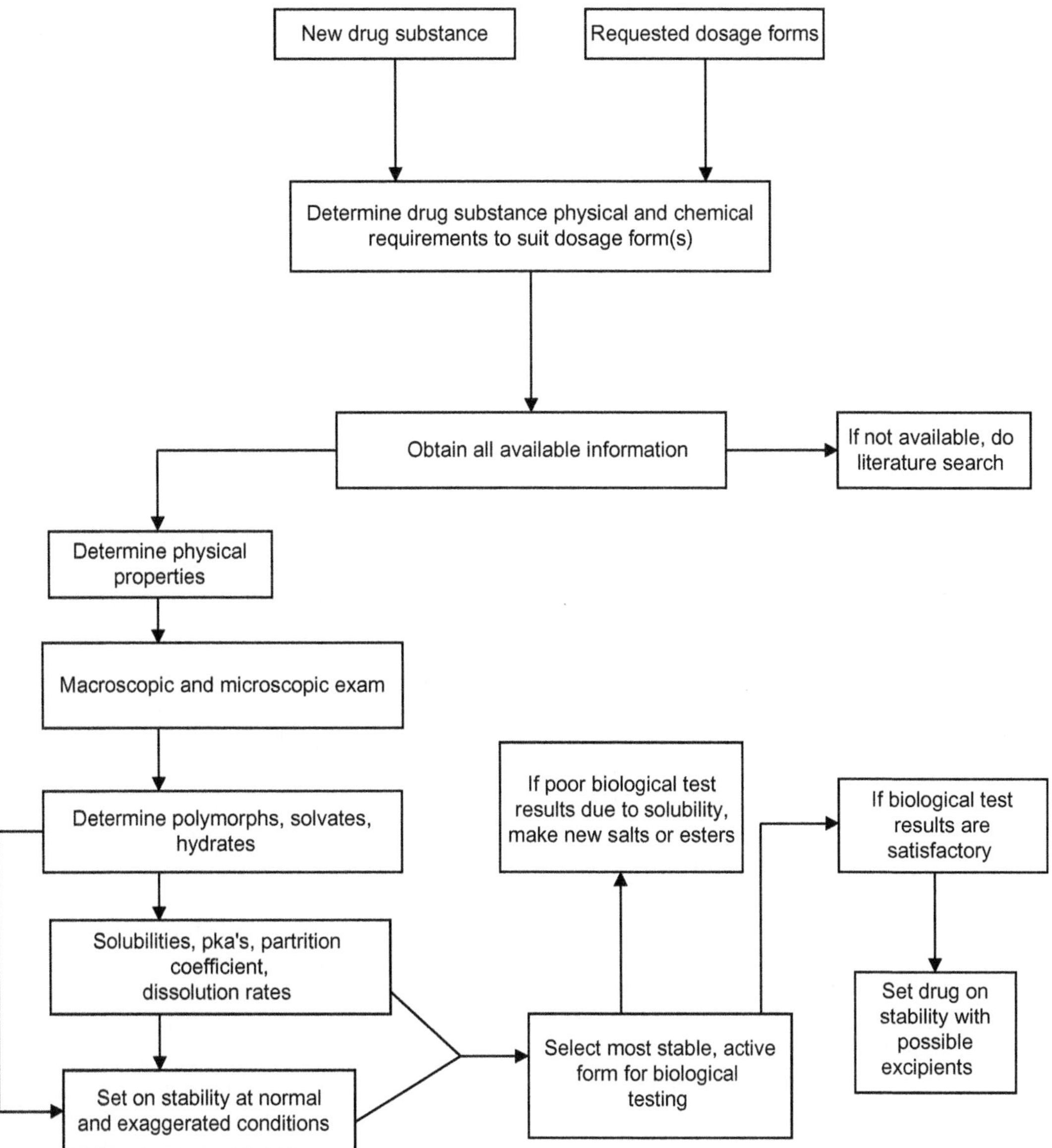

FIGURE 7.1 The preformulation process flow sheet.

Following are some formulation problems for liquid dosage forms:

1. Many liquids are volatile and also flammable. Therefore, they should be physically sealed in ampoules (for example, amyl nitrate)
2. Liquids cannot be formulated into tablet forms intended for oral administration. An exception to this is nitroglycerin tablet triturates, which disintegrate within seconds when placed under the tongue. Two approaches are generally used to deliver liquid orally as a solid formulation:
   a. Liquid drug delivered in soft gelatin capsules (for example, Paramethadione and Ethchlorvynol)
   b. Liquid drug converted to a solid salt or ester (for example, liquid scopolamine is converted to a scopolamine hydrobromide solid)
3. Stability difficulties arise less frequently with solid dosage forms than with liquid preparations.

Besides the preceding disadvantages, liquid drugs also pose certain advantages, as follows:

1. Large doses can be administered orally (for example, a 15 mL dose of mineral oil).
2. Topical application becomes easy and effective (for example, undecylenic acid in the local treatment of a fungal infection).
3. Liquid doses are convenient for administration to pediatric and geriatric populations.

7.6. SOLID DOSAGE FORMS

Tablets and capsules comprise the dosage forms dispensed more than 70% of the time by community pharmacists, with tablets dispensed twice as frequently as capsules [3].

7.6.1 Solid-State Properties

Following are properties of solid dosage forms:

- **Macroscopic properties:** Appearance, color, and odor of a drug substance should be recorded. Bulk density and true density of the material need to be determined at this stage if not available to a preformulation scientist.
  - **True density:** This is the density of the actual solid material. For nonporous material, density is measured by displacement in an insoluble liquid. For porous solids, a helium densitometer is generally used to determine density.
  - **Bulk density:** This density is defined by mass of the powder divided by its bulk volume. (About 50 cc of powder passed through a U.S. standard sieve #20 is weighed and placed in a 100 cc volumetric cylinder. The cylinder is dropped at 2-second intervals three times from a distance of 1 inch on a wooden table. The weight of powder is divided by bulk volume to give the bulk density.)
- **Flow properties:** Angle of repose is a measure of the flow properties of a powder or a granule. Powders are allowed to pass through a funnel until the angle of inclination is large enough to balance the frictional forces and form a heap. The *angle of repose* or, more precisely, the *critical angle of repose* is the steepest angle of dip of the slope relative to the horizontal plane when a material on the slope face is on the verge of sliding. This angle is given by the number (0°–90°). The tangent of the angle of repose is a measure of the internal friction of the powder bed:

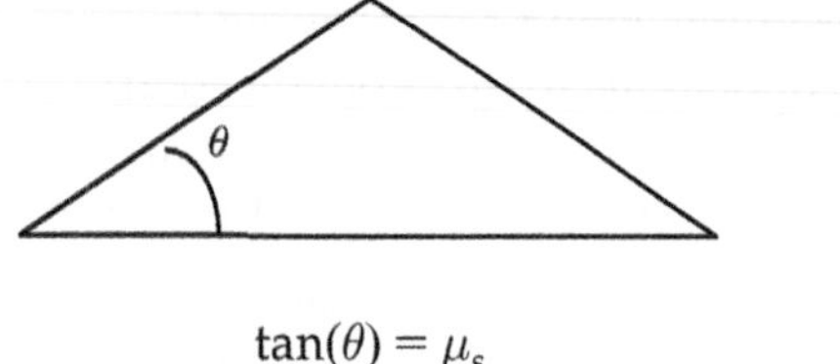

$$\tan(\theta) = \mu_s$$

where μ_s is the coefficient of static friction, and θ is the angle of repose.

7.6.2 Microscopic Examination

A microscopic examination provides information on particle size, size distribution, and crystal habit (shape) of a drug. These properties can be best identified through the use of a *polarizing* microscope. Crystal shape may be of prime importance and a deciding factor for certain formulations. Needle-like crystals, for example, are not suitable for parenteral formulations. A microscope attached to a hot stage may be utilized to determine

- The purity of a drug sample semi-quantitatively (the melting point)
- The presence of any hydrates or solvates in the crystal
- Physical changes that may occur during heating

7.6.3 Particle Size

Particle size and size distribution can affect various important properties of drug substances that may affect dissolution, absorption, solubility, content uniformity, taste, texture, color, and stability. The following methods can be used to determine the particle size of powders:

- **Sieving:** Sieving and screening are generally used for particle size analysis when the particles are approximately 44 microns and greater. The only disadvantage of this method is that relatively large sample size is required. This method is very simple both in technique and equipment requirements.
- **Microscopy:** The optical microscopy can be utilized to determine the particle size, size distribution, and shape of new drug substances. This method is tedious and time-consuming.
- **Sedimentation:** The sedimentation technique utilizes the relationship between rate of sedimentation and their size as described by Stoke's equation (Eq. 7.1). This method is generally used for particles within a range of 3–250 microns. The following precautions must be observed with this method: proper particle dispersion, good temperature control of the settling medium, and appropriate particle concentration.

$$v = \frac{d^2(\rho_s - \rho_0)g}{18\,\eta} \tag{7.1}$$

where
v = the velocity of sedimentation (cm/sec)
d = the diameter of the particle (cm)
ρ_s = the density of the particle (gm/cc)
ρ_0 = the density of the medium (gm/cc)
g = the acceleration due to gravity (cm/sec^2)
η = the viscosity of the medium (poise)

- **Stream scanning:** This technique utilizes a fluid suspension of particles that pass the sensing zone where individual particles are electronically sized, counted, and tabulated (for example, a Coulter counter). The main advantage of this method is that a large volume of data can be generated in a relatively short period of time. However, it has the shortcoming of not providing information relative to particle shape.

7.7. PARTITION COEFFICIENT AND pKa

To produce a biological response, a drug molecule must cross the biological membrane. Biological membranes are made up of lipid and protein material and act as a lipophilic barrier to the passage of many drugs. The oil/water (octanol/water, chloroform/water) partition coefficient is a measure of a molecule's lipophilic nature. It has been demonstrated that the hypnotic activity of a series of barbiturates is closely related to their octanol/water partition coefficient. The octanol-water partition coefficient (*P*) of a drug can be determined as follows:

$$P = \frac{(\textit{Concentration of drug in octanol})}{(\textit{Concentration of drug in water})}$$

For an ionizable drug:

$$P = \frac{(\textit{Concentration of drug in octanol})}{(1-\alpha)(\textit{Concentration of drug in water})}$$

where α is the degree of ionization.

From the preceding equation, it is clear that determination of the dissociation constant in preformulation work is important because it may be an indicator of a drug substance's absorption characteristics. The dissociation constant is usually determined by potentiometric pH titration.

7.8. SOLUBILITY

Relatively insoluble compounds (in water) sometimes exhibit either incomplete or erratic absorption. In such situations, preformulation work would include preparation of more soluble salts or esters, solubilization through use of a surfactant, complexation, micronization, and solid dispersion.

- **Equilibrium solubility:** This is determined by dispersing excess of a drug into 0.9% NaCl solution, water, 0.1 N HCl, or pH 7.4 buffer in a suitable container and agitating in a constant temperature bath (37°C). Samples are withdrawn and assayed until the concentration is constant. One must take into account the common ion effect (for example, hydrochloride salts are less soluble in 0.9% NaCl and 0.1 N HCl as compared to water).

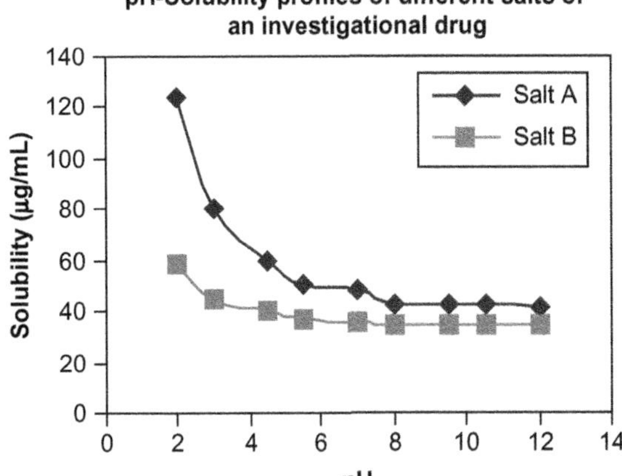

FIGURE 7.2 pH solubility profiles.

- **pH solubility profile:** Molecules having polybasic functional groups (for example, triamterene) may form complex salts at varying pH values. pH solubility profiles of two salts of a new drug are shown in Figure 7.2.

7.9. DISSOLUTION

Dissolution rate of a drug substance, when combined with the solubility, partition coefficient, and pKa results, provide some insight into the potential *in vivo* absorption characteristics.

Dissolution rate may be affected by chemical form, crystal form, particle size, and surface properties of a drug:

- **Chemical form:** Acid, base, and salt forms have significant differences in dissolution rate. (For example, the dissolution rate of sodium sulfathiazole in 0.1 N HCI is 5,500 times faster than sulfathiazole.)
- **Crystal form:** The metastable form has a greater dissolution rate compared to the stable form. (For example, sulfathiazole II has a higher dissolution rate than stable sulfathiazole I.)
- **Particle size:** A reduction in particle size increases the surface area of the particles and the dissolution rate.
- **Surface properties of drug:** High surface energy of micronized powder may result in poor wettability and agglomeration. In this case, dissolution rate decreases because total surface area of the material is unavailable to the fluid.

7.10. POLYMORPHISM

Polymorphism is the existence of at least two different crystal structures, known as polymorphs of the same chemical substance. Different polymorphs are different in their crystal structures but identical in the liquid and vapor state. They have differences in their physical properties, such as solubility, melting point, density, hardness, crystal shape, optical properties, electrical properties, and vapor pressure. The occurrence of polymorphism in pharmaceutics is important because of differences in rate and extent of absorption by the body. Different polymorphs of the same compound might give entirely different therapeutic responses. Some drugs and excipients showing polymorphism include progesterone, warfarin sodium, enalapril maleate, ranitidine HCl, nicotinamide, and theobroma oil.

In addition to the polymorphic forms in which compounds exist, they also can occur in noncrystalline or amorphous forms. The amorphous form of a compound is always more soluble than the corresponding crystal forms.

Evaluation of crystal structure, polymorphism, and solvate form is an important preformulation activity. The most widely methods used to characterize these properties are hot-stage microscopy, thermal analyses, infrared spectroscopy, spectroscopy (infrared, Raman, solid-state NMR) and X-ray powder diffraction (XRPD).

7.11. STABILITY

Prediction of stability of a new drug (both physical and chemical) is to be evaluated during the preformulation process. Validated stability indicating assay is commonly used for this evaluation. Thin layer chromatography, thermal analyses, and diffuse reflectance spectroscopy have also been used in preformulation development. During preformulation studies, more attention is provided to address factors such as light, heat, oxygen, moisture, pH, and excipients that can affect drug quality rather than the degradation mechanisms and pathways. Since drug stability and factors affecting it are described in detail in a separate chapter, we suggest the reader refer to Chapter 5.

7.12. CONCLUSIONS

Preformulation is an important first step in the dosage form design process. Its overall importance is underscored when one sees a successful dosage form in the market for a long time without any formulation challenges. Preformulation helps in identifying the best salt with ideal solubility and stability for a drug substance. Based on the knowledge gained from understanding all the physicochemical properties of drugs in a therapeutic group, the preformulation process can help the processing chemist identify ideal candidates with the best biological activity and select the best salt forms of the API with the needed particle size, compression properties, etc., to minimize processing problems during scale-up and future manufacturing.

CASE STUDIES

Case 7.1

The label of a pharmaceutical liquid formulation contains the following information:

Formulation Name: Chloraseptic Sore Throat Spray
Phenol 1.4%, Blue #1, Flavor, Glycerine, Purified Water, Saccharin Sodium

Answer the following questions:

1. Identify the active pharmaceutical ingredients (APIs) in this preparation
2. Identify the dosage form and a drug from this example.
3. Name at least two inactive ingredients (pharmaceutical ingredients) and the purpose of their inclusion in the formulation.

Approach:

1. The active pharmaceutical ingredient in this preparation is phenol 1.4% (drug).
2. The dosage form is a liquid spray that contains phenol 1.4% as the drug and many more inactive ingredients such as water, coloring agent, and flavor.
3. Saccharin sodium is a sweetener used to enhance sweetness of the product, and purified water is used as a solvent for this solution dosage form.

Case 7.2

If one assumes the pH of the stomach to be 1 to 3 and that of the small intestine to be 5 to 8, in most cases a drug substance with a p*K*a of 3 (salicylic acid) will be more rapidly absorbed in the stomach. On the other hand, a drug with p*K*a of 8 (quinine) will be absorbed more rapidly in the intestine. Can you explain this to a healthcare colleague of yours without a pharmacy background?

Approach: This can be explained if one has a better understanding of pH partition theory and ionization of acids and bases and p*K*a:

- Absorption of drug via GI membrane requires that the drug should be lipophilic, which has a better permeability as compared to a drug that is more water soluble.

- Ionization of the drug can be affected by both pH and p*Ka*.
- Ionized drugs are more water soluble as compared to the un-ionized portion. In other words un-ionized drugs are more lipophilic.

Once these three concepts are well understood, one can explain the scenarios presented in this case without any difficulty. Since p*Ka* of salicylic acid is 3, in acidic conditions like the first scenario, the drug will be in the un-ionized state and will be more lipid soluble and will have a better membrane permeability. Since the surface area of the stomach is much less than intestine, that may limit some of the drug absorption. In the case of quinine, the basic drug with a p*Ka* of 8, more of the drug will be present in the un-ionized state in the intestine; therefore, it is more lipophilic and has higher permeability and better membrane absorption from the intestine.

Case 7.3

Abbott laboratory stopped sales of Norvir, an approved novel protease inhibitor for HIV [4].

Facts: Norvir contained Ritonavir as the API, discovered by Abbott in 1992. In December 1995, Abbott filed a New Drug Application (NDA). In January 1996, commercial start-up of the drug began operation. In March 1996, the U.S. FDA approved Norvir as a semisolid capsule and also as a liquid formulation. In early 1998, final product lots failed the dissolution test and were seen to be precipitated out from the semisolid formulated product. As a pharmacovigilance person, how can one explain these facts?

Approach: One has to identify the precipitate by IR and powder XRD, etc. In this case, the precipitate was identified as a new polymorph of ritonavir (Form II). Form II was thermodynamically more stable and much less soluble than Form I. After 2 years of intensive research, the Abbott scientists found a way to control the formation of either Form I or Form II polymorphs. Abbott received FDA approval on the reformulated Norvir soft gelatin capsule in June 1999. This is a classic case in which a pharmaceutical company took a serious look at the polymorphism of solids in 1998.

References

[1] Wells FI, Aulton ME. Preformulations. In: M.E. Aulton, editor. Pharmaceuticals, the science of dosage form design. Churchill and Livingstone; 1994. p. 223–53.

[2] Fiese EF, Hagen TA. Preformulation. In: Lachman L, Lieberman HA, Kanig JL, editors. The theory and practice of industrial pharmacy. 3rd ed. Lea & Febiger; 1986. p. 171–96.

[3] Allen Jr. LV, Popovich N, Ansel HC. Ansel's pharmaceutical dosage forms and drug delivery systems. Wolters Kluwer/ Lippincott Williams & Wilkins; 2011. p 190–142.

[4] Saurabh G, Kaushal C. Pharmaceutical solid polymorphism in abbreviated new drug application (ANDA)-A regulatory perspective. J Chem Pharm Res 2011;3:6–17.

CHAPTER

8

Solid Dosage Forms

Alekha K. Dash

Department of Pharmacy Sciences, School of Pharmacy and Health Professions, Creighton University, Omaha, NE, USA

CHAPTER OBJECTIVES

- Define and describe the various solid dosage forms commonly used in pharmacy practice.
- Explain and understand the application of basic pharmaceutics principles necessary to prepare these dosage forms.
- Identify the applications of these dosage forms in practice, including powder, tablet, and capsule dosage forms.
- Identify the methods used for the manufacture of solid dosage forms including powder, tablet, and capsule dosage forms.
- Describe the various methods used to evaluate the quality of these solid dosage forms including powder, tablet, and capsule dosage forms.

Keywords

- Effervescent powder
- Granules
- Hard gelatin capsule
- Powder
- Soft gelatin capsule
- Tablet

8.1. INTRODUCTION

Pharmacists are regarded as the experts on drugs in healthcare teams. They deal with these entities every day in their professional practice. Drugs, irrespective of their sources, are available in three physical forms of matter, including solid, liquid, and gases. These physical forms can be used as such, or in formulations. Such formulations are also known as drug products or dosage forms that contain a drug or drugs and inactive ingredients called excipients. Many drugs and dosage forms that are used today in practice are solid. The solid dosage form is the preferred dosage form in the United States. Approximately one-third of the dosage forms dispensed by community pharmacists are solid dosage forms, usually tablets or capsules [1]. The solid dosage form encompasses the largest group of dosage forms used in clinical practice. This high acceptance is probably due to many factors, including convenience of handling and self-administration, chemical and physical stability, high-throughput production in a nonsterile environment, relatively inexpensive manufacture, and a long history of understanding of their manufacturing processes. The dosage forms that are most commonly used in practice are powders, tablets, and capsules. Other solid dosage forms that are less frequently used are implants, lozenges, suppositories, and plasters.

8.2. POWDERS

Powders are intimate mixtures of dry, finely divided drugs with or without excipients and can be used either internally or externally. Powders consist of particles ranging from about 10,000 μ to 0.1 μ. The USP describes powder in terms such as *very coarse, coarse, moderately coarse, fine,* and *very fine* depending on their particle size. Antacids, laxatives, dietary supplements, dentifrices, dusting, and douche powders are some commonly dispensed powders. Medicated powders are intended either for oral use or for external application. Many oral powder dosage forms are available as fine powders or as granules, usually administered orally with a glass of water or juice. Since granules have less surface area compared to fine powder, their dissolution in water or juice is much less.

Examples:

Internal use:

- Sodium bicarbonate powder (antacid)
- Psyllium (Metamucil) powder (laxative)

Pharmaceutics. DOI: http://dx.doi.org/10.1016/B978-0-12-386890-9.00008-X

- Massengill powder (douche powders)

External Use:

- Bacitracin zinc and polymyxin B sulfate (anti-infective)
- Tolnaftate powder (antifungal)

8.2.1 Advantages of Powders

- There is a wide choice of ingredients, and the dose can easily be achieved for patient administration.
- Powders have increased stability compared to solutions.
- A large dose that cannot be administered in other forms can be administered as powder.
- A rapid dispersion of drugs occurs in the stomach when given in powder forms rather than in compressed form.
- A powder can be dispersed in water or another liquid and more easily swallowed.

8.2.2 Limitations

- Due to unpleasant taste, drug powders are not the dosage form of choice.
- Drugs that deteriorate rapidly with exposure to atmosphere or acidic pH should not be dispensed as powders.
- Powders are bulky and inconvenient to carry.

Example: Ferrous iron salts are easily oxidized and should not be administered as powders.

8.2.3 Mixing of Powders

Powders do not mix spontaneously; therefore, effective mixing requires a thorough understanding of the materials to be mixed, as well as the science of mixing. Effective mixing of powders poses the greatest challenge when the amount of one of the components of the mix is relatively small compared to the other components. There are four main methods of mixing powders in small-scale operations [2]:

- Trituration
- Spatulation
- Sifting
- Tumbling

8.2.3.1 Trituration

The trituration process involves direct rubbing or grinding of hard powder in a mortar and pestle. The trituration method is used for both pulverization and mixing. Two different types of mortar and pestle are commonly used:

- A *Wedgewood mortar* is used for pulverization and grinding because of its rough inner surface.
- A *glass mortar* is used for simple mixing and for mixing of colored materials and dyes.

8.2.3.2 Spatulation

A powder spatula is used in the spatulation method, and the powders are mixed on a pill tile (ointment slab) or in a mortar. This method is adequate for mixing small amounts of powders and combinations of powders having the same densities. The possible loss during transfer is minimal in this method, and mixing does not reduce the particle size. This method is used when there is a possibility of liquefaction during the mixing of two solid powders.

8.2.3.3 Sifting

The sifting method is helpful for powders that resist mixing by trituration. Very light powders, such as magnesium oxide and charcoal, can be completely mixed by shaking them through a sieve. Standard-size prescription sieves are available, but an ordinary household flour sifter can be used effectively for this purpose. This process allows the removal of any large foreign bodies and agglomerates from the powder mix.

8.2.3.4 Tumbling

Tumbling is a process of mixing powders by shaking or rotating them in a closed container. This method is used when two or more powders have considerable density differences. This mode of mixing does not yield particle size reduction and compaction. Wide-mouthed closed containers or zip-locked bags can be used when the powder volume should be within one-third to one-half field. The powder mixture should flow freely in the air and avoid sliding the powder through the side of the container.

Homogeneity in large-scale mixing is achieved through the use of an appropriate mixer, which ensures the correct speed and sufficient time for mixing. Homogenous mixing is ascertained in a mixture when the concentration of each component in any region of the mixture is identical.

The mixing of pharmaceutical powders generally requires low shear rates; the mixers used for this purpose are planetary bowl mixers, high speed mixers, V blenders, ribbon/trough mixers, and rotating drum mixers.

8.2.3.5 Problems Encountered During Mixing

Most of the problems encountered during mixing of pharmaceutical powders can be minimized using special techniques, assuming that the cause of the problem is clearly understood.

8.2.3.6 Problems Encountered During Trituration

Crystalline salts are mixed well by trituration in a mortar. The inner surface of Wedgewood mortars grows smooth with long-term use. When this happens, powders do not mix well. In such instances, the surface of a mortar can be made rough by triturating with a little powdered pumice or pharmaceutical sand.

8.2.3.6.1 ELECTRIFICATION

Electrification is a phenomenon in which some substances repel each other during mixing. This might be due to simple resistance to admixture, or it may be due to electrical charges. This problem can be eliminated by moistening the powders very slightly with a few drops of alcohol or mineral oil.

8.2.3.6.2 PACKING

A packing problem is encountered when powders are pressed heavily during trituration. This problem can be avoided by triturating lightly and scraping the sides of the mortar frequently with a spatula.

8.2.3.6.3 PHYSICAL IMMISCIBILITY

The phenomenon of physical immiscibility may occasionally present minor problems. Mixing resinous materials with granular salts and mixing heavy powder (starch) with a light one (zinc stearate) may lead to this incompatibility issue. This problem can be minimized by triturating each substance separately to a fine state and then mixing by sifting or tumbling.

8.2.3.6.4 DAMPENING OR LIQUEFACTION

Dampening, or liquefaction, is the most troublesome problem in powder mixing and can happen for three different reasons:

- *Absorption of moisture from the air (deliquescent/hygroscopic)*: A substance that absorbs moisture from the air is termed *hygroscopic* (e.g., ephedrine sulfate, lithium bromide, ammonium chloride). A hygroscopic material that absorbs the moisture from the air to such an extent that it liquefies partially or fully is termed *deliquescent*. Hygroscopic materials should not be ground finer than is necessary and should be wrapped in close containers.
- *Giving up moisture to the air and liquefying during the process (efflorescent)*: Some examples include atropine sulfate, quinine HCl, and scopolamine hydrobromide.
- *Lowering the melting point of the mixture (eutectic mixture)*: Eutectic mixtures result when certain organic compounds (phenol, aldehydes, and ketones) are mixed in varying proportions. The melting point of a fixed composition of a mixture is considerably below that of any of the individual ingredients, and forms a damp mass or even liquefies when mixed together. When mixed in a definite composition from the following ingredients, some drug substances may form a eutectic mixture and liquefy:
  - Acetylsalicylic acid
  - Aminopyrine
  - Camphor
  - Menthol
  - Phenol
  - Salol
  - Thymol

There are three ways to handle this problem:

1. Separately dispense the individual components.
2. Mix each compound with an equal amount of inert diluents (lactose, starch, talc) and finally combine the diluted powders with light trituration.
3. Mix the materials together and allow them to liquefy, and then add sufficient amounts of adsorbents to adsorb the eutectic liquid mixture and remain as a free-flowing powder.

8.2.3.6.5 THREE BASIC RULES FOR MIXING OF POWDERS

- When mixing powders with different particle sizes (granular salt and fine powders), reduce each powder separately to fine particles before mixing.
- When mixing powders with different densities, put the light powder first and then put the heavier one on top of it.
- When mixing small amounts of a drug to a large volume of bulk powder, use the principle of geometric dilution (see below).

8.2.3.6.6 GEOMETRIC DILUTION

When two powders with unequal quantities are mixed, the small weight (least weight) of the powder, usually the active ingredient, is first triturated with an equal bulk of the diluting powder. This first dilution is then mixed with an equal portion of diluents. This process is repeated until all the powders are intimately mixed.

Example:

One gram of a potent drug to be mixed with 20 g of the diluent lactose.

- First dilution: Mix 1 g drug with $\sim$1 g lactose ($\sim$2 g mixture).
- Second dilution: Mix 2 g of the first dilution with 2 g of lactose with trituration ($\sim$4 g mixture).
- Third dilution: Mix 4 g of the second dilution with 4 g of lactose with trituration ($\sim$8 g mixture).
- Fourth dilution: Mix 8 g of the third dilution with 8 g of lactose with trituration ($\sim$16 g mixture).

This process continues until the lactose is fully mixed with the blend.

8.2.3.7 *Classification of Powders*

Powders can be classified by the way they are presented to the user. This may be given as bulk or divided powders.

8.2.3.7.1 BULK POWDERS

Doses of bulk powders are measured out by the patient; they are limited to nonpotent drugs. The patient should be educated regarding the appropriate handling, storage, and solvent to be used if needed for reconstitution, etc.

Examples:

- Dusting powder
- Powders used internally (a teaspoonful at a time)
- Powders used for making solution
- Powders used for inhalation

8.2.3.7.2 DIVIDED POWDERS

Divided powders, or chartulae, refer to single doses of powdered drug mixtures individually enclosed in paper, cellophane, or metallic foil wrappers or packets. *Chartula*, which is abbreviated as *chart*, is the Latin word for powder paper. Some divided powders are commercially available in folded papers or packets.

Example: Cholestyramine resin powder

8.2.3.8 *Special Powders*

- Effervescent salt
- Dentifrices
- Dusting powders
- Insufflations
- Powder aerosols

8.2.3.8.1 EFFERVESCENT SALTS

Powders or granules containing sodium bicarbonate, a suitable organic acid (citric or tartaric), or inorganic (sodium biphosphate) acid and medicinal agents are known as effervescent salts. When mixed with water, the acid and the base react to form carbon dioxide, which produces the effervescence.

8.2.3.8.1.1 ADVANTAGES

- Effervescent salts mask the unpleasant taste of many drugs.
- Carbon dioxide stimulates the flow of gastric juice and accelerates the absorption of many drugs.
- Effervescent salts have a favorable psychological effect on the patient.
- They have enhanced stability since they are stored in low moisture-content packages.

A representative formula for an effervescent salt:

Sodium bicarbonate (dry powder)	477 g
Tartaric acid (dry powder)	252 g
Citric acid crystals	162 g

8.2.3.8.1.2 PREPARATION Effervescent salts can be prepared using two methods:

- *Heat method*: This method requires blending of all the components, with 15%–20% of the acid ingredients as citric acid monohydrate, and heating on a bath (about 100°C). The mole of water released from citric acid during heating moistens the powder, and granules are formed from this moistened powder mass.
- *Wet method*: The citric acid is moistened and added to sodium bicarbonate. Granules are then formed from this partially fused mass, using a suitable granulator.

8.2.3.8.2 DUSTING POWDERS

Dusting powders are used for external use only and should have the following properties:

- Homogenous
- Free from local irritation
- Free-flowing
- Uniform spreading and covering capability
- Good adsorptive and absorptive capability

Medicated dusting powders are applied onto intact skin, open wounds, or even to mucous membranes. Highly adsorptive dusting powders should be avoided in areas with high liquid exudates because a hard crust may form. Starch and talc are commonly used as excipients for dusting powder formulations. Being organic, starch may support bacterial growth. On the other hand, talc is inert but can easily be contaminated and may be a potential source of infection. Therefore, sterilized talc is commonly used in medicated dusting powder formulations.

8.2.3.8.3 DENTIFRICES

Fine powders that are used to clean teeth are called dentifrices. Cleaning properties of these powders are achieved through incorporation of detergents. Besides the detergent, a small amount of mild abrasive (precipitated calcium carbonate or hydrous dibasic calcium phosphate) is also included. Dentists usually use dentifrices with high abrasive properties that are not suitable for daily use. In such instances, dentists use pumice powder.

8.2.3.8.4 INSUFFLATIONS

Insufflations are finely divided powders intended for application into body cavities, such as tooth sockets, ears, nose, vagina, and throat. An applicator known as an insufflator is used to deliver a stream of finely divided powder to the target organ. Intranasal insufflation is preferred over oral use if the therapeutic efficacy of the drug is lost upon oral use. It can be utilized for both local application and systemic absorption.

8.2.3.8.5 POWDER AEROSOLS

Powders can be dispensed as aerosols from pressurized containers that have a push-button actuator. They are easy to apply, can be evenly applied to a larger surface, and provide protection against harmful external exposure. The major disadvantages of powder aerosols include valve clogging, agglomerative sedimentation, and leakage.

Examples:

Antiperspirants and deodorants as powder aerosols
Tinactin powder aerosol

8.3. CAPSULES

Capsules are solid dosage forms designed to contain drug(s) for administration. Two types of capsules are commonly used in pharmacy: hard (two-piece) gelatin capsules and soft (one-piece) gelatin capsules [3].

8.3.1 Hard Gelatin Capsules

Hard-shell gelatin capsules are solid dosage forms in which one or more medicinal agents and/or inert materials are enclosed within a small shell. Hard gelatin capsules consist of two parts: the body designed to contain the drug and the diluent, and the cap that is approximately half as long as the body. Hard capsules are available in a variety of standard sizes and are designated by numbers from 000 to 5. The size of the 000 capsule is the highest and that of the number 5 capsule is the smallest, as shown in Table 8.1.

The large range of weights of powders that can be filled into different sized capsules depends on their bulk densities and compressibility. Mixtures of dry powdered materials may be incorporated in capsules as loose powders, granules, slightly compressed plugs, or tablets.

8.3.1.1 Advantages of Capsules

- There are fewer steps compared to the wet granulation method of tablet manufacture.
- Certain bioavailability problems encountered in the case of tablet formulations can be avoided by capsule formulation.
- Capsules completely mask unpleasant taste and odor.

TABLE 8.1 Various Sizes of Hard Gelatin Capsules

Capsule Size Designation	Usual Range of Powder Size
5	60–130 mg
4	95–260 mg
3	130–390 mg
2	195–520 mg
1	225–650 mg
0	325–920 mg
00	390–1300 mg
000	650–2000 mg

- They are easier to swallow than tablets.
- They can be made opaque and offer advantages for photosensitive drugs.
- They do not deposit powder or small fragments into the containers in which they are stored.
- They are difficult to counterfeit.

8.3.1.2 Disadvantages of Capsules

- Extremely soluble materials cannot be administered in capsules.
- Capsules are not suitable for efflorescent or deliquescent materials.
- They require specialized manufacturing equipment.

8.3.1.3 Capsule Shell Components

The major component of a capsule shell is gelatin. Other than gelatin, it may contain 10%–15% moisture, dyes, plasticizer, and opacifying agents. Starch and hydroxypropylmethyl cellulose are being investigated as possible capsule shell materials. Gelatin is a mixture of protein derived from animal collagen by irreversible hydrolytic extraction. Depending on the method of extraction, two types of gelatin can be produced. Type A gelatin is prepared by treating pig skin with acid, and has an isoelectric point between 7 and 9. Type B gelatin is prepared by base treating bovine bones, and has isoelectric points between 4.7 and 5.3. Because of this difference in isoelectric points, both gelatins show solubility differences at different pH values. Gelatin grade is further specified by bloom strength. This is defined as the weight in grams that is required to depress a cylindrical plunger of 12.7 mm diameter a depth of 4 mm with an aged gelatin gel of 6.6% (w/w) in water.

8.3.1.4 Capsule Filling

Capsules are generally filled by hand by placing the powder to be filled on paper or on a pill tile and pressing the open end of the capsule downward until it is filled. The cap is then placed to close the capsule.

Semiautomatic and fully automated filling machines are available for large-scale operations.

8.3.1.5 Storage Conditions

Capsules contain 10%–15% moisture. Under high humidities, capsules absorb moisture. Above 16% moisture, they lose their mechanical strength and may become sticky. Storage under extremely dry conditions will result in brittle capsules due to moisture loss. The best storage and process conditions for capsules are within a temperature range of 10°C–25°C and relative humidity of 35%–45%.

8.3.1.6 Filling of Hard Gelatin Capsules

The powders to be filled in hard gelatin capsule shells should be homogeneous and have excellent flow property. Flow property of a powder mix can be determined by the angle of repose, which is the angle the powder makes with the horizontal plane when it flows from a funnel onto a flat surface. The tangent of this angle is a measure of the internal friction of the powder bed. If the measured angle is around 25°, the flow is considered to be excellent; if it is 50° or more, the flow is considered to be poor. In such instances, use of a glidant will enhance powder flow by reducing particle-particle cohesion. During filling of hard gelatin capsules, the following problems may be encountered:

- *Improper flow of the powder mixture during the filling operation*: This problem can be overcome by incorporation of suitable amount of glidants or lubricants into the powder mixture.
- *Segregation and homogeneity*: This problem is generally encountered when semiautomatic or automatic machines are used for filling the capsules. The vibration during operation of these heavy-duty machines can cause segregation of particles and inhomogeneity. This segregation can be minimized by keeping particle sizes and densities of the powders as uniform as possible.
- *Incompatibility*: In some instances, incompatibility between formulation ingredients, formulation components, and the capsule shell may create problems. A proper understanding of the physicochemical properties of each ingredient may avoid such incompatibility issues. Some of the excipients commonly used in the filling of hard gelatin capsules may include the following:
  - Diluents to increase the overall working mass of the powder for easy and accurate handling during filling operations. These diluents include lactose, corn starch, and microcrystalline cellulose.
  - Disintegrants to break up the powder mass when exposed to a liquid medium. Corn starch, microcrystalline cellulose, sodium starch glycolate, and croscarmellose are disintegrants used in hard gelatin capsules.
  - Glidants to lower the interparticle attraction and thereby reduce agglomeration and enhance the flow of powder. Colloidal silicon and talc are commonly used for this purpose.
  - Lubricants to reduce the interaction between powders and components of the filling machine handling the powder. Magnesium and other metallic stearates are generally used as lubricants.
  - Surface-active agents incorporated into the powder mix to decrease surface tension and enhance wetting of the powder with the release medium when hydrophobic components are present in higher amounts. Sodium lauryl sulfate is commonly used for this purpose.

8.3.1.7 Finishing

Filled capsules may have small amounts of powder formulation adhering to the outside of the capsule. Therefore, the filled capsules require dusting and polishing to remove powder from the surface of these capsules. For small-scale operations, clean cloths or scientific cleaning wipes (e.g., Kimwipes®) may be used to de-dust the capsules. However, in large-scale operations, the following methods are generally used:

- *Pan polishing*: Accela-Cota® pan coating machines lined with a polyurethane or cheese cloth are used.
- *Cloth dusting*: Capsules are rubbed with a cloth that may be impregnated with an inert oil.
- *Brushing*: Capsules are fed under rotating soft brushes that remove the dust from the capsule surface, followed by the use of a vacuum system for dust removal.

8.3.2 Soft Gelatin Capsules

Soft gelatin capsules are made from shells of gelatin to which plasticizers such as glycerol and polyols (sorbitol, propylene glycol) have been added. The distinctive feature of this capsule is its one-piece construction. The feeding and sealing are achieved by only one machine. Hard gelatin capsules are manufactured in a two-step process, in which shells are manufactured by one type of machine and the filling is achieved by a different machine. Soft gelatin capsules are usually produced from two thin sheets of gelatin suitably molded and sealed together after the amount of drug to be encapsulated is inserted between them, as shown in Figure 8.1. Soft gelatin capsules are available in various sizes, shapes, and colors. Soft gelatin capsules have grown in popularity in recent years because they enable administration of a liquid in a

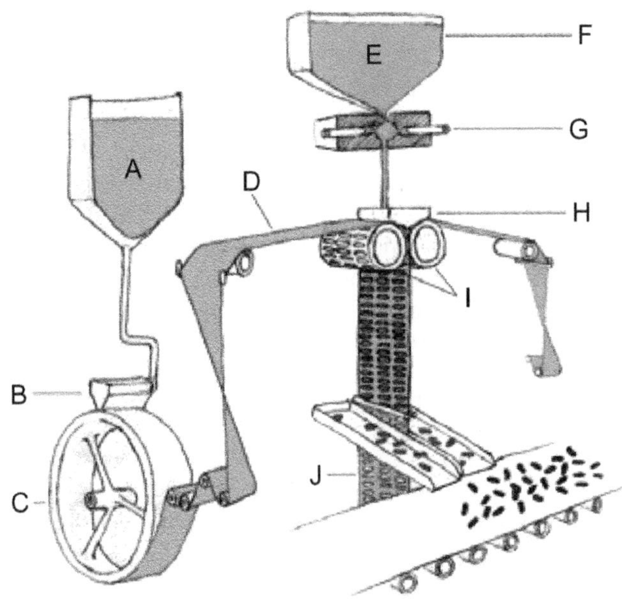

FIGURE 8.1 Schematic drawing of a rotary die process of making soft gelatin capsules. (A) Gelatin mix, (B) spreader, (C) cooling drum, (D) gelatin ribbon, (E) fill material, (F) fill tank, (G) fill pumps, (H) injection wedge, (I) die, and (J) gelatin net.

solid dosage form with a bioavailability advantage over other commonly used solid dosage forms (e.g., tablets).

8.3.2.1 *Advantages of Soft Gelatin Capsules*

- Soft gelatin capsules permit liquid medication to be easily transportable and administered as a solid dosage form.
- They provide accuracy and uniformity of the dose to be administered.
- They provide better drug availability than tablets and hard gelatin capsules.

8.3.2.2 *Pharmaceutical Applications of Soft Gelatin Capsules*

- Soft gelatin capsules are available as an oral dosage form.
- They are available as a suppository dosage form.
- They are available as a single-dose application of topical and ophthalmic preparations.
- They are extensively used in the cosmetic industry to dispense bath oil, perfume, skin creams, breath fresheners, etc.

8.3.2.3 *Basic Components of a Soft Gelatin Capsule*

The major components of soft gelatin capsule shells are gelatin, plasticizer (Glycerin USP, Sorbitol USP), and water. Besides these three components, they may contain other ingredients such as preservatives, coloring, flavoring, opacifiers, and sweetening agents. Type B gelatin is commonly used in the preparation of soft gelatin capsules; however, type A gelatin can also be used. The presence and the amount of plasticizer used in the preparation of the capsule shell determines its flexibility. In general, 20%−30% (w/w) of plasticizer is recommended. If the plasticizer concentration is less than 20%, the shell becomes very brittle. When the amount is above 30%, it becomes very tacky. The ratio of plasticizer and gelatin determines the overall hardness of the finished product. The ratio of 0.4:1.0 produces extremely hard shell capsules; when this ratio is 0.8:1.0, the capsules become very flexible. The ratio of water (on weight basis) to dry gelatin varies from 0.7−1.3 (water) to 1.0 (dry gelatin). Commonly, a 1:1 (water:gelatin) ratio is used. Since water is lost during the drying and manufacturing process, the final water content of the capsule shell lies in between the range of 5%−8%. Some of the other additives used in soft gelatin capsules are listed in Table 8.2.

TABLE 8.2 Other Ingredients Added to Soft Gelatin Capsule Shells

Ingredients	Concentration	USED AS
Methylparaben and propylparaben (4:1 ratio)	0.2%	Preservative
Titanium dioxide	0.2%−1.2%	Opacifier
Sugar (sucrose)	Up to 5%	Sweetener
Ethyl vanillin	0.1%	Flavoring agent
Cellulose acetate phthalate (CAP)	4%	Enteric coating agent
Fumaric acid	Up to 1%	Solubility enhancer and reduce aldehydic tanning of gelatin

8.3.2.4 *Capsule Content in a Soft Gelatin Capsule*

The fill material for soft gelatin capsules is mostly liquids, but solids and semisolid materials can be dispensed in this dosage form. Solutions of solids in liquid and suspensions of solids in liquid are also filled in soft gelatin capsules.

8.3.2.5 *Liquids*

Several categories of liquids can be used as fill material. This includes lipophilic liquid, self-emulsifying liquids, and water-miscible liquids. Some water-miscible and volatile liquids, such as ethyl alcohol, cannot be incorporated as major constituents since they can migrate to the capsule shell and volatilize from the surface. A high proportion of plasticizers such as glycerol and propylene glycol cannot be incorporated due to their softening effects on the shell. Lipophilic materials such as vegetable oil and esters of fatty acids are mostly used. Since these solvents have limited solubility to many solutes, other pharmaceutics techniques, such as co-solvent and solubilization by the use of a surfactant, are commonly used. Self-emulsifying systems consist of lipophilic liquids containing nonionic surfactants. When these liquids come into contact with GI fluid instantaneously from emulsions with high surface areas, they aid in rapid dissolution and absorption of hydrophobic drugs. Water-miscible liquids, such as high-molecular-weight alcohols like polyethylene glycols (PEG 400 and 600), nonionic surfactants like Tweens, and polyoxyethylene-polyoxypropylene block co-polymers (Pluronics), could be used as fill materials in soft gelatin capsules. The formulation of the capsule content is individually selected according to the product specification and end use of the product.

Examples of liquids for human use:

- Oily active ingredients (clofibrate)
- Vegetable oils (soybean oil)
- Mineral oil
- Nonionic surface active agents (polysorbate 80)
- Oil-soluble vitamins

8.3.2.6 Liquid Solutions and Suspensions as Fill Material

Before being filled into soft gelatin capsules, these fill materials should be homogenous, free of air, and flow freely under gravity at room temperature but not at the sealing temperature, which is around 37°C–40°C for soft gelatin capsules. The pH of the liquid fill should be in the range of 2.5–7.5. Highly acidic solution may cause hydrolysis of gelatin and leakage of the gelatin shell. Highly alkaline pH may lead to tanning of gelatin, which can affect its solubility.

Examples of commercially available drugs prepared as soft gelatin capsules include the following:

- Ethchlorvynol (Placidyl, Abbott)
- Chlorohydrate (Noctec, Squibb)
- Vitamin A, vitamin E, etc.

8.3.2.7 Soft Gelatin Capsule Manufacturing

The original patent for the manufacture of soft gelatin capsules was granted to R.P. Scherer in 1933. A schematic representation of the manufacturing process is shown in Figure 8.1. The first step is the preparation of the gelatin ribbons. The wet mass containing gelatin, water, plasticizer, and other needed ingredients is prepared. This gelatin solution is spread over two drums using a spreader box. The formed gelatin ribbons with controlled thickness are fed through a mineral oil lubricating bath, over guide rolls, and fed in between two rotary dies that are lubricated with mineral oil. The pump accurately meters the filled material through the leads and the wedge and into the gelatin ribbons between the die rolls. The two halves of the capsule containing the fill material are sealed by temperature (37°C–40°C) and pressure. The capsules are removed from the ribbon, subjected to a naphtha wash unit to remove the mineral oil, and exposed to an infrared drying unit to remove 60%–70% of the water. Capsules are equilibrated with forced air conditions of 20%–30% RH at 21°C–24°C, and the water content of the shell is within 6%–10%.

8.3.2.8 Quality Control of Capsules

Quality control and inspection for both hard and soft capsules are almost the same as for other solid dosage forms and must follow good manufacturing practices. Some of the additional steps needed for capsules are outlined here:

- *Empty capsules*: For hard gelatin capsules, care should be taken to evaluate and control the physical dimensions, wall thickness, length, and overall join length. Visual inspections for air bubbles, dents, cracks, loose caps, etc., are essential in the quality assurance protocols.
- *Filled capsules*: In the case of filled capsules, content uniformity, moisture content, fill weight, disintegration, dissolution, and stability evaluation are essential to maintain quality capsules and compare batch-to-batch variation and control. However, in the case of soft gelatin capsules, some additional quality control measures are used, including evaluation of seal thickness, total or shell moisture content tests, and effect of freezing and high temperature on the capsule shell. In the case of capsules containing liquids, leaking and other defects need to be determined.

8.4. TABLETS

Tablets are solid dosage forms containing medicinal agents, with or without any diluents. Based on the method of manufacture, tablets can be classified into two groups [3]:

- Molded tablets or tablets triturates
- Compressed tablets

Compressed tablets are solid dosage forms prepared by compaction of a formulation containing a drug and certain excipients selected to aid in processing and to improve product properties.

8.4.1 Advantages of Tablets as a Dosage Form

- Tablets are convenient and easy to use.
- They are less expensive to manufacture than other oral dosage forms.
- They are physically and chemically stable.
- Special release profiles, such as enteric or sustained release, can be achieved.
- There is high patient acceptance because of their portability and compact form.
- Tablets are the most tamper-proof of all oral dosage forms.
- They provide economy and convenience of production, storage, and transportation.

8.4.2 Disadvantages

- Some individuals experience psychological difficulties in swallowing tablets.
- Preparing tablets extemporaneously is impractical.

8.4.3 Essential Properties of a Good Tablet

- Tablets must be sufficiently strong to maintain their shape during manufacture, packing, shipping, and use.
- The drug in tablets should be bioavailable and released in a reproducible and predictable manner.
- Tablets should be accurate and uniform in weight.
- They should be elegant in appearance and easily identifiable.
- They should have reasonable physical and chemical stability during average storage conditions.
- They should be free of cracks, chipped edges, discoloration, and contamination.
- They should provide ease of manufacture and economy of production.

8.4.4 Types of Tablets

Tablets are generally classified according to their method of manufacturing (molded versus compressed) and their intended use.

8.4.4.1 Conventional Compressed Tablets

The majority of tablets used today in clinical practice are conventional compressed tablets. They are manufactured by a single compression cycle using powders or granules of both active and inactive agents. Disintegration and dissolution of the tablet after oral administration in the GI tract aid in the absorption of the drug via the gastric mucosa.

Examples: Tylenol® tablet, metformin tablet

8.4.4.2 Molded Tablets

Molded tablets are not manufactured by compression. They are prepared by molding and are very soft and disintegrate quickly. One example of molded tablets is tablet triturates. Tablet triturates are administered sublingually, or by placing them on the tongue followed by swallowing with a small volume of water. Lactose and sucrose are the common diluents used for tablet triturates.

Examples: Nitroglycerin tablet triturates

8.4.4.3 Buccal Tablets

Buccal tablets are designed to dissolve slowly in the mouth between the cheek and the gingiva. These tablets are manufactured so that the release of drug happens slowly in the mouth without disintegration. The drug is absorbed into the blood circulation directly through oral mucosa. Direct absorption through oral mucosa avoids first-pass metabolism.

Example: Fentanyl buccal tablet

8.4.4.4 Sublingual Tablets

Sublingual tablets are placed beneath the tongue and dissolve rapidly. This mode of administration also avoids first-pass metabolism.

Example: Glyceryl trinitrate sublingual tablet

8.4.4.5 Chewable Tablets

Chewable tablets are chewed in the mouth before swallowing. They are not intended to be swallowed intact. These tablets are intended for children, the elderly, and patients who have difficulty swallowing. Mannitol is commonly used as an excipient in chewing tablets because of its cooling effect during dissolution in the mouth.

Examples: Pepcid® chewable tablet, chewable aspirin tablet

8.4.4.6 Effervescent Tablets

Effervescent tablets are produced from compression of effervescence granules that contain an organic acid (citric) and sodium bicarbonate. When such tablets are placed in water, the chemical reaction of acid with the base produces carbon dioxide in the form of gas bubbles. Quick disintegration of these tablets helps in quick dissolution and absorption.

Example: Alka-Seltzer™ tablet

8.4.4.7 Lozenges and Troches

Lozenges and troches are intended to be sucked and held in the mouth, where they exert a local effect in the mouth or throat. These dosage forms are most commonly used in sore throat and cough remedies for common colds. Lozenges are made by fusion, compression, or a candy-molding process. Troches are made by a compression process. These dosage forms do not disintegrate in the mouth but slowly dissolve or erode with time.

Examples: Clotrimazole troches, Chloraseptic® lozenges, Nicorette® lozenges

8.4.4.8 Multiple Compressed Tablets

Multiple compressed tablets are designed to enable the separation of incompatible ingredients or make sustained release products, or they are merely designed for appearance. There are two classes of multiple compressed tablets: layered tablets and compression-coated tablets.

Examples: Phenylephedrine HCL, ascorbic acid with acetaminophen

8.4.4.9 Sugar-Coated Tablets

Conventional compressed tablets are coated with successive coats of sugar solution with or without a color to produce elegant, glossy, and easy-to-swallow tablets for oral use.

Example: Perphenazine tablet, sugar-coated

8.4.4.10 Enteric-Coated Tablets

Enteric-coated tablets are conventionally compressed tablets coated with a polymer that does not dissolve in the acidic condition of the stomach but readily dissolves in the alkaline pH of the small intestine. Such a coating can protect drugs from the degradative effects of gastric acidity. They also protect gastric mucosa from irritation from certain drugs. Polymers that have enteric-coating ability include cellulose acetate phthalate (CAP), cellulose acetate butyrate (CAB), hydroxypropylmethylcellulose succinate, and methacrylic acid co-polymers (Eudragit).

Examples: Enteric-coated aspirin tablet, naproxen enteric-coated tablet

8.4.4.11 Film-Coated Tablets

Film-coated tablets are compressed tablets coated with a colored polymeric coating that forms a thin skin-like film around the tablet core. The film coating is more durable than sugar coating and can be formed quickly. Polymers used in film coatings include hydroxypropylmethyl cellulose, hydroxypropylcellulose, and Eudragit® E100, etc.

Example: Glyburide/metformin (5 mg/500 mg) film-coated tablets

8.4.4.12 Sustained-Release Tablets

Sustained-release tablets are designed to release an initial therapeutically effective amount of a drug followed by maintaining this effective level over an extended period of time. This is achieved by design approaches. The advantages of sustained-release tablets include maintenance of therapeutic effect for a longer time, reduced frequency of administration, and enhanced patient compliance.

Example: Wellbutrin SR® (bupropion hydrochloride) tablet

8.4.4.13 Vaginal Tablets

Vaginal tablets are ovoid- or pear-shaped conventional compressed tablets that are inserted into the vagina using a plastic inserter. Antibacterial drugs, antifungal drugs, and steroids are generally administered using this dosage form. Lactose and sodium bicarbonate are used as diluents for vaginal tablets. After insertion, the drug is released by slow dissolution. Disintegration of these tablets must be avoided for proper retention inside the vagina. Both systemic and local delivery of drugs can be achieved by using this dosage form.

Examples: Vagifem® (estradiol vaginal tablets), nystatin vaginal tablets, USP

8.4.4.14 Orally Disintegrating Tablets (ODTs)

Orally disintegrating tablets are a solid dosage form containing medicinal substances that disintegrate rapidly, usually within a matter of seconds, when placed on the tongue. They are produced by dry granulation and compression, have a hardness of 40 N or more, a disintegration time of 30 seconds or shorter, a friability of 0.1% or less, and an excellent feeling upon ingestion that is capable of disintegrating with a small amount of water.

Example: Zofran ODT (Ondansetron ODT); Imodium Instant melts (Loperamide HCI ODT)

8.5. MANUFACTURE OF COMPRESSED TABLETS

Tablets are manufactured by compression using a tablet press. A compressed tablet is composed of two basic groups of ingredients: the medicaments, also known as the active pharmaceutical ingredients (APIs; always present except when it is a placebo tablet for investigational use), and excipients (all other materials needed to make the tablet except the medicament), which may or may not be present. Therefore, a tablet excipient is an inert substance used to give a preparation a suitable form or consistency and, in some instances, is present in higher amounts than the API. The choice of excipients depends on the process used for the manufacturing of compressed tablets. Some common excipients used in tablet formulations include diluents or fillers, binders, disintegrants, lubricants, glidants, coloring agents, and flavoring agents. Each of these excipients serves a unique function and, in some instances, may serve more than one function [3].

8.5.1 Diluents

Diluents are needed in all methods of tablet manufacturing when the active mass per each tablet is not sufficient for processing. Diluents can be categorized into insoluble and soluble. Some commonly used soluble diluents include lactose, sucrose, dextrose, and mannitol. Calcium sulfate dihydrate, dibasic and tribasic calcium phosphate, starch, and microcrystalline cellulose (MCC) are insoluble diluents that are mostly used as fillers.

8.5.2 Binders

Binders are adhesive materials used to hold powders together to form granules and assist in holding the tablet together after compression with adequate hardness (see Table 8.3).

8.5.3 Disintegrating Agents

Disintegrating agents are an important component of tablet dosage forms. They are added to a tablet formulation to break apart the compressed tablet (disintegrate) when placed in aqueous environments. Disintegration of conventional compressed tablets must occur within 15 minutes. Disintegrants may work by one of the following mechanisms (see Table 8.4):

- Disintegrants can increase the porosity and wettability of compressed tablets. In doing so, they enhance the penetration and uptake of GI fluids into the tablet matrix and disintegrate. Starch and microcrystalline cellulose act by this mechanism.
- Disintegration can happen due to the effervescence properties of granules, which can break the tablets very quickly when they come into contact with water.
- Swelling of the disintegrant in the presence of water can increase the internal pressure of the tablet matrix and cause eventual disintegration of the tablet. Sodium starch glycolate, croscarmellose, and pregelatinized starch work according to this mechanism.

Disintegrants can be added to formulations before compression by three different methods:

- *Internal addition*: The disintegrant is mixed with other powders before granulation.
- *External addition*: The disintegrant is added to the granules before compression (mixing prior to compression).
- *Combination method*: Both internal and external additions of disintegrants are used. This is the most efficient way of adding a disintegrant to a tablet formulation before compression. These agents swell when exposed to gastric fluids and exert sufficient mechanical pressure from within the tablet to cause it to break apart into small segments.

8.5.4 Lubricants and Glidants

Lubricants are added to granules before compression to achieve many functions. They enhance the flow of granules, reduce adhesion to punches and dies, facilitate ejection through the die wall, and reduce die and punch wire. Two types of lubricants are commonly used, depending on their aqueous solubility. The amount of lubricant used may adversely affect the disintegration and dissolution of tablets and should be carefully monitored. Some of the insoluble lubricants used in tablet formulations include magnesium stearate (0.25%–0.5% w/w), stearic acid (1%–3% w/w), and glycerylpalmitostearate (1%–3% w/w). Soluble lubricants are used to minimize the adverse effect of insoluble lubricants on tablet disintegration and dissolution. However, the lubricative powers of soluble

TABLE 8.3 Examples of Binders

Binder	Usual Concentration (% w/v)
Corn starch USP	5%–10% aqueous paste
Starch 1500	5%–10% aqueous paste
Gelatin	2%–10% aqueous solution
Acacia	5%–20% aqueous solution
PVP	5%–20% aqueous, alcoholic or hydroalcoholic
Methyl cellulose	2%–10% aqueous solution
Sodium carboxymethyl-cellulose	2%–10% aqueous solution

TABLE 8.4 Examples of Disintegrating Agents

Disintegrants	Concentration (% w/w) in Granulation
Starch USP	5–20
Starch 1500	5–15
Microcrystalline cellulose (Avicel)	5–15
Alginic acid	5–15
Guar gum	2–8
Methylcellulose, sodium carboxymethylcellulose	5–10

lubricants are inferior to their insoluble counterparts. Some soluble lubricants include polyethylene glycol (PEG) 4000, 6000, and 8000; polyoxyethylene stearate (1%–2% w/w); and sodium or magnesium lauryl sulfate (1%–2% w/w).

Glidants are added to enhance the flow properties of powders in the hopper and the feed frame into the die in the tablet press. Glidants act in between the particle and the surface of the hopper or dies to reduce the friction and aid in enhanced flow. Since glidants are hydrophobic, they can adversely affect disintegration and dissolution. Therefore, their amount in the tablet should be carefully monitored. Talc and silicon dioxide are used as glidants in tablet formulations.

8.5.5 Flavoring Agents and Sweetening Agents

Flavoring agents are mostly used in chewable tablets. Flavors can be available as oils and spray-dried beadlets. Oils can be sprayed onto dry granules as an alcoholic solution or incorporated in the lubricant. FD&C color is normally used to add appropriate color to a tablet. Color can be added to a binding solution or can be sprayed onto the granules. Dye can also be mixed with the dry powder blend before the wet granulation process.

8.6. METHODS USED FOR MANUFACTURE OF COMPRESSED TABLETS

A tablet granulation must be prepared first in a form suitable for compression on a tablet press. Such a procedure is called *granulation*. The granules used for tablet compression must have good flow properties, be compressible to form the compact, and have lubricant properties for ejection of the tablet from the die [3]. Three processes are used for making tablets by compression:

- Wet granulation
- Dry granulation (slugging)
- Direct compression

The wet and dry granulation processes are designed to improve the flow and compressibility of powders that would otherwise be unsuitable for compression. When the formulation has a satisfactory flow and compressibility, the ingredients can be mixed and directly compressed.

8.6.1 Wet Granulation

Wet granulation is the process in which a liquid is added to a powder with agitation to produce agglomeration or granules. Wet granules are prepared using oscillating granulators, high-speed mixers, or even fluidized-bed granulators. The wet granules are properly dried and mixed with other essential excipients and finally pressed in a tablet press. This is the oldest and most conventional method of making tablets. It is also the method of choice when large-dose drugs are to be compressed.

8.6.1.1 Advantages of Wet Granulation

- Wet granulation modifies the properties of formulation components to overcome their tableting deficiencies. Granules are relatively more spherical than the powders and have better flow properties. During compaction, granules are fractured, exposing new surfaces; this improves compressibility. Improved compressibility allows lower pressure to be used, which improves the life of the machine.
- This process ensures better content uniformity, especially for soluble low-dose drugs.
- It prevents segregation of components.
- It may improve the dissolution rate of an insoluble drug by proper choice of solvent and binder.

8.6.1.2 Limitations

- The cost of wet granulation is higher because of the space, time, and equipment involved.
- This process is not suitable for moisture- and heat-sensitive materials.
- Migration of soluble materials, including dyes, in the solvent to the surface of the granules may occur during the drying process.
- Incompatibilities between formulation components will be aggravated by the granulating solvent, bringing them into close contact.
- There is a possibility of material loss during processing due to the transfer of material from one unit operation to the other.

8.6.2 Dry Granulation

Dry granulation involves compacting the components of a tablet formulation by means of a tablet press and then milling the compact to obtain the granules. Compaction for the dry granulation process is generally achieved either by slugging or roller compaction. No water or heat is needed for this granulation process. In the slugging process, large tablets are compressed in a heavy-duty tablet press. These tablets are then broken into granules in a conventional mill. In the case of a roller compacter, the powders are pressed in a roller mill, and the thin sheet of compacted materials is further broken into granules with a conventional mill.

8.6.2.1 Advantages of Dry Granulation

- Dry granulation eliminates the use of binder solutions and can be used for moisture-sensitive materials (e.g., aspirin, effervescent tablets).
- No drying step is involved, so this process can be used for heat-sensitive materials.
- This process improves solubility.
- It improves blending since there is no migration.

8.6.2.2 Disadvantages of Dry Granulation

- Dry granulation requires a heavy-duty press.
- It does not permit uniform color distribution.

8.6.3 Direct Compression

The direct compression process involves the compression of mixed powder components into tablets without an intermediate granulating step. Recently, there has been a great deal of research to develop diluents for direct compression. Some available direct compression diluents include lactose, spray-dried lactose microcrystalline cellulose, calcium sulfate, dibasic calcium phosphate, and starch 1500.

8.6.3.1 Advantages of Direct Compression

- Direct compression is less expensive (labor, time, equipment, space, etc.).
- This process eliminates heat and moisture.
- It increases surface area for rapid drug dissolution once the tablet disintegrates.
- It creates more stable tablets.

8.6.3.2 Limitations of Direct Compression

- Differences in particle size and density in direct compression may lead to segregation in the hopper.
- Low-dose drugs may not be uniformly blended.
- High-dose drugs that have poor flow and compressibility characteristics cannot be used for direct compression.

8.6.4 Comparison of Methods Used for Manufacture

It is evident from Table 8.5 that direct compression has the least number of steps, as compared to other two methods. Therefore, direct compression is more economical and is currently the preferred method of preparation for compressed tablets.

8.7. TABLET COMPRESSION AND BASIC FUNCTIONAL UNITS OF A TABLET PRESS

The final step in the manufacture of a conventional tablet is the compression step. Powders and granules are compressed in a tablet press, and two types of presses are used: single-punch presses and rotary presses. A schematic diagram of a single tablet press with its essential parts is shown in Figure 8.2. The basic functional units of these presses are outlined here:

- *Hopper* for storing material to be compressed
- *Feed frame* for distributing the materials into dies
- *Dies* for controlling the size and shape of the tablet (as shown in Figure 8.3)

TABLE 8.5 Comparison of Various Steps Used in Different Methods of Tablet Manufacturing Processes

Wet Granulation	Dry Granulation	Direct Compression
1. Milling of all solid ingredients	1. Milling of all solid ingredients	1. Milling of all solid ingredients
2. Mixing of powders	2. Mixing of powders	2. Mixing of powders
3. Preparation of binder solution	3. Primary compression to make slugs	3. Tablet compression
4. Mixing of binder solution to powder mixture to form wet mass	4. Screening of slugs	
5. Screening of wet mass through 6- to 12-mesh screen to form granules	5. Mixing with lubricant and disintegrating agent	
6. Drying of moist granules	6. Tablet compression	
7. Screening of dry granules through 14- to 20-mesh screen		
8. Mixing of screened granules with lubricant and disintegrant		
9. Tablet compression		

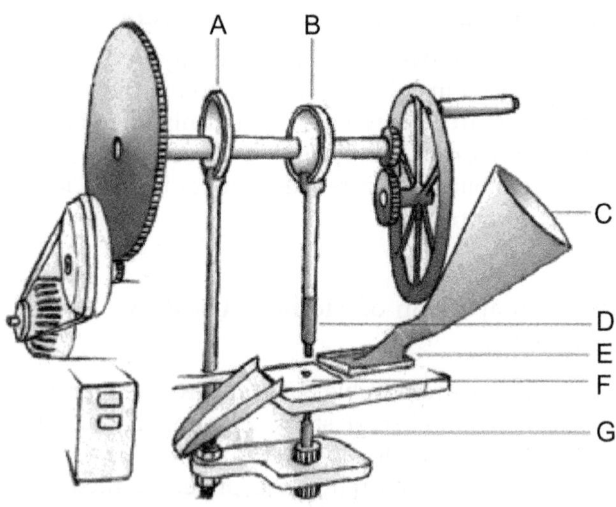

FIGURE 8.2 Schematic drawing of a single punch tablet press. (A) Lower lifting cam, (B) upper lifting cam, (C) hopper, (D) upper punch, (E) feed shoe, (F) die, and (G) lower punch.

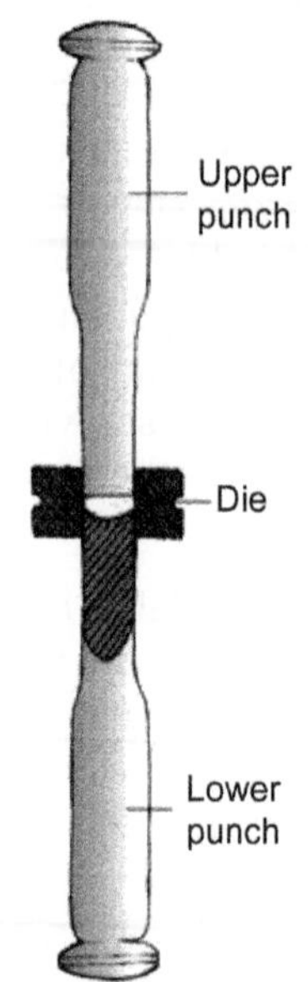

FIGURE 8.3 Schematic representation of punch and die assembly.

- *Punches* for compacting the materials within dies (as shown in Figure 8.3)
- *Cams* for guiding the punches for tablet ejection from the dies

8.7.1 Common Processing Problems during Tablet Compression [3]

8.7.1.1 Capping and Lamination

Capping is the partial or complete separation of the top or bottom layer of a tablet from the main body. Lamination is the separation of a tablet into two or more layers.

8.7.1.1.1 CAUSES

- Entrapped air in the granules
- Improper setting of the tablet press
- Plastic deformation to produce die wall pressures greater than can be relieved by elastic recovery on removal of punch

8.7.1.1.2 REMEDIES

- Change granulation procedures.
- Increase binder concentration.
- Increase or change the lubricant in the formulation.
- Add dry binder to the formulation.
- Use tapered dies.

8.7.1.2 Picking and Sticking

Sticking refers to tablet materials adhering to the die wall. Sticking may be due to slight dampness of the granulation.

Picking is a form of sticking in which a small portion of granulation sticks to the punch face. Picking may result from compressing granules that are not properly dried or when scratched punches are used in the compression of tablets.

8.7.1.2.1 REMEDIES

- Decrease moisture content of the granules.
- Add an adsorbent (microcrystalline cellulose).
- Polish the punch face.
- Clean and coat the punch face with light mineral oil or plate punch faces with chromium.
- Reduce the fraction of low-melting tablet components.

8.7.1.3 Mottling

Mottling is defined as an unequal distribution of color on a tablet with light and dark areas.

8.7.1.3.1 CAUSES

- Drug color different from other components
- Migration of colors during drying
- Uneven distribution of color when using a colored adhesive gel solution

8.7.1.3.2 REMEDIES

- Reduce drying temperature.
- Grind to smaller particle size.
- Change the binder system.
- Change the solvent system.

8.7.1.4 Weight Variation

Variations in the ratio of small to large granules and differences in granule size may lead to filling dies with the same volume but different weight of filling materials. Sporadic flow by granules may lead to unequal filling and weight variations. Segregation due to vibration of a tablet press may lead to weight variation in tablets.

8.7.1.5 *Hardness*

The same causes responsible for weight variation may cause hardness variation. Besides the concentration of binders used and the compression force, the hardness of a tablet depends on the weight of the material to be compressed and the space between the upper and lower punches at the time of compression. If the volume of the material to be compressed and the distance between punches varies, this will lead to variation in tablet hardness.

8.7.1.6 *Double Impression*

A double impression involves only lower punches that have a monogram or other engraving on them. The punch can make double impressions on a tablet surface during the ejection process. This can be avoided by incorporating antiturning devices for the punches.

8.8. QUALITY CONTROL OF TABLET DOSAGE FORM

During the manufacturing of tablet dosage forms, routine quality control tests are performed to maintain product quality. Some of these tests include thickness, hardness, disintegration, tablet weight, and elegance.

8.8.1 Thickness

Factors that can affect tablet thickness at a constant compression load include changes in die fill, particle size distribution, and packing of the particle mix during compression. Tablet thickness becomes very important in packing operations. Use of micrometer calipers to measure the thickness of tablets is common in practice. Variations in tablet thickness should not be more than ±5%.

8.8.2 Hardness and Friability

Although hardness is not an official test, diametral crushing is most frequently used in process control because of its simplicity. Hardness is generally expressed as the force required to break a tablet in a diametric compression test; it is often called breaking strength or tablet crushing strength. Various instruments are used to measure the breaking strength of tablets, including the Monsanto Tester, Strong–Cobb Tester, Pfizer Tester, Erweka Tester, and Herberlein Tester. Tablet hardness depends on compression load. Hardness increases with an increase in pressure, as this causes the tablet to laminate or cap.

Friability is a measure of the tendency of a tablet to powder, chip, and fragment during handling and is another measure of tablet strength. A Roche friabilator is used to measure the friability of a tablet. A preweighed tablet sample is placed in the friabilator and dropped over a distance of 6 inches during each revolution and operated for 4 minutes (100 revolutions). The tablets are dusted and reweighed. Accepted tablets are those that do not lose more than 0.5%–1.0% of their weight. The friability of tablets may be influenced by moisture content. Chewable tablets show a high friability weight loss compared to conventional compressed tablets.

8.8.3 Disintegration

The first thing that happens to a compressed oral tablet before absorption is disintegration, or breaking down of the tablets to granules and powders before dissolving in the gastric fluid. The time it takes to disintegrate is called disintegration time and is measured by a USP disintegration apparatus, as described in the USP NF. The USP disintegration apparatus uses six tubes (3 inches long) open at both ends with a 10-mesh screen at the bottom of the tube. Baskets are reciprocated up and down a distance of 5–6 cm at a frequency of 28–32 cycles per minute. The medium can be water or simulated gastric or intestinal fluid, and the volume of the medium is 1000 mL. The temperature is 37 ± 2°C.

The tablet must disintegrate and all particles pass through to 10-mesh screen in the specified time. For ordinary compressed tablets, the disintegration time should be within 5–30 minutes. For enteric-coated tablets, no disintegration should occur within 1 hour in simulated gastric fluid, but the same tablets have to disintegrate in 2 hours plus the time stated in the USP monograph when they are placed in simulated intestinal fluid. Many factors can affect the disintegration time of compressed tablets. Some of the major factors include media and the temperature of the disintegration test media, the nature of the drug, the diluent used in the formulation, the type and amount of binder and disintegrant used, and the compression load.

8.8.3.1 *Dissolution*

When a tablet is administered, disintegration results in the breaking down of the tablets into granules and

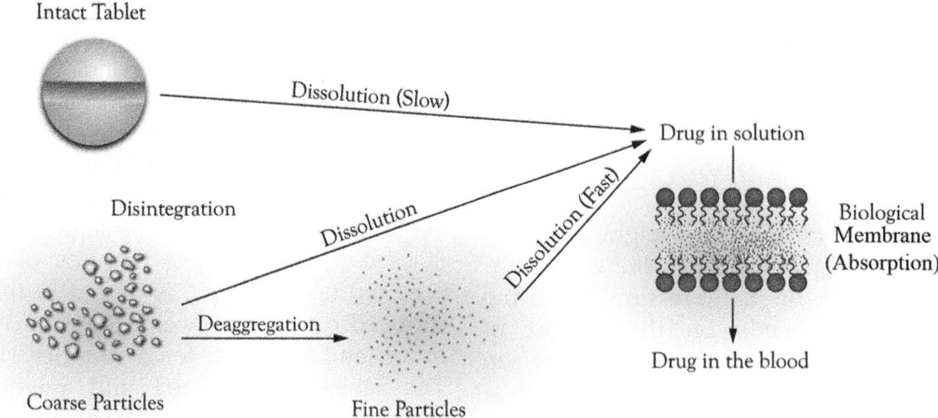

FIGURE 8.4 Absorption of a drug from an intact tablet.

primary particles (see Figure 8.4). For absorption to take place, dissolution of the drug in the gastrointestinal fluid has to occur, since only the drug in solution is absorbed.

8.8.3.2 *Objectives of a Dissolution Study*

The objectives of a dissolution study are to ensure that the drug is completely released or close to 100% release from the tablet, and that the rate of drug release is uniform from batch to batch and is the same as the release rate from batches proven to be bioavailable and clinically effective.

The rate at which a solid dissolves in a solvent is given by the Noyes and Whitney (1897) equation:

$$\frac{dc}{dt} = \frac{DA}{Vh}(C_s - C)$$

where dc/dt is the dissolution rate, D is the diffusion coefficient of the solute in dissolution medium, A is the surface area of the exposed solid, h is the thickness of the diffusion layer, C_s is the solubility of the solid in the dissolution medium, C is the concentration of the solute at any time t, and V is the volume of the release medium.

8.8.3.3 *Factors Affecting Dissolution Rate*

Various factors can affect the dissolution of a drug; they are classified under three categories as follows:

1. Physiochemical properties of the drug
   a. *Polymorphic form*: A metastable form of a solid has higher solubility and dissolution compared to its stable counterpart.
   b. *Particle size*: The smaller the particle size of a solid, the larger the particle surface area and the higher the dissolution.
   c. *Salt form*: A salt form of a drug has a higher aqueous solubility compared to its conjugate acid or base, as well as higher dissolution.
   d. *Hydrates versus anhydrates*: The anhydrous form shows higher dissolution than hydrates due to their solubility differences.
2. Factors related to tablet manufacturing
   a. The amount and type of binder can affect the hardness, disintegration, and dissolution of tablets.
   b. The method of granulation, granule size, and size distribution can affect tablet dissolution.
   c. The amount and type of disintegrants used, as well as the method of their addition, can affect disintegration and dissolution.
   d. Compression load can influence density, porosity, hardness, disintegration, and dissolution of tablets.
3. Factors related to method of dissolution study
   a. Composition of the dissolution medium, pH, ionic strength, viscosity.
   b. Temperature of the medium.
   c. Intensity of agitation.
   d. Volume of dissolution medium.
   e. Sink or nonsink conditions (under a sink condition, the concentration of the drug should not exceed 10%–15% of its maximum solubility in the dissolution medium in use).
   f. Type of dissolution equipment.
   g. Sensitivity of analytical method used to determine drug concentration in the release medium.

8.8.3.4 *Dissolution Testing Method*

According to USP 30, there are many dissolution apparatuses used to determine the dissolution profiles

TABLE 8.6 Comparison of Different USP Dissolution Apparatuses

USP Apparatus	Description of the Apparatus	Rotation Speed	Dosage Forms to be Tested
I	Basket	50–120 rpm	Immediate-release tablets Delayed-release tablets Extended-release tablets
II	Paddle	25–50 rpm	Immediate-release tablets Delayed-release tablets Extended-release tablets
III	Reciprocating cylinder	6–35 dpm (dips per minute)	Immediate-release tablets Extended-release tablets
IV	Flow-through cells	N/A	Extended-release tablets Poorly soluble drug
V	Paddle over disk	25–50 rpm	Transdermal
VI	Cylinder	N/A	Transdermal
VII	Reciprocating disk	30 rpm	Extended-release tablets

of drugs from different dosage forms. Some of them are outlined in Table 8.6.

USP dissolution conditions are maintained as close as possible to the *in vivo* situation:

Temperature:	37° ± 0.5°C
Medium:	0.1 N HCl, pH 7.4 buffer
	Simulated gastric fluid
	Simulated intestinal fluid, water
Agitation:	Mild
Volume of the Medium:	Enough to maintain sink condition (1000 mL)

USP Apparatus #1 (rotating basket) and USP Apparatus #2 (paddle method) are commonly used to evaluate the dissolution profile of solid dosage forms (see Figure 8.5). The dissolution testing may be repeated three times for a batch if necessary. First, the dissolution of six tablets is tested and accepted if all six tablets are not less than the USP monograph tolerance limit plus 5%. If they fail, another six tablets will be tested. The tablets will be acceptable if the average of the 12 tablets is greater than or equal to the USP monograph tolerance limit and no unit is less than this limit minus 15%. If this fails, an additional 12 tablets will be tested. The tablets will be acceptable if the average of the 24 tablets is greater than or equal to the USP monograph tolerance limit and not more than two tablets are less than the USP monograph limit minus 15%. Dissolution results are plotted as concentration versus time, and values such as $t_{50\%}$ and $t_{90\%}$ or the percentage dissolved in 30 minutes are used for comparison purposes. A value of $t_{90\%}$ in 30 minutes is considered satisfactory during a dissolution study.

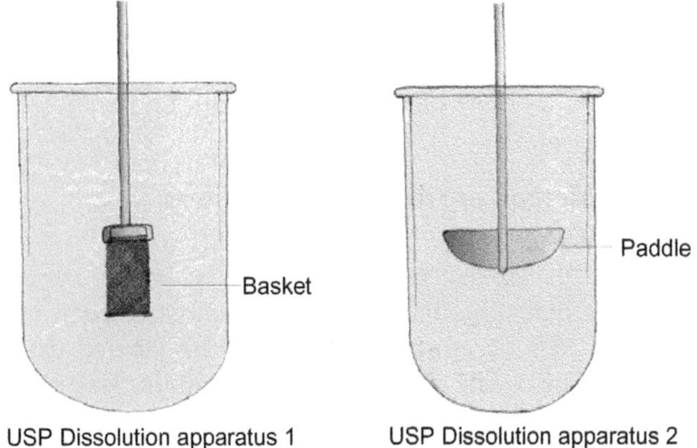

FIGURE 8.5 USP Dissolution Apparatus 1 and 2.

8.8.4 Weight Variation

Tablets generally are manufactured to contain a certain amount of active ingredients in a certain weight of tablet. A weight variation test is essential to ensure that this is satisfied. In this test, samples of 10 tablets are removed from a batch from time to time during compression, and then are weighed to determine whether they conform to the required weight criteria. There still may be a difference in the individual weights even when 10 tablets show the expected total weight.

TABLE 8.7 USP Weight Variation Test

Average Weight of Tablet (mg)	Maximum (%) Weight Difference Allowed
130 or less	10
130–324	7.5
More than 324	5.0

8.8.4.1 *USP Weight Variation Test*

Twenty tablets are weighed individually. Individual weights are compared with the average weight. If no more than two tablets are outside the percentage limit, and if no tablet differs by more than two times the percentage limit, the tablets pass the USP weight variation tests (see Table 8.7).

8.8.4.2 *USP Potency and Content Uniformity Test*

For tablets in which the active ingredients make up about 90% of the tablet weight, the weight variation test will give a good measure of content uniformity. The acceptable potency range for low-dose, highly potent drugs is 90%–110%. For large-dose drugs, the range is 95%–105% of the labeled amount.

8.8.4.3 *Method of Determining Content Uniformity*

Select 30 tablets randomly from a batch. Assay 10 tablets individually. Nine of them must contain not less than 85% or more than 115% of the labeled drug content. The tenth tablet may not contain less than 75% or more than 125% of the labeled drug content. If the preceding conditions are not met, the 30 remaining tablets are assayed individually and none may fall outside the 85%–115% range. Various factors are responsible for the variable content uniformity in tablets. This may include nonuniform distribution of the drug in the powder or granules, segregation of the powder mixture or granulation during manufacturing processes, and tablet weight variation.

8.9. TABLET COATING

Tablet coatings are essential to achieve certain tasks, as follows:

- An enteric coating is used to protect the drug from GI irritation and from acidic degradation in the stomach.
- Film and sugar coatings are used to mask unpleasant taste and improve pharmaceutical elegance of the tablet.
- A film coating can be used to protect the drug from environmental degradation and to provide sustained action dosage forms.
- Special tablet coatings may help in targeting the drug to a certain area of the GI tract (e.g., colon delivery).

Four different coatings are commonly used in tablets: sugar coating, film coating, compaction coating, and air suspension coating [4].

8.9.1 Sugar Coating

Sugar is one of the oldest forms of tablet coatings. In this process, successive layers of sugar coatings are applied by spraying sugar solution into pans in which tablets are rotated and tumbled. Coating pans are supplied with air blowers to admit cold or hot air as needed during the coating operation. Exhaust ducts are attached to these pans to remove dust and moisture. For this type of coating, a convex surface tablet is preferred because flat tablets are difficult to coat. The following steps are commonly used in sugar coating operations:

- Dusting of tablets to remove excess dust
- Application of a waterproofing seal (shellac, ethylcellulose, silicones)
- Subcoating to fill the edge (heavy sugar solutions containing acacia with occasional dusting with starch and powder sugar)
- Smoothing (addition of heavy syrup followed by drying with warm air)
- Application of color coat
- Polishing

8.9.2 Film Coating

Sugar coatings are time consuming. To avoid the extra time required for sugar coatings, formulation scientists introduced film coatings. A polymer solution is sprayed on the tablet surface with constant rotation and tumbling. Film coatings avoid the need for the subcoating and smoothing operations needed for sugar coating. Similar coating pans that are used for sugar coating are used for film coating. The polymers used for this coating operation include carboxymethylcellulose, ethyl cellulose, hydroxyl propyl methylcellulose, cellulose acetate phthalate, povidone, and acrylate polymers.

8.9.3 Compression Coating

Compression coating is also termed dry coating. In this process, very fine coating materials are compressed over the tablet surface by compression in a die with the aid of punches. This coating process is beneficial for those drugs that cannot withstand heat and moisture during the coating operation. Multiple layer tablets can also be produced by this compression coating to separate two incompatible drugs. Repeat action and sustained action tablets are produced by this coating method.

8.9.4 Air Suspension Technique

The air suspension technique is a very rapid and efficient method of coating tablets or granules. The tablets to be coated are suspended in a vertical chamber with an upward stream of warm air. A coating solution is spread from the bottom of the fluidized-bed coating chambers. This process is repeated until a uniform coating is achieved. In this coating, operation efficiency and quality are controlled by fluidized air volume, specific humidity of the warm air chamber, solvent evaporation rate, and the coating spray rate and duration.

8.9.5 Enteric Coating

Enteric coating of tablets starts with a waterproof coating with shellac in a coating pan, followed by several coats with the enteric-coated material. In some instances, a sugar coat is applied over the enteric coating. Materials that are used in enteric coating include shellac, cellulose acetate phthalate, cellulose acetate butyrate, lipids (mixture of myristic acid, hydrogenated castor oil, castor oil, cholesterol, and sodium taurocholate), hydroxypropylmethyl cellulose succinate, and methacrylic acid co-polymers (Eudragit®).

Problems associated with coating of tablet formulations may include poor adhesion of coating material to the tablet surface, blistering, color variation, cracking, abrasion, roughness, and filling of tablet markings.

Quality control of coated tablets must include testing of their appearance and performance. Checking for color, size, appearance, and physical defects in coating that can affect the release or stability of the drug in the dosage form is essential for quality assurance. The *in vitro* disintegration and dissolution methods of the coated tablets in appropriate media need careful evaluation. Other tests such as evaluation of mechanical strength and resistance to chipping and cracking during handling need careful evaluation.

8.10. CONCLUSIONS

The solid dosage form, the most established and most preferred route of administration, still offers many opportunities and challenges for a future formulation scientist. Some of the recent innovations in solid dosage form development include use of novel pharmaceutical excipients obtained from innovative material science research, more efficient ways of manufacturing, and advancement of oral sustained-release formulations. The availability of quick disintegrants and taste-masking technology has made orally disintegrating tablets (ODT) more cost effective and an attractive alternative. Although the solid dosage form still has a promising future, it is not free from many challenges and hurdles. Some of these challenges may include improving the oral bioavailability of poorly soluble drugs, oral delivery of biologics, and size limitation of oral dose via a tablet or a capsule and controlling the release characteristics of the active drug from the dosage form and site-specific delivery of the drug to a definite part of the GI tract. Some of these challenges will be overcome in the future by innovative drug delivery, which may require an interdisciplinary approach of many fields, including material science, molecular biology, biochemistry, physiology, computer technology, and pharmaceutics.

CASE STUDIES

Case 8.1 (Capsules)

In a rural community pharmacy, you receive a prescription for an older patient for 0.2 mL of peppermint oil to be dispensed as a solid dosage form. What do you, as the only pharmacist in the pharmacy, decide regarding this prescription?

Approach: Peppermint is available in the pharmacy as a viscous oily liquid. To dispense oil as a solid dosage form, you need to dispense it in a soft gelatin capsule. This approach is not feasible in a pharmacy. The other possible alternative is dispensing 0.2 mL of oil via a syringe into the body of an appropriately sized hard gelatin capsule, followed by sealing and locking the cap of the capsule carefully with a thin band of water near the outer rim of the body and replacing the cap for sealing.

You must address the following concerns regarding quality assurance:

1. The weight of oil dispensed in capsule should be carefully determined and documented.
2. Leakage of oil, if any, from the filled capsule should be evaluated by placing the filled capsules on a Kimwipe.

Case 8.2 (Powder)

An herbal resinous product is supposed to be diluted with an appropriate filler and dispensed as divided powder for a patient who is lactose intolerant. What do you do?

Approach: Since the patent is lactose intolerant, you cannot use lactose as a diluent. The other alternatives are microcrystalline cellulose (MCC) or calcium phosphate. Since calcium phosphate is too granular, you may have a problem mixing it with resinous material in a pestle and mortar. Therefore, MCC may be a better choice. If the patient is not diabetic, dextrose or mannitol can be the other alternatives.

Case 8.3 (Tablets)

As the director of clinical pharmacy, you are discussing with a pharmacy intern the reported *in vitro* dissolution profile of an investigational drug from the pharmaceutical literature. Following is some of the information available for this new drug:

In vitro dissolution data:

Solubility of drug in simulated gastric fluid is 100 μg/mL.

Concentration of the drug in the dissolution medium at the end of 4 hours = 34 mg/mL.

In vivo data:

Concentration of drug in the blood after 4 hours of oral administration = 6 μg/mL.

Total volume of blood in the patient = 4.8 L.

Solubility of the drug in the plasma at body temperature = 100 μg/mL.

At the end of 4 hours, does the dissolution follow the sink condition? At the end of 4 hours, does the oral absorption follow the sink condition?

Approach: To answer the first question, you have to understand the concept of the sink condition. At the sink condition, the concentration of drug in the release medium at any time during dissolution should not exceed 10%–15% of the solubility. Since the concentration at 4 hours of dissolution is 34 mg/mL, which is 34% of the solubility (100 mg/mL), the concentration exceeds 15% of the solubility limit; therefore, it does not maintain the sink condition.

The second part of the *in vivo* question can be answered similarly. The solubility of drug in the plasma is 100 μg/mL and the drug concentration is 6 μg/mL = (6/100) × 100 = 6%. Concentration of the drug is below 10%–15% of the solubility limit; therefore, absorption happens under the sink condition.

References

[1] Allen Jr LV, Popovich N, Ansel HC. Ansel's pharmaceutical dosage forms and drug delivery systems. Walters Kluwer/ Lippincott Williams & Wilkins; 2011. p. 184–271.

[2] Hoover JE, Ed. Dispensing of medication. 8th ed. Mack Publishing Company; 1976. p. 98–146.

[3] Lachman L, Lieberman HA, Kanig JL. The theory and practice of industrial pharmacy. 3rd ed. Lea & Febiger; 1986. p. 293–429.

[4] Jones D. Pharmaceutics dosage forms and design. Pharmaceutical Press; 2008. p. 203–271.

CHAPTER

9

Liquid Dosage Forms

Hari R. Desu[1], *Ajit S. Narang*[2], *Laura A. Thoma*[1] *and Ram I. Mahato*[3]

[1]Department of Pharmaceutical Sciences, University of Tennessee Health Science Center, Memphis, TN, USA

[2]Drug Product Science and Technology, Bristol Myers Squibb Co., New Brunswick, NJ, USA

[3]Department of Pharmaceutical Sciences, University of Nebraska Medical Center, Omaha, NE, USA

CHAPTER OBJECTIVES

- Identify and classify various liquid dosage forms.
- Describe factors that can affect drug solubility in liquids.
- Explain various formulation aspects of liquid dosage forms.
- Recognize various solution dosage forms, additives used, and their formulation aspects.
- Recognize various suspension dosage forms, additives used, and their formulation aspects.
- Recognize various emulsion dosage forms, additives used, and their formulation aspects.
- Appraise the manufacturing, packaging, and storage of liquid dosage forms.
- Recognize the importance of quality assurance and regulatory considerations for liquid dosage forms.

Keywords

- Co-solvent
- Elixir
- Emulsion
- Liquid dosage forms
- Self-emulsifying drug delivery
- Solubilization
- Solution
- Suspension
- Syrup

9.1. INTRODUCTION

A dosage form is a combination of drug substance and excipients to facilitate dosing, administration, and delivery of medicines to patients. The design of a dosage form is determined by physical, chemical, and pharmacological properties of the drug substance, as well as the administration route. Dosage forms can be classified as solid, semisolid, liquid, and gaseous forms at room temperature. Liquids are pourable dosage forms and can be solutions or dispersions. Pharmaceutical solutions are clear, homogeneous, and single-phase systems containing one or more drug substances dissolved in one or more solvents, while liquid dispersions can be two-phase or multiphase systems, composed of one phase dispersed through another phase(s). The dispersed phase can be composed of solid particles (suspensions), oil droplets (emulsions), micelles (surfactant solutions), and lipid vesicles (liposomes). For convenience, dispersions can be classified as molecular (e.g., solutions), colloidal (micelles, nanoemulsions, and nanosuspensions), and coarse dispersions (suspensions), whose particle sizes are in the range of <1 nm, 1–500 nm, and >500 nm, respectively.

Liquid dosage forms can be administered by oral and parenteral (injectable, inhalation, ophthalmic, otic, nasal, and topical) routes. Oral liquids are nonsterile, whereas liquids administered by the parenteral route are available as sterile and nonsterile formulations. The liquid formulations can be supplied as ready-to-use liquids or reconstitutable powders. This chapter details physicochemical factors that determine formulation aspects of liquid formulations, manufacturing processes, quality control and assurance, and regulatory guidelines for the manufacture of both sterile and nonsterile liquid dosage forms.

Pharmaceutics. DOI: http://dx.doi.org/10.1016/B978-0-12-386890-9.00009-1

9.2. SELECTION OF LIQUID DOSAGE FORMS

The solubility in gastrointestinal (GI) fluids, coupled with biologic membrane permeability, plays a critical role in eliciting a biological response when administering a dosage form [1]. Both these parameters formed the basis for the Biopharmaceutics Classification System (BCS) [2,3]. According to BCS, drugs whose highest administered dose strength dissolves in ≤250 mL of water between pH 1 and 7.5 are considered to be highly soluble drugs; those not meeting this criterion are considered to be poorly soluble. Permeability is measured using bioavailability with a "high-permeability" drug, defined as ≥90% absorption of the administered dose; those compounds not meeting this specification are considered low-permeability compounds.

Figure 9.1 illustrates four classes of BCS classification [1]. The low-water solubility compounds (class II and IV) and low-permeability compounds (class III and IV) often suffer from limited oral bioavailability. A challenge for pharmaceutical scientists is to formulate these drug molecules into oral dosage forms with sufficient bioavailability. A wide variety of solubility-enabling formulation approaches have been developed (e.g., use of surfactants, buffer compositions, cyclodextrins, and co-solvents). However, an apparent solubility increase often decreases intestinal membrane permeability. This trade-off goes back to the definition of permeability (i.e., intestinal permeability is equal to the diffusion coefficient of a drug through a membrane times the membrane/aqueous partition coefficient of a drug divided by membrane thickness). Accordingly, increasing the apparent solubility of a drug in the aqueous medium via formulation will decrease the membrane/aqueous partition coefficient of the drug, leading to decreased apparent intestinal permeability. The opposing effects of apparent solubility and permeability must be taken into account in order to fully understand the impact on the overall fraction of drug absorbed when solubility enhancement approaches are employed to increase the oral exposure of poorly soluble drugs. The interplay between solubility increase and permeability decrease is applicable to drugs with low aqueous solubility and high membrane permeability (i.e., BCS class II drugs). Indeed, solubility enhancement approaches, such as co-solvents/surfactant micelles, may increase the membrane permeability of drugs with poor intrinsic intestinal membrane permeability (e.g., BCS class III and IV drugs). This may

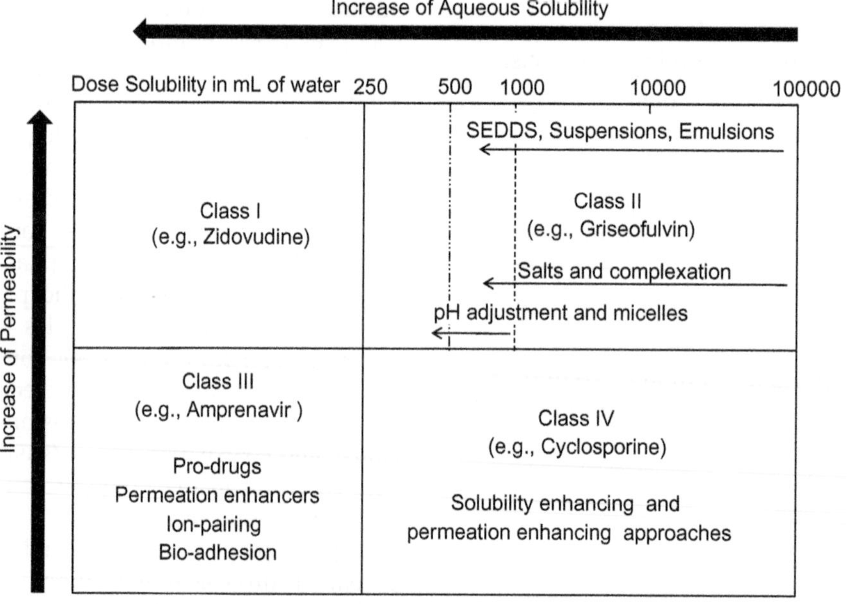

FIGURE 9.1 Demonstrates possible formulation approaches for BCS-classified drugs. Formulation approaches are applied to overcome solubility and permeability limitations. Based on solubility and permeability parameters, orally administered drugs are classified into four classes (I, II, III, and IV). With a decrease in the solubility of drugs (class II and IV), drug delivery approaches, such as dispersions (suspensions, emulsions, nanoparticles, SEDDS) and chemical modification (salts) are viable, while approaches such as pH adjustments and surfactant micelles are deemed to be suitable for drugs with solubility limits approaching class I levels (i.e., highest dose strength solubilized in ≤250 mL of water). For permeability-limited drugs (class III and IV), inclusion of absorption enhancers and drug efflux transporters increase drug absorption. Drug solubility is expressed as 'parts of solvent needed to dissolve 1 part of solute, i.e., grams of solute in milliliters of water.' Some of the examples of formulation approaches for drugs include: BCS class II (griseofulvin (suspension), sodium valproate (salt-form); risperidone (pH adjustment)); BCS class III (valacyclovir (prodrug), amprenavir (permeation enhancer)); BCS class IV (Cyclosporin (SEDDS formulations)).

occur through inhibition of efflux transporters or membrane disruption to increase paracellular transport (e.g., tight junction opening) of drugs.

With many drug compounds, the solubility-permeability relationship may be an overwhelming barrier to achieve bioavailable concentrations, which otherwise are possible with injectable routes. Various solubility enhancement approaches are used for administering drug substances through injectable routes. Particulate approaches, such as emulsions, liposomes, and lipid complexes, can be developed to achieve specific objectives, such as sustained drug release, reduced drug toxicity, minimized drug degradation, or even provision of calories. For large molecules, such as proteins and polysaccharides, which are permeability limited, the injectable route is still the only viable route.

9.3. TYPES OF LIQUID DOSAGE FORMS

9.3.1 Solutions

Solutions are defined as a mixture of two or more components that form a homogeneous molecular dispersion (i.e., a one-phase system). The components of a solution are referred to as the *solute* and the *solvent*. For example, when a solid is dissolved in a liquid, the liquid is usually considered as solvent and the solid as solute, irrespective of the relative amounts of constituents. Solutes are classified as nonelectrolytes and electrolytes, with the latter substances yielding ions when dissolved in water. Electrolytic substances are strong or weak electrolytes, depending on whether the substance is completely or partially ionized in water. For example, hydrochloric acid and sodium hydroxide are strong electrolytes, whereas ephedrine and phenobarbital are weak electrolytes. Compared to electrolytes, nonelectrolytes (e.g., docetaxel) are less polar and exhibit poor solubility in water. In addition to polarity of drug substances, molecular weight and functional groups play a role in their solubility.

9.3.1.1 Approaches to Enhance Solubility

The aqueous solubility of a drug substance may not always be sufficient for its pharmacological purpose. In such cases, solubility can be altered in a number of ways, including chemical modification, complexation, co-solvency, micelle solubilization, and self-emulsifying drug delivery systems (SEDDS). In the majority of cases, the goal is to enhance solubility, thereby increasing bioavailability of a drug substance. Table 9.1 lists representative examples of solubility-enhancing approaches to form solutions.

9.3.1.1.1 CHEMICAL MODIFICATION

The physicochemical properties of a drug substance may be improved by chemical modification of parent drug moieties. Ester formation, salt-form, and drug-adduct formation are some of the common chemical modifications employed to improve stability, solubility, and depot action, and to avoid formulation difficulties. *In vivo*, the modified drug (prodrug) transforms back to the active parent drug moiety. Ester prodrugs can be prepared by chemical reaction of amine and carboxylic acid functional moieties [5]. Examples of ester prodrugs include benzathine penicillin, procaine penicillin, triptorelin pamoate,

TABLE 9.1 Representative Examples of Solubility Enhancement Approaches for Solutions Administered by Oral Route [4]

Approach	Examples	Solubilizing Ingredients
Chemical modification	Hydromorphone HCl (Dilaudid®), Atropine sulfate (Atropine care®)	Hydrochloride salt form Sulfate salt form
pH adjustment	Risperidone (Risperdal®) Hyoscyamine sulfate (Hyoscine)	Tartaric acid, sodium hydroxide
Co-solvents	Digoxin (Lanoxin®) Phenobarbital	20% v/v alcohol Ethanol, propylene glycol (PG) 23% v/v ethanol
Co-solvent/surfactant micelle	Cetylpyridinium chloride (Colgate mouthwash) Fluphenazine HCl (Prolixin®)	Propylene glycol, polysorbate 20 14% v/v alcohol, polysorbate 40
Complexation	Itraconazole (Sporanox®)	Hydroxypropyl-β-cyclodextrin (HPβCD) TPGS, poly(ethylene glycol) (PEG) 400, PG
SMEDDS	Amprenavir (Agenerase®) Calcitriol Cyclosporin (Sandimmune®) Cyclosporin (Neoral®) Saquinavir	Medium chain triglycerides (MCTs) Alcohol, olive oil, labrafil 1944 CS Cremophor EL, alcohol Medium chain mono- and di-triglycerides and dl-tocopherol
Syrups	Amantadine HCl (Symmetrel®) Docusate sodium (Docqlace®)	Sorbitol solution Sucrose solution

fluphenazine decanoate, and olanzapine pamoate. For instance, the amine functional group of procaine reacts with the carboxylic acid group of penicillin to yield procaine penicillin. In recent years, prodrug derivatization-targeting transporters (e.g., amino acid, peptide, nucleoside and nucleobase, bile acid, and monocarboxylic acid) and receptors have been developed to enhance bioavailability.

A number of drug substances exist in a range of salt forms, each form exhibiting different aqueous solubility [6]. The phenomenon of salting-in may be used to increase the solubility of a drug substance through formation of ion-pairs. The appropriate choice of counter-ion is dictated by the nature of functionality, so acidic solutes will require the use of a cation, whereas basic solutes will require an anion. The pharmaceutical salt-form with adequate solubility and stability that meets dose requirements is incorporated into the dosage form. Some of the representative examples of salt-form approaches include methylprednisolone sodium succinate, dexamethasone phosphate, and chloramphenicol acetate.

9.3.1.1.2 CO-SOLVENTS

Co-solvents are liquid components incorporated to enhance the solubility of poorly soluble drugs [7]. Common co-solvents in liquid formulations include glycerol, propylene glycol, ethanol, and polyethylene glycols. Co-solvents are partially polar due to presence of hydrogen bond donors and/or acceptors, thus ensuring miscibility with water. Co-solvents improve the solubility of nonpolar drugs because small hydrocarbon regions of co-solvents reduce the ability of water to squeeze out nonpolar solutes. High drug solubilities can be achieved by co-solvents or co-solvent mixtures with similar polarity to the drug substance. Yalkowsky has shown that the solubility of a drug substance in a co-solvent mixture (Sm) can be estimated through the log-linear solubility relationship, as shown in Eq. 9.1 [7]:

$$\log \frac{Sm}{Sw} = f\sigma \tag{9.1}$$

where Sw is solubility of a drug substance in water, f is volume fraction of co-solvent, and σ is the slope of f versus log (Sm/Sw) plot, which indicates an enhanced solubility effect of the co-solvent for ionized and unionized forms. The selection of a co-solvent depends on a number of factors, including the solubility and stability of drug substance in the vehicle and toxicity of the vehicle. Each co-solvent is characterized by an acceptable concentration range, which cannot be exceeded without incurring biological damage [8]. In parenterals, uncontrolled precipitation of the drug substance upon dilution in aqueous/biological media/co-solvents results in embolism or necrosis at the injection site. Toxicity of co-solvents and uncontrolled precipitation of the drug substance upon injection has limited this approach in parenteral formulations. *In vitro* and *in vivo* models are available to evaluate the safety of co-solvent excipients [9].

9.3.1.1.3 MICELLAR SOLUBILIZATION BY SURFACTANTS

Surfactants possess both hydrophilic and hydrophobic groups that may associate in aqueous media to form dynamic aggregates, known as micelles [10]. According to the nature of the hydrophilic group, surfactants can be anionic (negative charge), cationic (positive charge), zwitter-ionic (positive and negative charges), or nonionic. Table 9.2 lists typical examples of surfactants in pharmaceutical liquid dosage forms. Due to hydrophilic functional groups, micelles can enhance the solubility of poorly water soluble drug compounds [13]. As surfactant concentration in aqueous medium

TABLE 9.2 Examples of Surfactants Used in Liquid Dosage Forms [11,12]

Range of HLB Value	Surfactant Category	Examples	Applications
1–3	Anti-foaming agents	Dimethicone, simethicone ethylene glycol distearate, sorbitan tristearate	Creams, lotions
3–6	W/O emulsifier	Propylene glycol monostearate, glyceryl monostearate, propylene glycol monolaurate, sorbitan stearate (Span 60), diethylene glycol monostearate, sorbitan monooleate (Span 80)	Creams, lotions
6–8	Wetting agent	Diethylene glycol monolaurate, sorbitan monopalmitate, sucrose dioleate	Suspensions
8–13	O/W emulsifier	Polyethylene glycol monooleate, sorbitan monolaurate (Span 20), polyoxyethylene sorbitan monostearate, polyoxyethylene sorbitan tristearate	O/W emulsions
13–14	Detergent	Polyethylene glycol (400) monolaurate, polyoxyethylene sorbitan monolaurate, triethanolamine oleate, PEG-8 laurate	Lotions
15–18	Solubilizer	Polyoxyethylene sorbitan monooleate (Tween 80), polyoxyethylene sorbitan monopalmitate (Tween 60), sodium oleate, polyoxyethylene stearate, potassium oleate	Solutions, O/W emulsions, lotions

increases, surface tension increases and reaches a constant value. The concentration at which such inflections occur is the critical micelle concentration (CMC), which is attributed to the self-association of surfactant molecules into small aggregates called micelles (Figure 9.2a). At CMC, there is a change from a solution containing single surfactant molecules or ions (monomers) to one containing monomers and micelles. Above CMC, surfactant molecules orient themselves with polar ends facing the aqueous solution and nonpolar ends facing the interior. A hydrophobic core is formed at the center of the micelle, with hydrophobic solute molecules residing in the core (Figure 9.2b). Solubilization in surfactant micelle solutions can be regarded as a partition phenomenon. The nonionized form of ionic compounds can partition and reside in the hydrophobic core of micelles. Buffer selection is made to achieve the nonionized form of drug substances, thus enabling partitioning into micelles. Depending on surfactant concentration, normal micelles can be spherical, cylindrical, or lamellar in shape. Nonionic surfactants, rather than ionic surfactants, are generally considered to be more suitable for pharmaceutical applications, not only because of their lower toxicity, but also because the surfactant's shell can confer stealth properties to the micelle, avoiding uptake by macrophages of the reticular endothelial system (RES), prolonging their lifetime in blood circulation [14]. Some of the surfactant-based formulations include docetaxel and paclitaxel formulations.

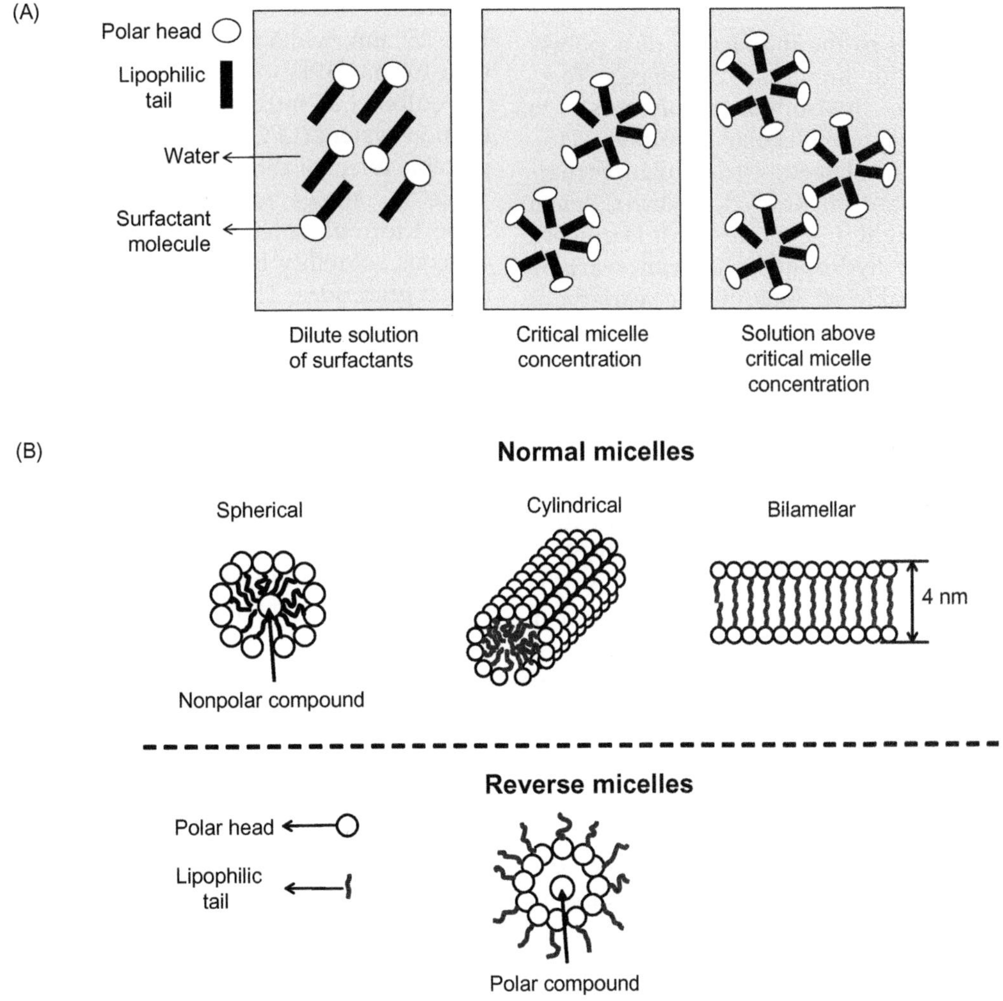

FIGURE 9.2 (A) Demonstrates the formation of normal micelles. The concentration at which amphiphilic surfactants start to self-associate into small aggregates called micelles is termed critical micelle concentration (CMC). In general, surfactant molecules exist as monomers and do not associate themselves below CMC or in very dilute solution. On the other hand, concentrations of surfactants above CMC yield strong (in terms of micelle number) micelle solutions. (B) Demonstrates types of micelles depending on the assembly of surfactant molecules. In normal micelles, polar head groups face the external aqueous phase, and lipophilic tails face the nonpolar interior. Normal micelles can assemble in spherical, cylindrical, and bilamellar forms depending on water content in the external phase. In reverse micelles, polar head groups face the interior polar phase, and lipophilic tails face the nonpolar solvent phase and the structure of the surfactant molecules. Normal micelles are capable of loading nonpolar drug compounds into their lipophilic core, while reverse micelles can incorporate hydrophilic drugs into their aqueous core.

TABLE 9.3 Lipid Formulation Classification System (LFCS) of Lipid-based Formulations [20]

Typical Composition	Type I	Type II	Type IIIA	Type IIIB	Type IV
Triglycerides/mixed triglycerides	100	40–80	40–80	0	–
Surfactants (%w/w)	–	0–20 (HLB < 12)	20–40 (HLB > 12)	20–50 (HLB > 12)	0–20 (HLB < 12) or 30–80 (HLB > 12)
Co-solvents (%w/w)	–	–	0–40	20–50	40–60
Particle size (μm)	> 250	100–250	100–250	50–100	<50
Significance of dilution	Limited importance	Solvent capacity unaffected	Some loss of solvent capacity	Significant phase changes	High risk of precipitation
Significance of digestion	Crucial requirement	Not crucial but likely to occur	Not crucial but may be inhibited	Not required	Not required

9.3.1.1.4 COMPLEXATION

Complexation refers to the interaction of a poorly soluble compound with an organic molecule (e.g., surface-active agents, hydrophilic polymers) to generate a soluble intermolecular complex [15]. Cyclodextrins are torus-shaped, cyclic oligosaccharides consisting of either six (α-cyclodextrin), seven (β-cyclodextrin), or eight (γ-cyclodextrin) D-glucose units. Owing to their hydrophobic interior, various cyclodextrins are capable of including a variety of solutes in their interior cavity. The predominant forces responsible for formation of host-guest complexes are hydrogen bonding and Van der Waals forces. A derivative of β-cyclodextrin, 2-hydroxypropyl-β-cyclodextrin (HPβCD) has been found to enhance the solubility of the antifungal compound, itraconazole (Sporanox®). Another β-cyclodextrin derivative, sulfobutylether-β-cyclodextrin (Captisol®), has been used to enhance the solubility of very insoluble, voriconazole (Vfend®). The application of another class of complexing agents, the drug-polymer resin complex, has been identified as extended-release oral suspensions [16].

9.3.1.1.5 SELF-EMULSIFYING DRUG DELIVERY SYSTEMS (SEDDS)

Self-emulsifying drug delivery systems (SEDDS) have attracted attention after the commercial success of HIV protease inhibitors, ritonavir (Norvir®) and saquinavir (Fortovase®), and cyclosporin (Neoral® or Sandimmune®) formulations. SEDDS encompass lipidic excipients to improve solubility and permeability of drug substances. These excipients emulsify when exposed to GI fluids to form oil-in-water emulsions or micro-emulsions [17,18]. Based on the droplet size, SEDDS can be termed as self-emulsifying drug delivery systems (SMEDDS) or self-nano-emulsifying drug delivery systems (SNEDDS). SMEDDS are transparent microemulsions with droplet size ranging between 100–250 nm, while the droplet size of SNEDDS is less than 100 nm [19].

Pouton et al. introduced the lipid formulation classification system (LFCS) on the basis of composition and possible effect of dilution on drug precipitation [17,20]. Table 9.3 shows four classes of lipid formulations. Type I formulations comprise drugs that exhibit poor aqueous solubility but are soluble in triglycerides and mixed glycerides. These formulations require digestion by pancreatic lipase/co-lipase in GI fluids to produce oil-in-water dispersion and promote drug absorption [21]. For example, valproic acid is solubilized in corn oil. Type II formulations are isotropic mixtures of lipids [e.g., lipophilic surfactants (hydrophilic lipophilic balance, HLB < 12) or co-surfactants] and drug substances. In GI fluids, these mixtures form oil-in-water emulsion under mild agitation. Self-emulsification is obtained at surfactant concentrations above 25% w/w. Type III formulations, referred to as SEDDS, comprise oils, hydrophilic surfactants (HLB > 12), and co-solvents (e.g., ethanol, propylene glycol, and polyethylene glycol). For example, Neoral consists of corn oil glycerides, cremophor RH40, glycerol, propylene glycol, and ethanol. Type IV formulations are hydrophilic formulations that are devoid of oils. These formulations produce fine dispersions with aqueous media. Amprenavir (Agenarase®) is an example of a type IV lipid formulation.

Lipidic excipients include vegetable oils and their derivatives [22,23]. Vegetable oils contain mixtures of triglycerides, fatty acids, phospholipids, and nonsaponifiable matter, such as pigments and sterols. According to carbon chain length, triglycerides are classified as short-chain (<5 carbons), medium (6–12 carbons), and long-chain (>12 carbons) compounds. Some of the vegetable oils include castor oil, coconut oil, corn oil, olive oil, and sesame oil. Vegetable oil derivatives are used as solubilizers or bioavailability enhancers. Some of the classes of vegetable oil derivatives include the following:

a. Hydrogenated vegetable oils are produced by partial or complete hydrogenation of long-chain triglycerides. Examples are hydrogenated castor oil (Lubritab®, Akofine®, and Cutina HM®) and soybean oil (Hydrocote®).
b. Partial glycerides are products of glycerolysis, and are produced by partial esterification of fatty acids and glycerol-yielding mono- or diglycerides. Examples include glyceryl monocaprylocaprate (Capmul MCM®), glyceryl monostearate (Imwitor® 191), and glyceryl monooleate (Peceol™).
c. Polyoxylglycerides (macrogolglycerides) are produced by polyglycolysis of vegetable oils with polyethylene glycols. These are derivatives of unsaturated fatty acids (Labrafil® M1944CS and Labrafil M2125CS), saturated medium-chain fatty acid esters (Labrosol®), Gelucire® 44/14), or long-chain fatty acids (Gelucire® 50/13).
d. Ethoxylated glycerides are castor oil derivatives. Classic examples include ethoxylated castor oil (Cremophor® EL) and ethoxylated hydrogenated castor oil (Cremophor® RH40 and Cremophor® RH60).
e. Esters of fatty acids and alcohols are the largest family of vegetable oil derivatives. Some of the examples include
   - Polyglycerol derivatives—e.g., polyglycerol oleate (Plurol™)
   - Propylene glycol derivatives—e.g., propylene glycol monocaprylate (Capryol™ 90)
   - Polyoxyethylene glycol derivatives—e.g., PEG-8 stearate (Mrij 45), PEG-40 stearate (Mrij 52), PEG-12 hydroxystearate (Solutol HS 15)
   - Sorbitol derivatives—e.g., sorbitan monooleate (Span 80), polyoxyethylene-20 sorbitan monooleate (Tween 80)

As discussed earlier, type III formulations contain co-solvents. Common co-solvents used in SEDDS include ethanol, propylene glycol, polyethylene glycol, glycerol, and sorbitol. In addition, SEDDS include preservatives and stabilizers to prolong the shelf-life of formulations. SEDDS are formulated in hard gelatin or soft gelatin capsules. Design and optimization of SEDDS formulations involve solubility and stability screening using phase diagrams. These diagrams are necessary to determine the concentration of excipients required for drug loading.

Advantages of SEDDS include:

- Improved oral bioavailability of drug substances belonging to BCS class II and IV drug substances
- Increased drug-loading capacity of formulations to deliver appropriate drug dose
- Reduced intersubject and intrasubject variability and negated food effects on drug absorption
- Inhibition of enzymatic hydrolysis of drug substances

9.3.1.2 Formulation Considerations

Solutions can be classified by route of administration as inhalation solutions, injectable solutions, oral solutions, ophthalmic solutions, otic solutions, mouthwashes and gargles, nasal solutions, topical solutions, enemas, and douches. Based on composition, solutions can be aqueous or nonaqueous. Aqueous solutions include simple solutions, syrups, dilute acids, aromatic waters, and dry powder mixtures for reconstitution. Nonaqueous solutions may include hydro-alcoholic solutions, such as mouthwashes, gargles, elixirs, and oily preparations (e.g., oil-soluble vitamins).

9.3.1.2.1 ORAL SOLUTIONS

Oral solutions are liquid preparations intended for oral administration. Oral solutions contain one or more active substances and inactive excipients, such as solubilizers, stabilizers, buffers, preservatives, flavoring agents, coloring agents, and sweetening agents. Table 9.4

TABLE 9.4 Excipients in Solution and Suspension Formulations [24]

		Concentration (% v/v)	
Inactive Ingredients	**Example**	**Solutions**	**Suspensions**
Solubilizers	Alcohol	0.05–35	0.1–52
	Propylene glycol	0.125–55	1–28.5
	PEG 400	1–60	1–5
	Glycerin	1–75	0.01–40
	Sorbitol	1–90	0.1–72

(Continued)

TABLE 9.4 (*Continued*)

Inactive Ingredients	Example	Concentration (% v/v)	
		Solutions	Suspensions
Surfactants	Docusate sodium	na	0.01–0.1
	Polyoxyl 35 castor oil (Cremophor EL)	1–51.5	0.01–0.05
	Polyoxyl 40 castor oil (Cremophor RH 40)	1–45	na
	Polysorbate 20 (Tween 20)	na	0.01–0.5
	Polysorbate 40 (Tween 40)	0.001	0.1–0.5
	Polysorbate 60 (Tween 60)	na	0.1–3
	Polysorbate 80 (Tween 80)	0.01–12.6	0.01–5
	d-α-tocopheryl polyethylene glycol 1000 succinate (TPGS)	1–20	na
	Sorbitan monooleate (Span 20)	1–15	0.01–0.05
	Sorbitan monostearate (Span 60)	na	0.1–2
	Tyloxapol	na	0.01–0.3
Buffers	Acetates, borates, citrates, phosphates		
Preservatives	Benzalkonium chloride	0.01–2	0.01–0.02
	Benzyl alcohol	0.1–5	0.1–5
	Methyl parabens	0.1–1.5	0.1–20
	Propyl parabens	0.02–36	0.01–0.1
	Butyl parabens	na	0.01–0.2
	Thimerosal	na	0.001–1
Antioxidants	Ascorbic acid	0.01–0.6	0.1–0.5
	Butylated hydroxy toluene (BHT)	0.001–0.02	na
	Butylated hydroxy anisole (BHA)	0.01–2.0	0.01–0.1
	Sodium bisulfite	0.01–0.1	0.001–0.05
	Sodium metabisulfite	0.1–0.2	0.01–0.30
Chelating agents	EDTA disodium	0.01–0.5	0.01–0.1
Viscosity modifiers	Microcrystalline cellulose	0.1–2.0	0.1–3.0
	Carboxymethylcellulose (CMC)	0.1–3.5	0.1–40
	Hydroxy ethylcellulose (HEC)	0.1–3.5	0.1–3
	Hydroxypropyl methylcellulose (HPMC)	0.1–2	0.1–2.5
	Carbomers	0.1–0.25	0.1–1.5
	Tragacanth	na	0.1–6.0
	Xanthan gum	0.1–4.0	0.01–19.0
	Gellan gum	0.1–0.6	na
	Guar gum	na	0.01–0.2
Sweeteners	Sucrose	85	1–55.5
	Sucralose	0.1–0.8	0.1–1
	Saccharin sodium	0.05–2	0.1–0.6
Coloring agents	FD&C colors	0.0001–2.5	0.0001–2.0

na—not available.

lists inactive ingredients and their concentration ranges in solutions. Purified water (USP) is a common vehicle used in the preparation of aqueous dosage forms. Solution formulations require solubilizing excipients when the active ingredient dose is large relative to its aqueous solubility. For water-insoluble drugs, solubilizing vehicles include water-miscible co-solvents, such as ethanol, glycerin, polyethylene glycol 300 or 400, and propylene glycol [25]. The maximum amount of solvent used can be up to 55% propylene glycol, 17% polyethylene glycol 400, and 42% ethanol. Among the alcohols, ethanol (USP, 94.9–96.0 %v/v), dehydrated ethanol (USP), or dilute ethanol (50/50 %v/v ethanol and water) is used. Together with water, ethanol forms a hydroalcoholic mixture that dissolves both alcohol and water-soluble substances.

Water-miscible surfactants are also common in solubilization of poorly water-soluble substances. Surfactants can be used either alone or mixed with co-solvents in aqueous solution. Nonionic surfactants are common in oral formulations. Some of the typical examples of nonionic surfactants include polyoxyl 35 castor oil (Cremophor EL), polyoxyl 40 hydrogenated castor oil (Cremophor RH40), polysorbate 20 (Tween 20), polysorbate 80 (Tween 80), tocopheryl polyethylene glycol succinate (TPGS), solutol HS 15, and sorbitan monooleate (Span 80).

The solubility of a vast number of drugs is pH-dependent, and may be compromised by small changes in the pH of the solution. The pH plays a critical role in the stability (e.g., hydrolysis and oxidation) of drug substances. Buffer solutions are employed to control the pH of the solutions. The pH range for oral solutions is usually in the range of 2–10 to maximize the chemical stability of drug substances. Examples of buffer salts in pharmaceutical solutions include acetates, citrates, and phosphates.

Preservatives in solutions control the microbial bioburden of formulations. Ideally, preservatives should exhibit properties, such as (1) broad spectrum of antimicrobial activity against gram-positive and gram-negative bacteria, as well as fungi; (2) stability over the shelf-life of drug products; and (3) low toxicity. Various preservatives in oral solutions include benzoic acid and salts, sorbic acid and salts, and alkyl esters of parahydroxybenzoic acid (parabens). Drug substances undergo oxidation when exposed to atmospheric air. Oxidation of a drug substance in a pharmaceutical preparation can be accompanied by change in color, odor, or precipitation of drug substance. The oxidative process can be prevented by inclusion of antioxidants in the formulation. In aqueous solution, antioxidants are oxidized in preference to the therapeutic agents, thereby protecting the drug substance from decomposition. Water-soluble antioxidants include sodium sulfite (Na_2SO_3, at high pH values), sodium bisulfite ($NaHSO_3$, at intermediate pH values), sodium metabisulfite ($Na_2S_2O_5$ at low pH values), and ascorbic acid; oil-miscible antioxidants include butylated hydroxytoluene (BHT), butylated hydroxyanisole (BHA), and propyl gallate. Certain pharmaceuticals require an oxygen-free atmosphere during preparation and storage. In such cases, atmospheric air can be replaced by inert gases, such as nitrogen and argon.

The viscosity of formulations can be controlled to ensure accurate measurement of volume to be dispensed and to increase palatability. The viscosity of solutions may be increased by addition of hydrophilic polymers (e.g., cellulose derivatives) and natural gums (e.g., sodium alginate, xanthan gum, and guar gum). Sweeteners, flavoring agents, and coloring agents are added to enhance the palatability and appearance of solutions. Common sweetening agents are sucrose, liquid glucose, glycerol, sorbitol, saccharin sodium, and aspartame. Artificial sweeteners replace sugars in formulations to meet the prescription requirements for children and diabetes patients. Coloring agents are added to impart preferred color to the formulation. When used in combination with flavors, selected color should "match" flavor of the formulation (e.g., green for mint-flavored solutions, red for strawberry-flavored formulations). Flavoring agents often are included in liquid formulations to mask the unpleasant taste of drug substances. In aqueous formulations, alcohol (USP) may be used in small portions to solubilize oil-based flavoring agents (e.g., orange oil). Flavor adjuncts (e.g., menthol) are also added to desensitize taste receptors. The flavor adjuncts may augment the taste-masking properties of conventional flavors.

Oral formulations are either formulated in a conveniently administered volume, 5 mL or a multiple, or filled into gelatin capsules in the size range of 0.19–5.0 mL. An adult full dose is contained within a reasonable upper volume, 30 mL, and the pediatric dose is contained within a measurable lower volume, 0.25–1.0 mL.

9.3.1.2.2 SYRUPS

Syrups are concentrated, aqueous preparations of sugar or sugar substitutes intended for oral administration of bitter-tasting drug substances. Syrups containing flavoring agents without drug substances are called nonmedicated or flavored vehicles (syrups). These syrups serve as pleasant-tasting vehicles for drug substances to be added later, either in the extemporaneous compounding of prescriptions or in the preparation of medicated syrups. A typical nonmedicated syrup formulation contains (a) sugar (sucrose) or sugar substitute to provide sweetness and viscosity, (b) an antimicrobial preservative (e.g., benzoates and parabens), (c) a buffering agent (e.g., citrates), (d) a flavoring agent, and (e) a coloring agent (e.g., FD&C colors) [11]. In addition, syrups may contain solubilizing agents, thickeners, or stabilizers to improve the stability of formulations. Medicated syrups contain drug substance and inactive ingredients. Examples of nonmedicated syrups include cherry, corn, and orange syrups, and medicated syrups include chlorpromazine hydrochloride, perphenazine, piperazine citrate, promazine hydrochloride, sodium valproate, ritonavir, and guaifenesin.

Syrup vehicles with appropriate viscosity and sweetness mask the taste of drug substances. Both these properties conceal the taste of bitter compounds, which otherwise is not possible with dilute aqueous preparations. Most syrup solutions contain sucrose, but it may be replaced in whole or part by sugars, such as dextrose, or nonsugars, such as sorbitol. In contrast to the unstable nature of dilute sucrose solutions, syrup vehicles containing a high proportion (60%–80%) of sugar impart desirable viscosity and stability [24,26]. The aqueous sugar medium of dilute sucrose solutions serves as a source for the growth of microorganisms, particularly yeasts and molds. Concentrated sugar solutions (e.g., syrup NF) are hyperosmolar and resistant to the growth of microorganisms. Under cold storage conditions, some sucrose may crystallize from solution, resulting in an unsaturated solution suitable for microbial growth. Many of the commercial syrups are not as saturated as syrup, NF, and therefore include preservatives to prevent microbial growth during shelf-life. In these syrup formulations, the amount of preservative required to protect syrup against microbial growth varies with the proportion of water available for growth and inherent preservative efficacy. In some instances, sugars are replaced by artificial sweeteners and viscosity modifiers, such as cellulose derivatives, which provide a syrup-like vehicle for medications intended for diabetic patients.

On a large scale, most of the syrup preparations are made by heating to dissolve the ingredients. In this method, sugar is added to purified water, and heat is supplied to form the syrup solution. Other heat-stable components are added to the hot syrup, and the mixture is allowed to cool. Final volume is adjusted by the addition of purified water. In some instances, heat-sensitive ingredients or volatile substances are added after the solution is cooled to room temperature. Uncontrolled heating hydrolyzes sucrose into dextrose and fructose. This hydrolytic reaction is referred to as inversion, which results in bitter taste and darkening of the vehicle. To avoid heat-induced inversion of sucrose, the syrup may be prepared without heat by agitation. Solid ingredients, except sucrose, are dissolved in a small portion of purified water by agitation, and the resulting solution is incorporated into the syrup. Preparation of syrup solutions by agitation is time-consuming but yields a stable syrup formulation.

Another method is addition of sucrose to vehicles containing fluid extracts or tinctures. However, direct addition of aqueous phase (containing sucrose) to alcohol containing fluid extracts or tinctures precipitates resinous material dissolved in alcohol. An alternative approach is to allow the mixture (fluid extract or tincture and water) to stand for a few hours. The mixture is then filtered to remove suspended resinous material and produce a clear solution. Sucrose is then added to the medicated vehicle to produce medicated syrup. This method is not preferable if the precipitated materials are expensive. Aromatic eriodictyon syrup (USP) is prepared using this method. The percolation method is employed to prepare ipecac syrup and syrup (USP) on a commercial scale. In this method, purified water or the aqueous phase is percolated through a bed of crystalline sucrose. A flow-meter (stopcock) can be used to regulate the aqueous phase flow, and thereby improve contact of the aqueous phase with the sugar bed. Precautions include use of a cylindrical or conical percolator to hold and direct the flow of the aqueous phase; use of coarse sugar to provide adequate porosity for the aqueous phase flow; and careful insertion of a cotton plug into the neck of percolator to avoid hindering (a tight plug) the flow or allowing turbid solution (a loose plug) to pass through. If the percolation process is adopted for preparing medicated syrups, plant parts, such as leaves or bark, are percolated with water; then the percolate is collected into a vessel containing the sucrose. The vessel is agitated to dissolve the sucrose and other ingredients, as well as facilitate the mixing operation to prepare the final syrup formulation.

Dry syrups are prepared to improve the stability of ingredients and minimize contamination. Dry syrups can be prepared as powders, whole granules, or partial granules. For dry powders, process and instrumentation requirements are minimal. However, powders exhibit segregation of ingredients, resulting in nonuniform syrup. Whole granules contain all the ingredients, and the granules are sieved or screened to obtain particular particle-size distributions. Whole granules offer advantages, such as better flow and minimal segregation properties. Partial granules are prepared to take advantage of granules and powders. In partial granules, stable ingredients are prepared as granules, while thermolabile ingredients (e.g., flavors) are added to dried granules. Before they are dispensed to patients, dry syrup powders or granules are mixed with purified water and shaken well to prepare liquid syrup.

9.3.1.2.3 MOUTHWASHES AND GARGLES

Mouthwashes are concentrated hydroalcoholic solutions containing one or more active ingredients and excipients. Mouthwashes can be used for therapeutic, diagnostic, and cosmetic purposes. Examples of therapeutic mouthwashes include allopurinol for treating stomatitis [27], pilocarpine for xerostomia (dry mouth) [28], and nystatin for oral candidiasis [29]. Toluidine blue mouth rinse is used for detection of oral cancer and lesions [30]. Cosmetic mouthwashes (e.g., phenol and mint mouthwashes) may be used for refreshing purposes. Other topical mouthwashes include antiplaque (e.g., cetylpyridinium chloride) and fluorinated mouthwashes (Oral-B rinse, Colgate Phos-Flur, and Fluoride dental rinse). In general, mouthwashes contain alcohol as a flavor, which enhances taste and masks the unpleasant taste of active ingredients. Alcohol may serve as a solubilizer for active and inactive ingredients. Common active ingredients in mouthwashes include thymol, eucalyptol, hexetidine, methyl salicylate, menthol, and chlorhexidine gluconate. Preservatives in mouthwashes and gargles include benzalkonium chloride, parabens, benzoates, and sorbates. Various surfactants are included as solubilizers for active and inactive ingredients. Humectants (e.g., glycerin and sorbitol) are used to improve the viscosity of mouthwash solutions. Other inactive ingredients include antioxidants, chelating agents, flavoring agents, and coloring agents.

Gargles are aqueous solutions containing antiseptics, antibiotics, or anesthetics, intended to relieve or treat sore throats. Gargles contain high concentrations of active ingredients and are diluted with warm water before use. Medicated gargles may be taken inside the mouth, swished around as long as possible, and then gargled and swallowed. Betadine (7.5% w/v povidine-iodine) and chlorhexidine gluconate are examples of gargles. Betadine aids in the treatment of sore throats caused by bacteria and viruses, and chlorhexidine gluconate reduces swelling, redness, and bleeding of gums.

9.3.1.2.4 ELIXIRS

Elixirs are clear, sweetened, hydroalcoholic (5%–40% v/v) solutions intended for oral use. Nonmedicated elixirs are employed as vehicles for medicated elixirs. Advantages of elixirs are (a) insoluble drug compounds can be incorporated into the hydroalcoholic vehicle; (b) drug concentrates can be prepared in high-alcohol-containing elixirs; (c) hydroalcoholic vehicles can be self-preserving; and (d) elixirs are less viscous and contain a lower proportion of sugar. Some of the disadvantages of elixirs are (a) they cannot be administered to pediatric patients and patients on antidepressant medication; (b) the concentration of active and inactive ingredients may vary if not preserved in cool places; and (c) water-insoluble drug compounds may precipitate due to alcohol evaporation.

Hydroalcoholic vehicles enhance the solubility of both water-soluble and -insoluble ingredients. The proportion of alcohol in elixirs can be varied with solubility requirements of active ingredients. In addition to alcohol and water, glycerin and propylene glycol can be used as adjunct solvents. Elixirs are sweetened with sweeteners, such as sucrose, sucrose-syrup, sorbitol, glycerin, and saccharin. Elixirs with a high alcohol content use artificial sweeteners, such as saccharin. All elixirs contain flavoring agents to increase their palatability and coloring agents to enhance their appearance. Elixirs are stored in cool, tight, and light-resistant containers due to the presence of alcohol and volatile oils in their formulations. Nonmedicated elixirs are useful as vehicles for extemporaneous filling of prescriptions and dilution of existing medicated elixirs. Common nonmedicated elixirs include aromatic and compound benzaldehyde; examples of medicated elixirs are dexamethasone, fluphenazine HCl, and hyoscyamine sulfate.

Elixirs are prepared by simple solution with agitation or by admixture of two or more liquid ingredients. Alcohol-soluble and water-soluble components are dissolved in alcohol and purified water, respectively. In general, aqueous solution is added to the alcoholic solution to avoid changes in alcohol strength and separation of alcohol-soluble ingredients. The final volume is made with a specified solvent vehicle. Elixirs are then allowed to stand for saturation of the hydroalcoholic mixture and to permit excess flavoring agent oil globules to coalesce. These coalesced oil globules are removed by filtration using talc as a filter aid. Talc absorbs excess oils. During filtration, presoaked filters (in solvent vehicles) are used to prevent loss of elixir ingredients.

9.3.1.2.5 INJECTABLE SOLUTIONS

The United States Pharmacopoeia (USP) and The National Formulary (NF) published public standards for formulating sterile preparations. The procedures outlined in USP chapter <797> are intended to prevent patient harm from ingredient errors and microbial contamination. The advantages of injectable sterile products include rapid onset of action, complete bioavailability, negation of variable drug absorption, and ease of administration for ill patients. Large-volume parenterals include intravenous admixtures, intravenous fluids and electrolyte solutions, irrigation solutions, and dialysis solutions. Some examples of small volume parenterals include injectable antibiotics and antineoplastic agents, available as solutions or reconstitutable powders. An increasing number of biotechnology drugs and critical nutritional mixtures are available for administration through various parenteral routes.

9.3.1.2.6 OPHTHALMIC SOLUTIONS

Ophthalmic liquid products are sterile preparations intended for application to the conjunctiva, conjunctival sac, or eyelids. Common categories of ophthalmic liquids are eye drops and irrigation solutions. Ophthalmic drops can be formulated as aqueous solutions, suspensions, emulsions, or reconstitutable powders. Irrigating solutions (e.g., intraocular and periocular solutions) maintain hydration and clarity of the cornea, providing a clear view of the surgical area.

A majority of instilled eye drops drain into the nasolacrimal duct due to the tendency of the eye to maintain precorneal fluid volume at 7–10 μL [31]. Various factors that influence drainage include instilled volume, viscosity, pH, and tonicity. Pharmaceutical excipients are added to ophthalmic solutions to maintain the stability and sterility of the formulation, as well as prolong solution precorneal residence time. A typical ophthalmic solution is composed of the ingredients described below [31].

9.3.1.2.6.1 VEHICLES Water for injection (WFI) is the most widely used solvent vehicle for ophthalmic and parenteral preparations. WFI is obtained by distillation of de-ionized water or a reverse osmosis procedure. Inorganic metal traces are removed by distillation, reverse osmosis, de-ionization, or a combination of these processes. Membrane filters are used to remove particulate contaminants, and charcoal beds may be used to remove organic materials. Filtration and autoclaving procedures reduce microbial growth and prevent pyrogen formation. The USP also lists sterile WFI and bacteriostatic WFI for use in sterile preparations. Sterile water for injection (USP) is sterilized and packaged in single-dose containers not exceeding 1000 mL. Bacteriostatic WFI (USP) must not be placed in containers larger than 30 mL to prevent administration of large quantities of bacteriostatic agents (phenol) that could become toxic. Aqueous isotonic vehicles are often used in sterile preparations. A common vehicle is sodium chloride solution, 0.9% w/v solution (also known as normal saline), which is sterilized and packaged in single-dose containers no larger than 1000 mL. Sodium chloride irrigation also is a 0.9% w/v solution; however, it has no preservatives. Other vehicles include boric acid solution (pH 5.0), which serves as vehicle for active ingredients, such as cocaine, neostigmine, procaine, tetracaine, atropine, homatropine, and pilocarpine. The boric acid vehicle contains benzalkonium chloride as the preservative.

9.3.1.2.6.2 BUFFERING AGENTS The physiological pH range of tears is 7.0–7.7 and is governed by substances in the tear fluids, including salts and proteins. Due to the small buffer capacity of tear fluids, acidic or basic pH solutions cause excessive secretion of tears and may cause damage to corneal epithelial cells. Hence, pH adjustments are made close to the pH of tears. Also, pH adjustments are made to maintain drug compounds in un-ionized form, which enables rapid penetration across the corneal epithelial barrier. The pH values of ophthalmic solutions are adjusted to a range in which an acceptable shelf-life of at least 2 years can be achieved. If buffers are required, their capacity is controlled to be as low as possible, enabling tears to bring the pH of the eye to physiological range. Common buffering agents in ophthalmic preparations are acetates, borates, citrates, and phosphates. The pH adjustments of ophthalmic solutions are usually made with hydrochloric acid, sulfuric acid, or sodium hydroxide.

9.3.1.2.6.3 PRESERVATIVES Antimicrobial preservatives are added in multidose ophthalmic solutions to inhibit the growth of microorganisms, but this is not intended to be a means of preparing a sterile solution. U.S. Food and Drug Administration (FDA) regulations also allow unpreserved ophthalmic solutions to be packaged in multidose containers only if they are packaged and labeled in a manner that affords adequate protection and minimizes microbial contamination. This can be accomplished by using a reclosable container with a minimum number of doses that is to be discarded 12 hours after initial opening. Unit-dose ophthalmic preparations do not contain preservatives.

Common preservatives in ophthalmic preparations include quaternary ammonium compounds (benzalkonium chloride), substituted alcohols and phenols (chlorobutanol), organic mercurials (phenyl mercuric acetate; thimerosal), esters of parahydroxy benzoic acid (methyl and propyl parabens), polyquad, chlorhexidine, and polyaminopropyl biguanide. Benzalkonium chloride is a typical preservative in more than 65% of ophthalmic products and is usually combined with disodium ethylene diamine tetra-acetic acid (EDTA). Benzalkonium chloride is cationic and is therefore incompatible with anionic drug compounds or inactive excipients. Despite its compatibility limitations, it has shown to be a most effective and rapid-acting preservative. Benzalkonium chloride is stable over a wide pH range and does not degrade even under high-temperature storage conditions. Chlorobutanol, an aromatic alcohol, is considered to be a safe preservative but has slow antimicrobial action and packaging and formulation limitations. Chlorobutanol indicates the use of glass containers, since it permeates polyolefin plastic ophthalmic containers. Methyl and propyl parabens have been used primarily to prevent mold growth. Paraben use is limited by its low aqueous solubility, ability to cause ocular irritation, and nonspecific binding to surfactants and polymer components.

9.3.1.2.6.4 TONICITY AGENTS The osmolarity of lacrimal fluid is between 280 and 320 mOsm/kg, which is dependent on the number of ions dissolved in the aqueous layer of tear film. Ophthalmic solutions need to be isotonic with tear secretions. A hypotonic solution results in excessive secretion of tears and causes irritation of the corneal epithelium. An osmotic pressure corresponding to normal saline solution is considered to be isotonic. Tonicity-adjusting agents employed in ophthalmic solutions include sodium chloride, dextrose, mannitol, and buffering salts.

9.3.1.2.6.5 VISCOSITY MODIFIERS Ophthalmic solutions may contain viscosity-imparting polymers to prolong the retention time of drug solution in the precorneal area and decrease the lachrymal drainage of drug substances. Polymers, such as methylcellulose, hydroxylmethylcellulose, hydroxylpropyl methylcellulose, polyvinyl alcohol, and carbomers are used in the concentration range of 0.2–2.5% to produce viscosities in the range of 5–30,000 cP. These polymers are also used as viscoelastic agents in artificial tear solutions for their lubrication and moistening properties in dry-eye therapy. The major commercial viscous vehicles are hydroxylpropyl methylcellulose (Isopto®) and polyvinyl alcohol (Liquifilm®).

9.3.1.2.6.6 SURFACTANTS Surfactants are used to solubilize or disperse drugs in solutions and dispersions. However, the use of surfactants is limited due to irritation and toxicity issues. Several nonionic surfactants are used in small concentrations to reduce irritation to eye tissues. Surfactants are also used to prevent drug loss to adsorption on the container walls. For example, polyoxyl hydrogenated castor oil (HCO-40) has been used to stabilize Travoprost®, indicated for reduction of elevated intraocular pressure in patients with glaucoma or ocular hypertension.

9.3.1.2.6.7 STABILIZERS Trace metal sources in drug materials, excipients, solvents, containers, or closures are a constant source of oxidation. The trace metals can be eliminated in free-form from labile preparations through chelation (complexation). Chelating agents are added to complex and inactivate metals, such as copper, iron, and zinc, that catalyze oxidation of drug substances. In some instances, chelating agents (e.g., metal complexing agents) and antioxidants are added together to stabilize ophthalmic solutions. Common chelating agents include edetate disodium, citric acid, and tartaric acid. Sulfur salts, such as bisulfate, metasulfite, and sulfite, are the most common antioxidants used in ophthalmic solutions. These antioxidants stabilize the products by acting as oxidizable substrates for free radicals and reactive oxygen species.

9.3.1.2.7 OTIC SOLUTIONS

Otic solutions, also termed ear or aural solutions, are administered in small volumes for treating ear ailments. Most otic solutions are nonsterile, while a few are sterile preparations (e.g., Floxacin®, Cortisporin®). The middle ear and tympanic membrane are commonly infected with bacterial pathogens, such as *Streptococcus pneumoniae, Hemophilus influenza, Moraxella catarrhalis,* and less commonly with *Streptococcus pyrogens, Pseudomonas aeruginosa,* and *Staphylococcus aureus,* causing otitis media (inflammation of the middle ear) and otic discharge. These ear infections can be treated by topical application of antibiotics, such as chloramphenicol, colistin sulfate, neomycin, polymyxin B sulfate, ofloxacin, gentamicin, and antifungal agents, such as nystatin.

Otic solutions contain vehicles, such as glycerol, propylene glycol, and polyethylene glycol 300 or 400. Propylene glycol in otic solutions also lowers surface tension and improves drug substance contact time with infected tissues. Some anti-infective otic solutions (e.g., acetic acid otic solution, USP) contain surfactants, such as benzethonium chloride, to promote contact of the solution with tissues. Dehumidifying agents, such as isopropyl alcohol, lower the moisture content needed for bacteria to survive, thus limiting the spread of infection. Solutions containing analgesics (e.g., antipyrine) and local anesthetics (e.g., benzocaine) are formulated in vehicles containing anhydrous glycerin or propylene glycol. Antipyrine and benzocaine solution combines the hygroscopic property of anhydrous glycerin and the analgesic action of antipyrine and benzocaine to relieve pressure, reduce inflammation and congestion, and alleviate pain and discomfort in acute otitis media. Multiuse otic solutions contain preservatives, such as benzyl alcohol and benzalkonium chloride. The pH of otic solutions is in the range of 2.0–7.5 and is adjusted using buffers, hydrochloric acid, or sodium hydroxide.

Over-the-counter otic solutions, such as cerumen cleansing solutions (e.g., carbamide peroxide, Debrox®) cleanse accumulated cerumen. Otic solutions containing surfactants, such as triethanolamine oleate, emulsify cerumen and aid in its removal. Light mineral oils, vegetable oils, and hydrogen peroxide have been used for cerumen removal. These cerumen-cleansing solutions are placed in the patient's ear canal and retained for a while; then they are flushed with a fine stream of warm water using applicators.

Commercial otic solutions available for relieving otic pain and infections include acetic acid; antipyrine and benzocaine; benzocaine (Americaine®); ciprofloxacin and dexamethasone (Ciprodex®); gentamicin sulfate and betamethasone valerate; hydrocortisone and acetic acid; and neomycin, polymyxin B sulfate, and hydrocortisone.

9.3.1.2.8 NASAL SOLUTIONS

Most nasal solutions are administered as nasal drops or sprays for local and systemic purposes. Rapid absorption and onset of action are major advantages of nasal administration. The nasal route may also be useful for administration of biologics (e.g., proteins and peptides) to avoid first-pass metabolism and GI degradation, and thus contribute to a rapid increase in therapeutic concentrations [32]. For example, 1-deamino-8-D-arginine-vasopression (DDVP; Desmospray®) is used in the treatment of pituitary diabetes insipidus. Nasal solutions are formulated to be isotonic to nasal secretions (equivalent to 0.9% w/v sodium chloride) and are buffered to the normal pH range of nasal fluids (pH 5.5–6.5) to prevent damage to ciliary transport in the nose [33]. The normal dose volume of nasal formulations is in the range of 25–200 μL.

Nasal solutions are usually formulated in water and co-solvents, such as ethanol, propylene glycol, and polyethylene glycol 400. Nasal solutions may contain excipients, such as preservatives (e.g., benzalkonium chloride, benzyl alcohol, parabens, phenylethylalcohol, and potassium sorbate), buffering agents (e.g., citrate and phosphate), antioxidants (e.g., sodium metabisulfite, sodium bisulfite, butylated hydroxytoluene, tocopherol, and disodium EDTA), isotonic adjusting agents (e.g., sodium chloride), viscosity enhancers (e.g., cellulose derivatives), absorption enhancers, flavoring agents (e.g., menthol, eucalyptol, camphor, and methylsalicyate), and sweetening agents (e.g., saccharin). Since nasal formulations are administered in small volumes, nasal secretions may alter the pH of the administrated dose. This can affect the concentration of the un-ionized drug available for absorption. Therefore, buffers with high buffer capacity (phosphates or citrates) are employed to maintain pH *in situ*. Nasal formulations without buffering agents are pH adjusted with hydrochloric acid or sodium hydroxide. The FDA requires that all nasal drug products be manufactured as sterile (e.g., unit-dose) or preserved (multidose) products [34]. Depending on the drug and formulation characteristics, sterility may be accomplished via aseptic filling processes, terminal sterilization, or both.

Numerous delivery devices are available for intranasal administration. Currently, nonpressurized metered-dose pumps provide dose accuracy and reproducibility. Delivery devices are important for delivering medication and protection from microbial contamination and chemical degradation. For most pumps, dispensed volume per actuation is set between 50 and 140 μL. Standard spray pumps will deposit most of the sprayed dose into the anterior region of the nasal cavity. Surface tension of the droplets and mucus layer will cause immediate spread of the spray. Afterward, mucociliary clearance will distribute the liquid layer within the nasal cavity.

Commercial nasal sprays include butorphanol tartarate (Stadol®) for relieving migraine pain; calcitonin salmon (Miacalcin®) for treating osteoporosis; cromolyn sodium (NasalCrom®) for relieving nasal allergy and eustachian tube congestion; tetrahydrozoline hydrochloride (Tyzine®) for relieving nasal congestion; and xylometazoline hydrochloride (Sinosil®) for relieving nasal congestion and respiratory allergies.

9.3.1.2.9 ENEMAS

Enemas are oily or aqueous solutions that are administered rectally. Examples include arachis oil and magnesium sulfate. Retention enemas are administered for local action (e.g., prednisolone), systemic absorption (e.g., diazepam), or topical irrigation purpose (e.g., sodium phosphate, sodium citrate, or docusate sodium). Enemas are packaged in plastic containers with a nozzle for insertion into the rectum. Large-volume enemas should be warmed to body temperature before administration. Extemporaneous enemas are packaged in amber, fluted-glass bottles, whereas manufactured enemas are packaged in disposable polyethylene or polyvinyl chloride bags. Patients are advised on how to use the enema if it is intended for self-administration. Enemas available for relieving constipation are saline laxative (Equaline®), mineral oil (GENT-L-TIP®), and bisacodyl (FLEET®). Mesalamine enema is available for treating ulcerative colitis and proctitis.

9.3.1.2.10 DRY MIXTURES FOR SOLUTION

A number of pharmaceutical compounds are instable in aqueous solution over shelf-life. The commercial manufacturers of these products provide them in dry powder or granule form for reconstitution with a prescribed volume of diluent or reconstitution fluid. Dry powders are available either as simple powders containing only the active pharmaceutical ingredient or manufactured by processes, such as lyophilization, crystallization, and spray drying. These processed dry powders may contain formulation ingredients, including stabilizers and buffer salts. Once reconstituted, the resulting solutions are either administered or further diluted according to packaging instructions. Some dry mixtures for reconstitution are alteplase (Activase®), azacytidine (Vidaza®), bortezomib (Velcade®), etoposide phosphate (Etopophos®), gemcitabine (Gemzar®), and temozolamide (Temodar®).

9.3.2 Suspensions

Suspension is a liquid dosage form of poorly water-soluble drug(s) dispersed in a liquid medium. In an ideal suspension, particles are uniformly dispersed, free from aggregation. Even if sedimentation occurs, particles should be resuspended upon mild agitation. Aqueous suspensions are intended for oral, ophthalmic, inhalation, and topical applications, while oil-based suspensions have parenteral applications (e.g., sustained-release depot formulations). Oral and topical suspensions contain a high concentration of solids in the range of 5%–50% solid particles, while parenteral suspensions incorporate 0.5%–25% solid particles. Based on particle size, suspensions are classified as coarse or colloidal dispersions, with the former containing particles of mean diameter in the range of 1–25 μM, and the latter containing particles with a mean diameter less than 1 μM [35].

Suspensions offer advantages, such as (a) water-insoluble drug compounds can be formulated as suspensions; (b) they prolong drug release rates; (c) they slow down the degradation rate of hydrolytic drug compounds; and (d) for patients with swallowing difficulties, suspensions can be formulated as palatable formulations. Some of the disadvantages include (a) aggregation of particles; (b) complex manufacturing processes; and (c) pourability and syringeability issues (e.g., injectable suspensions).

9.3.2.1 Applications

Suspensions have a number of therapeutic applications across different routes of administration. Most suspensions are available in ready-to-use form from the manufacturer. In cases of physical or chemical incompatibility, the pharmacist will have to reformulate a tablet or a capsule into a suspension (e.g., oral suspension). Table 9.5 lists representative examples of pharmaceutical suspensions and their therapeutic indications. Some of the specific applications of pharmaceutical suspensions administered through various routes are detailed below.

9.3.2.1.1 ORAL SUSPENSIONS

- Drugs with poor solubility and poor bioavailability are formulated as fine colloidal suspensions to increase their bioavailability (e.g., megestrol acetate oral suspension, Megace ER).
- Drugs for patients with difficulties in swallowing solid dosage forms can be formulated as palatable suspensions (e.g., megestrol acetate oral suspension, Megace®).
- Drugs unstable in aqueous media are prepared as powder granules and reconstituted in water to form suspension before administration to patients (e.g., ampicillin suspension).

9.3.2.1.2 OPHTHALMIC/OTIC/NASAL SUSPENSIONS

- Drug substances can be formulated as suspensions to prolong therapeutic action [e.g., brinzolamide suspension (Azopt®), ciprofloxacin (Ciprodex®)].
- Despite poor aqueous solubility, drug substances administered to nasal mucosa are suspended in aqueous vehicles to avoid mucosa irritation (Rhinocort® Aqua)].
- Drugs unstable in aqueous media are prepared in nonaqueous media to overcome stability issues (e.g., tetracycline hydrochloride in coconut oil for ophthalmic use).

9.3.2.1.3 PARENTERAL SUSPENSIONS

- Drug substances, which show poor oral absorption or extensive first-pass metabolism can be formulated as parenteral suspensions to improve bioavailability.
- Drug substances can be formulated as parenteral suspensions to prolong drug release rates (e.g., naltrexone extended-release injectable suspension, Vivitrol®).

9.3.2.1.4 PULMONARY SUSPENSIONS

Antiasthmatic drugs (e.g., steroids and antibiotics), which have poor solubility in water, are delivered as suspensions to treat pulmonary diseases. Most pharmaceutical aerosol suspensions have been propelled with chlorofluorocarbons, but current global regulations require pharmaceutical aerosols to be reformulated to contain non-ozone-depleting propellants [36]. Alternatives to chlorofluorocarbon propellants are hydrofluorocarbon (HFC) 134a [also known as hydrofluoroalkane (HFA) 134a or 1,1,1,2-tetrafluoroethane] and HFC-227ea (HFA-227ea or 1,1,1,2,3,3,3-heptafluoropropane) [37,38]. However, eliminating chlorine from HFCs has added a significant solvency challenge. The lower solvency of HFC fluids has turned attention from solution-based aerosols to suspension-based metered-dose inhalers (MDIs) [39].

9.3.2.1.5 TOPICAL SUSPENSIONS (LOTIONS)

Many topical suspensions (lotions) are available for treating acne and fungal and viral infections. Cosmetic applications of lotions are numerous, ranging from sun protectors to antiperspirants. Examples include calamine lotion, ciclopirox lotion, and sodium sulfacetamide lotion. Calamine lotion contains 8% each of zinc oxide

TABLE 9.5 Examples of Suspension Products Administered by Various Routes [4]

Active Ingredient (Brand Name)	Suspending Agents	Indication
ORAL SUSPENSIONS		
Acyclovir (Zovirax®)	Carboxymethylcellulose sodium (CMC sodium) and microcrystalline cellulose	Herpes simplex virus infections
Indomethacin (Indocin®)	Tragacanth	Moderate to severe arthritis and spondylitis
Megestrol acetate (Megace®)	Xanthan gum	Anorexia, cachexia, significant weight loss in patients with AIDS
Megestrol acetate (Megace ES)	Hydroxypropyl methylcellulose	Anorexia, cachexia, significant weight loss in patients with AIDS
Cefpodoxime proxetil (Vantin®)	Carboxymethylcellulose sodium, microcrystalline cellulose, carrageenan, croscarmellose sodium, hydroxypropylcellulose, and propylene glycol alginate	Bacterial infections
Pantoprazole sodium (Protonix®)	Crospovidone, hypromellose, methacrylic acid copolymer, microcrystalline cellulose, and povidone	Short-term treatment of erosive esophagitis associated with gastroesophageal reflux disease (GERD)
Oxcarbazepine (Trileptal®)	Cellulose	Epilepsy
Ampicillin for oral suspension (Principen®)	Lecithin	Bacterial infections
Griseofulvin (Grifulvin V)	Sodium alginate	Fungal infections
OTIC SUSPENSIONS		
Ciprofloxacin and dexamethasone (Ciprodex®)	Hydroxyethyl cellulose	Acute otitis media/externa
Neomycin sulfate and hydrocortisone (Cortisporin®)	Cetyl alcohol	Acute otitis externa
OPHTHALMIC SUSPENSIONS		
Brinzolamide (Azopt®)	Carbomer 974P	Elevated intraocular pressure
Loteprednol etabonate (Lotemax®)	Povidone	Allergic conjunctivitis
NASAL SUSPENSIONS		
Budesonide (Rhinocort® Aqua)	Microcrystalline cellulose and CMC sodium	Seasonal and perennial allergic/nonallergic rhinitis
Triamcinolone acetonide (Nasacort® AQ)	Microcrystalline cellulose and CMC sodium	Seasonal and perennial allergic rhinitis
Beclomethasone dipropionate (Beconase® AQ)	Microcrystalline cellulose and CMC sodium	Seasonal allergic rhinitis
TOPICAL SUSPENSIONS		
Sulfacetamide topical suspension (Plexion®)	Xanthan gum NF	Topical treatment of acne vulgaris

and calamine, the latter composed of zinc oxide and a small amount of ferric oxide. In the preparation of a lotion, powders are levigated with a small portion of glycerin (levigating agent); the mixture is diluted with a combination of bentonite magma and calcium hydroxide solution. The product is made to volume with additional calcium hydroxide solution. The bentonite magma can be used to suspend zinc oxide and calamine; however, on standing, the powders do settle. Calamine lotion relieves itching, pain, and skin irritation.

9.3.2.2 Flocculated and Deflocculated Suspensions

Particle interactions and their settling properties in a suspension vehicle determine the suspension's rheological behavior, and render suspensions into deflocculated or flocculated suspensions. In flocculated suspensions, particles tend to agglomerate to form loose structures (floccules). In contrast, a deflocculated suspension consists of drug particles that do not agglomerate into floccules. Given that flocculated and deflocculated suspensions have the same drug particle-size distribution, drug crystal habit, drug particle density, and vehicle viscosity, drug particles in deflocculated suspensions exhibit rapid sedimentation than in flocculated suspension. Sedimented flocculated drug particles can be redispersed upon mild agitation, whereas sediments in deflocculated suspensions are difficult to redisperse. In deflocculated suspensions, no clear boundary between sedimented cake and supernatant liquid is formed. The supernatant remains turbid for a long period of time due to varied sedimentation rates by different particle sizes. Formation of a clear supernatant liquid or a turbid layer during settling is a good indication of flocculated and deflocculated suspensions, respectively.

The selection of a suspension (flocculated versus deflocculated) is dependent on the physicochemical properties of drug substances and their compatibility with excipients. Therefore, selection of a suspension should be treated as specific to drug substances. Sedimentation can be minimized with structured vehicles (viscous) as opposed to unstructured vehicles, where rapid sedimentation occurs. Structured vehicles exhibit pseudoplastic and plastic flow behavior. These vehicles reduce particle settling by entrapping particles. It is preferred that thixotropy be associated with these two types of flows. At steady state, thixotropic vehicles are physically stable and readily pourable upon mild agitation. The shear thinning property of these vehicles facilitates uniform dispersion and pourable characteristics when shear is applied.

In many instances, deflocculated suspensions in structured vehicles are also desirable. For example, in a structured vehicle in which large particles (floccules) sediment faster than smaller particles, a deflocculated suspension in which drug particles exist as separate entities (as opposed to floccules) is desirable. Another aspect is that deflocculated suspensions are devoid of flocculating agents, which can catalyze chemical degradation of drug compounds and excipients. On the contrary, physical and chemical incompatibility of drug substances with excipients could result in rapid sedimentation and hard cake formation. It is for these reasons that flocculated suspensions are preferred over deflocculated suspensions.

Flocculated suspensions can fulfill the requisites of an ideal pharmaceutical suspension (i.e., sedimentation volume being equal to one). In practice, some sedimentation occurs; therefore, suspending agents are added to retard sedimentation of floccules. For example, a dispersion of positively charged drug particles can be flocculated by addition of an anionic electrolyte. The physical stability of the suspension can be increased further by addition of anionic protective colloids, which are compatible with anionic flocculating agents. However, if a negatively charged suspension is flocculated with positively charged electrolytes, the subsequent addition of anionic colloids may result in strong ionic interactions between oppositely charged ions, forming a mass, which has little or no suspending action. Therefore, it is necessary to include a protective colloid with the same charge (i.e., positively charged) as flocculating agents, to preclude ionic interactions.

9.3.2.3 Stability Aspects

9.3.2.3.1 PHYSICAL STABILITY

Often, rapid sedimentation and hard cake formation in suspensions are a result of physical characteristics of drug particles. Some of the key particle features that determine the stability of suspensions include size distribution, hydrophobicity, crystal habit, and density. Solids are milled to reduce particle size before dispersing in a vehicle. Reduction in particle size leads to an increase of both surface area and surface free energy, resulting in an unstable thermodynamic system. In an energy compensation phenomenon, particles tend to regroup/flocculate to decrease surface area and, thus, surface free energy. The formation of aggregates/floccules is considered a suspension's tendency to form a stable thermodynamic system. Surface free energy and total surface area can be correlated by Eq. 9.2:

$$\Delta F = \gamma_{SL} \times \Delta A \tag{9.2}$$

where γ_{SL} is the interfacial tension between solid particles and liquid vehicle in dyne/cm, F is the surface free energy in dyne × cm (erg), and A is the surface area in cm^2. Since suspension of solid particles in a liquid vehicle is an interfacial phenomenon, intermolecular forces at the particle surface affect the degree of flocculation and agglomeration in a suspension. In particular, weak Van der Waals attractive forces and repulsive forces arising from interaction of electric double layers surrounding each particle influence the degree of flocculation [40,41]. In a flocculated suspension, the energy barrier between approaching particles is high enough (>1000 Å) to be surmounted. However, when the approaching distance between particles is less than 1000 Å, attractive forces become dominant, leading to sedimentation.

Although it is not possible to prevent settling completely, it is necessary to consider factors that influence sedimentation and adopt formulation strategies to minimize it. The velocity of sedimentation can be expressed by Stoke's law as shown in Eq. 9.3:

$$\nu = d^2(\rho_s - \rho_o)g/18\eta_o \quad (9.3)$$

where ν is terminal velocity in cm/sec; d is diameter of the particle in cm; ρ_s and ρ_o are densities of dispersed phase and dispersion medium, respectively; g is acceleration due to gravity in cm^2; and η_o is viscosity of dispersion medium in poise. From the equation, it can be concluded that the rate of fall of a suspended particle in a vehicle of a given density is greater for larger particles than for smaller particles. Also, the greater the difference in density between particles and vehicle, the greater the sedimentation rate. Increase of viscosity of the dispersion medium can reduce the sedimentation rate. Thus, a decrease in the sedimentation rate in a suspension could be achieved by reducing the size of particles and by increasing the density and viscosity of the dispersed phase.

Stoke's equation can be applied only in conditions such as (a) suspensions contain spherical particles in a very dilute suspension (0.5–2% suspension); (b) particles do not collide with each other; and (c) free settling of particles may occur. However, in most pharmaceutical suspensions, the concentration of suspended particles is > 5% and they exhibit slow settling. Even a corrected Stoke's equation could not represent the mass rate of settling of irregular particles in concentrated suspensions. However, two parameters that are useful to measure the velocity of sedimentation are sedimentation volume and degree of flocculation [42]. The sedimentation volume, F, is defined as the ratio of the final volume, Vi, of the sedimented suspension to the original volume of the suspension, Vo, as shown in Eq. 9.4:

$$F = Vi/Vo \quad (9.4)$$

Figure 9.3 demonstrates that sedimentation volume can have values ranging from less than 1 to greater than 1. In a settled deflocculated suspension, $F < 1$, where the final volume of sediment is smaller than the original volume of the suspension. In a stable suspension, $F = 1$, where the final volume of sediment in a flocculated suspension equals the original volume of the suspension. It is possible that $F > 1$, when the final volume of the suspension is greater than the original suspension volume. This increase in volume could be due to an expanded structure formed due to slow swelling of excipient polymers.

Another parameter is the degree of sedimentation (β), which is more of a quantitative estimate of sedimentation. The degree of sedimentation is defined as the ratio of the final sedimentation volume of a flocculated suspension (V_f) to the final sedimentation volume (V_d) of a deflocculated suspension, as shown in Eq. 9.5:

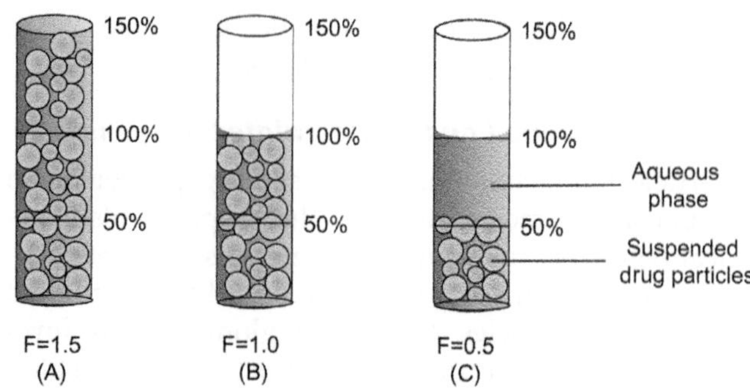

FIGURE 9.3 Demonstrates the three cases of sedimentation volumes: (A) swollen suspension, (B) flocculated suspension, and (C) deflocculated suspension. In a settled deflocculated suspension, $F < 1$, where the final volume of the sediment is smaller than the original volume of the suspension. In a stable suspension, $F = 1$, i.e., final volume of the sediment in a flocculated suspension equals the original volume (100%) of the suspension. It is possible that $F > 1$, where the final volume of the suspension is greater than the original suspension volume. This increase in volume could be due to an expanded loose structure. For example, excessive concentrations of polymer swell over a period of standing, resulting in expansion of suspension volume.

$$\beta = (V_f/V_o)/(V_d/V_o) \quad (9.5)$$

9.3.2.3.2 INTERFACIAL PHENOMENON AND ELECTROCHEMICAL STABILITY

In suspension medium, particles become charged due to ion adsorption onto the particle surface or ionization of functional groups at the particle surface. Selective adsorption of ions could be due to ions from excipients (e.g., electrolytes), hydronium, and hydroxyl ions of water. The overall charge is dependent on the pH of the liquid medium. For a description of an electric double layer, consider suspended particles in contact with a polar liquid medium (Figure 9.4) [12]. Assuming an inherent negative charge of the solid surface, some cations (hydronium or cations from ionic excipients) are adsorbed onto the surface. The adsorbed ions that imparted cationic charge are referred to as potential-determining ions ($\alpha\alpha'$ layer). This cationic layer attracts anions (counter-ions) of the suspension medium and repels cations (vice versa, if the potential determining ion is negative, positive counter-ions may present in the layer). The limit of this region is termed line $\beta\beta'$, whose potential is still positive due to fewer anions than cations bound to the solid surface. In the region $\beta\beta'$–$\gamma\gamma'$, the concentration of anions is higher; at $\gamma\gamma'$, anion concentration

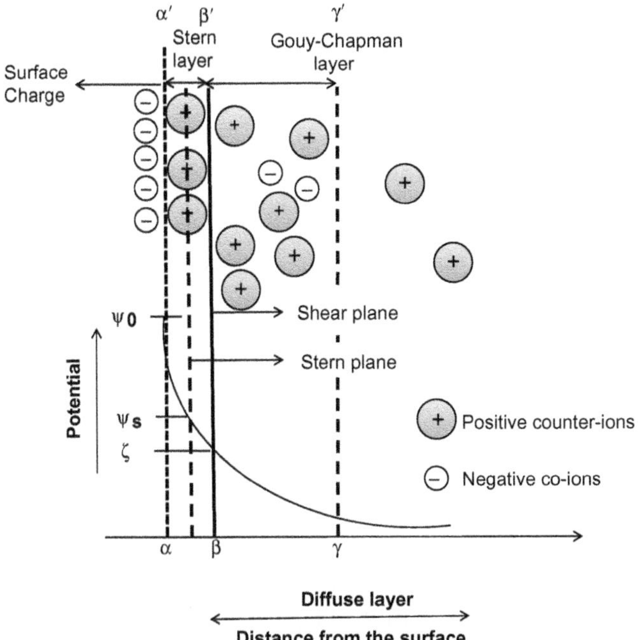

FIGURE 9.4 Represents changes in potentials with distance from the particle surface.

becomes equal to cations (i.e., the system becomes electroneutral); and beyond $\gamma\gamma'$, anion concentration decreases. Despite uneven distribution of charged regions, the system as a whole is considered neutral.

Due to formulation composition (e.g., high concentration of ionic excipients, such as flocculating agents, suspending agents), changes in the electroneutral region occur. For example, if the total charge of counter-ions in the region $\alpha\alpha'-\beta\beta'$ exceeds potential determining ions, then the net charge at $\beta\beta'$ will be negative rather than positive. Instead of electric neutrality at the $\gamma\gamma'$ boundary, an excess of positive ions must be present in the region $\beta\beta'-\gamma\gamma'$. Also, electrical neutrality may occur at the $\beta\beta'$ boundary itself, if the concentration of counter-ions equals potential determining ions.

Figure 9.4 represents changes in potential with distance from the solid surface. The electric distribution at the interface is equivalent to the charge of the first double layer, $\alpha\alpha'-\beta\beta'$, which is termed the stern layer or Helmholtz layer. The diffused double layer $\beta\beta'-\gamma\gamma'$ is termed the Gouy–Chapman layer. The potential at the solid surface ($\alpha\alpha'$) due to potential determining ions is termed the Nernst potential (ψ_0), defined as the potential difference between the solid surface and neutral region ($\gamma\gamma'$) of the dispersion medium. The potential at the shear plane (where counter-ions diffuse away) is considered the zeta potential (ζ),which can be defined as the potential difference between the shear plane and neutral region ($\gamma\gamma'$) of the dispersion medium.

When a suspended particle moves (e.g., gravity or Brownian motion), Stern and Gouy–Chapman layers move along and ions beyond the Gouy–Chapman layer boundary remain in the bulk dispersion medium. While moving, particles undergo Van der Waals attractive and electrical double-layer repulsive forces. The repulsive forces between particles prevent them from approaching each other and adhering to each other. However, particle collisions could overcome the repulsive force energy barrier, resulting in the adherence of particles. Often, zeta potential measurements are made to determine the magnitude of interactions between colloidal particles and assess the stability of colloidal systems. If the suspended particles have a large negative or positive zeta potential, then particles tend to repel each other. However, if the particles have low zeta potential values, then attractive forces exceed repulsive forces, and the particles come together, triggering settling of particles. In general, stable and unstable suspensions are on either side of +25 or −25 mV (i.e., particles with zeta potentials more positive than +25 mV or more negative than −25 mV are considered stable). It is important to remember that particles whose density is different from the dispersion medium will also undergo sedimentation, forming a hard cake.

Various factors, such as pH, ionic strength, and concentration of formulation components, influence the zeta potential value of suspended particles. Imagine a weak acid drug being suspended in a dispersion medium (pH > p*K*a). Drug particles undergo ionization and exhibit negative zeta potential. If more alkali is added to this suspension, then particles tend to acquire more negative charge. If acid is added to this suspension, neutralization occurs at a certain pH of the medium. Further addition of acid will result in a positive zeta potential. For a weak acid, a zeta potential versus pH plot exhibits a negative potential at high pH and a positive potential at low pH of the dispersion medium. The point of zero potential is termed the isoelectric point, at which the suspension is unstable. The concentration of ions in suspension determines the thickness of the double layer. The higher the ionic strength, the more compressed the double layer and greater the magnitude of interactions on the particle surface. Also, high valence of ions causes compression of double layers.

9.3.2.3.3 CHEMICAL STABILITY

In suspensions, a kinetic equilibrium exists between the suspended insoluble drug form and the soluble form. At a particular temperature, the drug concentration of the soluble form remains constant with time; therefore, the rate of formation of the soluble form in suspensions follows zero-order kinetics. Although insoluble, the suspended drug substances have intrinsic solubility, which triggers chemical reactions, such as hydrolysis, leading to degradation. From these observations, it is assumed that decomposition of drug substances in suspensions is due to the amount of drug dissolved in the aqueous phase. Despite decomposition, the concentration of drug solution remains constant with time (i.e., zero-order kinetics).

The kinetics of formation of a soluble drug concentration in a suspension is also referred to as apparent zero-order because the soluble form follows zero-order only as a result of the suspended drug reservoir. If the suspended particles are converted into a drug solution, the entire system changes from zero-order to first-order, and degradation then depends on solution concentration. However, most suspension dosage forms are stable (shelf-life period) enough for the soluble drug fraction to exhibit zero-order kinetics. It is also uncommon to design and manufacture suspension dosage forms, in which the soluble fraction undergoes rapid degradation, triggering first-order kinetics. In such a case, there is the potential to produce degradants at greater than acceptable thresholds.

9.3.2.4 Formulation Considerations

Drugs are formulated as suspensions due to their low aqueous-soluble nature. Different categories of inactive ingredients are required for suspending drug particles in aqueous vehicles. The inactive ingredients are intended to alter drug physicochemical characteristics, such as particle-size distribution, surface tension, and surface charge, to produce a stable suspension. Some excipients are added to modulate the rheological behavior of suspensions and minimize irreversible sedimentation of particles. Table 9.4 lists common inactive ingredients and their concentration ranges in pharmaceutical suspensions, which include wetting agents (surfactants), viscosity modifiers, buffers, taste-masking agents, flavoring agents, and coloring agents.

9.3.2.4.1 VEHICLES

De-ionized water is a common suspending medium in pharmaceutical suspensions. In a few instances, viscous nonaqueous solvents, such as propylene glycol and polyethylene glycols, are used as vehicles to impart stability to suspended drug particles.

9.3.2.4.2 WETTING AGENTS

The foremost requirement to produce a pharmaceutical suspension is to achieve adequate wetting of solid particles by the liquid vehicle. Wetting of solids is related to a phenomenon in which the solid-air interface is instantly replaced by a solid-liquid interface when the drug is suspended in a vehicle. The wetting phenomenon (spreading) can be expressed in terms of surface tension, W^s, given by Eq. 9.6:

$$W^s = \gamma_S - \gamma_L - \gamma_{SL} \tag{9.6}$$

where γ_S is the surface tension of the solid, γ_L is the surface tension of the solid, and γ_{SL} is the solid-liquid interfacial surface tension. The surface tension of liquids is readily measured by well-established methods, such as Wilhelmy plate or du Nuoy ring [43]. In the case of solids, only indirect methods are available to estimate γ_L and γ_{SL} based on Young's equation (9.7) [43]:

$$\gamma_L \cos(\theta) = \gamma_S - \gamma_{SL} \tag{9.7}$$

where θ is the contact angle between the solid surface and tangent to the liquid phase. Wettability of hydrophobic drugs can be achieved by reducing the contact angle of water on solid surfaces. Surfactants are added to wet the solid surfaces. The adsorption of surfactants can increase the stability of particles against aggregation. The solid-liquid interfacial interactions of adsorbed surfactants can be one of the following [44]: (a) ion-exchange (i.e., substitution of previously adsorbed ions on the solid by surfactant ions of identical charge); (b) ion-pairing (i.e., adsorption of surfactant ions on the surface sites of opposite charge not occupied by counter-ions); (c) acid-base interactions, mainly hydrogen bonds; (d) adsorption by polarization of π electrons; (e) adsorption by dispersion forces occurs via Van der Waals forces between solid surface and liquid; and (f) hydrogen bonding.

Typical examples of surfactants in pharmaceutical suspensions include docusate sodium, sodium dodecyl sulfate, and ammonium lauryl ether sulfate (anionic); benzalkonium chloride, benzethonium chloride, and cetyl trimethylammonium bromide (cationic); and polyoxyethylene alkylphenylethers (e.g., nonoxynol 9 and nonoxynol 10), poloxamers, polyoxyethylene fatty acid glycerides (e.g., Labrasol®), polyoxyethylene (35) castor oil, polyoxyethylene (40) hydrogenated castor oil, polyoxyethylene sorbitan esters (e.g., polysorbate 20 and polysorbate 80), propylene glycol fatty acid esters (e.g., propylene glycol laurate), glyceryl fatty acid esters (e.g., glyceryl monostearate), and sorbitan esters (e.g., sorbitan monolaurate, sorbitan monooleate, sorbitan monopalmitate, and sorbitan monostearate) (nonionic). Nonionic surfactants whose HLB is in the range of 6–9 are often used in low concentrations to wet solid surfaces [45]. Nonionic surfactants minimize sedimentation through steric hindrance of particle interactions. Polysorbate 80 is the most widely used nonionic surfactant in parenteral and oral suspensions [46].

Adequate concentration of surfactants should be used for wetting of insoluble powder. Excessive surfactant concentration in suspensions leads to undesirable dissolution of drugs. Since the dissolved fraction of a drug is susceptible to chemical degradation and interaction with other ingredients, suspensions comprising free drugs can be chemically unstable. Also, high free-surfactant concentration could result in more rapid sedimentation of flocculated particles than deflocculated particles. High surfactant concentration could result in air entrainment inside the particles, leading to lowered wetting and nonuniform doses. In addition to surfactants, hygroscopic substances can be used as wetting aids. For example, glycerin flows into voids between particles to displace air and, during the mixing operation, coats the material so that water can penetrate and wet individual particles.

9.3.2.4.3 FLOCCULATING AGENTS

In flocculated suspensions, agents are added to produce controlled flocculation of wetted particles to prevent formation of compact sediments, which are difficult to redisperse. Substances such as salts, surfactants, and polymers act as flocculating agents. Salts reduce the electric barrier between particles to link them to form floccules. One example of an electrolyte is monobasic potassium phosphate. Surfactants, such as docusate sodium, sodium dodecyl sulfate, benzalkonium chloride, and cetyl trimethylammonium bromide, have been used as flocculating agents. However, it is critical to maintain low surfactant concentration, which otherwise may hinder flocculation. Polymers (e.g., xanthan gum, carbopols, and cellulose derivatives) also function as flocculating agents because part of the chain is adsorbed onto the particle surface, with the remaining parts projecting out into the dispersion medium. Bridging between these portions leads to formation of floccules. Hydrophilic polymers (e.g., clays) act as protective colloids, and particles coated with polymers are less prone to caking than uncoated particles. These polymers exhibit pseudoplastic flow, which serves to promote physical stability of suspensions.

9.3.2.4.4 VISCOSITY MODIFIERS

According to flow behavior, liquids are classified as Newtonian and non-Newtonian. Simple liquids follow Newtonian behavior, in which stress is proportional to shear. Emulsions and suspensions follow a non-Newtonian (e.g., plastic, pseudoplastic, dilatant flow behaviors) [47,48]. In concentrated suspensions, it is difficult to control particle-particle collisions, which affect the flow properties of suspensions. An increase of viscosity of the dispersion medium will reduce the frequency of collisions, while simultaneously hindering particle sedimentation. Viscosity modifiers are added to impart physical stability to suspensions. It is desirable that these viscosity modifiers be associated with thixotropic features (i.e., physically stable at the steady state and pourable upon mild agitation). Viscosity modifiers must have the following properties: (a) water-soluble or swell in aqueous media; (b) stable; and (c) compatible with other suspension components. Common viscosity modifiers are cellulose derivatives (e.g., methylcellulose, microcrystalline cellulose, and hydroxypropyl methylcellulose), clays (e.g., bentonite and kaolinite), natural gums (e.g., acacia, guar gum, tragacanth and xanthan gum), synthetic polymers (e.g., polyvinylpyrrolidone), and miscellaneous compounds (e.g., colloidal silicon dioxide and silicates). Each of the viscosity modifiers has its own mechanism of action. It is common to use more than one category of viscosity modifier to exert a synergistic effect on rheological behavior, as well as improve the stability of suspensions. For example, magnesium aluminum silicate and xanthan gum are used in nystatin oral suspension. The silicate exerts a synergistic effect with xanthan gum, enhancing the thixotropic characteristic of the suspension.

9.3.2.4.5 BUFFERS

In an ideal situation, pharmaceutical suspensions should be stable in a wide pH range. Citrates and phosphates are commonly used buffers in pharmaceutical suspensions. Citrate buffers are used to stabilize suspensions in the pH range of 3–5, while phosphate buffers are used in the pH range of 7–8.

9.3.2.4.6 TONICITY-ADJUSTING AGENTS

Tonicity-adjusting agents are added to produce osmotic pressure comparable to biological fluids when the suspension is intended for ophthalmic or parenteral purposes. Common tonicity-adjusting agents for ophthalmic suspensions are dextrose, mannitol, and sorbitol, while tonicity-adjusting agents used in parenteral suspensions are sodium chloride, sodium sulfate, dextrose, mannitol, and glycerol.

9.3.2.4.7 OTHER ADDITIVES

A number of additives are needed for preparation of an elegant and stable suspension. A few of them include preservatives, complexing agents, colorants, and flavoring agents. In colloidal formulations, trace metals may trigger aggregation and an oxidation reaction. Complexing agents hinder formation of large aggregates responsible for the caking phenomenon. Flavoring agents, cellulose derivatives, and natural gums (viscosity modifiers) are a source of microbial growth. Preservatives are added to prevent microbial growth in suspensions. Common preservatives in suspensions are parabens, alcohol, glycerin, propylene glycol, and sorbates. Preservatives lose antimicrobial action due to one of several factors, such as oxidation, solubility in oils, incompatibility with ions or container, and closures. In general, ionic preservatives are active in the un-ionized form; therefore, suitable buffers are chosen to maintain preservatives in un-ionized form and exert antimicrobial action. In a few instances, a combination of two or more preservatives is used to exert a wide spectrum of antimicrobial action.

9.3.3 Emulsions

Emulsions are liquid disperse systems consisting of two immiscible phases, one of which is dispersed as globules in the other liquid phase [49]. The two phases of emulsions are stabilized by the presence of an emulsifier. The droplet diameter of the dispersed phase extends from about 0.1 to 10 μM, although particle diameters as small as 0.01 μM and as large as 100 μM are not uncommon [50]. The consistency of emulsions ranges from that of a liquid (e.g., fat emulsions) to a semisolid (e.g., ointments and creams).

As illustrated in Figure 9.5, one liquid phase of an emulsion is polar (e.g., aqueous), and the other is relatively nonpolar (e.g., oil). When an oil phase is dispersed as globules through an aqueous continuous phase, the system is referred to as an oil-in-water (o/w) emulsion. When an oil phase serves as the continuous phase, the emulsion is referred to as a water-in-oil (w/o) emulsion. Pharmaceutical emulsions are usually the o/w type and require the use of an o/w emulsifier. Topical emulsions may be o/w or w/o emulsions; the latter is currently popular. Other special classes of emulsions include multiple and micro-emulsions.

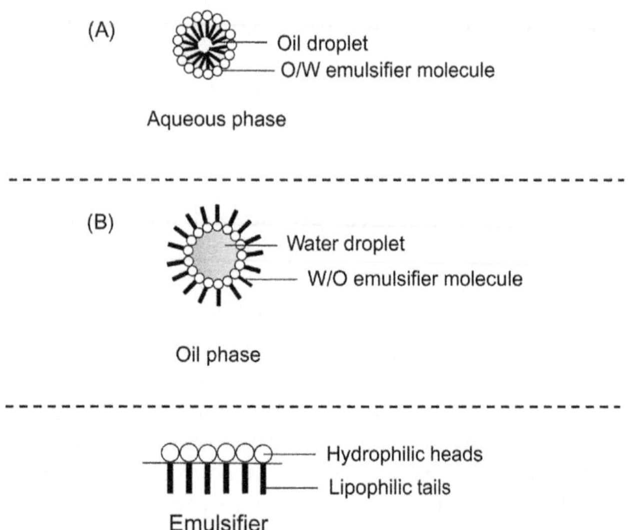

FIGURE 9.5 Demonstrates (A) oil-in-water dispersion, where o/w emulsifier disperses the oil phase in a continuous aqueous phase; (B) water-in-oil emulsion, where w/o emulsifier disperses water in a continuous oil phase.

Multiple emulsions may be water-in-oil-water, in which the aqueous phase is in between two oil phases, or oil-in-water-oil, in which the internal and external oil phases are separated by an aqueous phase. Multiple emulsions are being investigated to prolong drug release rates through incorporating drug substances in the inner aqueous or oil phase of an emulsion [51]. Micro-emulsions are another class of emulsions that consist of large or swollen micelles in the internal phase, much like that of a solubilized solution [52]. Micro-emulsions appear as clear transparent solutions and are thermodynamically stable. Micro-emulsions contain droplet diameters of about 0.01 to 0.2 μM.

9.3.3.1 Applications

In general, oil-in-water emulsions are designed for oral (e.g., cod liver emulsion), injectable, ophthalmic, and topical purposes. Table 9.6 lists representative examples of pharmaceutical emulsions. Intravenous fat emulsions employed for total parenteral nutrition (TPN) are formulated using vegetable oils as the dispersed phase and phospholipids as the emulsifier, with an objective to provide calories and essential fatty acids. The fat emulsions are particularly indicated in cases of GI tract traumas, cancer, infections, burns, radiation exposures, and psychological disorders (e.g., bulimia). Fat emulsions are oil-in-water emulsions with mean droplet diameters in the range of 0.2 to 0.5 μM [53,54]. For intravenous applications, it is necessary that there be no droplets larger than the diameter of blood capillaries (~5 μM) to avoid blockage [55]. Intravenous fat emulsions can be used as drug carriers. Emulsions containing hypnotics, such as diazepam, etomidate, or propofol, are available. A number of drug-containing emulsions are in preclinical and clinical trials. Advantages that favor the use of fat emulsions as drug carriers [56] are (1) poor solubility of drugs in water, but excellent solubility in oil; (2) stabilization of drugs that are sensitive to hydrolysis; (3) reduction of side effects associated with drugs; and (4) drug targeting. Although injectable emulsions present a number of potential advantages, the number of approved products is relatively low. Some of the major issues preventing a broader application of injectable emulsions are (1) oil phase compositions (e.g., long- and medium-chain triglycerides) approved by the regulatory agencies are not necessarily good solvents for lipophilic drugs; (2) the oil phase should not exceed 20–30% of the emulsion, which possibly limits the required solubility of drug substances; an increase of the oil phase over 20% poses challenges to concentration limits of the emulsifier and processing conditions to obtain a droplet diameter less than 5 μM; and (3) drug crystallization out of emulsions.

Emulsions have applications for ophthalmic purposes; they transfer drug substances in an effective concentration to ocular disease sites and prolong drug release. Cyclosporin (Restasis®) and Difluprednate (Durezol®) are the available topical ophthalmic emulsions. Cyclosporin, an immunosuppressant, is indicated for treating keratoconjunctivitis sicca (dry-eye syndrome), while difluprednate is indicated for treating postoperative inflammation and pain associated with ocular surgery. Because both cyclosporin and difluprednate have such a low solubility in water, it is difficult to prepare ophthalmic drops in a concentration effective to produce therapeutic efficacy. Cyclosporin and difluprednate exhibit better solubility in oils than in aqueous phase, and therefore are administered as oil-in-water emulsions.

The use of emulsions for oral application is limited since other alternatives, such as SEDDS, are popular. Emulsions containing contrast agents have been used in computed tomography, magnetic resonance imaging, and radionuclide imaging. Perfluorochemical emulsions serve as vehicles for respiratory gas (e.g., oxygen). Fluosol-DA (Green Cross and Alpha Therapeutics, Japan), which consists of perfluorodecalin and perfluorotripropylamine, has been marketed as an artificial blood substitute for tissue oxygenation. Topical emulsion formulations include creams and lotions.

9.3.3.2 *Theories of Emulsions*

Several theories have been proposed to explain the stability of emulsions. Some of the theories are related to the functional role of emulsifiers and others to processing conditions. The most important theories are the surface tension, oriented-wedge, and interfacial film theories. According to surface-tension theory, emulsifiers lower interfacial tension between two immiscible liquids, thus allowing the miscibility of phases [57]. The oriented-wedge theory assumes formation of a monomolecular layer of emulsifier around the droplet of the internal phase of an emulsion [58]. Certain emulsifiers orient themselves around a liquid droplet in a manner reflective of their solubility in a particular phase. The interfacial theory describes that the emulsifier is located at the interface between oil and water phases, forming a thin film by being adsorbed onto the surface of internal phase droplets [59]. The surfactant film must be sufficiently rigid to stabilize the interface, but also needs to be flexible enough that the collision of emulsion droplets does not lead to the rupture of the film, resulting in coalescence.

TABLE 9.6 Examples of Marketed Emulsion Products [4]

Product (Approved Market)	Composition	Indication
Liposyn® (USA)	10%/20% soy oil/safflower oil, egg phospholipid, water for injection	Total Parenteral Nutrition
Intralipid® (USA)	10%/20%/30% soy oil, egg phospholipid, water for injection	Total Parenteral Nutrition
Lipofundin® (USA)	10%/20% soy oil, egg phospholipid, water for injection	Total Parenteral Nutrition
Cleviprex® (USA)	Clevidipine butyrate, soy oil, egg phospholipid, glycerol, water for injection	Reduction of blood pressure
Diazemuls® (USA)	Diazepam, acetylated glycerides, egg phospholipid, glycerol, sodium hydroxide	Anxiolytic or sedative
Disoprivan® (Worldwide)	Propofol, soybean oil, egg lecithin, disodium edetate, glycerol, sodium hydroxide, water for injection	Induction and maintenance of anesthesia, conscious sedation for surgical procedure
Etomidate-Lipuro® (Germany)	Etomidate, soy oil, MCT, egg lecithin, glycerol, sodium oleate	Induction of anesthesia
Fluosol-DA® (Worldwide)	Perfluorodecalin, perfluorotripropylamine, egg phospholipid, glycerol, pluronic F68, potassium oleate	Blood substitute
Restasis® (USA)	Cyclosporine, glycerin; castor oil; polysorbate 80; pemulens, sodium hydroxide, and purified water	Keratoconjunctivitis sicca (dry eye syndrome)
Durezol® (USA)	Difluprednate, boric acid, castor oil, glycerin, polysorbate 80, sodium acetate, sodium EDTA, and sodium hydroxide, sorbic acid, and purified water.	Postoperative inflammation

None of the theories of emulsification is of universal application, and though each may cover a particular class of emulsifiers, different classes of emulsifiers exert a slightly different mechanism of action from one another. Emulsifiers may be divided into three groups as follows:

a. Surface-active agents, which are adsorbed at oil-in-water interface to form monomolecular films and reduce interfacial tension
b. Hydrophilic colloids, which form a multimolecular film around the dispersed droplets of oil-in-water emulsion
c. Finely divided solid particles, which are adsorbed around dispersed globules

An important property of emulsifiers that determines their type is their hydrophilic-lipophilic-balance (HLB) value [60]. In general, an oil-in-water emulsion is formed when the HLB value of an emulsifier is within the range of about 9–12, whereas water-in-oil emulsions are formed with emulsifiers in the HLB range of 3–6. The type of emulsion is also a function of the relative solubility of surfactants (i.e., the phase in which it is more soluble being the continuous phase). This sometimes is referred to as the Bancroft rule. Thus, an emulsifier with a high HLB value is preferentially soluble in water and results in the formation of an oil-in-water emulsion. The reverse is true with surfactants of low HLB, which tend to form water-in-oil emulsions.

Emulsions may undergo a wide variety of shear stresses during preparation or use. In many of these processes, the flow properties will be vital for the proper performance of an emulsion [48,61]. For example, the flow of a parenteral emulsion through a hypodermic needle, removal of an emulsion from a bottle or tube, and flow behavior of an emulsion in various milling operations employed in manufacturing require correct flow characteristics. Flow properties of emulsions are influenced by factors such as phase volume ratio, droplet-size distribution, and viscosity of the internal phase. Most emulsions, except dilute ones, exhibit non-Newtonian flow. When the phase volume of the dispersed phase is low (less than 0.05 or 5%), the system is Newtonian. As the volume is increased, the system becomes more resistant to flow and exhibits pseudoplastic flow. When the phase volume approaches 0.74 or 74%, phase inversion may occur with marked viscosity changes. Droplet-size distribution is another factor that affects the viscosity of emulsions. Reduction in mean droplet size increases viscosity; however, polydisperse emulsions exhibit lower viscosity compared to monodisperse systems (i.e., narrower particle-size distribution). Another factor is the emulsifier and its concentration. The higher the concentration of an emulsifier, the greater the viscosity of an emulsion.

9.3.3.3 Stability Aspects

The stability of pharmaceutical emulsions can be characterized by absence of the aggregation of emulsion droplets, separation of phases, and maintenance of elegance with respect to appearance, color, and odor. As shown in Figure 9.6, the stability of emulsions is governed by different mechanisms (i.e., flocculation, creaming, and coalescence), which may lead to irreversible destabilization (cracking).

9.3.3.3.1 FLOCCULATION

Flocculation may be subdivided into two general categories: sedimentation aggregation and Brownian motion aggregation. In sedimentation aggregation, droplet paths are vertically linear. High-density droplets (e.g., water droplets of water-in-oil emulsions) settle at the bottom, leading to aggregation. In Brownian aggregation, emulsions consisting of droplets of different sizes cream at different rates, with large droplets moving faster and colliding with slow-moving small droplets. These collisions lead to the aggregation of droplets. Flocculation is a precursor phenomenon to

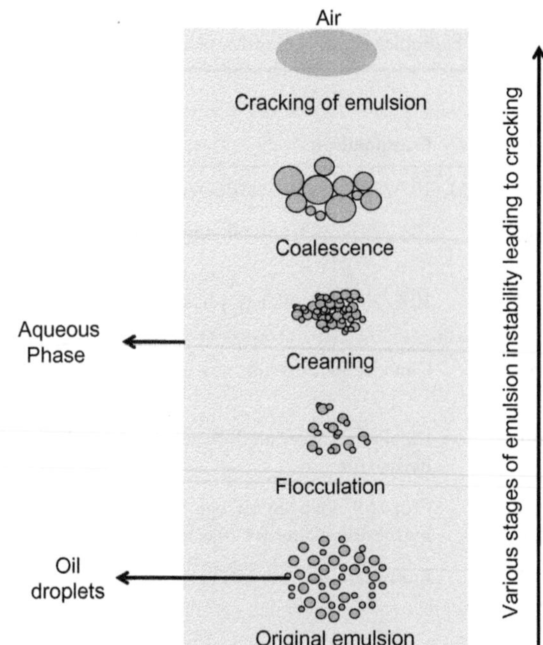

FIGURE 9.6 Schematic representation of various mechanisms leading to cracking of oil-in-water emulsion. Primary mechanisms of an unstable emulsion are flocculation, creaming, and coalescence. In some instances (e.g., unoptimized formulation composition or processing conditions), emulsion exhibits the cracking phenomenon without showing signs of flocculation, creaming, and coalescence.

creaming. An estimate of the relative rates of each type of flocculation can be made from Eq. 9.8 [62]:

$$\tau_{\max} = \frac{2\pi(\rho - \rho_0)gr4}{3K_bT} \tag{9.8}$$

where ρ is the density of the droplet, ρ_0 is the density of the dispersion medium, r is the droplet radius, K_b is the Boltzmann constant, and T is the absolute temperature. When $\tau\max > 10$, Brownian aggregation is negligible; when $\tau\max < 0.1$, sedimentation aggregation is negligible.

9.3.3.3.2 CREAMING

Creaming is a process by which the disperse phase separates from an emulsion, and is typically the precursor of coalescence. The creaming rate can be estimated from Stoke's equation. According to Stoke's law, if the dispersed phase is less dense than the continuous phase, which is the case of oil-in-water emulsions, the velocity of sedimentation becomes negative (i.e., upward creaming results). If the internal phase is heavier than the external phase (e.g., water-in-oil emulsions), the globules settle, which is referred to as creaming in the downward direction. The greater the difference between the densities of the phases, the greater the creaming rate. The size of the globules is also a determining factor in the creaming rate. As per Stoke's law, doubling the diameter of oil globules increases the creaming rate by a factor of four. The rate of creaming can be reduced by adding viscosity enhancers, such as methylcellulose, and droplet-size reduction.

9.3.3.3.3 COALESCENCE AND BREAKING

Creaming is a reversible process, whereas breaking is irreversible. The cream floccules may be redispersed, and a uniform mixture can be obtained by agitation. When breaking occurs, the emulsifier film surrounding the globules will be destroyed, and the oil droplets tend to coalesce. In such a case, simple mixing fails to resuspend globules. The coalescence phenomenon could be the result of numerous factors, such as inappropriate selection of emulsifier, inadequate emulsifier concentration, errors in the manufacturing process, phase volume ratio, viscosity of emulsion, and droplet size. Viscosity alone does not produce stable emulsions; however, viscous emulsions may be more stable than dilute ones by virtue of retardation of flocculation and coalescence. The phase volume ratio, which refers to the relative volume of the internal phase to the external phase in an emulsion, also influences the stability of the emulsion. Incorporation of more than 74% of oil in oil-in-water emulsion results in coalescence of oil globules [63]. This value, known as the critical point, is defined as the concentration of the internal phase above which the emulsifier cannot produce a stable emulsion.

9.3.3.4 *Formulation Considerations*

Emulsion formulation contains a number of inactive ingredients, such as oil phase-soluble lipids, emulsifiers, preservatives, pH-adjusting agents, and antioxidants. The selection of inactive ingredients depends on their approved use, route of administration, concentration limits, stability, and nontoxic nature. Lipids (e.g., triglycerides) approved by regulatory agencies, alone or in combination, are generally the first choice for developing emulsions [64]. Long-chain triglycerides include soybean oil, safflower oil, sesame oil, and castor oil, while medium-chain triglycerides include Miglyol 810 and 812. The solubility and stability of active ingredients govern the selection of the lipid phase. The oil phase must be of high purity and free of undesirable components, such as peroxides, pigments, degradation products, and unsaponifiable matter (e.g., sterols). Lipid peroxides of the oil phase can serve as initiators of oxidation and destabilize compounds susceptible to oxidation. The oxidation of oil can be minimized by the addition of antioxidants.

Emulsifiers are a class of emulsion stabilizers that reduce interfacial tension between oil and aqueous phases to produce a stable colloidal dispersion. Egg and soy lecithins have been used extensively as emulsifiers in injectable emulsions. These emulsifiers are biocompatible and nontoxic [65]. However, hydrolysis of lecithin during emulsification, sterilization, and storage leads to formation of lysophospholipids, with detergent-like properties, and causes hemolysis. Process optimization (e.g., cold homogenization) and storage conditions (e.g., mild temperatures) could reduce the hydrolysis of emulsions. Other potential emulsifiers in injectable emulsions include PEGylated phospholipids (e.g., polyethylene glycol phosphatidylethanolamine) and nonionic surfactants (e.g., Pluronic® F68).

The aqueous phase includes additives such as antioxidants, preservatives, tonicity modifiers, and pH-adjusting agents. Antioxidants that impart protection in the aqueous phase include sodium metabisulfite, ascorbic acid, thioglycerol, and cysteine. Oil-soluble antioxidants include α-tocopherol, propyl gallate, ascorbyl palmitate, and butylated hydroxytoluene. Microbial organisms degrade emulsifiers and glycerin, with a consequential deterioration of emulsion, and therefore require adequate concentration of preservatives to resist microbial growth. Due to the heterogeneous nature of emulsions, partitioning of preservatives will occur between oil and water phases.

In general, bacteria grow in the aqueous phase of emulsions, and preservatives with a tendency to partition into the oil phase may be useless because of low concentration remaining in the aqueous phase. In addition, the preservative must be in an un-ionized state to penetrate the bacterial membrane. Finally, preservative molecules must not bind to other components of the emulsion, since the complexes are ineffective as preservatives. Antimicrobial agents, such as benzalkonium chloride, benzyl alcohol, EDTA, parabens, and sodium benzoate, are added to the aqueous phase to prevent microbial growth. Tonicity can be achieved with glycerol and sorbitol. Buffering agents, which consist of weak or strong electrolytes, interact with phospholipids and cause catalysis of lipids, leading to destabilization of the emulsion. Instead, small amounts of sodium hydroxide are used to adjust the pH of the emulsion to around 8.0 before sterilization.

Ophthalmic emulsion compositions differ from injectable emulsions, specifically surfactants and thickening agents. Water-soluble and oil-soluble ingredients are solubilized in aqueous and oil phases, respectively. Different oils used in ophthalmic emulsions include castor oil, soybean oil, safflower oil, olive oil, arachis oil, and mineral oil. In ophthalmic emulsions, emulsifiers, such as polysorbates, glyceryl esters, and acrylate crosspolymers are used to form stable dispersion [66]. Acrylate polymers include carbomers and pemulens, which also act as viscosity agents. The pH of emulsions can be adjusted using sodium hydroxide to a near ocular pH level (7.2–7.8). In general, buffering agents are not required; if they are required, suitable buffers may include phosphates, citrates, acetates, and borates.

Emulsion-based topical lotions are low- to medium-medicated or nonmedicated topical preparations. Most lotions are oil-in-water emulsions; these are preferred due to their water washable and nonabsorptive nature. It is not uncommon for the same active pharmaceutical ingredient to be formulated into lotion, cream, and/or ointment dosage forms. Lotions are less viscous than creams and may be readily spread to affected regions. Some of the emulsion-based lotions are lindane, metronidazole (Metrolotion®), clotrimazole and betamethasone dipropionate (Lotrisone®), and ivermectin (Sklace®).

Typically, lotions include one or more of the following: a surfactant, thickener, emulsifier, emollient, perfuming agent, coloring agent, preservative, or buffer. Due to functional requirements, excipients used in topical lotions are extensive, and their concentration limits are higher than those administered through other routes. Emulsifiers used in lotions are derived from natural or synthetic sources. Natural emulsifiers in lotions are egg or soy lecithins and gelatin. Among the synthetic emulsifiers are anionic, cationic, and nonionic surfactants. Predominantly, nonionic surfactants contain the following classes: polyoxyethylene sorbitan fatty ester derivatives (e.g., polysorbate 80); glycerin fatty acid ester derivatives (e.g., glyceryl monocaprylate); polyethylene fatty acid ester derivatives (e.g., polyoxyethylene 40 monostearate); and fatty acid mono- or diglycerides (e.g., caprylic acid diglyceride); they may be used alone or in combination. Emulsifier concentration ranges from about 0.01% to 2.5% w/w. Auxiliary emulsifiers are added to improve the emulsifying capacity of primary emulsifiers. Examples of auxiliary emulsifiers are agar, pectin, and cholesterol. Some of the primary emulsifiers are also used as auxiliary emulsifiers.

Emollients or skin conditioning agents can be included in lotions to provide a softening or soothing effect on skin. Emollients also help control the rate of evaporation and the tackiness of the lotion. Emollients are used in concentrations of 0.1%–10% w/w. Suitable emollients include hydrocarbons, such as petrolatum and mineral oil, and fatty acid alcohols or their esters, such as myristyl alcohol, cetyl alcohol, stearyl alcohol, cetostearyl alcohol, glyceryl monostearate, glyceryl monooleate, isopropyl myristate, isopropyl palmitate, cholesterol, lanolin alcohols, and glycerin. Among the preceding, oleaginous hydrocarbons are widely used for occlusive properties. Fatty acids, fatty acid alcohols, or their esters are used for multifunctional roles, such as primary or auxiliary emulsifiers, emollients, and thickening agents. Thickening agents or viscosity agents in lotions aid in the attainment of the desired texture and spreadability. Thickeners from natural, semisynthetic, and synthetic sources can be used. Natural thickeners include acacia, tragacanth, carrageenan, clay, and magnesium aluminum silicate. One or more fatty acids, fatty acid alcohols, or their esters of the series C_{14}–C_{20} may be used in combination to obtain a particular consistency of lotion. For example, in sufficient concentration, stearyl alcohol produces a firm consistency, which can be softened with cetyl alcohol. Suitable preservatives include phenoxyethanol, parabens, benzyl alcohol, chlorhexidine gluconate, imidurea, and hydantoin derivatives. Preservative concentrations range from 0.01%–5% w/w. Antifoaming and antiwhitening agents may be included in lotions to increase elegance and inhibit formation of a white soapy appearance upon rubbing the lotion onto the skin. Antifoaming agents are used in the concentration range 0.2–3% w/w of the total weight of lotions. Some examples include silicone fluid, dimethicone, and simethicone.

Typical antioxidants in lotion formulations are butylated hydroxy toluene, butylated hydroxy anisole, sulfite salts, sodium ascorbate, and propyl gallate.

Optionally, chelating agents may be included in the continuous phase of lotion to inactivate metals during processing, and thereby increase the stability of formulation. Suitable chelating agents include dipotassium ethylene diamine tetraacetate (EDTA), diethylenetriamine (DETA), and aminoethylethanolamine (AEEA). Chelating agents are used in the concentration range 0.25–1% w/w. Perfume agents may sometimes be included in lotions to impart a soothing olfactory sensation. Common perfume agents are cocoa butter and floral oil fragrances, such as rose oil, lilac, jasmine, wisteria, and apple blossom. Coloring agents improve the aesthetic appearance of lotions. Colorants suitable for lotions may be derived from water-soluble synthetic organic food additives (FD&C colors), water-insoluble lake dyes (e.g., aluminum salts of water-soluble dyes), and natural pigments (e.g., beta-carotene). Approximately 0.0075–1% w/w of colorant is included in lotions. Common buffer salts are gluconate, lactate, acetate, oleate, citrate, phosphate, and/or carbonate salts, as well as triethanolamine or 2-amino-2-methyl-1-propanol. The liquid media used as the continuous phase in lotions are water, lower alcohols (e.g., ethanol, isopropyl alcohol), glycols (e.g., ethylene glycol and propylene glycol), glycerin, and mixtures thereof. Liquid medium ranges from about 50% to 95% w/w of the total weight of lotions.

9.4. GENERAL ASPECTS OF LIQUID DOSAGE FORMS

In general, ease-of-swallowing, palatability, and convenience of administration constitute the advantages of liquid dosage forms. However, liquid dosage forms may deteriorate and lose potency more quickly than solid and semisolid dosage forms if not designed and tested during product development studies. A testing protocol must consider not only physical and chemical but also biological properties of the dosage form. Table 9.7 summarizes general aspects, including physicochemical stability, antimicrobial stability, taste masking, and bioavailability considerations, that may be required to meet some of the target product quality features of liquid dosage forms.

9.4.1 Physicochemical Stability

The stability of a drug substance may be the major criterion in determining the suitability of dosage forms. Drug substances undergo chemical and physical degradation, leading to loss of potency, production of toxic degradation products, and decrease in bioavailability. These degradation reactions may result in substantial changes in the physical appearance of dosage forms (e.g., discoloration or precipitation). Different degradation pathways could be triggered by incompatibility between ingredients of the dosage form, incompatibility with primary packaging material (container and closure), vehicles, and storage conditions (temperature, humidity, light, and headspace).

Common chemical degradation reactions manifested in dosage forms include solvolysis, oxidation, photolysis, dehydration, and racemization. Drug substances with functional groups, such as esters (e.g., aspirin), lactones (e.g., spironolactone), amides (e.g., chloramphenicol acetate), lactams (e.g., penicillins), oximes, imides, and nitrogen mustards, are prone to hydrolysis. Oxidation is one of the most prominent degradation pathways for many drug substances. Mechanisms of oxidation reactions are complex and involve multiple pathways for initiation, propagation, branching, and termination steps. Many oxidation reactions are initiated by trace amounts of impurities, such as metal ions or free radicals. Oxidation reactions are manifested as changes in the appearance of the dosage form. Drug substances with functional groups, such as phenols, catechols, ethers, thiols, and carboxylic acids, are prone to oxidation. Photolytic reactions may be mediated by normal sunlight, which causes an increase in the energy of absorbed molecules sufficient to achieve activation. Photolysis is often associated with oxidation and is a common reaction in steroids. Racemic mixtures of drug substances would result in different absorption, distribution, metabolism, and elimination profiles. These racemization reactions can be catalyzed by either acid or base.

Physical degradation reactions of drug substances in solutions include polymorph generation, vaporization of actives or vehicles, and adsorption to containers. Due to differences in physicochemical characteristics, polymorphs exhibit different bioavailability profiles. Volatile actives and inactives (e.g., flavors) with high vapor pressures at room temperature permeate through the container and result in the loss of desirable characteristics of drug products. Similar to solutions, drug molecules in disperse systems exhibit similar physical degradation processes. For more details on degradation of drug substances in disperse systems, readers are suggested to refer literature [67]. Suspensions manifest agglomeration of particles, sedimentation, and caking phenomena, while emulsions exhibit flocculation, creaming, and coalescence.

During drug product development studies, experimental designs include thorough study of factors affecting the stability of drugs. These study conditions include pH, humidity, temperature, container, and compatibility studies with potential inactive

TABLE 9.7 Summary of General Considerations for Oral Liquid Dosage Forms

Dosage Form	Taste-masking Approaches	Stability Considerations	Antimicrobial Stability	Factors Affecting Bioavailability
Solutions	1. Sweeteners and flavors are added.	1. Oxidation: Antioxidants and packing under inert gas or vacuum	Preservatives added to control bioburden	1. Solubility and permeability of drugs
	2. In general, flavors that match colors are added	2. Hydrolysis: Buffers		2. Inclusion of permeability affecting excipients
		3. Photolysis: Amber-colored primary packages		
Mouthwashes, gargles, and elixirs	1. Sweeteners and flavor adjuncts added to mask the unpleasant tastes.	1. Vaporization of volatile ingredients: Store in cool place and tight packaging containers	1. Alcohol components of the formulation are self-preservative	na[c]
	2. Flavor adjuncts augment taste-masking properties of conventional flavors.	2. Chemical degradations (oxidation, hydrolysis and photolysis): As listed under solutions	2. Additional preservatives may be added	
Syrups	1.Syrup vehicle acts as sweetener.	1. Inversion of sugars: Thermal control and processing under nonthermal mixing conditions	1.High concentration of solids impede growth of microbes	1. Solubility and permeability of drugs
	2. Artificial sweetener may be added to nonsugar vehicles.	2. Crystallization of ingredients: Store in controlled thermal conditions	2. Preservatives may also be included	2. Palatability
				3. Viscosity
Suspensions[a]	1. Sweeteners are added to mask the taste of actives and high-concentration inactive solids.	1. Flocculation	Preservatives added to	1. Particle size
			1. Protect stabilizers, suspending agents, and thickening agents	
	2. Flavors are added to reduce the cloying taste of inorganic solids.	2. Sedimentation	2. Control bioburden	2. Particle-size distribution
		3. Caking		3. Particle shape
				4. Viscosity
Emulsions[b]	1. Nonreducing sugars (sucrose, trehalose) are added as sweeteners.	1. Flocculation	Preservatives added to	1. Droplet size
			1. Protect oil phase, stabilizers/emulsifiers, and thickening agents	
			2. Control bioburden	
	2. Lecithins and fruit flavors are added.	2. Creaming		2. Oil phase content
		3. Coalescence		3. Emulsification
		4. Cracking		4. Viscosity

[a]*Similar particle-size distribution, good wetting properties of solids, minimal density difference between the suspended drug particles and vehicle, and viscosity form a stable suspension formulation;*
[b]*Similar droplet-size distribution, low oil phase content, good emulsification with GI fluids, viscous, and wide range of pH stability impart stability to emulsions;*
na[c]—not applicable (localized actions)

ingredients (buffers, surfactants, complexing agents, antioxidants) to be included in formulations. ICH guidelines (Q1A(R)) provide guidance for conducting the stability testing of a drug substance or drug product under a variety of environmental factors, such as temperature, humidity, and light, and establish a retest period for the drug substance or a shelf-life period for the drug products.

9.4.2 Antimicrobial Stability

The presence of microorganisms in nonsterile preparations may have the potential to reduce or even inactivate the therapeutic activity of drug products. Therefore, manufacturers need to ensure a low bioburden of finished dosage forms by implementing cGMP during the manufacture, storage, and distribution of pharmaceutical preparations. Antimicrobial preservatives are added to nonsterile dosage forms to protect drug products from microbiological growth or microorganisms that may be introduced during or subsequent to the manufacturing process. In the case of sterile products packaged in multidose containers, antimicrobial agents are added to inhibit the growth of microorganisms that may be introduced during repeated withdrawal of doses.

The efficacy of antimicrobial agents varies with the physicochemical characteristics of the preservative, concentration, spectrum of activity against microbes, and temperature. Antimicrobial agents are toxic substances, and the concentration of preservative shown to be effective in the final packaged product should be below a level that may be toxic to human beings. Antimicrobial preservative efficacy must be demonstrated in products packaged in multidose containers. In all cases, antimicrobial agents must not be used as a substitute for good manufacturing practice of sterile products. USP <51> enumerates criteria and methods for determination of antimicrobial preservative effectiveness.

9.4.3 Bioavailability Considerations

The definition of bioavailability focuses on processes by which active ingredients or moieties are released from an oral dosage form and move to the site of action. From a pharmacokinetics perspective, bioavailability data provide an estimate of the relative fraction of an administered dose (e.g., oral solution or suspension) that is absorbed into systemic circulation when compared to bioavailability data for an intravenous dosage form. In addition, bioavailability studies provide information related to absorption, distribution, and elimination. Bioavailability data can also provide information indirectly about the properties of a drug substance before entry into the systemic circulation, such as permeability, influence of presystemic enzymes, and transporters (e.g., p-glycoprotein).

The absorption of drugs from liquid dosage forms is governed by various physicochemical properties (pH, solubility, permeability, stability, and absorption potential) of drug substances. Drug movement from an oral dosage form into blood circulation is a multistep process (i.e., GI membranes and absorption into blood circulation). The slowest of these steps, termed as the rate-limiting step, will determine the rate and extent of drug absorption. Among oral dosage forms, the solution form should have the maximum bioavailability, but the drug substance may precipitate from solution owing to changes in the pH of GI fluids.

For drugs in suspension, the rate-limiting step could be disintegration of aggregates, if any; dissolution of fine particles into drug solution; and then absorption across GI membranes. Factors influencing the aggregation phenomenon of suspensions could be particle size, particle surface area, particle-size distribution, wetting properties of solid particles, density difference between suspended particles and suspension medium, and viscosity of the suspending medium. The aggregation phenomenon could be a rate-limiting step for disintegration, which in turn could become a rate-limiting step for dissolution of drug substance.

In comparison to solutions and suspensions, oral administration of emulsions is not popular due to the unpalatability of the oil phase and unpredictable drug release profiles. Emulsions also pose challenges to drug release due to a complex solubility and partitioning phenomena. In oil-in-water emulsions, the drug may partition from the internal oil phase to its own continuous aqueous phase or emulsify directly with GI fluids. This equilibrium is dependent on oil phase composition and partitioning equilibrium between the oil and aqueous phases, emulsification with GI fluids, and external emulsifier concentration. Emulsification with GI fluids may increase drug absorption across GI membranes.

Bioavailability of oral liquid dosage forms can be obtained by developing a systemic exposure profile. A profile can be obtained by measuring the concentration of drug substances and its active metabolites over time in samples collected from systemic circulation. Systemic exposure patterns reflect the release of drug substance from the dosage form and a series of possible presystemic/systemic actions on the drug substance after its release from the dosage form. The systemic exposure profiles of clinical trial batches can be used as a benchmark for subsequent formulation changes and can be useful as a reference for future bioequivalence studies.

9.4.4 Taste Masking

Taste is one of the most important parameters governing patient compliance. Oral administration of bitter drugs with an acceptable degree of palatability is a key issue for healthcare providers, especially for pediatric patients. Several oral liquid dosage forms and bulking agents have unpleasant and bitter-tasting components. In particular, oral liquid dosage forms have the drug in solubilized form, which may further enhance the unpleasant taste of drug substances. Improved palatability in these products has prompted the development of numerous palatable formulations. Inactive excipients available for taste making include aromatic flavors, sweeteners, amino acids, ion-exchange resins, gelatin, gelatinized starch, lecithin, surfactants, salts, and polymers. Taste masking is achieved using techniques such as polymer coating, conventional granulation, spray congealing, cyclodextrin complexation, freeze-drying process, and emulsification (e.g., multiple emulsions).

Taste masking with flavors, sweeteners, and amino acids is the simplest approach, especially in the case of pediatric liquid formulations. The flavor adjuncts may augment taste-masking properties of conventional flavors. For example, the unpleasant taste of mouthwashes containing medicinal and bitter-tasting substances, such as eucalyptus oil, can be masked by adding flavor adjuncts (e.g., fenchone, borneol, or isoborneol), which suppress unpleasant organoleptic sensations of volatile oils. Clove oil has been found to mask the bitter taste of a number of drugs, particularly analgesics, expectorants, antitussives, and decongestants.

For suspensions, taste-masking agents are added to mask the bitterness of the solubilized fraction of drug substances and other unpleasant sensations of inactive ingredients. Several of the sweeteners used in oral suspensions are ionic and have the potential to interact with other components of suspensions. Some of the sweeteners in suspensions include acesulfame, aspartame, sodium cyclamate, dextrose, fructose, galactose, sorbitol, xylitol, sucrose, and trehalose. Oral suspensions produce a cloying sensation in the mouth due to high levels of inorganic excipients. Flavors reduce the cloying taste and improve palatability of oral suspensions. One problem with flavors in oral suspensions is adsorption onto finely divided suspending agents, thus reducing their effectiveness. Flavor preferences vary with age, but citrus flavors are acceptable to most age groups.

Coating with hydrophilic polymers is one of the common methods to achieve taste masking. Polymeric coating acts as a physical barrier to drug particles, thereby minimizing interaction between the drug substance and taste buds. A specialized technique (i.e., micro-emulsification) has been used for taste masking of powders and liquid suspensions. Ion-exchange resins (IERs) are another class of polymers (high molecular-weight polymers with cationic and anionic functional groups) used in liquid suspensions. The most widely used resin in liquid dosage forms is a copolymer of styrene and divinylbezene. Quinolones and their derivatives are formulated using ion exchange resins, such as methacrylic acid polymer crosslinked with divinylbenzene as a carrier. The formation of quinolone-resin complex (resinate) eliminates the extreme bitterness of quinolones to make liquid orals palatable.

9.4.5 Over-the-Counter Agents

Drugs that do not require a physician's prescription and are bought off the shelf in stores are termed as over-the-counter (OTC) medications. All OTC medications are regulated by the FDA through OTC monographs. Products conforming to the monographs may be marketed without further FDA clearance, while those that do not conform must undergo review and approval through the new drug approval system. Due to convenience and cost-effectiveness, and to avoid physician's appointments, many patients prefer OTC medications. As OTC treatment options can be overwhelming, it is important that physicians, manufacturers, and regulatory agencies provide appropriate information about treatment regimens and potential drug interactions, which enable patients to select the correct medication and its dose. Some of the important considerations for OTC medication for consumers include

- Always follow the printed directions and warnings. It is important to talk to your physician before starting a new OTC drug. Administration procedures should be strictly followed. For example, nasal sprays should be administered through the nasal route.
- Check the expiration date before administration.
- Women should consult their physicians before taking OTC medication while pregnant or breastfeeding. Any medicine may have a different effect in children. People who are in these age groups should take special care when taking OTC products.

OTC medications comprise solids, semisolids, and liquid dosage forms. Liquid dosage forms administered for otic, ophthalmic, dental, cough and allergic rhinitis, diarrhea, and heartburn purposes include solutions, syrups, elixirs, enemas, douches, sprays, lotions, and suspensions. As per FDA guidance, orally administered liquid products should be provided with appropriate devices that are marked with calibrated units of liquid measurements. These markings should be clearly visible when the liquid product is added to the device to avoid dosing errors. Table 9.8 lists some of the examples of OTC medications administered for different medical conditions.

9.5. MANUFACTURING PROCESSES AND CONDITIONS

As per good manufacturing practice (GMP) requirements, manufacturing of solutions includes procurement of raw materials, compounding, filling, and packing [68]. Each stage of the process is critical to ensure the safety and stability of dosage forms. In general, raw materials, semifinished drug products (bulk solutions), and finished drug products are handled in

TABLE 9.8 List of Over the Counter (OTC) Medications [4]

Therapeutic Class	Medical Use	Dosage Form	Marketed Products
OTIC AGENTS			
Earwax-softening agents	Removes excess cerumen	Solution	Carbamide peroxide, 6.5% (Murine®, Debrox®), hydrogen peroxide, olive oil, mineral oil, and docusate sodium
Water-clog removal solutions	Avoids otitis owing to tissue maceration	Solution	95% isopropyl alcohol and 5% anhydrous glycerin
DENTAL AGENTS			
Dental irrigation	Cleans gum and dental infection areas	Solution	Interplak Water Jet, Hydro-Pik, and Waterpik
Mouthwash	Debris removal	Solution	Biotene, Sensodyne, Rembrandt Natural
	Anti-plaque removal	Solution	Cepacol, Scope, Oral-B rinse, Crest Pro-Health rinse, Colgate PerioGard, Fluorigard
	Gingivitis treatments	Solution	Listerine®, 1.5% peroxide solution
Artificial saliva	Relieves xerostomia (dry mouth)	Solution	Moi-Stir and Xero-Lube
Wound-cleansing agents	Cleans oral wounds	Solution	Carbamide peroxide, 10%–15%; hydrogen peroxide, 3%
Cosmetic whitener	Teeth whitener	Solution	Carbamide peroxide, 10% (Gly-Oxide®)
OPHTHALMIC AGENTS			
Artificial tears	Relieves dry eye	Solution	Advanced Eye Relief™, Bion tears®, Murine® tears, Viva-Drops®
Antihistamines	Relieves itching from allergic conjunctivitis	Solution	Zaditor®
Vasoconstrictor and antihistamines	Allergic conjunctivitis	Solution	Naphcon A, Opcon A, Visine-A
Contact lens solution	Maintains moisture for contact between contact lenses and eyes	Solution	Opti-Free®, Opti-Free Express®
DERMATOLOGICAL AGENTS			
Retinoids	Acne	Solution	Differin®, Retin-A®
Antibiotics	Acne	Solution	Clindamycin, Erythromycin
Others	Acne	Lotion	Sulfacetamide (Klaron®)
Antihistamines	Relieves itching from contact dermatitis	Spray solution	Benadryl®
Inorganic salts	Relieves itching	Solution	Domeboro®
Corticosteroids	Relieves eczema	Lotion	Cortizone
ANALGESICS, ANTIPYRETICS, AND DECONGESTANTS			
Oxymetazoline	Relieves nasal discomfort caused by cold, allergies, and hay fever	Spray solution	Afrin®
Naphazoline HCl	Nasal decongestion	Spray solution	Privine®
Xylometazoline	Nasal decongestion	Spray solution	Otrivin®
Phenylephrine	Nasal decongestion	Spray solution	Neo-Synephrine®
Local anesthetics	Oral decongestant (relieves sore throat)	Spray solution	Chloraseptic®, Cepacol®

(Continued)

TABLE 9.8 (*Continued*)

Therapeutic Class	Medical Use	Dosage Form	Marketed Products
GASTROINTESTINAL AGENTS			
Saline laxative	Relieves constipation	Solution	Fleet Phospho-Soda
Osmotic laxative (glycerin, lactulose)	Relieves constipation	Solution, Syrup	Fleet Babylax, Chronulac®
Emollient laxative (docusate salts)	Relieves constipation	Syrup, Suspension	Colace®, Kaopectate®
Anti-diarrheal agents	Relieves upset stomach	Suspension	Pepto-Bismol®
OTHERS			
Astringents	Lessens mucous secretions and protects underlying tissue	Solution	Witch hazel
Antacids	Relieves heartburn, acid indigestion	Suspension	Mylanta®

batches. Batch management of production simplifies the process and makes it easier to control the status of transformation between starting materials and final products. For scale-up, it is necessary to divide the process into stages, batches, and unit operations. These units operations are coordinated together in the manufacturing of final dosage forms.

9.5.1 Solutions

Flow properties of liquids rarely vary due to their constant density at a constant temperature. Solutions are formulated on a weight basis (gravimetric) in order to measure the final volume by weight before filling and packaging [69]. The importance of selecting the gravimetric method instead of the volumetric method to measure liquids is illustrated by volume contraction of water-ethanol liquid mixtures. The National Formulary diluted alcohol is a typical example of volume contraction of liquid mixtures [70]. This solution is prepared by mixing equal volumes of alcohol and purified water (USP). The final volume of this solution is about 3% less than the sum of the individual volumes because of contraction during mixing.

Temperature control during compounding is important because heat supports mixing and filling operations. Uncontrolled thermal operations may cause chemical and physical instabilities, such as potency loss of drugs in solutions, oxidation of components, and activation of microbiological growth after degradation of preservatives. Oxidation-prone materials are protected from oxygen by methods such as nitrogen purging through solution stored in sealed tanks or overlaying headspace of tanks with nitrogen atmosphere.

The low-solubility drugs or preservatives in the "dead leg" at the bottom of the tank result in a loss of potency [69]. When there is inadequate solubility of a drug in the chosen vehicle, the dose will not contain the correct amount of the drug substance. Therefore, processing parameters should be optimized to obtain a uniform and accurate dosage form. Whenever possible, ingredients should be added together, and an impeller mixer often should be located near the bottom of the vessel for an efficient mixing process. The mixing of high-viscosity materials requires higher velocity gradients in the mixing zone than in regular mixing operations. During the filling and sampling process, constant mixing of bulk solution to ensure solution homogeneity is indispensable to ensure an acceptable quality level for finished products.

The preparation of sterile products requires a number of manufacturing processes and classified environments intended to control bioburden and reduce particle levels. All these activities are conducted in controlled environments and are subject to qualification. Materials and components must be transferred from a warehouse environment into a classified area. Material containers are disinfected and passed through air locks into different zones of operation within the aseptic area. Raw materials may be weighed in ISO 7 areas, while sterile ingredients are opened only in aseptic environments. The majority of parenteral formulations are solutions, which require tanks, stirrers, filtration-related equipment and accessories, transfer tubings, washing accessories for containers, and closures. Process equipment and accessories are subjected to washing/rinsing to remove particles and reduce bioburden and endotoxin levels. Following cleaning, items for sterilization are dried, wrapped, and staged for steam sterilization. Washed containers are placed in trays or boxes for depyrogenation in ovens or tunnels. It is a common practice to protect all washed items with ISO 5 air, from completion of washing through wrapping and placing into a sterilizer.

The scale of manufacturing varies from in excess of 5000 L (LVPs) down to less than 50 mL (e.g. for radiopharmaceuticals). The majority of the equipment is composed of 300-grade stainless steel lined with tantalum or glass. The vessels can be equipped with external jackets for controlling thermal operations. Compounded formulations are subjected to sterilization procedures depending on the stability requirements of formulation ingredients. The USP recognizes six methods of sterilization: (a) steam sterilization, (b) dry heat sterilization, (c) gas sterilization, (d) sterilization by ionizing radiation, (e) sterilization by filtration, and (f) aseptic processing. In general, sterile product holding and filling operations are conducted in ISO 5 areas. The holding vessels are often steam sterilized along with product transfer tubings prior to use. A number of times, filling is performed from the compounding vessel using in-line filtration, eliminating the intermediate vessel. When this approach is used, a small moist heat sterilized surge tank or reservoir tank may be required for pressure-assisted filling. An inert gas (nitrogen/argon) is overlaid into the headspace of the container or purged into an empty container to protect oxygen-sensitive formulations.

9.5.2 Suspensions

Pharmaceutical suspensions have a characteristic particle-size distribution, which is dependent on mean particle size, particle size distribution, drug crystal habit, dissolution characteristics, and temperature. Particle size reduction can be accomplished by using a ball mill, jet mill, or hammer mill. Ball milling is used at the preformulation stage to reduce the particle size of small amounts of a drug substance through a combined process of impact and attrition. Ball-milled micronized particles are typically less than 10 μM in diameter. The efficiency of the milling process is affected by the rotation speed, number of balls, mill size, wet or dry milling, amount of powder, and milling time. On a large scale, the hammer mill is preferable. Powder is bled into the mill house via the hopper, and rotating hammers impact the powder. The minimum particle size range is about 50 μM. Heavy-duty hammer mills may give 20 μM-size particles. For particles less than 10 μM, micronizers are preferred [12].

For injectable nanosuspensions, particles in the size range of 0.1–5 μM are required to avoid thrombophlebitis. A popular approach to produce nanosuspensions is a combination of micronization and high-pressure homogenization [71]. The drug powder can be micronized using a jet mill or colloid mill, and dispersed in a surfactant-added buffer solution. The micronized drug suspension (<25 μM) is passed through a homogenizer. High-pressure homogenizers are available with different capacities ranging from 40 mL (lab scale) to a few thousand liters (large-scale production). During the homogenization process, the drug suspension is subjected to cavitation and high-shear forces in the homogenization gap to achieve nano-size. Both homogenizer pressure and number of homogenization cycles play a critical role in the reduction of the particle size of hard drug substances. A high-pressure homogenizer can handle pressures ranging from 1,000 to 20,000 pounds per square inch (psi). Typically, multiple cycles are required to achieve the desired particle size. If nanosuspensions are intended for oral administration, two homogenization cycles often are necessary to obtain a product of sufficient quality for oral administration. If nanosuspensions are intended for the parenteral route, 5–10 homogenization cycles are anticipated to obtain a fine particle size.

Sterile suspensions need to be sterile, which can be accomplished by approaches such as termination sterilization (autoclaving, sterile filtration, and gamma irradiation) of finished products or aseptic processing [12,72]. In a number of cases, termination sterilization procedures are not possible due to drug chemical instability, surfactant aggregation (e.g., autoclaving), and physical incompatibility (e.g., sterile filtration) of the suspension. Along with sterilization validation concerns, gamma irradiation may generate impurities. Therefore, the aseptic processing of suspensions is of high importance. In some cases, a combination of one of the terminal sterilization procedures and aseptic processing is employed to produce a sterile suspension. For example, preparation of brinzolamide (Azopt®) suspension involves autoclaving and aseptic processing. A milling slurry comprising brinzolamide (active ingredient), milling beads, and surfactant is autoclaved, followed by bill milling in aseptic conditions to obtain the desired particle size range. Filling, capping, and sealing operations are carried out in ISO 5 rooms to obtain a sterile suspension.

9.5.3 Emulsions

Emulsions may be prepared by using different methods, depending on the nature of the emulsion components and instrumentation available for use. On a small scale, as in the laboratory or pharmacy, emulsions may be prepared using equipment such as a porcelain mortar and pestle, mechanical blenders, and homogenizers. In small-scale extemporaneous preparation of emulsions, four methods may be used: the (a) continental, or dry gum, method; (b) English, or wet gum, method; (c) *in situ* soap method; and (d) mechanical method. The dry gum method is also referred to as the "4:2:1" method because for every 4 parts (volumes) of oil, 2 parts of water and 1 part of gum are added in preparing the primary emulsion. About 1 minute of trituration is required to produce a creamy white primary emulsion, during which the oil phase is converted into oil droplets, producing a cracking sound. In the wet gum method, the proportions of oil, water, and emulsifier are the same (4:2:1), but the order and techniques of mixing are different. Emulsifier (1 part) is triturated with 2 parts water to form a viscous mass; then 4 parts of oil are added slowly in portions while triturating. After all the oil is added, the mixture is triturated for several minutes to form the primary emulsion.

On a large scale, injectable and ophthalmic emulsions are manufactured using the mechanical method. Water- and oil-soluble ingredients are dissolved in the aqueous and oil phases, respectively. With the aid of co-solvents, water-insoluble drugs can be incorporated into the oil phase of emulsions prior to emulsification (*de novo* method) or added to prepared emulsions (extemporaneous addition). For drugs that are highly oil-soluble, the *de novo* method is popular. Alternatively, oil-soluble drugs that are liquid at room temperature, such as halothane and propofol, can be extemporaneously added to preformed emulsions in which the drug substance preferentially partitions into the oil phase. Another approach involves dissolving drugs and phospholipids in organic solvents, followed by evaporation of the organic phase under vacuum. Emulsifiers, such as lecithins, can be dispersed in the oil or aqueous phase. It is preferred to solubilize in the aqueous phase due to ease of dispersion, while heating may be required for dispersing in the oil phase. The oil phase is added to the aqueous phase under controlled temperature and agitation (using high-shear mixers) to form a homogeneous coarse emulsion with a droplet size in the range of 20–30 μM. The coarse emulsion is then homogenized using a high-shear homogenizer or microfluidizer at optimized pressure, temperature, and cycles to reduce droplet size. The pH of the fine emulsion can be adjusted to a designated value and filtered through 1–5 μM filters. Sterilization of emulsions can be achieved by terminal heat sterilization (e.g., steam sterilization) or aseptic filtration. For heat-labile emulsions, sterile filtration can be used. However, sterile filtration requires droplet (>95% of droplet population) diameters less than 0.2 μM. Alternatively, aseptic processing may be adopted for heat-labile emulsions whose droplet diameters are greater than 0.2 μM.

Ophthalmic emulsions are produced on a large scale in aseptic conditions. Due to the heat-labile and viscous nature of ophthalmic emulsions, heat sterilization and sterile filtration methods may not be employed to obtain a sterile formulation. Drugs incorporating the oil phase and aqueous phase (containing emulsifier and tonicity-adjusting agents) are subjected to aseptic homogenization (with or without heating aid) to produce a fine emulsion. The fine emulsion is then subjected to pH adjustment using sodium hydroxide. The final emulsion can be clarified before filling. Ophthalmic emulsions whose mean droplet diameters are less than 0.2 μM and whose viscosity is close to water (~1 cP) can be subjected to sterile filtration.

Lotions are manufactured using homogenizers. The oil phase, consisting of preservatives, emulsifiers, auxiliary emulsifiers, antioxidants, emollients, antifoaming agents, and fatty acid-derived thickeners, is maintained at a temperature of 65°C–70°C. Similarly, water-soluble ingredients, such as preservatives, buffers, antioxidants, and thickeners, are dissolved in the aqueous phase and maintained at a temperature of 65°C–70°C. The oil phase is added to the aqueous phase slowly and homogenized until the desired droplet-size distribution and consistency are obtained. Drug suspension is added during homogenization. The product is cooled under slow stirring, and water is adjusted as necessary.

9.6. PACKAGING

Pharmaceutical packaging is a combination of components necessary to contain, preserve, protect, and deliver safe and efficacious drug products. From the contemporary definition, primary packaging is composed of packaging components and subcomponents that come into contact with product or those that may have a direct effect on product shelf-life. Typical packaging components are containers (e.g., ampoules, vials, bottles), closures (e.g., screw caps, stoppers), closure liners, stopper overseas, container inner seals, administration ports (e.g., on large-volume parenterals), overwraps, and administration accessories. The outer packaging components are referred to as secondary and tertiary packaging, and include items such as outer labels, wrappers, cartons, corrugated shipments, and pallets. cGMP regulations titled "Drug Product Containers and Closures" provide the statements most relevant to packaging [73].

Each component must have adequate prior testing to ensure appropriateness of the chosen packaging system. Subsequently, shelf-life tests (to ensure expiration date) and specifications (to ensure quality of components) are required for packaging systems in which the product will be marketed. The package evaluation is performed for characterization of the package material, and is performed together with the drug product system. Characterization procedures include physicochemical and biological procedures to evaluate glass and plastic bottles, metal closures, elastomeric closures, and syringe components. For example, USP tests (<661> for containers; <381> for elastomeric closures for injections; <87> for biological reactivity *in vitro*, and <88> for biological reactivity *in vivo*) are generally required for containers and closures to address protection. Testing for properties other than those described in USP (e.g., gas transmission) may also be necessary. For drug products, such as injection, inhalation, and ophthalmics, a comprehensive study is appropriate. This involves leachable and extractable studies on packaging components to determine the migration of chemical species into the dosage form from container and closure, and toxicological evaluation of substances extracted to determine the safety level of exposure.

The evaluation studies include the effect of packaging components on finished products during accelerated, intermediate, and long-term stability studies. Stability study protocols also include photo-stability studies. Light can act as a catalyst to oxidation reactions, transferring its energy (photons) to drug molecules, making the latter more reactive. Most photo-degradation reactions occur in UV (190–280 nm) and visible (320–380 nm) light ranges. As a precaution against the acceleration of oxidation, sensitive drug formulations are packaged in light-resistant containers (e.g., amber glass, aluminum foil wraps).

It is a common practice to store liquid dosage forms inverted and upright to assess the effect of long-term contact with the closure. Such studies provide detailed information on absorption or adsorption of the drug substance or degradation of the drug substance induced by a chemical entity leached from a packaging material, reduction in the concentration of excipients, precipitation, pH changes, discoloration of dosage form or packaging components, or increase in the brittleness/softening of packaging components. Package evaluation studies result in setting up specifications for each of the packaging components. The specifications serve as a guideline for the qualification of containers and closures.

9.6.1 Oral Liquids

The primary packaging components for oral liquids (solutions, syrups, elixirs, emulsions, and suspensions) include pouches, cups, and bottles. Bottles are usually made of glass or plastic, often with a screw cap and liner, and possibly with a tamper-resistant seal. Glass offers the following advantages: they (a) are inert to most medicine, (b) are impervious to air and moisture, (c) can be amber-colored to protect light-sensitive medicine contents, and (d) provide ease of inspection of the contents. Disadvantages include the following: they (a) are fragile, (b) release alkali into container contents, and (c) are heavy, resulting in increased transportation costs. Plastics made of resin have been used as primary and secondary packaging materials. Bottles made of low-density polyethylene (LDPE), high-density polyethylene (HDPE), PVC, or polypropylene (PP) are used as primary packaging materials. Plastic bottles are available as plain or amber-colored bottles to protect photosensitive contents. Advantages of plastic packaging include these: they (a) release few particles into the container, (b) are flexible and lightweight for transportation, and (c) can be heat sealed and molded into various shapes.

Along with the container, it is essential to assess the interactions of closures with formulation components. Loss of moisture (leakage or permeation losses) is another important factor to be considered when a closure is applied to a container. Closures are made of aluminum, polypropylene, or high-density polyethylene. For the pediatric population, several designs of child-resistant containers are used for pharmaceutical packaging under the assumption that children are unable to coordinate opening of containers. These designs include cap-bottle alignment systems, push-down-and-turn caps, and squeeze-and-turn caps. The closures in common use with dispensed medicines are the Snap-safe® alignment and Clic-loc® closures. Various tamper-evident closure designs are also available for avoiding unlawful access of containers. These closures cannot be opened until the tamper-evident band connecting the cap to the skirt of the container is torn away.

9.6.2 Injectables and Ophthalmics

The packaging of parenteral and ophthalmic dosage forms presents a major challenge because package, product, and package-product interactions must all be characterized in greater detail than nonsterile liquid dosage forms. For each major type of parenteral product, the investigator should consider the effect of the drug manufacturing process on the integrity of packaging materials. For example, if the product is subjected to terminal sterilization, the effect of the sterilization method must be evaluated. Various packaging materials are available for parenteral containers;

thus, the range of potential interactions has multiplied, requiring advanced analytical methods for characterizing interactions.

For parenterals, glass containers made by blowing and tubing methods are common packaging materials. Blown containers have a seam line running from the top finish to the bottom of the sidewall. The tubing container has smooth seamless sidewalls and no bottom markings. Blown glass is used for making vials and bottles, while tubing glass is used for packaging forms such as ampoules, vials, and prefilled syringes. The glass used for pharmaceutical packaging has been primarily classified by USP/NF into four types based on the capacity of hydrolytic resistance to aqueous solutions: type I (highly resistant borosilicate glass), type II (treated soda-lime glass), type III (soda-lime glass), and type IV (general-purpose soda-lime glass). Because of the chemical differences in glass, it is important to take these compositional factors into account when choosing containers. Although glass is considered to be inert material, leaching and corrosion of glass surfaces in contact with water or buffered solutions are common phenomena. As a result, glass containers are surface-treated (e.g., ammonium sulfate) to avoid reactions with formulation compositions. These treatments enhance three things: the durability of glass during handling, resistance to chemical corrosion of filled products, and the lubricity of glass on production lines. Some of the treatments are temporary and removable before product filling. Advanced test methods are available to discriminate among glass types and find the best suitable glass for a particular application.

Injectable solutions, suspensions, and fine emulsions are packaged in type I glass containers. Siliconized glass containers may be used to prevent droplet-size growth (e.g., emulsions) or particle aggregation (e.g., suspensions). Lyophilized powders for reconstitution are packaged in type II glass containers. Low-density polyethylene (LDPE) and high-density polyethylene (HDPE) are also widely used as packaging material for small-volume and large-volume parenterals, such as plastic infusion bags (LDPE), vials (LDPE or HDPE), form-fill-seal containers (LDPE), plastic syringes (HDPE), and tubing for infusions (LDPE). Intralipid emulsions are supplied in PVC bags. However, it is advisable to observe for any oiling out on the surface of the emulsion bag and discoloration of the emulsion formulation. With the exception of ampoules, all glass and plastic parenteral containers require a closure made of rubber elastomeric material. Typically, the stopper formulation consists of ingredients such as elastomer, vulcanizer, plasticizer, filler, emulsifier, and coloring agents. Teflon-coated stoppers may be used to prevent oxygen permeation and softening on contact with the oil phase (e.g., emulsions). Stoppers used for lyophilization are designed to facilitate lyophilization (i.e., vacuum evaporation of solvents).

Ophthalmic drops (solutions and suspensions) are frequently packaged in multidose containers ranging from 4–60 mL. Ophthalmic drops are marketed in LDPE bottles with a dropper built into the neck (sometimes referred to as DROP-TAINER®). The main advantages of DROP-TAINER and similar designs are ease of use, decreased contamination potential, low weight, and low costs. The patient removes the cap, turns the bottle upside down, and then squeezes gently to form a single drop that falls into eye. The dispensing tip can deliver a single drop or a stream of fluid for irrigation. When the plastic bottle is squeezed, the solution or suspension is minimally exposed to airborne contaminants; thus, it will maintain very low to nonexistent microbial content as compared to glass bottles with a separate dropper assembly. The caps of primary packaging components are made of hard plastic materials, such as HDPE or polypropylene. The major disadvantage of plastic containers is permeation of formulation components through the container. Volatile ingredients, such as preservatives (e.g., chlorobutanol and phenylethyl alcohol), can migrate into plastic and permeate through the walls of the container. In such cases, a safe and reasonable excess of the permeable component may be added to balance the loss over shelf-life. Another means of overcoming permeation effects is to employ a secondary package, such as peel-apart blister or pouch composed of nonpermeable materials (e.g., aluminum foil or vinyl). The plastic bottles are also permeable to water and contribute to weight loss by water vapor transmission. The consequences of water vapor transmission must be taken into consideration during analysis of components.

A few ophthalmic solution products use glass containers due to stability (e.g., oxidation) and permeation concerns of plastic packaging components. Powders for reconstitution also use glass containers due to heat-transfer characteristics necessary during lyophilization. Ophthalmic glass containers are usually made with type I glass materials, and are sterilized by dry heat or steam. The dropper assembly is made of glass or plastic and is usually gas sterilized in a blister composed of a vinyl and Tyvek package. Large-volume intraocular solution (for irrigation) may be packaged in a glass or polyolefin (polyethylene and/or polypropylene) container. Some of the heat-labile and nonfilterable ophthalmic products use the blow-fill-seal process, whereas plastic containers are blow-molded, filled, and sealed in one continuous aseptic operation. The blow-fill-seal process is applied to packaging unit-dose ophthalmic products in the volume range of 0.3–1 mL or multidose products in the range of 5–15 mL.

9.6.3 Nasals, Otics, and Topicals

Otic solutions and suspensions are supplied in type II glass bottles with a dropper built into the neck. Droppers made of glass or plastic are used to pull out medication from the bottles. Nasal formulations are filled into bottles made of type II glass or plastic materials (e.g., HDPE), which are closed by attaching a spray pump, including a dip tube. The pump may be fixed by a screw closure, crimped on, or simply snapped onto the bottle. Safety clips are included in pump units to prevent accidental discharge of the spray. Due to convenience and cost-effectiveness, multidose dispensers are widely used for the administration of nasal formulations. Bottles made of hydrolytic glass types I and II are used for sterile nasal drops, while bottles made of plastic material are necessary because a bottle-squeeze is needed to dispense spray solutions. Topical liquids, including solutions, suspensions, and lotions, are packaged in type III glass containers or HDPE plastic bottles.

9.7. LABELING

All the finished dosage forms are labeled to serve the following functions: (a) identify contents of the container, (b) ensure patients have clear and concise information on how to use the medicine, and (c) satisfy legal requirements. The details that appear on the label of a finished dosage form include (a) name of the preparation, strength, and form; (b) quantity; (c) instructions for use; (d) precautions on handling and usage of the product; (e) warning or advisory labels; (f) batch number or lot number; (g) storage conditions; (h) manufacturing and expiration date; and (i) manufacturer or distributor. In the case of extemporaneously dispensed medicines, identification information of patients for whom the medicine is dispensed, name and address of the pharmacy, and expiry date indicating the shortened shelf-life should be included.

In general, solutions are stored in the temperature range of 2°C–25°C. Photosensitive medications are usually labeled with the instruction "protect from light or store in tight and light-resistant containers." Oral suspensions are labeled with the instruction "shake well before use," as some sedimentation is expected. Shaking the bottle will redisperse contents and ensure an accurate dose. In addition, suspensions are labeled with instructions such as "store in cool place" to slow down degradation reactions. The stability of suspensions is affected by extreme variations of temperature. Extemporaneously prepared and reconstituted suspensions will have a relatively short shelf-life (7–14 days). The manufacturer's packaging insert literature for reconstituted products will provide recommended storage conditions. Intralipid emulsions are labeled with the instruction "should not be stored above 25°C/77°F to avoid creaming and breaking phenomena." Ophthalmic emulsions are stored in the temperature range of 15°C–25°C. If frozen, refrigerated products need to be discarded.

9.8. QUALITY ASSURANCE AND QUALITY CONTROL

9.8.1 Quality Assurance

The terms *quality assurance* and *quality control* are sometimes used interchangeably, but quality assurance is a broader term that includes quality control, written operating procedures, personnel training, record keeping, facility design, and monitoring. The objective of quality assurance is to build quality into products, rather than relying on final product testing to identify defective products.

9.8.2 Quality Control

The capacity of drug products to remain within specifications to ensure their identity, strength, quality, and purity is referred to as stable drug products. The manufacturing and storage conditions pose challenges to the stability of drug products, resulting in the degradation of drug substances and excipients. Therefore, it is important to assess the quality of products. Quality control testing is performed in two stages to evaluate the actual performance of final products against product and process specifications. The two stages include (a) in-process quality control and (b) final product quality control.

9.8.2.1 In-process Quality Control

In-process quality control involves monitoring of critical variables during the manufacturing process to assess the quality of final products and give necessary instructions if any deviations are observed. The process manufacturing controls are established and documented by quality control and production personnel to ensure that a predictable amount of each cycle's output falls within the acceptable standard range. Common product characteristics that are evaluated in-process include the assay and degradation products' profile of drug substances, pH, and appearance. In-process controls during production of sterile preparations may also include monitoring of environmental conditions (especially with respect to particulate and microbial contamination) and pyrogens (e.g., limulus amebocyte lysate, or LAL, test).

9.8.2.2 Finished Products Testing

In addition to in-process testing parameters, finished products require additional tests, such as antimicrobial preservative efficacy and particulate matter. Testing specifications change with drug formulation, intended use, and device characteristics. For example, drop size and plume geometry (spray pattern) are critical for ophthalmic and nasal products, respectively. Both drop size and spray pattern determine the dose delivered to respective tissues/organs; any changes in these respective parameters will likely result in change of dose. The USP recommends sterility testing for all sterile products.

For suspensions and emulsions, parameters such as rheological properties, electrical properties, and particle-size distribution play a critical role. Suspensions are observed for color, air globules, and separation of phases. The color changes could result from oxidative degradation of active or inactive ingredients. Caution should be exercised for the presence of air bubbles during sampling of suspensions because these bubbles may lower assay of drug compounds and even produce erroneous particle-size distribution results. Photon correlation spectroscopy or dynamic laser diffraction particle-sizing measurements can be made to assess particle-size distribution of suspensions. Any deviation in particle-size distribution from specifications may lead to physical instability of suspensions. The quantitative procedures for particle-size distribution testing should be appropriately validated, in terms of sensitivity and ability to detect shifts that may occur in size distribution. In case of technologies that cannot be validated, qualitative and semiquantitative methods (e.g., microscopy) for particle-size distribution can be used.

Electrophoretic mobility or zeta potential measurements of suspensions indicate changes in adsorption or desorption of chemical species from the particle surface. During zeta potential measurements, electric field strength is applied to obtain the electrophoretic mobility parameter, which is converted to zeta potential in millivolts (mV) using the Helmholtz–Smoluchowski equation. As a rule of thumb, suspensions with a zeta potential on either side of $-30\,\text{mV}$ and $+30\,\text{mV}$ are physically stable. Suspensions with a zeta potential close to the isoelectric point undergo pronounced aggregation [74].

The stability of a suspension is dependent on the sedimentation rate of the dispersed phase, which is dependent on the viscosity of the dispersion medium. The viscosity measurements can be made with the Brooke field viscometer. Sedimentation volume is also a good measure of rate of settling of suspended particles in a dispersion medium. An increase in the sedimentation volume may indicate formation of particle aggregates. Syringeability and pourability of suspensions also characterize the flow properties of suspensions. In the case of flocculated suspensions, syringeability may become difficult due to large floccule size. Pourability is performed to determine whether the final preparation is pourable.

Release studies of suspensions can be performed using type II or IV USP dissolution apparatus to determine the release rates of a drug substance. Release rates are modeled to describe the behavior of suspensions. According to the Nernst–Brunner and Levich modification of the Noyes–Whitney dissolution model, the rate of dissolution of nanosuspensions is described as Eq. 9.9 [75–77]

$$dX/dt = (DA/h) * (Cs - C/V) \tag{9.9}$$

where dX/dt is rate of dissolution, D is the diffusion coefficient, A is the particle surface area, h is the diffusion distance, Cs is the saturation solubility of the drug substance, C is the concentration of the drug substance in surrounding liquid, and V is the volume of the dissolution medium. For a suspension consisting of monodisperse spherical particles, the rate of dissolution is given by the Hixon–Cromwell cube root equation (9.10) [77]:

$$\sqrt[3]{Mo} - \sqrt[3]{\text{M}} = kt \tag{9.10}$$

where Mo is the original mass of drug particles, M is the mass of drug particles at time t, and k is the dissolution rate constant.

Emulsions exhibit creaming, flocculation, and coalescence before phase separation becomes visible. The phase separation processes are dependent on electrical, rheological, and droplet-size distribution. The USP specifies light-scattering and light-obscuration methods for determining mean droplet diameter. On the other hand, for determination of the amount of fat globules comprising larger diameters of size $\geq 5\,\mu\text{M}$, use of the light-obscuration or light-extinction method is recommended.

Any variation in droplet-size distribution, degree of flocculation, or phase separation results in viscosity changes. Flocculation of emulsions will increase viscosity during storage, and is important for assessing stability and shelf-life. Since most emulsions are non-Newtonian, a cone-plate type viscometer can be used to determine viscosity changes. The surface charge and zeta potential of emulsified droplets can be a useful indicator of the stability of emulsions because electrostatic repulsion can contribute to avoidance of flocculation and coalescence. A number of factors, such as pH, ionic strength, type and concentration of emulsifiers, and presence of electrolytes, can affect the zeta potential of emulsions.

Characterizing *in vitro* drug release from emulsions is a challenging task because of the submicron size of droplets and difficulty in separating the disperse and continuous phases. A number of experimental techniques, such as the dialysis bag method, diffusion cell method, and centrifugal ultra-filtration technique, have been investigated to measure drug release from colloidal emulsions [79]. However, caution should be exercised because the surface area of emulsion droplets available for the diffusion of drug substance from submicron emulsion droplets is considerably larger than the surface area of the dialysis membrane available for diffusion of drug substance. Drug released from oil droplets accumulates and leads to high concentration inside the dialysis bag, rather than maintaining equilibrium between drug release from oil droplets and drug diffusion across the dialysis membrane.

For emulsions, water washability tests can be performed to distinguish oil-in-water and water-in-oil emulsions. Water-in-oil emulsions are immiscible with water; therefore, they are not washable with water. Also, water-in-oil emulsions are occlusive and greasy due to the external oil phase. Oil-in-water emulsions are washable with water, nonocclusive, and nongreasy due to an external water phase.

9.9. REGULATORY CONSIDERATIONS

The manufacture and sale of dosage forms is regulated by federal and state laws, as well as the USP. The USP provides specifications, test procedures, standards, and training programs. In addition to individual monographs, the USP and the FDA limit the dose administered to patient populations, use of excipients, and size of multidose containers. The chemistry, manufacturing, and controls (CMCs) guidance documents prepared by the FDA recommend inclusion of information regarding drug product components, manufacturing processes and associated controls, and labeling. The guidance only suggests approaches that are appropriate for submitting CMC-related regulatory information. Also, CMC recommendations may vary depending on specific drug products (e.g., sterility requirements for sterile drug products).

A new drug application or abbreviated new drug application should include a statement of the quantitative composition of the unit formula of the drug product and the names and amounts of active and inactive ingredients. The amounts are expressed in concentration (i.e., amount per unit volume or weight), as well as amount per container. Similarly, a production batch formula representative of the one to be employed in the manufacture of the drug product is included. Any intended change in the formulation of the commercial product from that used in the submitted batches (e.g., critical clinical, biobatch, primary stability, production) is indicated in the CMC documentation.

9.9.1 Drug Substance

Comprehensive characterization of physical and chemical properties of the drug substance must be included in the CMC documentation. Appropriate acceptance criteria and routine control tests (i.e., release, stability, and retests) are adopted for evaluating key physicochemical properties of the drug substance. Any impurity found in the drug substance at a concentration of 0.10% or 1.0 milligram (mg) per day intake (whichever is lower) relative to the drug substance should be identified. Justification of acceptance criteria for drug substance impurities should be based on toxicological considerations. For suspension formulations, drug substance specifications include controls for particle-size distribution, surface area, and drug crystal morphology.

9.9.2 Excipients

Depending on the route of administration and sensitive nature of various patient populations, a thorough characterization of excipients used in drug products is considered to ensure safety and effectiveness. Critical excipients are those that can affect the quality, stability, and performance of drug products. The source of excipients is assessed and materials supplied should meet appropriate acceptance criteria based on test results from a minimum of one batch used to prepare submitted batches of drug products (e.g., critical clinical, biobatch, primary stability, production). For noncompendial excipients, a drug master file is prepared by the excipients' manufacturer. The drug master file information includes analytical procedures, acceptance criteria, and a brief description of manufacturing controls. When a USP or NF monograph material is used, associated specifications may not always provide adequate assurance regarding the assay, quality, or purity of the material or its performance in drug products. In these cases, monograph specifications are supplemented with appropriate controls (e.g., particle-size distribution, crystal forms, amorphous content, foreign particulates) to ensure batch-to-batch reproducibility of the components.

9.9.3 Manufacturers

The name, street address, and, if available, registration number of each facility involved in the manufacture of a drug substance is listed, along with a statement of each manufacturer's specific operations and responsibilities. The same information is provided for each facility involved in the manufacturing, processing, packaging, controls, stability testing, or labeling of drug products, including all contractors (e.g., testing laboratories).

9.9.4 Manufacturing Process and Controls

A detailed description of the manufacturing, processing, and packaging procedures for drug products is included. A copy of the actual (executed) batch record containing process controls is submitted, as appropriate, for representative batches (e.g., critical clinical, biobatch, primary stability). A schematic diagram of the proposed production process, a list of process controls, and a master batch production and controls record also are submitted. The manufacturing directions include control procedures on process variables (mixing time, mixing speeds, and temperature) to reduce batch-batch variability of drug products. These controls are performed at specified production steps and can include assay, osmolarity, and pH.

9.9.5 Drug Product Description

Comprehensive and well-defined *in vitro* performance characteristics should be established before initiating critical clinical or bioequivalence studies. Appropriate, validated test procedures and corresponding acceptance criteria that are reflective of the test results for submitted batches (e.g., critical clinical, biobatch, primary stability, and production) are critical to define and control these characteristics.

9.9.6 Containers and Closures

The composition and quality of materials used in the manufacture of containers and closures is carefully selected. For safety considerations, materials are chosen that minimize or eliminate leachables without compromising integrity or performance of drug products. The identity and concentration of recurring leachables in drug products or placebo formulations (i.e., drug product formulation without drug substance) are determined through the end of the drug product's shelf-life. The following information is included in the application so that the applicant can ensure continued product quality with respect to the container closure system:

- Manufacturers of container, closure, and the assembled pump, if any
- Engineering drawings of container and closure
- Composition and quality of materials of container and closure and pump components
- Control extraction methods and data for elastomeric and plastic components
- Toxicological evaluation of extractables
- Acceptance criteria, test procedures, and analytical sampling plans
- Qualitative and quantitative extractable profiles from container and closures

9.9.7 Stability Data

Stability studies provide a means for evaluating the physical and chemical stability of drug products at various storage conditions, including the compatibility of the formulation device, as well as the performance of drug products. The application should contain a complete, detailed stability protocol; stability report and data; and information regarding the suitability of employed test procedures. The protocol includes drug product specifications and acceptance criteria, test time points, container storage orientations (upright and inverted, upright and horizontal), and test storage conditions (accelerated, intermediate, long-term, and photo-stability studies) for protective packaged products, semipermeable containers without protective packaging (e.g., ophthalmics), and refrigerated products.

9.9.8 Patient Population

9.9.8.1 Pediatrics

In a continuing effort to improve the safety and efficacy of drugs in the pediatric population, the FDA has defined five subgroups of this population by age. Each subgroup has similar characteristics that are considered milestones in the growth and development of children. Accurate pediatric doses are determined by both weight and age. Age affects the capacity of physiological functions, such as drug absorption, distribution, metabolism, and elimination, resulting in differences in drug responses. Because of immature metabolic pathways, infants and children may have metabolic patterns different from those of adults.

When one is selecting excipients for drug products intended for use in the pediatric population, additional cautions must be taken. Several subgroups of the pediatric population have been identified as being susceptible to excipient reactions. Many of these reactions are related to the quantity of excipients found in the dosage form. Benzyl alcohol, propylene glycol, and polysorbates are associated with dose-related toxic reactions, which are of concern in infants because of immature hepatic and renal functions. Sucrose is a popular sweetener in oral liquid formulations. The sucrose content of oral liquids may cause significant problems (asthma, seizure control, recurrent infections) when these products are administered long-term in infants. Oral liquid preparations containing sucrose can pose a substantial carbohydrate load to children with juvenile diabetes. In another example, ethanol is employed as a solubilizer, preservative, and flavoring agent in pharmaceuticals. Young children have a limited ability to metabolize and detoxify ethanol. The American Academy of Pediatrics Committee on Drugs recommended that pharmaceutical formulations intended for use in children should not produce ethanol blood levels > 25 mg/dl after a single dose. Another major problem in pediatrics is dosing errors in intravenous administration. Due to unavailability of stock solutions for pediatric doses, errors in dilution have resulted in errors in administered doses.

Parents have to be educated about package insert instructions to improve compliance to prescribed dosing regimens for pediatric patients. The FDA issued guidelines recommending that pediatric safety and efficacy studies be completed before marketing a new drug [80] for use in children.

9.9.8.2 Geriatrics

Elderly patients constitute the largest segment of consumers of drug products. In older patients, the aging process contributes to a significantly larger interindividual variation in drug responses than is observed in younger populations. Aside from alteration of pharmacokinetic and pharmacodynamic processes, elderly patients tend to suffer from a number of chronic conditions, which may result in complex dosing regimens. To overcome the decreased rate of drug absorption resulting from GI-associated problems (a rise in stomach pH and decreased gastric emptying rate), geriatric patients are recommended liquid dosage forms. They may also require dose adjustment.

Liquid dosage forms may not be packaged in unit-dosage forms, and therefore require withdrawal of the required amount of medication from the container. Visual impairments and neurologic disorders may impair the accuracy of withdrawal of dosage, resulting in dosing errors. Errors in the dispensed amount of suspension medications may occur when a patient cannot see or disregards labeling instructions (e.g., "shake well before use"). This may result in either under- or overdosing. These errors may precipitate with concentrated solutions because small errors represent large dosing errors. The compliance issues can be mitigated to some extent by using alternative drug delivery systems or using packaging and labeling designs that enable accuracy in dosing administration.

9.10. CONCLUSIONS

Liquid dosage forms encompass numerous dosage forms for treating a variety of diseases. Special techniques are required to solubilize or disperse poorly soluble drugs. Drug-delivery technologies, such as micelles, suspensions, emulsions, and liposomes, have been developed to meet therapeutic challenges. These dosage forms pose formulation challenges to manufacturing scientists and extemporaneous compounding challenges to compounding pharmacists. A greater degree of understanding of formulation composition, processes, and regulatory guidance is essential for manufacturing stable drug products.

LIST OF ABBREVIATIONS

Acronym	Abbreviation
BA	Bioavailability
BCS	Biopharmaceutics Classification System
BE	Bioequivalence
CFCs	Chlorofluorocarbons
DMF	Drug Master File
EDTA	Ethylene Diamine Tetra-acetic Acid
FDA	Food and Drug Administration
CGMP	Current Good Manufacturing Practices
HLB	Hydrophilic-Lipophilic Balance
ICH	International Conference on Harmonization
NDA	New Drug Application
NF	National Formulary
OTC	Over-the-Counter
RES	Reticular Endothelial System
TPN	Total Parenteral Nutrition
USP	United States Pharmacopeia
WFI	Water for Injection

CASE STUDIES

Case 9.1

The stability of a drug in a solid dosage form and the stability of the same drug in solution dosage form of the same strength were compared. Stability data at room temperature revealed that the drug in solution degrades much faster than in the solid dosage form.

How can one explain this fact? If the same drug solution is kept in a refrigerator, the degradation is shown to be slower as compared to keeping it at room temperature.

Approach: Chemical degradations are due to collision between two reactants to give products. From the collision theory, it is evident that the rate of a chemical reaction depends on the rate of collision between reactant molecules. In a solid state, the rate of collision between reactants is much slower as compared to the solution. This explains that the rate of degradation in a solid is much slower as compared to the same drug in solution.

The rate of a reaction increases about two- to threefold for every 10°C rise in temperature. Since the temperature difference between a refrigerator (2°C–8°C) and room temperature (23°C–25°C) is at least 20°C, one can expect a four- to six-fold increase or decrease in the rate of degradation depending on the storage condition. It is one of the reasons that refrigerated products have a better shelf-life.

Case 9.2

The bioavailabilities of griseofulvin from three different oral dosage forms were compared and shown in Figure 9.7. Explain why the emulsion dosage form has a larger area under the curve (AUC) than the other dosage forms?

Approach: The same dose of the drug in corn oil emulsion showed the highest AUC as compared to the suspensions. High bioavailability of griseofulvin from emulsion dosage form could be due to greater partitioning of hydrophobic oil phase containing griseofulvin and higher surfactant content.

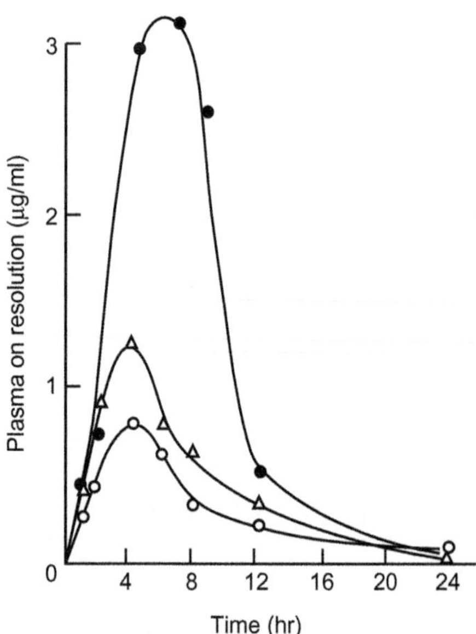

FIGURE 9.7 Administration of griseofulvin in different dosage forms (30 mg/kg of micronized griseofulvin in rats). (o) Aqueous suspension; (Δ), corn oil suspension; and (●), corn-oil-in-water emulsion containing suspended griseofulvin.

References

[1] Amidon GL, Lennernas H, Shah VP, Crison JR. A theoretical basis for a biopharmaceutic drug classification: the correlation of *in vitro* drug product dissolution and *in vivo* bioavailability. Pharm Res 1995;12:413–20.

[2] Dahan A, Miller JM, Amidon GL. Prediction of solubility and permeability class membership: provisional BCS classification of the world's top oral drugs. AAPS J 2009;11:740–6.

[3] Martinez M, Amidon GL. A mechanistic approach to understanding the factors affecting drug absorption: a review of fundamentals. J Clin Pharmacol 2002;42:620–43.

[4] The Internet Drug Index. 2012 (Accessed at <www.rxlist.com>.)

[5] Rautio J, Kumpulainen H, Heimbach T, et al. Prodrugs: design and clinical applications. Nat Rev Drug Discov 2008;7:255–70.

[6] Berge SM, Bighley LD, Monkhouse DC. Pharmaceutical salts. J Pharm Sci 1977;66:1–19.

[7] Jeffrey W, Millard JW, Alvarez-Núñez FA, Yalkowsky SH. Solubilization by cosolvents: establishing useful constants for the log–linear model. Int J Pharma 2002;245:153–66.

[8] Trivedi JS, editor. Solubilization using cosolvent approach. Boca Raton, FL: CRC Press; 2008.

[9] Fu RC, Lidgate DM, Whatley JL, McCullough T. The biocompatibility of parenteral vehicles—*in vitro/in vivo* screening comparison and the effect of excipients on hemolysis. J Parenter Sci Technol 1987;41:164–8.

[10] Rosen MJ, editor. Micelle formation by surfactants. 3rd ed. Hoboken, NJ: John Wiley & Sons, Inc.; 2004.

[11] Rowe RC, Sheskey PJ, Owen SC, editors. Handbook of pharmaceutical excipients. Washington, DC: American Pharmacists Association and Pharmaceutical Press; 2006.

[12] Gonzalez-Caballero F, Lopez-Duran JDG, editors. Suspension formulation. New York: Marcel Dekker; 2000.

[13] Rangel-Yagui CO, Pessoa Jr A, Tavares LC. Micellar solubilization of drugs. J Pharm Pharm Sci 2005;8:147–65.

[14] Lee JH, Lee HB, Andrade JD. Blood compatibility of polyethylene oxide surfaces. Prog Polymer Sci 1995;20:1043–79.

[15] Brewster ME, Loftsson T. Cyclodextrins as pharmaceutical solubilizers. Adv Drug Deliv Rev 2007;59:645–66.

[16] Mehta K, Yu-hsing T, inventors. Tris Pharma, assignee. Modified release formulations containing drug-ion exchange resin complexes. U.S.A. patent 20100166858. 2010.

[17] Pouton CW. Formulation of poorly water-soluble drugs for oral administration: physicochemical and physiological issues and the lipid formulation classification system. Eur J Pharm Sci 2006;29:278–87.

[18] Constantinides PP. Lipid microemulsions for improving drug dissolution and oral absorption: physical and biopharmaceutical aspects. Pharm Res 1995;12:1561–72.

[19] Chakraborty S, Shukla D, Mishra B, Singh S. Lipid—an emerging platform for oral delivery of drugs with poor bioavailability. Eur J Pharm Biopharm 2009;73:1–15.

[20] Pouton CW. Lipid formulations for oral administration of drugs: non-emulsifying, self-emulsifying and 'self-microemulsifying' drug delivery systems. Eur J Pharm Sci 2000;11:S93–8.

[21] Porter CJ, Pouton CW, Cuine JF, Chapman WN. Enhancing intestinal drug solubilisation using lipid-based delivery systems. Adv Drug Deliv Rev 2008;60:673–91.

[22] Jannin V, Musakhanian J, Marchaud D. Approaches for the development of solid and semi-solid lipid-based formulations. Adv Drug Deliv Rev 2008;60:734–46.
[23] Mullertz A, Ogbonna A, Ren S, Rades T. New perspectives on lipid and surfactant based drug delivery systems for oral delivery of poorly soluble drugs. J Pharm Pharmacol 2010;62: 1622–36.
[24] Inactive Ingredients Guide, 2012. (Accessed at <www.accessdata.fda.gov/scripts/cder/iig/index.cfm>.)
[25] PDR Network L. Physician's desk reference. Montvale, NJ: Medical Economics Company, Inc.; 2003.
[26] U.S.P-N.F. The United States Pharmacopeia and National Formulary USP 32-NF 27. In: USP, editor. Rockville, MD; 2009.
[27] Hanawa T, Masuda N, Mohri K, Kawata K, Suzuki M, Nakajima S. Development of patient-friendly preparations: preparation of a new allopurinol mouthwash containing polyethylene(oxide) and carrageenan. Drug Devel Ind Pharm 2004;30:151–61.
[28] Nieuw Amerongen AV, Veerman EC. Current therapies for xerostomia and salivary gland hypofunction associated with cancer therapies. Support Care Cancer 2003;11:226–31.
[29] Ellis ME, Clink H, Ernst P, et al. Controlled study of fluconazole in the prevention of fungal infections in neutropenic patients with haematological malignancies and bone marrow transplant recipients. Eur J Clin Microbiol Infect Dis 1994;13:3–11.
[30] Joseph BK. Oral cancer: prevention and detection. Med Principles Pract 2002;11(Suppl. 1):32–5.
[31] Lang J. Ocular drug delivery conventional ocular formulations. Adv Drug Deliv Rev 1995;16:39–43.
[32] Illum L. Nasal drug delivery—possibilities, problems and solutions. J Control Release 2003;87:187–98.
[33] Arora J. Development of nasal delivery systems: a review. Drug Deliv Technol 2002;2:70–3.
[34] FDA. Nasal Spray and Inhalation Solution, Suspension, and Spray Drug Products—Chemistry, Manufacturing, and Controls Documentation. Rockville, MD: CBER, FDA; 2002:1–45.
[35] Zimmer A, Kreuter J. Microspheres and nanoparticles used in ocular delivery systems. Adv Drug Deliv Rev 1995;16:61–73.
[36] Molina MJ, Rowlands FS. Stratospheric sink for chlorofluoromethanes: chlorine atomcatalysed destruction of ozone. Nature 1974;249:810–2.
[37] Partridge MR, Woodcock AA, editors. Propellants. New York: Marcel Dekker; 2002.
[38] McDonald KJ, Martin GP. Transition to CFC-free metered dose inhalers: into the new millenium. Int J Pharm 2000;201:89–107.
[39] Newman SP. Principles of metered-dose inhaler design. Respir Care 2005;50:1177–90.
[40] Haines Jr BA, Martin AN. Interfacial properties of powdered material; caking in liquid dispersions. II. Electrokinetic phenomena. J Pharm Sci 1961;50:753–6.
[41] Martin AN. Physical chemical approach to the formulation of pharmaceutical suspensions. J Pharm Sci 1961;50:513–7.
[42] Hiestand EN. Theory of coarse suspension formulation. J Pharm Sci 1964;53:1–18.
[43] Couper A, editor. Surface tension and its measurement. 2nd ed. New York: John Wiley & Sons; 1993.
[44] Rosen MJ, Kunjappu JT, editors. Adsorption of surface-active agents at interfaces: the electrical double layer. 4th ed. Hoboken, N.J.: John Wiley & Sons, Inc.; 2012.
[45] Rieger MM, editor. Surfactants. New York: Marcel Dekker; 1988.
[46] Duro R, Gómez-Amoza JL, Martínez-Pacheco R, Souto C, Concheiro A. Adsorption of polysorbate 80 on pyrantel pamoate: effects on suspension stability. Int J Pharm 1998;165:211–6.
[47] Shijie Liu S, Masliyah JH, editors. Rheology of suspensions. Washington, DC: American Chemical Society (ACS); 1996.
[48] Derkach SR. Rheology of emulsions. Adv Colloid Interface Sci 2009;151:1–23.
[49] Everett DH. Definitions, terminology and symbols in colloid and surface chemistry. Washington DC: International Union of Pure and Applied Chemistry; 1972.
[50] Martin A, Swarbrick J, Cammarata A, Chun AHC, editors. Physical pharmacy: physical chemical principles in the pharmaceutical sciences. 3rd ed. Malvern, PA: Lea and Febiger; 1983.
[51] Vaziri A, Warburton B. Slow release of chloroquine phosphate from multiple taste-masked W/O/W multiple emulsions. J Microencapsul 1994;11:641–8.
[52] Lawrence MJ, Rees GD. Microemulsion-based media as novel drug delivery systems. Adv Drug Deliv Rev 2000;45:89–121.
[53] Muller RH, Heinemann S. Fat emulsions for parenteral nutrition II: characterisation and physical long-term stability of Lipofundin MCT LCT. Clin Nutr 1993;12:298–309.
[54] Collins-Gold LC, Lyons RT, Bartholow LC. Parenteral emulsions for drug delivery. Adv Drug Deliv Rev 1990;5:189–208.
[55] Koster VS, Kuksa PFM, Langea R, Talsmab H. Particle size in parenteral fat emulsions, what are the true limitations? Int J Pharm 1996;134:235–8.
[56] Prankerd RJ, Stella VJ. The use of oil-in-water emulsions as a vehicle for parenteral drug administration. J Parenter Sci Technol 1990;44:139–49.
[57] Roon L. The physical significance of emulsions. J Am Pharm Assoc 1916;5:496–505.
[58] Harkins WD, Beeman N. The oriented wedge theory of emulsions. Proc Natl Acad Sci U S A 1925;11:631–7.
[59] Serrallach JA, Jones G, Owen RJ. Strength of emulsifier films at liquid-liquid interfaces. Ind Eng Chem 1933;25:816–9.
[60] Griffin WC. Calculation of HLB values of non-ionic surfactants. J Soc Cosmetic Chem 1954;5:259.
[61] Pal R. Effect of droplet size on the rheology of emulsions. AIChE J 1996;42:3181–90.
[62] Reddy SR, Fogler HS. Emulsion stability—experimental studies on simultaneous flocculation and creaming. J Colloid Interface Sci 1981;82:128–35.
[63] Taylor P. Ostwald ripening in emulsions. Adv Colloid Interface Sci 1998;75:107–63.
[64] Driscoll DF. Lipid injectable emulsions: 2006. Nutr Clin Pract 2006;21:381–6.
[65] Floyd AG. Top ten considerations in the development of parenteral emulsions. Pharm Sci Technol Today 1999;4:134–43.
[66] Shulin D, inventor. Allergan, CA, assignee. Nonirritating emulsions for sensitive tissue. U.S.A. patent US5474979. 1995.
[67] Carstensen JT, Rhodes CT, editors. Drug stability: principles and practices. 3rd ed. New York, NY: Marcel Dekker Inc; 2000.
[68] FDA. Pharmaceutical cGMPs for the 21st Century—A Risk-Based Approach. In: HHS, editor. Rockville, MD: US FDA; 2004.
[69] FDA. Guide to Inspections Oral Solutions and Suspensions. In: HHS, editor. Rockville, MD: US FDA; 1994.
[70] Crowley MM, editor. Solutions, emulsions, suspensions, and extracts. Philadelphia, PA: Lippincott, Williams & Wilkins; 2005.
[71] Krause K, Muller RH. Production and characterisation of highly concentrated nanosuspensions by high pressure homogenization. Int J Pharm 2001;214:21–4.
[72] FDA. Sterile drug products produced by aseptic processing—current good manufacturing practice. In: HHS, editor. Rockville, MD: CBER, FDA; 2004:1–59.

[73] FDA. Guidance for Industry - Container and closure systems for packaging human drugs and biologics. Chemistry, manufacturing, and controls documentation. In: HHS, editor, Rockville, MD: CBER and CDER, FDA; 1999:1-56.
[74] Muller RH. Zetapotential and partikelladung in der laborpraxis–einfuhrung in der theorie, praktische mebdurchfuhrung dateninterpretation. Wissenschaftliche Verlagsgesellschaft; 1996.
[75] Brunner E. Reaktionsgeschwindigkeit in heterogenen Systemen. Z Phys Chem 1904;43:56–102.
[76] Nernst W. Theorie der Reaktionsgeschwindigkeit in heterogenen Systemen. Z Phys Chem 1904;47:52–5.
[77] Levich V, editor. Physicochemical hydrodynamics. Eagle Cliffs, NY: Prentice-Hall; 1962.
[78] Hixson AW, Crowell JH. Dependence of reaction velocity upon surface and agitation (I) theoretical consideration. Ind Eng Chem 1931;23:923–31.
[79] Washington C. Drug release from microdisperse systems: a critical review. Int J Pharm 1990;58:1–12.
[80] FDA. Guidance for Industry - Qualifying for pediatric exclusivity under section 505A of the federal food, drug, and cosmetic act. In: HHS, editor. Rockville, MD: CBER and CDER, FDA; 1999:1-26.

CHAPTER

10

Aerosol Dosage Forms

Pulmonary Drug Delivery

Justin A. Tolman and Megan Huslig
Department of Pharmacy Sciences, Creighton University, Omaha, NE, USA

CHAPTER OBJECTIVES

- Describe lung anatomical and physiological barriers to pulmonary drug delivery.
- Relate physiological lung volumes with breathing patterns for appropriate patient counseling on proper pulmonary drug administration.
- Describe the factors that affect pulmonary drug deposition in the lungs.
- Explain the role, mechanisms of aerosol generation, and parts/components of devices used for pulmonary drug delivery.
- Compare and contrast the properties of inhaled gases, nebulizers, pressurized metered-dose inhalers, and dry powder inhalers.
- Anatomical and physiological considerations for pulmonary drug delivery.
- Formulation requirements and factors that affect gas inhalation or aerosol production.
- Device design and relationship to inhaled formulations.

Keywords

- Aerosols
- Dry powder inhaler
- Lung anatomy
- Lung physiology
- Metered-dose inhaler
- Nebulizer
- Pulmonary drug deposition

10.1. INTRODUCTION

The inhalation of substances for pharmacologic effects has been reported throughout history [1]. Substances have been inhaled for localized effects in the treatment of pulmonary disorders or conditions. Systemic effects are also possible due to the extremely large absorptive surfaces and capillary networks present in the lungs. However, substances were principally inhaled either as suspended particulates in smoke or fumes from burning or heating materials. Few substances were able to retain pharmacological activity following incineration in order to exert localized or systemic action.

Scientific advances in the 1700s and 1800s saw the development of the first medicinal uses of inhaled anesthetic gases and vapors, including nitrous oxide, chloroform, and ether—the forerunners to modern anesthesia. Specialized medical devices were also developed from the 1600s through the 1800s to facilitate the delivery of vapors and dispersions and have been categorized as inhalers. These early inhalers ranged from simple pots that passed inspiratory airflow through moistened and heated medicinal solutions to devices that atomized medicinal liquids or powders. In 1867, the British Pharmacopeia included several inhaled medications as formal recognition of therapeutic drug delivery to the lungs [18]. Since that time, pulmonary drug administration has advanced for rational delivery of gases and vapors, solid particles, and liquid droplets by a variety of devices. Inhaled drug delivery devices include vaporizers, nebulizers, pressurized metered dose inhalers (pMDIs), and dry powder inhalers (DPIs). However,

Pharmaceutics. DOI: http://dx.doi.org/10.1016/B978-0-12-386890-9.00010-8

pulmonary drug delivery is predicated on the mechanisms by which a device interacts with the lung anatomy and physiology.

10.2. LUNG ANATOMY

The pulmonary system is principally designed to support the process of respiration—the exchange of gases between a cell with functioning metabolic processes and the external environment [23]. In humans, respiration first occurs through air movement and gas exchange in the lungs, followed by distribution of dissolved gases through the systemic circulation, concluding with utilization of dissolved gases for biological processes in cells and tissues. The first stage of respiration, focused on air movement and gas exchange, is dependent on anatomical structures of the nose, nasal cavity, mouth, and throat; the trachea and conducting airways; and the lungs composed of alveoli and the pulmonary vasculature (Figure 10.1).

The nose and nasal cavity warms, moistens, and serves as a coarse particle filter for inhaled air. The mouth also serves as a separate airway for inhaled air but has less efficient warming, moistening, or filtering capacity than the nose/nasal cavity. The throat, or pharynx, is the anatomical structure that unifies airflow from the nasal and mouth airways. The pharynx redirects the inhaled air down into the thorax through the trachea by way of a sharp angle change of approximately 90°. The back of the throat also serves as a principal impaction surface for inhaled particles and reduces large particle deposition deeper in the conducting airways. These deposited particles are then ingested or expectorated.

The trachea is the first generation airway, or principal conducting airway, in the lungs [12]. At the base of the trachea, the airway then asymmetrically bifurcates into the left or right main bronchi. The right bronchus is slightly larger in diameter and shorter in length compared to the left. This initial point of bifurcation changes airflow direction as inhaled air encounters the second generation of airways and is drawn deeper into the lungs. The bronchi further subdivide into conducting airways of narrowing diameters through successive generations of bifurcations. Conducting airway generations 3 through approximately 16 are classified as bronchioles. These airways are covered with a pseudostratified epithelium composed of ciliated or mucous-producing cells. The specialized epithelial linings of conducting airways form a mucociliary escalator to entrap and then physically translocate particles up to the throat for eventual ingestion or expectoration for particles that deposit on conducting airway surfaces.

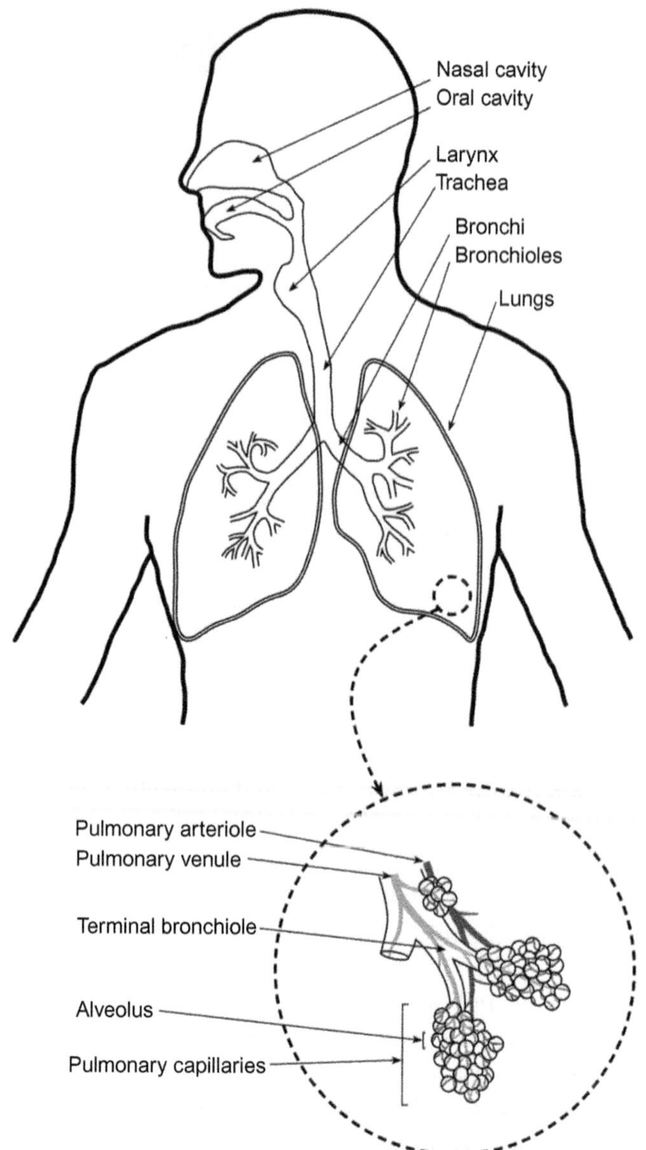

FIGURE 10.1 Schematic representations of the lungs. (A) The respiratory system, (B) the alveolar region of the lungs.

Starting in approximately airway generation 17, terminal bronchioles begin and contain a small number of alveolar structures. At approximately airway generation 20, alveolar structures become more prevalent, and respiratory bronchioles can be found. Final airway generations occur at approximately generation 23 and terminate in porous alveolar sacs where principal gas exchange can occur. Collateral ventilation throughout alveolar regions is facilitated by holes or pores between adjacent alveoli. Alveoli are specialized pulmonary structures designed for efficient gas exchange. They are composed mainly of very thin Type I cells with membrane thicknesses of 0.1 μm–0.2 μm with some larger surfactant-producing Type II cells that

TABLE 10.1 Inhaled Anesthetic Agents Physicochemical Properties of Inhaled Anesthetic Agents

						Partition Coefficient at 37°C		
Inhaled Anesthetic	**Molecular Weight (g/mol)**	**Specific Gravity**	**Boiling Point (°C)**	**Vapor Pressure (mm Hg)**	**MAC (%)**	**Blood: Gas**	**Brain: Blood**	**Fat: Blood**
Desflurane	168.04	1.47	23	669	6.0	0.42	1.3	27
Enflurane	184.49	1.52	56	175	1.6	1.8	1.4	36
Isoflurane	184.49	1.50	48	250	1.2	1.4	2.6	45
Halothane	197.38	1.87	50	243	0.75	2.5	2.9	51
Sevoflurane	200.05	1.52	58	160	2.0	0.65	1.7	48

MAC: minimum alveolar concentration.

help maintain alveolar integrity. Alveoli are surrounded by a vast network of pulmonary capillaries to facilitate gas diffusion into and out of the blood. The alveolar-capillary interface is then the principal site of gas exchange and respiration. Ventilation and respiration as well as pulmonary drug deposition are dependent on pulmonary epithelial surfaces.

Airway and alveolar epithelial membranes are sensitive to potential irritation and inflammation caused by inhaled drugs. Pulmonary inflammatory processes are often immune-mediated if inhaled substances have antigenic potential. Additional inflammatory processes can be triggered by airway irritation caused by the drug chemical structure, functional groups, and reactivity as well as the drug product tonicity, ion content (e.g., chloride ion concentration), and pH. Additionally, the lungs do not have significant levels of biometabolism, which require that inhaled drugs, drug products, and degradation by-products be biodegradable, bioabsorbable, and/or biocompatible with the lung epithelia. The FDA has approved only a limited number of excipients for use in the lungs and inhaled drug products (Table 10.1). Often, airway irritation and inflammation produce bronchospasms or coughing in attempts to eliminate or expel the cause of irritation. Bronchospasms are involuntary responses and substantially interfere with normal breathing and drug delivery to the lungs.

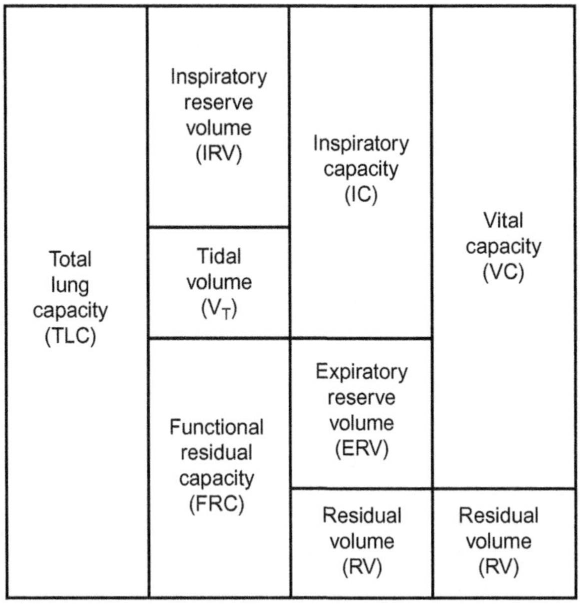

FIGURE 10.2 Standardized lung air volumes and lung capacities.

10.3. LUNG PHYSIOLOGY

Breathing is defined as the physiological process that facilitates gas exchange [9]. Specifically, breathing is composed of two different actions that cause air movement in the lungs. Inspiration or inhalation is the movement of air into the lungs, whereas expiration or exhalation is the expulsion of air from the lungs. A breath is then a single set of paired air movements: inspiration and expiration. Breathing is highly variable between patients based on numerous factors (e.g., age, gender, activity level, body position, pathological processes, etc.). However, comparisons between physiologic or pathologic differences can be made based on a standardized set of lung volumes and lung capacities (Figure 10.2) [15].

Normal breathing causes a volume of air referred to as the tidal volume (V_T) to be exchanged per breath. Under resting conditions, patients do typically have conscious control over the tidal volume. This air volume represents the baseline levels for passive inspiration and expiration. Patients have an additional inspiratory reserve volume (IRV) of air that can be inhaled into the lungs during maximal forced inspiration. The inspiratory capacity (IC) is then the V_T plus the IRV. A separate air volume that can be forcibly expired from the lungs following maximal inspiration is the vital capacity (VC) of the lungs. This vital capacity represents the maximal air volume that can be exchanged per breath. An expiratory reserve volume (ERV) represents the air volume that is not normally exhaled but can be forcibly exhaled and is represented by the VC minus the V_T and the IRV. A residual volume (RV) represents the dead air space that cannot be exhaled and is necessary to prevent the lungs from collapsing under low air volumes. A functional residual capacity (FRC) represents air volumes that are present in the lungs during normal breathing (breaths that only utilize tidal volume) and not exhaled. The FRC is equal to the ERV plus the RV. The total lung capacity (TLC) then represents the maximal air volume a patient can contain within the lungs following the greatest inspiratory effort possible and is equal to the sum of the IRV, V_T, ERV, and RV.

With an understanding of various lung volumes and capacities, one can use objective measures to both evaluate lung function and train patients on proper breathing techniques for optimal drug delivery. A patient's respiration rate is defined as the number of breaths, usually tidal breaths, which an individual takes per unit time. Basal respiration rates for healthy adults are typically 8–12 breaths per minute but highly variable based on physiologic and pathologic factors. Assessment of a patient's vital capacity is also possible through a forced vital capacity (FVC) test where maximal expiratory effort is made following maximal inspiratory effort. During this test, the forced expiratory volume in the first second (FEV_1) represents the maximal volume of air the body is able to initially forcefully exhale. It is often used as a measure of lung inflammation because FEV_1 is particularly sensitive to impaired airflow resulting from altered airway epithelial pathologies that impair air movement out of the lungs. Patients with sufficient cognition can therefore affect the respiration rate, breath volume (to some degree), breath holding, force of inspiration and expiration, and position and posture to influence pulmonary drug deposition and delivery.

10.4. PULMONARY DRUG TARGETS

The majority of inhaled medications are used in modern medicine for their therapeutic use in localized lung conditions (e.g., asthma, emphysema, pneumonias, etc.) [6]. Targeted lung delivery via inhalation of active pharmaceutical ingredients (APIs) continues to be investigated for cancers, gene therapy, and other therapeutic applications. These uses of pulmonary drug delivery are essentially topical and use patients' inspiration or breathing only to get the drug to the site of action. Dependent on the clinical application, it could be therapeutically optimal for the drug to be delivered to the upper airways, conducting airways, and/or alveoli.

The pulmonary route of administration can also be utilized for systemic drug delivery if drugs are delivered to the highly vascularized alveolar regions of the lungs [14]. To reach the alveoli, inhaled APIs must be able to avoid deposition in the upper airways or conducting airways but then deposit on the alveolar epithelium. Once a drug is deposited, it can potentially be absorbed across the very thin alveolar cell membrane and into the systemic circulation. Clinical decisions and patient counseling points are then informed through an understanding of the physics that govern drug deposition in the lungs.

10.5. PULMONARY DRUG DEPOSITION

Drugs administered to the lungs can be inhaled as drug molecules mixed in a gas or as dispersions, coarse or colloidal, of drug or particles containing drug in a gaseous continuous phase [26]. Drug deposition in the lungs is principally influenced by three mechanisms: inertial impaction, gravimetric sedimentation, and diffusion (Figure 10.3 [10,19]). Additional deposition mechanisms include interception for fibrous particles and electrostatic deposition for charged particles [25].

The principal deposition mechanism for many inhaled particles is inertial impaction and can be illustrated using a simplified model of bifurcating tubes to represent the conducting airways (Figure 10.2 [7]). Air movement in the conducting airways is a complex

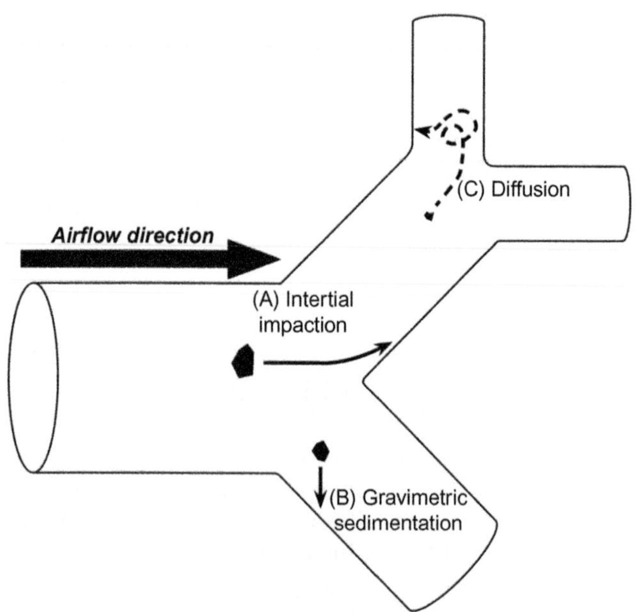

FIGURE 10.3 Schematic model of particle deposition mechanisms in the airways.

physiologic process that is affected by numerous physiologic and pathologic factors [24]. In this simplified system, air is assumed to have laminar flow through the start of the conducting airways. Laminar flow is the smooth ordered movement of parallel layers of air and can occur in this model due to the circular tube, smooth walled sides, unidirectional airflow, and constant air velocity. When moving layers of air encounter an airway bifurcation, turbulence is induced as airflow is redirected into new airflow paths (Figure 10.4). This airflow redirection causes chaotic air subcurrents while retaining overall unidirectional flow through the airways. Turbulent airflow becomes predominant in lung regions where bifurcations become more prevalent (especially in airway generations through 16), in airways that are not smooth, when air velocity is not constant throughout the airways, and when air direction changes due to breathing [27]. Laminar flow can be reinstated in airway generations greater than 16 as ordered airflow is imposed by small-diameter airways. Modeling drug deposition by impaction, sedimentation, and diffusion in the lungs is a complex process and is described by each component process.

Inertial impaction occurs when a drug particle suspended in an airstream resists a change in air direction induced by airway bifurcations and collides with the airway walls. The Stoke's number (S_t) is a dimensionless parameter that a particle's likelihood to follow an initial trajectory due to high inertial energy or change trajectory based on redirected airflow:

$$S_t = \frac{\nu_a \rho_p d^2}{18R\eta}$$

where v_a is the air velocity, ρ_p is the particle density, d is the particle diameter, R is the airway radius, and η is the viscosity of air. Systems that have large Stoke's numbers will likely have substantial particle deposition by impaction. Impaction can also occur due to chaotic airflow patterns in regions of turbulence that induce particle collisions with airway surfaces. The magnitude of a particle's inertia is directly proportional to the force imparted by the air velocity. Particles with large sizes and/or densities will have more inertial energy in an airstream and have higher probabilities of collisions with pulmonary surfaces. Particle impaction is much more probable in the tortuous air pathways of the central lungs or conducting airways. However, inhaled particles can also impact in alveolar regions if their size and density are small enough to avoid impaction in the central airways.

Gravimetric sedimentation is another deposition mechanism by which particles settle in the lungs [21]. Spherical particle sedimentation in airflow is described by Stoke's Law. This law states that the particle velocity (v_p) is defined by

$$\nu_p = \frac{d^2(\rho_p - \rho_a)g}{18\eta}$$

where d is the particle diameter, ρ is the particle density, ρ_a is air density, g is the force of gravity, and η is the viscosity of air. The sedimentation velocity is proportional to the size and density of the particle. The residence time of inhaled particles represents the average time a suspended particle is retained within the respiratory system before either deposition or expiration. Eventually, inhaled particles will settle and come in contact with the lung epithelium if particles are unperturbed by air movement. Deposition by sedimentation is then more probable if inhaled particles have long residence times in a space unperturbed by air movement.

Diffusion is another deposition mechanism by which inhaled particles can collide with epithelial linings in the lungs. Particle diffusion in air is due to the random and chaotic collision of particles with gas molecules. Diffusion is governed by the Stokes–Einstein Equation. The diffusivity of a particle (D) is described by

$$D = \frac{k_B T}{3\pi\eta d}$$

where k_B is Boltzmann's constant, T is the temperature (in Kelvin), η is the viscosity of air, and d is the particle

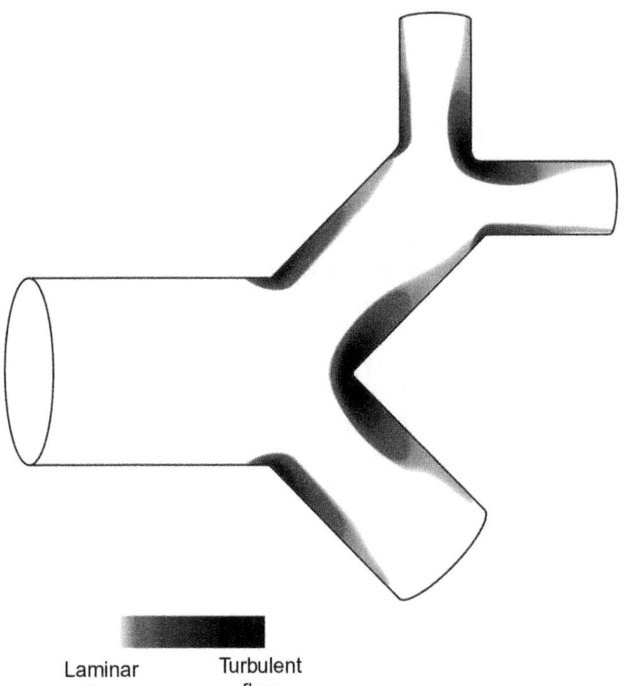

FIGURE 10.4 Schematic diagram that represents airflow patterns in simulated airway bifurcations.

diameter. Diffusion is inversely proportional to particle size. Particle diffusion will be more pronounced under physiological conditions (e.g., 37°C, standard air viscosity, and normal breath-holding times) for particles with diameters <100 nm. Drug deposition by diffusion is also more probable when the diffusional distance is short or the particle residence time in the lungs is long.

These three main mechanisms for drug deposition in the lungs are all influenced by the size of an inhaled particle. Particle density also is significant for deposition by impaction and sedimentation. The nominal particle size does not adequately describe how an inhaled particle behaves in the airstream. An aerodynamic particle size is used to describe and relate the size and density of a suspended particle intended for pulmonary delivery with its behavior in moving air. The Mass Median Aerodynamic Diameter (MMAD) is the average diameter of a sample of particles that have the same aerodynamic behavior as spheres of a known size (Figure 10.5). The MMAD is not necessarily a "true" diameter but suggests that large non-dense particles can behave aerodynamically like smaller but denser particles. Specifically, a particle's aerodynamic diameter (d_a) is described by

$$d_a = d\sqrt{\frac{\rho_p}{\rho_0}}$$

where d is the true diameter, and $\sqrt{\frac{\rho_p}{\rho_0}}$ is the particle-specific gravity. MMAD values have been associated with region-specific drug deposition (Figure 10.5) [6]. For therapeutic purposes, inhaled particles with MMAD values of >5 μm tend to be deposited in the conducting airways while particles <5 μm tend to be deposited in the alveolar regions. This 5 μm "cutoff" diameter is also used to describe the dose fraction below this size and is referred to as either the Fine Particle Dose (FPD) with mass units or the Fine Particle Fraction (FPF) expressed as a percentage of the delivered dose below this diameter.

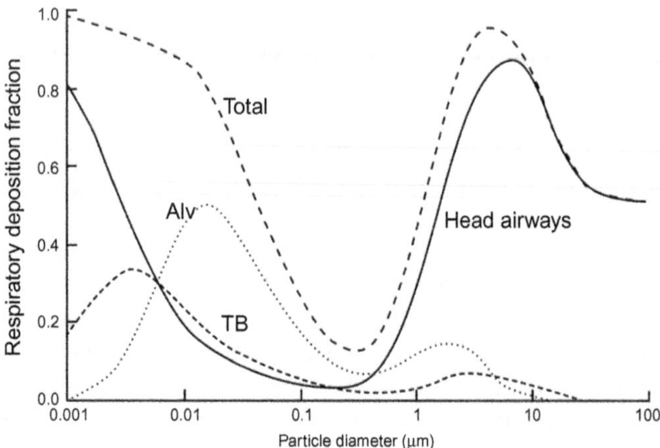

FIGURE 10.5 Average predicted total and regional lung deposition based on International Commission on Radiological Protection (ICRP) deposition model for nose-breathing males and females engaged in light exercise. Alv: alveolar region; TB: tracheobronchial region. *(Reproduced with permission from [6]).*

Ultimately, pulmonary drug deposition patterns of inhaled medications are influenced by impaction, sedimentation, and diffusion to varying degrees [2]. Many patients can be trained to have breathing parameters conducive to optimal drug deposition for varying clinical needs based on patient and formulation factors. For example, patients can alter the rate and extent of inspiration to induce fast airflow velocities to promote particle deposition in the conducting airways by inertial impaction. This could be beneficial for drugs used to treat central airway conditions (e.g., asthma). Conversely, slow airflow rates can be induced through slow inspiration to minimize the energy imparted to particles and thereby minimize inertial impaction. Patients can refrain from breathing for short periods of time through breath-holding to promote sedimentation and diffusion of smaller particles. The "depth" of a breath can also be varied to recruit alveolar regions during maximum ventilation and utilization of the total lung capacity. "Shallow" breathing can also be used to reduce alveolar availability if breathing is restricted to the tidal volume or less. These breathing techniques can be used to alter the drug deposition patterns and are important considerations for achieving optimal drug therapy outcomes for inhaled medications.

10.6. THERAPEUTIC GASES

A relatively small portion of inhaled pulmonary drugs are delivered as gases or vapors. This is due to the limited number of drug molecules that are physically in a gaseous state at standard temperatures and pressures or which have very low vapor pressures. Therapeutic gases typically have low molecular weights, very weak intermolecular interactions, and are nonpolar and highly lipophilic (Table 10.1, Figure 10.6). However, once inhaled, therapeutic gases utilize normal lung physiology for rapid therapeutic effects and efficient systemic drug delivery.

Systemic delivery is possible following inhalation due to the physiologic structure of the lungs. Fick's Law of Diffusion states

$$-\frac{dC}{dt} = \frac{DAK(C_L - C_B)}{h}$$

where $\frac{dC}{dt}$ is the rate of concentration change with respect to time, D is the diffusion coefficient, A is the surface area across which diffusion is occurring, K is the partition coefficient, C_L is the drug concentration in the lung, C_B is the drug concentration in the blood, and h is the membrane thickness. Drug diffusion across the alveolar-capillary interface is then highly likely due to the enormous alveolar surface area, a very thin alveolar membrane thickness, and good molecular diffusivity due to the nonpolar or mildly polar nature of these APIs. Additionally, the concentration gradient (C_L-C_B) of gas across the diffusional membrane can usually be regulated to ensure sufficient therapeutic effects are obtained while also allowing for exhalation of drug. Inhaled gases are almost always administered as gaseous mixtures, often with varying concentrations of oxygen. Assuming these gaseous mixtures have minimal intermolecular interactions, the fractional pressure of each component in these mixtures can be described by Dalton's Law:

$$p_T = p_1 + p_2 + \cdots p_n$$

where p_T is the total pressure of the system and is equal to the summation of each individual component's partial pressure (p_n) in the mixture. The partial pressure for each gas in the mixture is determined by the mole fraction of each component, and the Ideal Gas Law states that

$$pV = nRT$$

where p is pressure, V is volume, n is the number of particles, R is Avogadro's number, and T is the temperature. The partial pressure of mixtures is also applicable to dissolved gases in liquids (e.g., blood) and can be used with Fick's Law of Diffusion to describe the process of gaseous drug distribution across a membrane. Once absorbed, dissolved gases distribute thoroughly into tissues in the body. Distribution equilibrium is reached when the partial pressure of the gas is equal in all tissues in the body. The concentration of inhaled gas in different regions of the body will not be equal during equilibrium due to tissue-specific API solubility in different tissues. Partition coefficients are used to describe the relative concentrations of gases in tissues (e.g., blood: gas, brain: blood, and fat: blood) (Table 10.1).

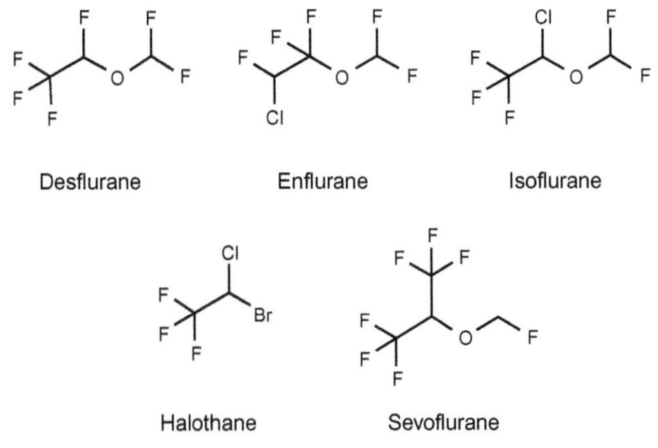

A class of drugs that are administered as gases is inhaled anesthetics, which induce general anesthesia (Table 10.1) [13]. These drugs often have very narrow therapeutic indices and must be used with extreme caution. Pharmacologic effects of these drugs are generally independent of patient breathing parameters but instead are affected by drug physicochemical properties and by the devices used for their administration.

Many but not all inhaled anesthetic drugs are short-chain halogenated ethers that are structural mimics of diethyl ether. These agents are mildly polar compounds with high hydrogen bonding potential. Halogen substitution alters drug solubility, boiling point, vapor pressure, flammability, and potency to varying degrees. Most inhaled anesthetics are commercially available as liquids that typically have low molecular weights and very low vapor pressures. These liquid APIs are used in drug-specific, specialized, and calibrated vaporizers that convert the drug liquid to a drug vapor. These anesthetic vapors are then mixed with varying concentrations of oxygen and possibly other agents based on clinical need before delivery to the patient. Anesthetic gas mixtures are then delivered directly to the lungs through equipment such as a complete face mask, an endotracheal tube, or a laryngeal mask airway (a specialized airway tube).

A key clinical mechanism to evaluate anesthetic gas potency is through the minimum alveolar concentration (MAC). The MAC is the gas concentration in the alveoli, as measured by the drug concentration during expiration that causes no pain response in 50% of patients. It is a relative pharmacodynamic measure and can be affected by numerous physiological or pathological conditions (e.g., age, temperature, pregnancy, and co-administration of drugs). Drug potency is inversely related to the MAC value for inhaled anesthetic agents because the relationship between the MAC and the anesthetic blood concentration is directly related to the concentration gradient across the alveolar-capillary interface. This concentration gradient is proportional to the partial pressure of the gas and inversely proportional to the concentration of the dissolved gas in the blood. Once dissolved, the drug will distribute throughout the body as determined by tissue: gas partition coefficients. The rate of anesthesia induction is controlled by the rate at which drug concentrations in the brain equal the MAC. This rate is also approximately equal to the rate at which the

Desflurane Enflurane Isoflurane

Halothane Sevoflurane

FIGURE 10.6 Chemical structures of inhaled anesthetic agents.

alveolar partial pressure reached the MAC value. Therefore, the rate of anesthesia induction is inversely proportional to the solubility of gas in the blood but directly proportional to the partial pressure of gas administered to the patient.

Desflurane is one example of an inhaled anesthetic that has special considerations for drug delivery. It is a moderately polar compound that readily diffuses across the alveolar-capillary interface. Desflurane has a blood: gas partition coefficient of 0.42 and a brain: blood coefficient of 1.3, indicating low relative blood solubility and rapid induction of anesthesia. It also has a relatively high vapor pressure but a low boiling point. This necessitates a specialized vaporizer for desflurane that utilizes heat to regulate vapor concentrations in gaseous mixtures administered to patients.

10.7. INHALED AEROSOLS

The majority of drugs delivered to the lungs are administered as disperse systems of solid particles or liquid droplets suspended in air [16,20]. These disperse systems are referred to as aerosols (*aero*—air and *sol*—solution) in the broadest sense of the term. "Aerosol" also has an official and more restrictive definition by the United States Pharmacopeia: a system under pressure. This definition is appropriate for inhaled medications formulated as pressurized systems that produce fine drug dispersions in air due to the rapid vaporization of volatile propellants from a metered volume of drug/propellant mixture (more information about these systems later). However, the broadest definition of an aerosol as solid or liquid particles dispersed in a gas will be used to describe inhaled aerosols.

All currently available aerosolized drug products are drug-device combinations or are drug products that require a separate device for proper therapeutic utilization. The reason is that aerosol creation is a device-specific process that is influenced by both patient and formulation factors. A discussion of inhaled aerosols then is typically centered around broad device categories of nebulizers, pressurized metered-dose inhalers (pMDIs), and dry powder inhalers (DPIs). Recent advances in inhaler technology have also led to breath-assisted devices that adapt drug delivery to the patient's inspiratory patterns. In each of these device categories, the aerosol is created at the time of inspiration. The aerosol's aerodynamic particle size distribution as measured by the MMAD and FPF (or FPD) in conjunction with the patient's breathing parameters will significantly affect how the aerosol particles navigate the anatomical and physiologic barriers of the lungs to reach their intended targets. Therefore, these broad categories do not supersede the device-specific aerosol creation processes or patient handling requirements for proper therapeutic use.

10.7.1 Nebulizers

Nebulizers are devices that continuously produce a dispersed cloud of liquid droplets in an air stream [5]. The aerosol cloud is then inspired and expired through normal tidal breathing. Most patients do not need to be compliant with breathing regulation or have the dexterity to manipulate the device. Indeed, nebulizers are often used to deliver inhaled medications to pediatric patients and intubated or mechanically ventilated patients. Nebulized aerosols are often delivered to patients through a face mask or mouthpiece and can often be delivered to mechanically ventilated patients through in-line junctions.

There are three principal types of nebulizers currently used for drug delivery: air-jet, ultrasonic, and vibrating-mesh nebulizers. All three produce an aerosol of drug-containing droplets from solutions or suspensions. However, the aerosol generation mechanisms differ between devices and result in varied clinical utility based on comparative advantages and disadvantages.

10.7.1.1 Air-jet Nebulizers

Air-jet nebulizers are the oldest type of nebulizer and consist of a diverse group of devices produced by a variety of manufacturers. All air-jet nebulizers produce an aerosol through the Bernoulli effect. That is, a reduction in pressure occurs as air velocity increases in a given space. When compressed air is passed through the air-jet nebulizer, a volume of liquid is drawn up from a liquid reservoir into a region of high-shear forces. This liquid is then forcefully dispersed into droplets that are then carried out of the nebulizer on a gentle stream of carrier air, usually produced by the patient's breathing (Figure 10.7). Generally, these nebulizers consist of a drug-containing fluid reservoir or cup that is connected by a tube to a region through which a high velocity airstream is directed. An external air source, often a compressor, is the source of the high velocity airstream. As the air moves across the mouth of the tube connected to the reservoir, a low-pressure region is created by the Bernoulli principle that draws fluid up into the high-velocity airstream. Droplet shear, air turbulence, and a series of impaction baffles then create a gentle aerosol cloud with a polydisperse particle size distribution. Some droplets coalesce and return to the fluid reservoir while other particles form an aerosol cloud above the drug reservoir. This aerosol can then be suspended in the inspired airstream and be inhaled by the patient.

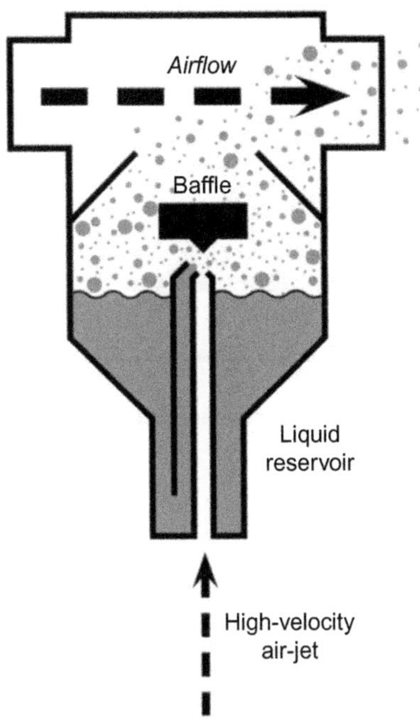

FIGURE 10.7 Schematic representation of an air-jet nebulizer.

A minimum volume within the reservoir cup is required for the Bernoulli effect to be effective. This often results in residual volumes that are retained within the nebulizer and cannot be nebulized through these devices. The chaotic environment of aerosol generation is also potentially wasteful because much of the dose fails to be nebulized initially. Aerosolized droplets often impact within the device and are further subjected to repeated shear stresses. Long nebulization times are often necessary due to these aerosolization inefficiencies. This turbulent aerosol generation mechanism is also potentially damaging to sensitive drug product formulations. Special considerations should be given to drug products that have possible sensitivity to repeated physical stresses (e.g., some suspensions or emulsions). Additionally, environmental exposure to exhaled drug aerosol is possible, especially for caregivers and healthcare workers and could be cause for concern based on possible drug effects.

Most air-jet nebulizers have a very broad aerodynamic particle size distribution due to the chaotic system of liquid shearing forces and droplet impaction prior to inspiration of the aerosol cloud. This broad distribution can lead to low FPF values for these nebulizers and inefficient drug delivery to the alveolar region of the lungs. Formulation factors such as surface tension, viscosity, osmolality, fluid reservoir volume, and temperature can affect the fluid dynamics within the nebulizer and ultimately droplet creation. Typically, those formulation factors that impede or inhibit droplet formation (e.g., increasing viscosity or increasing surface tension) would tend to create larger-sized droplets. Conversely, smaller droplets would be more prevalent for formulations that stabilize or induce droplet formation (e.g., surfactants or co-solvents that reduce surface tension). The air velocity, air composition, temperature, and humidity can also affect droplet creation and aerodynamic particle size distribution changes of the aerosol cloud. Typically, commercial products for nebulization are approved for use with specific air-jet nebulizers due to the variability in drug product aerosolization between different systems.

Despite the small nebulizer size, air-jet nebulizers are not typically very portable due to the need for a large external compressor. Some newer models integrate a small compressor with the nebulizer and are substantially smaller and quieter than older models. However, the compressor needed for proper functioning of air-jet nebulizers is a limitation for these systems because they are typically loud and bulky. Some compressors have variable pressure regulation, whereas others lack any regulation ability. Familiarity with the air compressor is a key requirement for the patient or caregiver for proper medication inhalation using air-jet nebulizers.

10.7.1.2 Ultrasonic Nebulizers

Ultrasonic nebulizers were developed much later than air-jet nebulizers and were designed to be more portable. These nebulizers incorporate a piezoelectric crystal at the bottom of the drug reservoir or cup. This crystal mechanically vibrates at a high frequency when subjected to an electric field. Crystal vibrations send shockwaves through the liquid-filled reservoir and cause droplet formation at the liquid surface through turbulence on the liquid surface and by cavitation in the liquid. Cavitation is the creation and implosion of voids in the liquid caused by crystal vibrations. The resulting droplets form a gentle aerosol cloud above the liquid reservoir. The aerodynamic particle size distribution of aerosols is also polydisperse due to the chaotic liquid surface environment but is generally less disperse than for air-jet systems. The aerosol cloud can then be mixed with inspiratory airflow for pulmonary drug delivery (Figure 10.8).

Ultrasonic nebulizers do not have a minimum volume for operation as do air-jet nebulizers and can indeed operate with relatively small volumes. These devices are often more efficient and require shorter nebulization times. The lack of a compressor allows hand-held ultrasonic nebulizers to be much more portable, quiet, and user-friendly. An electric source is required for operation and can often be supplied by battery power. The crystal vibrations can induce large temperature elevations in the liquid. Heat-labile drugs

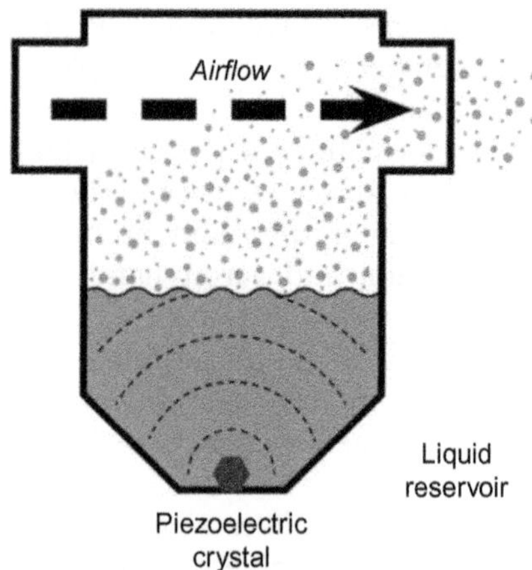

FIGURE 10.8 Schematic representation of an ultrasonic nebulizer.

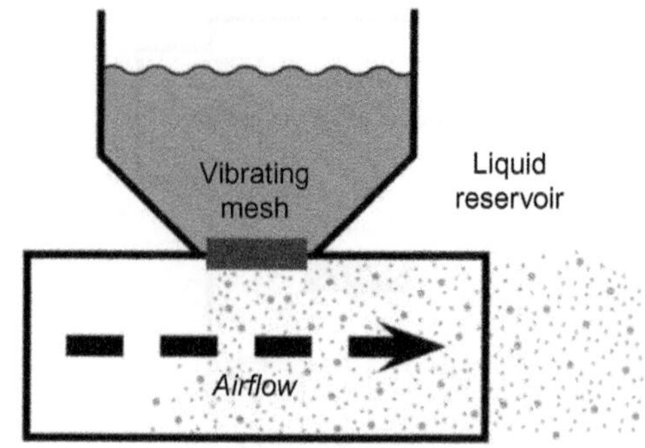

FIGURE 10.9 Schematic representation of a vibrating mesh nebulizer.

should be used with caution in ultrasonic nebulizers. As with air-jet nebulizers, formulation factors such as viscosity and surface tension can influence aerosol generation in ultrasonic nebulizers. Sensitive drug formulations have varied responses in ultrasonic nebulizers but are typically more stable through the aerosolization process than air-jet nebulizers.

10.7.1.3 *Vibrating-mesh Nebulizers*

The vibrating-mesh nebulizer is a relatively new nebulizer system that was designed to have more consistent aerosol particle size distributions and operate with a wider variety of formulations. These nebulizer systems attach a piezoelectric crystal to a laser-drilled metal mesh at the bottom of a drug reservoir or cup. When the crystal is subjected to an electric field, the metal mesh rapidly oscillates and forces the drug liquid through the holes in the mesh. A gentle aerosol is then produced with a uniform aerodynamic particle size distribution due to the uniform nature of the laser-drilled holes in the metal membrane. This aerosol is generated below or to the side of the liquid reservoir and can be delivered to a patient through a mouthpiece, face mask, or in-line junction for mechanically ventilated patients (Figure 10.9).

Vibrating-mesh nebulizers are relatively compact and portable systems that require a small nebulizer unit and a companion controller unit that houses the system electronics. These nebulizers are operationally silent and do not produce fluid heating as do ultrasonic nebulizers. They can aerosolize a wide range of liquid drug formulations. Specifically, low-stability formulations and sensitive drug products have been reported to be well aerosolized with these systems. Vibrating-mesh nebulizers have generated inhalable aerosols with formulations of higher viscosities and surface tensions than other nebulizers. However, the cost for vibrating mesh nebulizers is typically high.

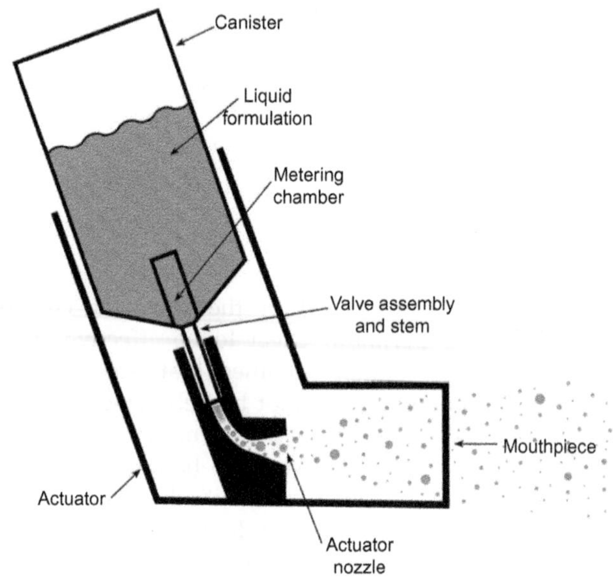

FIGURE 10.10 Schematic representation of a pressurized metered-dose inhaler (pMDI).

10.7.2 Pressurized Metered-dose Inhalers

A pressurized metered-dose inhaler (pMDI) is a self-contained aerosol device that is composed of (1) a drug-containing canister; (2) a valve assembly and metering chamber; and (3) an actuator that activates and directs drug formulation aerosolization and serves as a mouthpiece for aerosol inhalation (Figure 10.10) [4,11,17]. The canister is pressurized with a liquefied compressed gas, termed a propellant, which is metered by the actuator. The propellant is rapidly volatilized when exposed to atmospheric pressure following actuation, which leaves behind a liquid or solid aerosol cloud that is then inspired by the patient.

pMDIs are compact and portable inhalation devices that have gained wide acceptance for pulmonary drug delivery in the treatment of a variety of conditions, most notably asthma. Despite wide clinical acceptance, a substantial degree of coordination is needed between physically manipulating the pMDI device and patient breathing for optimal inhaled aerosol delivery. Each component in pMDI systems affects aerosol generation and inhaled aerosol delivery.

10.7.2.1 *Canister and Drug Formulation*

The canisters used for pMDIs must be able to withstand high pressures and compatible with the drug formulation. Aluminum, stainless steel, and glass have all been used for creation of canisters, with aluminum being the most common. Occasionally, inert coatings are applied to the canister interior to ensure compatibility with the formulation, prevent drug adhesion to the container, and ensure the formulation is able to be metered appropriately. The canister must be able to contain the pMDI formulation as well as headspace to compensate for formulation pressurization and allow for propellant vapor equilibrium.

pMDI formulations contain a propellant, the API, and excipients with varied functions (e.g., surfactants, solubilizers, stabilizers, lubricants, pH/tonicity adjustment agents). Based on API properties and excipient use, these formulations could be drug solubilized in propellant, drug solution mixed with propellant, drug suspended in propellant, and drug suspensions mixed with propellants. The resulting aerosol following pMDI actuation could then be liquid droplets or solid particles suspended in air. This versatility for inhaled aerosol formulation is an additional reason pMDI use is so prevalent for inhaled aerosol systems. Key formulation limitations then are based on the propellant properties and excipient acceptability. Currently formulated propellants include hydrofluoroalkane compounds (HFA) (Table 10.2) [8].

Only a limited number of excipients have been approved for use in inhaled delivery systems (Table 10.3). The FDA has expressed concerns for the pulmonary biocompatibility and clearance of inhaled excipients. Additionally, many excipients that are generally regarded as safe (GRAS) are not approved for pulmonary systems due to the potential for safety, toxicity, and irritation concerns when inhaled. Therefore, pharmaceutical companies must complete additional exhaustive toxicological and safety studies on any unapproved excipients that are formulated in new drug approval applications. Despite these limitations, several excipients have been approved as co-solvents, surfactants, lubricants, antioxidants, flavoring agents, and agents to adjust pH and tonicity.

TABLE 10.2 HFA Propellants Physicochemical Properties of some Hydrofluoroalkane (HFA) Propellants

Property	HFA134$_a$	HFA227
Molecular Formula	$C_2H_2F_4$	C_3HF_7
Molecular weight (g/mol)	102.0	170.0
Boiling point (°C)	−26.3	−16.5
Vapor pressure (psig at 20°C)	68.4	56.0
Liquid Density (g/cm^3)	1.21	1.41
Solubility in Water (%w/w)	0.193	0.058

TABLE 10.3 Excipients Selected FDA-Approved Excipients for Inhaled Drug Products

FDA-approved Function in Inhaled Formulations	Excipient
Co-solvents	Water
	Ethanol
	Glycerin
	Propylene glycol
	PEG 1000
Surfactants/Lubricants	Sorbitan trioleate
	Soya lecithin
	Lecithin
	Oleic acid
	Magnesium stearate
	Sodium lauryl sulfate
Carrier Particles	Lactose
	Mannitol
	Dextrose
Preservatives/Antioxidants	Methylparaben, propylparaben
	Chlorobutanol
	Benzalkonium chloride
	Cetylpyridinium chloride
	Thymol
	Ascorbic acid
	Sodium bisulfite, sodium metabisulfite, sodium bisulfate
	EDTA
Buffers, pH Adjustment, or Tonicity Adjustment	NaOH, Tromethamine, Ammonia
	HCl, H_2SO_4, HNO_3, Citric acid
	$CaCl_2$
	$CaCO_3$

(*Continued*)

TABLE 10.3 (*Continued*)

FDA-approved Function in Inhaled Formulations	Excipient
	Sodium citrate
	Sodium chloride
	Disodium EDTA
Flavoring	Saccharin
	Menthol
	Ascorbic Acid
Others	Glycine
	Lysine
	Gelatin
	Povidone K25
	Silicone dioxide
	Titanium dioxide
	Zinc oxide

Note: Some products might have multiple functions in a given formulation.

10.7.2.2 *Valve Assembly*

All pMDI valves contain a metering chamber and a valve stem despite numerous valve assembly designs. The valve assembly in pMDI devices is the key mechanical determinant for drug dosing because the metering chamber volume capacity and drug concentration within the formulation limit the potential dose a patient can receive. Most metering chambers have 25–100 μL volume capacities and are surrounded by a reservoir of liquid drug formulation to promote complete chamber filling. Some devices require priming of the metering chamber before patient dosing can begin.

Valve assemblies mechanically operate based on actuation of the device by depressing the canister so that the valve stem is depressed against the actuator. When the valve stem is depressed, a valve opens to connect the metering chamber to the channel in the valve stem. The pressurized metered dose expands through a channel in the valve stem. This channel directs the pressurized formulation into the actuator where rapid propellant vaporization produces a high-velocity aerosol cloud. Actuation then allows formulation to refill the metering chamber in preparation for the next dose.

10.7.2.3 *Actuator*

The actuator is a molded or formed plastic component that performs several functions for proper pMDI use. It holds the canister in the proper orientation for device use, serves as a surface against which the valve stem can depress, provides a space for principal propellant vaporization, redirects the high-velocity aerosol cloud toward the patient, and has a mouthpiece for patient use. Canisters are typically operated in an inverted position where the valve assembly is in contact with the pressurized liquid formulation to allow for proper metering. The valve stem is in contact with a specialized plastic component that contains an expansion chamber and the actuator nozzle. The expansion chamber receives the metered dose and acts as a space for the propellant to vaporize and induce droplet shear. The actuator nozzle restricts formulation movement out of the expansion chamber to form a spray cone and induces substantial particle turbulence. The actuator nozzle hole diameter is a key determinant for the aerosol particle size distribution.

10.7.2.4 *Patient Use of pMDI Devices*

The high-velocity aerosol cloud produced by most pMDI devices imparts a substantial amount of momentum to aerosolized particles. This tends to produce high levels of inertial impaction in the back of the throat unless optimal breathing technique is employed or particles decelerate before inhalation. A spacer is often a static air-volume particle deceleration chamber that allows particles to lose velocity prior to inhalation. Many spacers fit on the actuator mouthpiece adapter and facilitate better drug deposition in the lungs than can be achieved following typical inhaler use. Another option some healthcare providers recommend to promote aerosol deceleration is for the patient to hold the pMDI close to and in front of the mouth for actuation.

Proper pMDI use requires a substantial degree of patient cognition and physical coordination. The patient must be able to physically handle and actuate the device while controlling breathing and timing inspiration with device actuation. Typical patient counseling for pMDI devices could contain the following steps: (1) take a few deep cleansing breaths and expel the breaths fully; (2) while holding the device in the proper orientation, slowly and deeply inspire; (3) during this inspiration, actuate the device and continue to inspire a full breath even after the device has been actuated; (4) hold your breath for a short period of time; (5) slowly expel the held breath; and (6) repeat steps 1–5 for the prescribed dose as instructed by the healthcare provider.

Thoroughly mixing the formulation before device actuation will promote inter-dose uniformity and homogenous metered doses. Mixing can be promoted by the patient before each dose by vigorously shaking the pMDI device. Dose uniformity can then be impaired by improper formulation mixing and over the life span of the device as the formulation is exhausted. Dose uniformity is also improved by consistent device priming but is unlikely in clinical settings due to dose wasting. It is critical that patients clean and maintain pMDI devices. Patients should not mechanically disturb the nozzle but instead use gentle cleaning procedures if the nozzle becomes obstructed.

10.7.3 Dry Powder Inhalers

Dry powder inhalers (DPIs) are a very diverse group of often portable inhaler devices that create an aerosol of solid particles suspended in air [3]. These devices generally have an air-inlet channel, a dose metering and holding chamber, and a mouthpiece adapter. Substantial differences exist between the various aerosolization mechanisms used by these inhalers for drug powder dispersion. DPIs can be single-dose devices where the drug dose is loaded into the machine prior to each use and multidose devices that contain either a drug reservoir or multiple unit doses. Once a dose is loaded into the holding chamber and prior to inspiration, all DPIs require a proper orientation to prevent the prepared and primed dose from leaking or spilling out of the device. A key limitation for these devices is the requirement of both physical dexterity and cognitive ability to manipulate the device in order to load, meter, prime, prepare, and/or actuate the dose.

10.7.3.1 Passive DPI Devices

The aerosolization mechanisms vary substantially between DPIs. Some devices use the patient's inspiratory airflow to disperse the dose. These mechanisms direct air from inlet channels in various device-specific pathways to inducing airflow turbulence, vibrations, and/or powder motion in the dose-holding chamber. A mesh or screen is also often placed in between the dose-holding chamber and the mouthpiece adapter to assist in aerosol dispersion and prevent the inhalation of large dose fragments or particles. These aerosolization mechanisms are generally passive and require very rapid and full patient inspirations to adequately aerosolize the dose. As a result, inter-and intra-patient pulmonary drug deposition can vary substantially based on inspiratory inconsistencies. Additionally, many patients are incapable of producing inspiratory airflows of sufficient velocity to adequately aerosolize the drug dose. Dose retention in the inhaler can be a significant problem in passive devices based on patient use and might require training and device cleaning.

10.7.3.2 Active DPI Devices

Other DPI devices utilize active aerosolization mechanisms by using external energy sources. Active devices can use compressed gases, induced pressure differences, and electronic or piezoelectric mechanisms to disperse the powder drug dose. For example, some DPI systems use pressurized air or vacuums to induce airflow through the device for drug powder aerosolization. Other devices induce vibrations or acoustic waves to aerosolize drug powders. Active aerosolization mechanisms separate inspiration from aerosol generation and can avoid the drug deposition variability of passive systems. Patients are then instructed to inspire slowly and deeply, often with breath-holding for active DPI use.

10.7.3.3 DPI Formulations

Drug powder formulations differ substantially from those used in nebulizers and pMDIs [22]. Often, the formulation has been prepared for maximum pulmonary particle deposition by having powder MMAD values between 1 and 5 μm. Significant efforts are expended to rationally engineer and prepare dry powder drug particles in this optimal aerodynamic size range. However, these fine particle sizes often have poor flowability and dispersibility in air. Some products are formulated as small-particle loose aggregates that will readily disperse under the DPI aerosolization mechanisms. Other systems employ small drug particles adhered to the surface of large, inert carrier particles that have improved aerosolization properties. Once adhered particles are dispersed in the airstream, the smaller particles can be inhaled deeper into the lungs.

10.7.4 Breath-assisted Inhalers

Newly developed technology has been incorporated into inhaler devices to better optimize drug delivery to the lungs. This technology synchronizes the device function with the patient's breathing for superior drug delivery compared to typical devices. Improved drug delivery can be achieved by avoiding drug retention within the device, minimizing drug waste by expiration, and ensuring appropriate inspiratory airflow will carry aerosols into the lung. These devices monitor the patient for changes in breathing pattern (e.g., respiration rate, peak flow, tidal volume) and only generate an aerosol timed for the beginning of inspiration. Breath-assisted inhalers can also assist and train patients in proper breathing techniques for optimized pulmonary drug delivery. Studies have demonstrated the drug delivery efficiency and benefit of these devices. However, a major disadvantage for these systems is a very high cost.

10.8. CONCLUSIONS

Aerosol dosage forms are becoming increasingly common as drug products are designed and developed for the pulmonary route of drug administration. However, lung anatomy and physiology impose challenges for the formulation, aerosol generation methods, and delivery of aerosols and gases to the lungs. Patient breathing and device manipulation and coordination can also impact pulmonary drug delivery. Current and future drug development has allowed the rational delivery of gases and vapors, solid particles, and liquid droplets through several devices. The most common aerosol dosage forms include liquid formulations delivered by air-jet, ultrasonic, or vibrating mesh nebulizers; solid or liquid propellant-based formulations delivered through pressurized metered-dose inhalers; and solid powders delivered through dry powder inhalers.

CASE STUDIES

Case 10.1

The vapor pressure of pure propellant 11 (MW = 137.4) is 13.4 pounds per square inch (psi), and the vapor pressure of propellant 12 (MW = 120.9) is 84.9. A mixture of 50:50 gram weight of two propellants was added to prepare an aerosol in a glass container. You, as a fourth year pharmacy student, are asked to find out the total pressure of this propellant mixture and advise the manufacturer whether he can use a glass container for this aerosol packaging.

Approach: Both Raoult's law and Dalton's law of partial pressure are used to calculate the total pressure:

Moles of Prop-11 = 50/137.4 = 0.364 moles, Moles of Prop-12 = 50/120.9 = 0.414.
Mole fraction of Prop-11 = 0.364/(0.364 + 0.414) = 0.468, Mole fraction of Prop-12 = 1 − 0.468 = 0.532.
Partial pressure of Prop-11 = 0.468 × 13.4 = 6.27 psi.
Partial press of Prop-12 = 0.532 × 84.9 = 45.2 psi.
Total pressure = 6.27 + 45.2 = 51.5 psi.

The second question is whether this mixture can be packaged in a glass container. The total pressure is more than 25 psi, which is the maximum pressure a glass container can withstand. Advise the manufacturer to use aluminum or plastic containers instead.

Case 10.2

One of the advantages of a pulmonary delivery system is that it is a noninvasive alternative for parenteral injection. Then why was Exubera, the first FDA-approved inhaled insulin, pulled from the market?

Approach: Inhaled insulin (brand name Exubera) was approved in January 2006. Upon its approval, Pfizer and market analysts predicted that Exubera would be a blockbuster drug since it was the first inhaled option on the market for people who needed to take insulin. However, Exubera's high price and bulky inhaler, as well as concerns about its effects on lung function, led to much lower sales than had been expected. The journal *Diabetes Care* reported on study in which 582 adults with Type 1 diabetes were tested for participants' lung function; the study found that both test groups experienced small declines within the first three months [28]. The decline observed in the inhaled insulin group was larger than that of the parenteral insulin users. However, neither group experienced a drop in lung function of more than 2%, and deterioration did not progress in either group for the rest of the study period (2 years). The inhaled insulin group also experienced more coughing than the injected insulin group (38% vs. 13%). Rates of other side effects were similar between the two groups.

In a statement on the Exubera product website (www.exubera.com), Pfizer emphasizes that Exubera was a safe and effective dosage form and was not discontinued because of any concerns in those areas. Rather, it says, "Pfizer has made this decision because too few patients are taking Exubera."

Acknowledgments

The authors wish to thank G. Scott Oldroyd, MD, for technical guidance regarding inhaled anesthetics.

References

[1] Anderson PJ. History of aerosol therapy: liquid nebulization to MDIs to DPIs. Respir Care 2005;50(9):1139–50.
[2] Carvalho TC, Peters JI, Williams III RO. Influence of particle size on regional lung deposition—What evidence is there? Int J Pharm 2011;406(1–2):1–10.
[3] Crowder TM, Donovan MJ. Science and technology of dry powder inhalers. In: Smyth HDC, Hickey AJ, editors. Controlled pulmonary drug delivery. Springer; 2011. p. 203–22.
[4] da Rocha SRP, Bharatwaj B, Saiprasad S. Science and technology of pressurized metered-dose inhalers. In: Smyth HDC, Hickey AJ, editors. Controlled pulmonary drug delivery. Springer; 2011. p. 165–202.
[5] Gibbons A, Smyth HDC. Science and technology of nebulizers and liquid-based aerosol generators. In: Smyth HDC, Hickey AJ, editors. Controlled pulmonary drug delivery. Springer; 2011. p. 223–36.
[6] Henning A, et al. Pulmonary drug delivery: medicines for inhalation. In: Schäfer-Korting M, editor. Drug delivery. Springer; 2010. p. 171–92.
[7] Kleinstreuer C, Zhang Z, Li Z. Modeling airflow and particle transport/deposition in pulmonary airways. Respir Physiol Neurobiol 2008;163(1–3):128–38.
[8] Leach CL. The CFC to HFA transition and its impact on pulmonary drug development. Respir Care 2005;50(9):1201–8.
[9] Levitzky MG. Pulmonary physiology. 7th ed. Chicago, IL: McGraw Hill; 2007. p. 280.

[10] McClellan RO. Particle interactions with the respiratory tract. In: Gehr P, Heyder J, editors. Particle-lung interactions. New York, NY: Marcel Dekker, Inc.; 2000. p. 3–63.

[11] Newman SP. Principles of metered-dose inhaler design. Respir Care 2005;50(9):1177–90.

[12] O'Donnell KP, Smyth HDC. Macro- and microstructure of the airways for drug delivery. In: Smyth HDC, Hickey AJ, editors. *Controlled pulmonary drug delivery*. Springer; 2011. p. 1–20.

[13] Patel PM, Patel HH, Roth DM. General anesthetics and therapeutic gases. In: Brunton LL, editor. The pharmacological basis of therapeutics. Chicago, IL: McGraw Hill; 2011.

[14] Patton JS, Byron PR. Inhaling medicines: delivering drugs to the body through the lungs. Nat Rev Drug Discov 2007;6(1):67–74.

[15] Peters JI, Levine SM. Introduction to pulmonary function testing. In: DiPiro JT, editor. *Pharmacotherapy: a pathophysiologic approach*. Chicago, IL: McGraw Hill; 2011.

[16] Pilcer G, Amighi K. Formulation strategy and use of excipients in pulmonary drug delivery. Int J Pharm 2010;392(1–2):1–19.

[17] Rubin BK, Fink JB. Optimizing aerosol delivery by pressurized metered-dose inhalers. Respir Care 2005;50(9):1191–200.

[18] Sanders M. Inhalation therapy: an historical review. Primary Care Respir J 2007;16(2):71–81.

[19] Schulz H, Brand P, Heyder J. Particle deposition in the respiratory tract. In: Gehr P, Heyder J, editors. Particle-lung interactions. New York, NY: Marcel Dekker, Inc.; 2000. p. 229–90.

[20] Sciarra JJ, Sciarra CJ. Aerosols. In: Allen LV, editor. The science and practice of pharmacy. Pharmaceutical Press; 2013. p. 999–1016.

[21] Sinko PJ. Colloids. Martin's physical pharmacy and pharmaceutical sciences. New York, NY: Lippincott Williams & Wilkins; 2006.

[22] Telko MJ, Hickey AJ. Dry powder inhaler formulation. Respir Care 2005;50(9):1209–27.

[23] Wang N-S. Anatomy and ultrastructure of the lung. In: Bittar EE, editor. Pulmonary biology in health and disease. New York: Springer; 2004. p. 1–19.

[24] Weibel ER. What makes a good lung? Swiss Med Wkly 2009;139(27–28):375–86.

[25] Xu Z, Hickey AJ. The physics of aerosol droplet and particle generation from inhalers. In: Smyth HDC, Hickey AJ, editors. Controlled pulmonary drug delivery. Springer; 2011. p. 75–100.

[26] Yeh HC, Phalen RF, Raabe OG. Factors influencing the deposition of inhaled particles. Environ Health Perspect 1976;15:147–56.

[27] Zhang Z, Kleinstreuer C. Airflow structures and nano-particle deposition in a human upper airway model. J Comput Phys 2004;198(1):178–210.

[28] Skyler JS, Jovanovic L, Klioze S, Reis J, Duggan W. Two-year safety and efficacy of inhaled human insulin (Exubera) in adult patients with type 1 diabetes. Diabetes Care 2007;30:579–85.

CHAPTER

11

Semisolid Dosage Forms

Shailendra Kumar Singh[1], *Kalpana Nagpal*[1] *and Sangita Saini*[2]

[1]Department of Pharmaceutical Sciences, G. J. University of Science and Technology, Hisar, India

[2]PDM College of Pharmacy, Sarai Aurangabad, Bahadurgarh, Haryana, India

CHAPTER OBJECTIVES

- Identify and classify the various types of semisolid dosage forms.
- Discuss the theory involved in the preparation of ointments, creams, pastes, and transdermal patches.
- Describe the clinical applications of semisolid dosage forms.
- Define percutaneous absorption.
- Discuss methods of enhancement of percutaneous absorption.
- Explain the evaluations of quality for ointments, creams, pastes, and transdermal patches.
- Discuss the mechanism of drug release from the transdermal system.

Keywords

- Cream
- Ointment
- Paste
- Percutaneous absorption
- Transdermal patch

11.1. INTRODUCTION

Semisolid preparations represent dosage forms that have properties in between solid and liquid dosage forms and possess characteristic rheological properties such that they can be easily applied on biological membranes and can be retained on the site of application for a prolonged time. Semisolid dosage forms may contain one or more active ingredients in suspended/dissolved forms, in inclusion complexes, or in a solubilized state and are applied topically to the skin or on the surface of the eye, nasally, vaginally, or rectally for local and/or systemic effects [1]. Semisolid systems are characterized as materials that retain their shape when unconfined [2] and are too viscous or thick to be considered as liquid dosage forms yet not rigid enough to be considered as solid dosage forms [3]. If the active ingredient is insoluble in the vehicle, then in addition to ensuring uniformity of the distribution in the mix, potency uniformity depends on the control of particle size. An increase in particle size causes a reduction in the surface area and absorption through the skin, and due to grittiness, it becomes more irritating to the skin [4]. Such forms may be applied directly to the skin or mucous membranes of the eye, or to body cavities nasally, vaginally, or rectally, which constitute about 8–10% of all dosage forms in the market [5].

The major advantages of semisolid dosage forms include their demonstrated ability to readily incorporate a wide variety of hydrophilic and hydrophobic drugs, to reduce the undesirable effects arising from the presystemic metabolism, and to minimize unnecessary fluctuations in drug concentration, which in turn will significantly enhance the efficacy of the incorporated drug. The semisolid classification is not based on any scientific criteria but can be divided into a range of different types of formulations based on their traditional usage. Creams, gels, ointments, pastes, suppositories, and transdermal drug delivery are examples of these dosage forms. The current U.S. Food and Drug

Pharmaceutics. DOI: http://dx.doi.org/10.1016/B978-0-12-386890-9.00011-X

Administration (FDA) Center for Drug Evaluation and Research (CDER) Data Standards Manual contributes the definition of a semisolid, which is the same as in the USP, BP, EP, and Japanese Pharmacopeia [6].

Creams are semisolid emulsion systems containing an emulsifying base used in dermatological treatments and in cosmetology. This preparation has good patient acceptability and can be safely applied on the skin. Creams are of two types: (i) oil-in-water (aqueous cream) and (ii) water-in-oil (oily cream) type emulsion systems. In the case of oil-in-water (o/w) creams, oil is dispersed in water. Oil is called the dispersed phase, and water is the continuous phase. These o/w creams are hydrophilic by nature, whereas in water-in-oil (w/o) creams, water is in the dispersed phase and oil forms the continuous phase. These w/o creams have a greasy appearance, but they moisturize the skin very effectively.

Examples:

Triamcinolone acetonide cream (0.1% Aristocort A cream, used in the treatment of inflammatory dermatoses)
Tolnaftate cream (1% Tinactin cream, used in the treatment of fungal infection)

Gels are semisolid systems in which a liquid phase is immobilized by a three-dimensional network, composed of a self-assembled, intertwined, net-like structure cross-linked by a suitable gelling agent. Despite their liquid composition, these systems demonstrate the appearance and rheological behavior of solids [7]. They are coherent masses generally composed of one phase (oil or water) or two phases (oil and water), one of which is a continuous (external) phase, and the other is a dispersed (internal) phase. The physical and chemical bonds between the molecules provide this system with a relatively stable and structured system that has decreased mobility and increased viscosity of the molecule [2].

Examples:

Aluminum hydroxide gel, USP
Lidocaine hydrochloride (2%) gel

Pastes are semisolid stiff preparations containing a high proportion (more than 20%) of finely powdered material to a conventional ointment base. Powders such as zinc oxide, titanium dioxide, starch, kaolin, and talc are incorporated in high concentrations into a preferably lipophilic, greasy vehicle. A clinically distinctive feature that is generally attributed to pastes is the quality to absorb exudates through the nature of the powder or other absorptive components [8]. Because of their stiffness, pastes are not suitable for application to hairy parts of the body.

Example:

Zinc oxide paste

Ointments are viscous semisolid preparations used topically on body surfaces. These surfaces include the skin and the mucous membranes of the eye, vagina, anus, and nose. Ointments may or may not be medicated. Medicated ointments contain a medicament dissolved, suspended, or emulsified in the base. Ointments are used topically for several purposes, e.g., as protectants, antiseptics, emollients, antipruritics, keratolytics, or astringents. Ointment bases are almost always anhydrous and generally contain one or more medicaments in suspension, solution, or dispersion. Ointment bases may be oligeanous (hydrocarbon), absorptive, water-removable, and water-soluble. On the basis of their level of action, they are classified as epidermatic, endodermatic, or diadermatic.

Examples:

Lidocaine ointment (2.5% Xylocaine ointment, used for relief of pain)
Mupirocin ointment (Bactroban 2% ointment, used for the treatment of skin infection)

Suppositories are solid bodies of various weights, sizes, and shapes suitable for insertion into a body cavity, which includes the rectum, vagina, or urethra, for both local as well as systemic effect. They usually melt, soften, or dissolve at body temperature.

Examples:

Bisacodyl suppository (Dulcolax, 10 mg, cathartic)
Indomethacin (Indocin, 50 mg, anti-inflammatory)

A chemically synthesized material or a plant extract can be used as a drug in semisolid formulations. The formulation of the dosage form is a combination of the drug and different types of inactive components called additives or excipients. The additives, such as emulsifiers, thickening agents, antimicrobial agents, antioxidants, or stabilizing agents, are added to the formulation. A suitable antimicrobial agent should be added in an appropriate concentration, if formulation is prone to the growth of microorganisms or the preparations themselves may have adequate antimicrobial properties. Assurance must be provided from the preformulation studies that active ingredients are compatible with the excipient used in the formulation. The base used in the preparation should be inert, odorless, and smooth. It should be physically and chemically stable, and it should be compatible with skin and the medicaments. It should be of such consistency that it can be applied easily on the skin. It should neither retard the healing of the wound nor produce any irritation on the skin.

11.2. CLASSIFICATION OF SEMISOLID DOSAGE FORMS

The traditional classification of various semisolid dosage forms cannot distinguish properly between two semisolid dosage forms. Moreover, the definitions are not based on any scientific principle. Physicochemical properties such as loss on drying; specific gravity, especially rheology; and composition of formulation are important parameters for the classification of semisolid dosage forms [6]. A decision tree can be used to design a new topical dosage form on the base of physicochemical properties, as shown in Figure 11.1. See also Figure 11.2.

11.2.1 Ointments

Ointment dosage forms are homogenous semisolid preparations intended for local or transdermal delivery of active substances for application to the skin [9]. These semisolid preparations are intended to adhere to the skin or certain mucous membranes and are usually solutions or dispersions of one or more medicaments in nonaqueous bases. Ointment bases are often anhydrous and include fats, oils, and waxes of animal, vegetable, or mineral origin; nonoleaginous and synthetic substances are also incorporated in the substance. Ointments are used as a vehicle for medicaments intended to produce a pharmacological effect at or near the application site; they are also applied as emollients and skin protectives. The ointment bases are soft hydrocarbon-based preparations, composed of fluid hydrocarbon (liquid paraffin) meshed in a matrix of higher melting solid hydrocarbon petrolatum (soft paraffin or paraffin wax). They can stain clothes because they are greasy in nature. Principal ingredients forming the system, generally hydrocarbon and silicon oil, are generally poor solvents for most drugs, seemingly setting a low limit on the drug delivery capabilities of the system.

The rate of diffusion from the ointment bases has been observed to be pH dependent [10]. The amount of drug release depends on the composition of the vehicle and the concentration of drug incorporated in it [11]. The use of ointments as an ocular drug vehicle adds an important dimension to topical therapy. Ointments are well tolerated and fairly safe; they also provide an excellent means for enhanced ocular contact time. In the case of certain antibiotics, this improved contact time yields increased ocular drug levels. Corticosteroid ointments as well as suspensions do not penetrate into the eye, which may be related to the binding of the drug to the ointment base and also to the physicochemical property of the particular drug. Like other ophthalmic preparations, ointments may become contaminated. Ophthalmic ointments should not be instilled into eyes with open wounds. Instillation of ointments into postoperative eyes where wound closure is secure appears to be safe and effective.

There are two main types of ointments:

- *Water-soluble ointments* include mixtures of polyethylene glycol 400 (a liquid) and propylene glycols 3350 (a solid) in which their consistency can be easily controlled. They are easily washed off and are used in burn dressings, as lubricants, and as vehicles that readily allow passage of drugs into the skin, e.g., hydrocortisone ointment.
- *Water-insoluble ointments* are further divided into two classes:
  - *Emulsifying ointments* are made from emulsifying wax (cetostearyl alcohol and sodium lauryl sulphate) and paraffins.
  - *Nonemulsifying ointments* do not mix with water. They adhere to the skin to prevent evaporation and heat loss; i.e., they can be considered a form of occlusive dressing, with increased systemic absorption where skin maceration may occur. Nonemulsifying ointments are helpful as vehicles in chronic dry and scaly conditions, such as atopic eczema; they are not appropriate where there is significant exudation. They are difficult to remove except with oil or detergent and are messy and inconvenient, especially on hairy skin. Paraffin ointment contains beeswax, paraffin, and cetostearyl alcohol [12].

Ointments may be medicated or nonmedicated, the latter type being commonly referred to as ointment bases. The ointment bases are used as emollients or lubricating agents or used as vehicles in the preparation of medicated ointments.

11.2.1.1 Classification of Ointment Bases

i. Hydrocarbon (oleaginous) bases

Examples:

a. Petrolatum, USP, is a mixture of semisolid hydrocarbons.
Melting point 38°C–60°C
Commercial Product: Vaseline

b. Yellow ointment, USP, 95% (w/w) petrolatum and 5% (w/w) yellow wax

c. White ointment, 95% (w/w) petrolatum and 5% (w/w) white wax

d. Paraffin, NF: It is a purified mixture of solid hydrocarbons obtained from petroleum. It is used to stiffen oleaginous semisolid ointment bases.

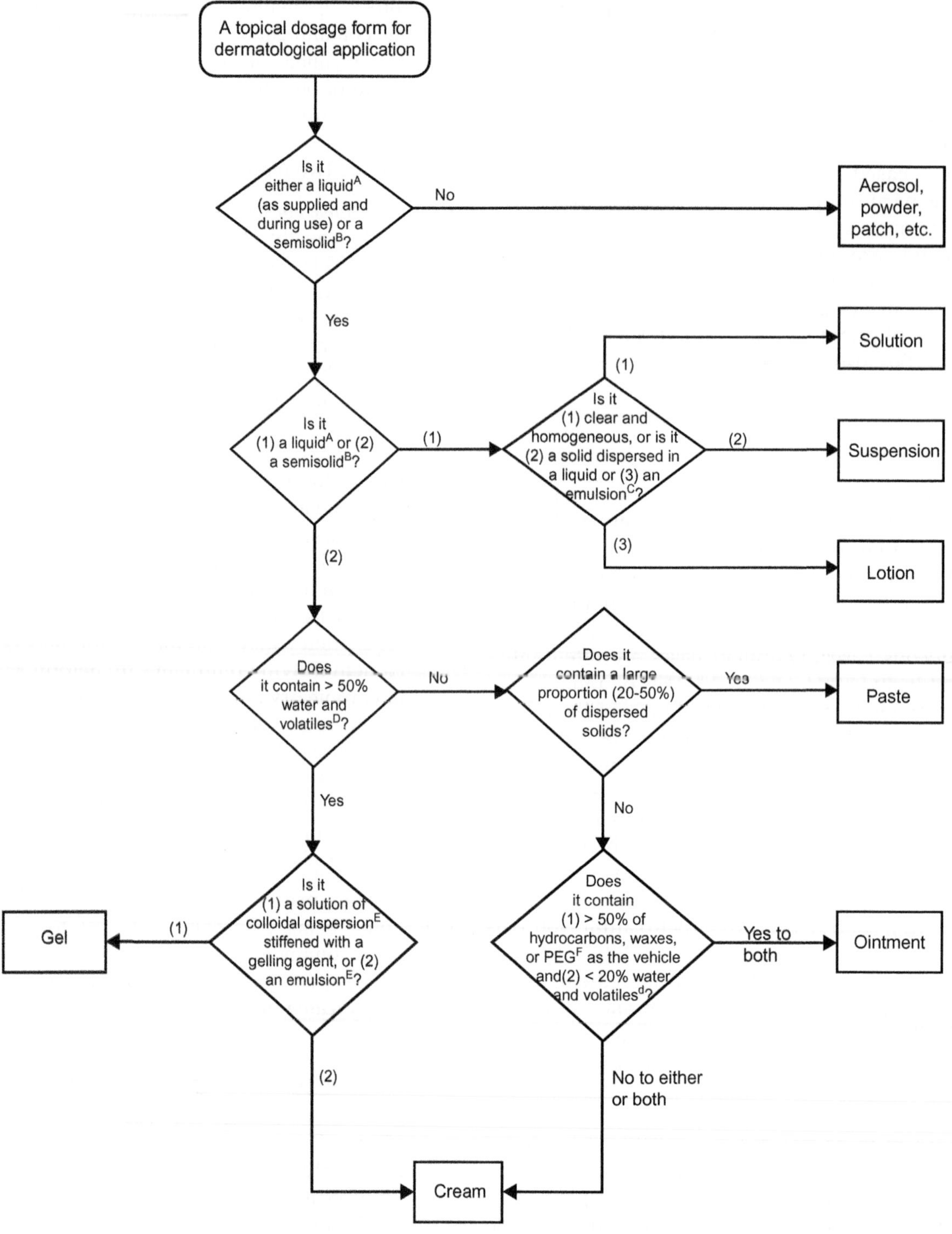

FIGURE 11.1 Decision tree on topical dosage form nomenclature. (A) A liquid is pourable; it flows and conforms to its container at room temperature. A liquid displays Newtonian or pseudoplastic flow behavior. (B) A semisolid is not pourable; it does not flow or conform to its container at room temperature. It does not flow at low shear stress and generally exhibits plastic flow behavior. (C) An emulsion is a two-phase system consisting of at least two immiscible liquids, one of which is dispersed as globules (internal or dispersed phase) within the other liquid phase (external or continuous phase), generally stabilized by an emulsifying agent. (D) Water and volatiles as measured by a loss on drying (LOD) test by heating at 105°C until constant weight is achieved. (E) A colloidal dispersion is a system in which particles of colloidal dimension are distributed uniformly throughout a liquid. (F) Polyethylene glycol, a vehicle for semi solid dosage forms.

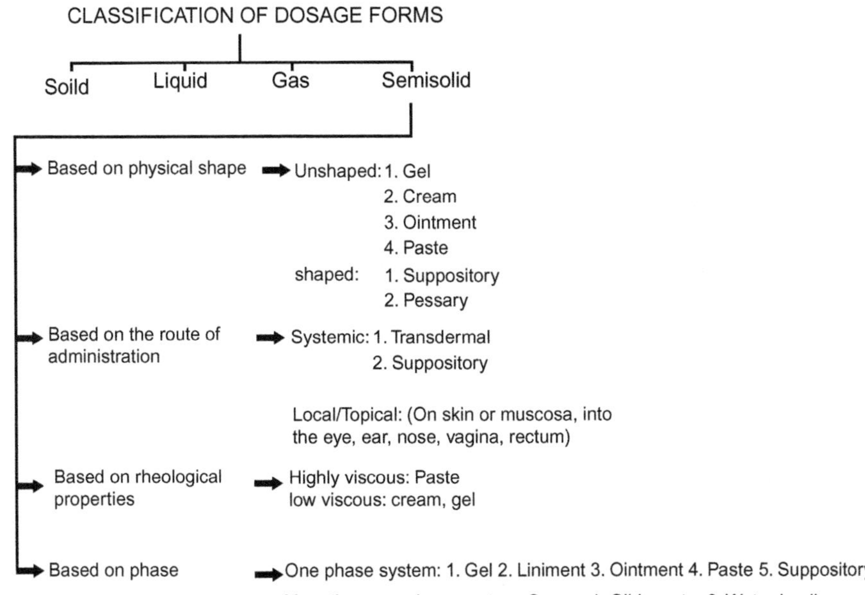

FIGURE 11.2 Classification of various semisolid dosage forms.

e. Mineral oil, USP: It is a mixture of liquid hydrocarbons obtained from petroleum. It is used as a levigating agent. Commonly known as liquid petrolatum.

ii. Absorption bases (anhydrous)

There are two types of absorption bases:

a. Those that permit the incorporation of aqueous solutions to become water-in-oil emulsions.

Examples:

i. Hydrophilic petrolatum, USP (3% cholesterol in white petrolatum)

ii. Anhydrous lanolin

iii. Aquaphor (6 parts wool-wax alcohols and 99 parts of aliphatic hydrocarbons)

b. Those that are already water-in-oil emulsions which have the capability to absorb additional water.

Example: Cold cream

iii. Water-removable bases

Water-removable bases can be washed from skin or clothing with water. These bases can be diluted with water or with an aqueous solution.

The water-removable bases consist of three parts: an oil phase, a water phase, and emulsifiers.

Example: Acid Mantle Cream®

iv. Water-soluble bases

Water-soluble bases contain only water-soluble substances; they are water-removable and "greaseless."

Example: Polyethylene glycol ointment, USP

11.2.1.2 Selection of the Appropriate Base

The following factors should be considered before selecting an ointment base:

- Release rate of the particular drug from the ointment base
- Enhancement of percutaneous absorption
- Stability and incompatibility of the drug in the ointment base
- Whether the drug influences the consistency or other features of the ointment base

11.2.1.3 Ideal Properties of an Ointment Base

- Nonirritating, nondehydrating, and nongreasy
- Compatible with common medicaments
- Stable
- Easily removable with water
- Good absorptive properties (water and other aqueous liquids)
- Good release properties of the drug from the base

11.2.1.4 Preparation of Ointments

Ointments can be prepared through two methods:

- Mechanical incorporation
- Fusion

The choice of method depends on the drug used and the physical properties of the constituents of the base.

11.2.1.4.1 PREPARATION BY MECHANICAL INCORPORATION

Incorporation involves mixing a drug to be incorporated into the ointment base. In a small-scale operation, it can be achieved by using either a mortar and pestle or a glass slab and a pair of spatulas. When ointments are to be prepared in large amounts (5 pounds or more), mechanical mixers are generally used.

Examples of Large-Scale Mixing Equipment:

Roller mill
Hobart mixer

When solid ingredients are incorporated, it is very important to bear in mind the particle size of the powder to be incorporated and that it is always kept as small as possible. The best result is obtained by mixing small amounts of the base with the powder to form a very smooth nucleus, which is eventually mixed with the remainder of the base. The ingredients can also be levigated with a levigating agent (mineral oil for oleaginous base or glycerol for oil-in-water bases) to form a smooth paste. The paste is then mixed with the remainder of the base.

11.2.1.4.2 FUSION METHOD

In the fusion method, the base is melted separately, starting with the highest melting point materials. Other oil phase ingredients are added in order of decreasing melting points. In this way, the whole base is not heated up to the highest temperature. Usually, heating is achieved by using a water bath to avoid excessive temperatures. The solid to be incorporated is also added to this melt, depending on its melting point. The ointment should be stirred until it congeals to ensure a homogeneous product.

11.2.1.5 Containers

Two different types of containers are most commonly used for packaging of ointments: ointment jars and tubes.

11.2.2 Creams

Creams are widely used in cosmetics; they are an essential part of daily make-up used to moisturize skin. These viscous semisolid emulsion systems have an opaque appearance in contrast to translucent ointments. This dosage form can penetrate the outer layer (keratinized layer) of the skin and provide emolliency.

Creams can be classified into two categories: medicated and nonmedicated. Medicated creams have active pharmaceutical ingredients with a particular pharmacological activity such as antibacterial, antifungal, or antipruritic, whereas nonmedicated creams are used for cosmetic purposes to moisturize, beautify, and nourish the skin. Skin cream reduces surface roughness and increases the hydrophilic properties of skin. The higher viscosity results in higher friction and longer durability. Cream-treated skin reduces charge build-up on the skin surface [13].

Creams, being semisolid emulsions, are also classified as oil-in-water (o/w) and water-in-oil (w/o) types depending on whether the continuous phase is oil or water. The consistency and rheological character depend on the type of cream. Properly designed o/w creams are an elegant drug delivery system, pleasing in both appearance and feel after application. Oil-in-water creams are nongreasy and can be easily removed by rinsing with water. Since the external phase is water, these creams can be easily diluted with water and therefore are water washable. They are good for most topical purposes and are considered particularly suited for application to oozing wounds because they have a tendency to absorb water. Water-in-oil creams are composed of small droplets of water dispersed in a continuous oily phase. Water-in-oil creams are more difficult to handle and are not water washable. Since many drugs that are incorporated into creams are hydrophobic, they are released more readily from water-in-oil creams than oil-in-water creams.

Water-in-oil creams are also more moisturizing because they provide an oily barrier that reduces water loss from the stratum corneum, the outermost layer of the skin, and are widely used as cold creams where the oil phase forms a protective covering and prevents excessive loss of moisture from the skin in the winter season.

Creams are semisolid emulsion systems with a creamy white appearance. Creams can be classified as follows:

- Oil-in-water (o/w) creams
  - Foundation creams
  - Hand creams
  - Shaving creams
- Water-in-oil (w/o) creams
  - Cold creams
  - Emollient creams

Properly designed (o/w) creams make a good topical drug delivery system for the following reasons:

- They have a pleasing appearance.
- They provide a good feeling after application.
- They are nongreasy and washable.
- They are suitable for oozing wounds.

11.2.3 Pastes

Pastes are semisolid preparations for topical use, into which a high percentage of an insoluble solid has been added. The higher amount of particulate matter stiffens the system through direct interactions of the dispersed particulates and by adsorption of the liquid hydrocarbon fraction of the vehicle on the particle surface.

Pastes are usually prepared by incorporating solids directly into a congealed system by levigation, with a portion of the base to form a paste-like mass. The remainders of the base are added with continued levigation until the solids are uniformly dispersed in the vehicle.

Pastes are less penetrating and less macerating than ointments and make a particularly good protective barrier when placed on the skin. Pastes are less greasy because of the absorption of the fluid hydrocarbon fraction into the particulates. In addition to forming an unbroken film, they can absorb serous secretions and thereby neutralize certain noxious chemicals before they ever reach the skin. Like ointments, pastes form an unbroken relatively water-impermeable film that is opaque; therefore, zinc oxide paste is an effective sun barrier. Skiers apply paste around the nose and lips to gain dual protection.

There are two types of pastes:

- Fatty pastes (e.g., zinc oxide paste)
- Nongreasy pastes (e.g., bassorin paste, which is also named tragacanth jelly since the hydrophilic component of tragacanth gels in water).

11.2.4 Gels (Jellies)

Gels are a semisolid system in which a liquid phase is constrained within a three-dimensional polymeric matrix having a high degree of physical or chemical cross-linking.

Gels are aqueous colloidal suspensions of the hydrated forms of an insoluble medicament. Gels may be a single-phase system or two-phase system based on the existence of an apparent boundary between the macromolecules and the liquid. Two-phase systems contain floccules of small, distinct particles with higher viscosity and are referred to as magma. Jellies are transparent or translucent non-greasy semisolid gels. Some are as transparent as water; others are turbid because the colloidal aggregates disperse light.

Gels are used for medication, lubrication, and some miscellaneous applications such as carriers for spermicidal agents to be used intravaginally with diaphragms as an adjunctive means of contraception.

11.2.5 Poultices

A poultice is a soft, viscous, paste-like preparation for external use, particularly for reducing inflammation. It is spread thickly on a dressing and applied to the skin while the preparation is hot. The poultice must retain heat for a considerable time because it is intended to supply warmth to inflamed parts of body, e.g., Kaolin poultice (BPC).

11.2.6 Plasters

Plasters are solid or semisolid masses that adhere to skin when spread upon cotton, felt, linen, or muslin as a backing material; they are mainly used to provide protection and mechanical support. They may provide an occlusive and macerating action and bring medication into close contact with the surface of the skin.

11.2.7 Rigid Foams

Foams are systems in which air or some other gas is emulsified in the liquid phase with sufficient viscosity to the point of stiffening, e.g., shaving creams, whipped creams, aerosolized shaving creams.

11.2.8 Suppositories

Suppositories are solid dosage forms containing medicinal agents intended for insertion into body cavities, including the rectum, vaginal cavity, or urethral tract but not through the oral cavity. While suppositories are frequently used for local action, they can also be used to achieve adequate systemic concentration of a drug. This dosage form is specifically useful where hepatic first-pass metabolism converts the drug into an inactive form. The following factors can affect drug absorption from rectal suppositories:

- Anorectal physiology
- Solubility of the drug
- Particle size and concentration of the drug
- Physiochemical properties of the base
  - Melting point
  - Solubility
  - Chemical reactivity
  - Polymorphism

The major inactive component of a suppository dosage form is the suppository base.

Properties of an ideal suppository base:

- Melts at rectal temperature 37.5°C
- Is nontoxic and nonirritating to sensitive and inflamed tissues
- Is physically stable and compatible with a variety of drugs
- Is convenient for the patient to handle and does not break or melt
- Does not leak from the rectum
- Is stable on storage and does not change color, odor, and drug release pattern

Suppository bases can be classified in three categories according to their physicochemical properties:

- Oleaginous
  - Cocoa butter (Theobroma oil)
  - Cocoa butter substitutes
- Water-soluble
  - Glycerinated gelatin
  - Polyethylene glycol mixtures
- Water-dispersible
  - Polyethylene glycol derivatives
  - Cocoa butter substituted with surfactants

Cocoa butter is the most widely used suppository base for rectal use. This is the base of choice when no suppository base is specified. It satisfies many of the requirements for an ideal base.

11.2.8.1 *Manufacture of Suppositories*

Earlier suppositories were prepared by using the rolling method, but presently, they are prepared either by using the fusion or cold compression method. In the fusion method, the molten mass of base and drug is poured into a lubricated mold kept over ice and made up of plastic/stainless steel, containing two halves that are fixed firmly by a screw. The mold is then cooled at room temperature for 10–15 minutes. The suppositories, when set, are removed, and each drug is wiped off with a clean cloth and wrapped individually in wax paper.

The cold compression method is used for thermolabile and insoluble drugs. It makes use of a mold and cylinder. The medicament, incorporated into theobroma oil, is placed into the mold and then is passed into the cylinder through a narrow opening, where it is compressed until it forms a homogenous fused mass. Before the suppository achieves its final form, the compression cylinder of the machine is chilled to prevent heating of suppositories. They are stored in a cool place to retain their shape at room temperature.

In large-scale manufacturing, automatic molding is commonly used. The suppositories can be poured, cooled, and removed from the mold by rotary automatic molding machines. The output of a typical rotary machine is from 3,500 to 6,000 suppositories per hour.

Disposable molds are more frequently used now, with some additional advantages over the conventional metal molds:

- Costly molds and wrapping materials are not required.
- Mold shapes can be changed with less expense.
- The costly and time-consuming wrapping process with aging and precooling is eliminated.

11.2.8.2 *Characterization and Evaluation of Suppositories*

11.2.8.2.1 MEASUREMENT OF HARDNESS OF BASE

A rheometer can be used to measure the hardness of base, which is determined by the peak value of the shearing stress at breaking under pressure of 30 cm/min.

11.2.8.2.2 MEASUREMENT OF THE MELTING POINT OF BASE

A differential scanning calorimeter is used to measure the melting point of a base at a heating speed of 3°C/min, which is shown by a DSC curve, and its peak shows the melting point of the base [14].

11.2.8.2.3 DETERMINATION OF DRUG RELEASE

It is essential to know the drug release rate from suppositories to study the absorption of the drug within a given period of time. *In vitro* drug release studies can be performed by using the rotating dialysis cell method. In this method, the rotating cell assembly is placed in a cylindrical vessel containing 900 mL dissolution media. It requires the placement of suppositories in a rotating cell that is continuously stirred by Teflon-coated stirring bar at 25 rpm (see Figure 11.3). A constant temperature is maintained through the dissolution process using a thermostat. The drug samples are withdrawn at a predetermined time interval and are replaced with fresh samples in order to maintain the sink condition. The drug concentration can be determined by using a suitable analytical technique [15].

11.2.9 Transdermal Drug Delivery Systems

Transdermal Drug Delivery Systems (TDDS) are used to facilitate transportation of drugs through skin for a systemic effect. This noninvasive method

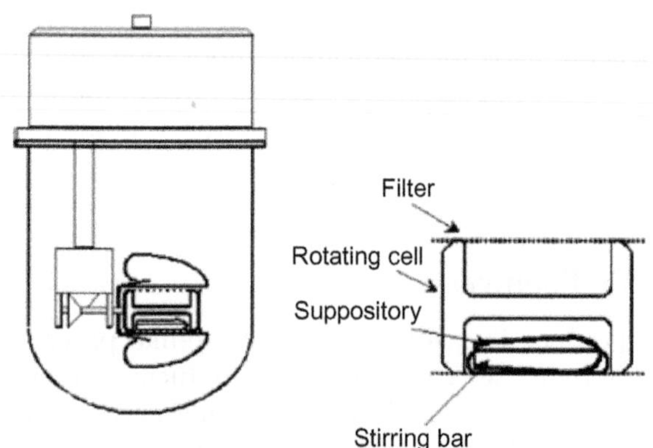

FIGURE 11.3 Schematic representation of *in vitro* release testing apparatus: PTSW-type rotating dialysis cell method with a stirring bar [15].

is ideal for drugs with a short biological half-life, and besides bypassing first-pass metabolism, it also avoids the unpredictability associated with gastrointestinal absorption and produces more uniform plasma levels. The required flux for a drug from transdermal patch is calculated using Eq. 11.1:

$$\text{Flux},\ J_{ss} = CL_t \times C_{pss}/A \qquad (11.1)$$

where CL_t is total body clearance, C_{pss} is steady-state plasma concentration, and A is surface area (cm^2).

Many transdermal drug delivery devices are now available in the market, and many are in the pipeline because patient acceptability for such systems is high. These are broadly classified as matrix systems, reservoir systems, or drug-in-adhesive systems. Transdermal drug delivery devices are usually prepared through the form-fill-seal method, solvent cast method, or extrusion method. With the advent of newer penetration enhancers, the scope of such delivery systems has widened, and now high-molecular-weight drugs and drugs with a varying degree of hydrophilicity or lipophilicity can be incorporated in such systems.

11.3. PERCUTANEOUS ABSORPTION

Despite the complex structure of skin, chemical agents and medicinal substances that are lipophilic in nature permeate through the skin. The skin forms the largest viable tissue with meticulous absorption characteristics. When a substance comes into contact with the skin, it penetrates into the keratinized *stratum corneum* containing lipid keratinocytes (when not massaged on the affected area). The stratum corneum behaves as a permeability barrier membrane because it contains extra cellular lipid composed of 50% ceramides, 25% cholesterol, and 15% free fatty acids [16], whereas viable epidermis is permeable to highly lipophilic compounds.

The lipids are delivered to the extracellular space by the secretion of lamellar bodies, which contain phospholipids, glucosylceramides, sphingomyelin, cholesterol, and enzymes. In the extracellular space, the lamellar body lipids are metabolized by enzymes to the lipids that form the lamellar membranes. The lipids contained in the lamellar bodies are derived from both epidermal lipid synthesis and extracutaneous sources. Inhibition of cholesterol, fatty acid, ceramide, or glucosyl ceramide synthesis adversely affects lamellar body formation, thereby impairing barrier homeostasis.

11.3.1 Structure of Skin

Skin is a flexible, self-repairing capsule that separates the internal environment of the body from the external environment. The cutaneous membrane covers the external surface of the body in surface area and weight. In adult humans, skin covers an area of about 2 square meters and is about 16% of total body weight. It ranges in thickness from 0.5 mm on the eyelids to 4.0 mm on the heels; however, it is 1–2 mm thick in other body parts. Skin acts as a protective barrier against the entry of foreign substances, pathogens, and radiation and prevents the loss of endogenous contents, including water. The advantages of drug delivery through the skin include easy accessibility, convenience, prolonged therapy, avoidance of liver first-pass metabolism, and availability of a large surface area [17].

Skin is composed of two layers, the epidermis and the dermis, separated by a basement membrane zone. Beneath the dermis, there is a layer of adipose tissue and sweat glands.

11.3.1.1 Epidermis

Keratinocytes, which are part of the epidermis (50–100 μm thick), migrate outward from the basal cell into highly differentiated nondividing cells. This forms 90% of epidermal cells. During proliferation, keratinocytes renovate from polygonal cells to spinous cells, flattened granular cells, and finally to flattened polyhedral dead corneocytes full of the protein keratin. The epidermis can be divided into the (a) stratum basale (SB), (b) stratum spinosum (SS), (c) stratum granulosum (SG), and (d) stratum corneum. The epidermal cell layers are interconnected by desmosomes [18].

The *stratum basale* is a thick layer made up of polygonal cells superficially, and columnar or cuboidal epithelial cells in the deeper parts. Here, new cells are constantly formed by mitotic division. Newly formed cells move continuously toward the stratum corneum. The stem cells, which give rise to new cells, are known as keratinocytes. From this, some projection extends downward to the dermis [19].

The *prickle cell* layer is composed of several layers of polygonal prickle cells or squamous cells. The layers become flat as they near the surface so that their long axis appears parallel to the skin surface. These cells possess intracellular bridges or tonofilaments. These intercellular cytoplasmic tonofilaments contain PAS-positive material that is a precursor of keratin.

The *granular cell* layer consists of one to three layers of flat cells containing keratohyaline basophilic granules, which are PAS-negative. The granular cell layer is much thicker in the palms and soles.

The *stratum lucidum* is present exclusively in the palms and soles as a thin homogenous, eosinophilic, non-nucleate zone.

The *horny layer* (stratum corneum) is also normally devoid of nuclei and consists of eosinophilic layers of keratin. Intraepidermal nerve endings are present in the form of Merkel cells, which act as touch receptors [20].

11.3.1.2 Dermis

The dermis is formed from connective tissue and a matrix containing collagen fibers interlaced with elastic fibers, making it tough and elastic. Rupture of the elastic fiber occurs when the skin is overstretched, resulting in permanent striae, which are generally observed in pregnancy and obesity. A collagen fiber binds water and gives the skin its tensile strength, but as this ability declines with age, wrinkles develop. Fibroblast, macrophage, and mast cells are found in the dermis. Underlying its deepest layer, there is areolar tissue and a varying amount of adipose fat.

The dermis consists of two parts: the superficial *pars papillaris* or *papillary dermis*, and the deeper *pars reticularis* or *reticular dermis*. The dermis is composed of fibrocollagenic tissue containing blood vessels, lymphatics, and nerves. In the skin of fingers, arteriovenous shunts or *glomera* are normally present. The specialized nerve endings present at some sites perform specific functions. They are as follows:

- *Pacinian corpuscles* concerned with pressure are present in deep layers of skin.
- *Meissner corpuscles* are touch receptors, located in the papillae of skin on palms, soles, tips of fingers, and toes.
- *Ruffini corpuscles* are cold receptors found in the external genitalia.
- *End-bulbs of Krause* are cold receptors found in the external genitalia.

Beside these structures, the dermis contains cutaneous appendages or adnexal structures, which include the following:

- *Sweat glands:* These are of two types: eccrine and apocrine.
  - *Eccrine glands:* These glands are present all over the skin but are more abundant on the palms, soles, and axillae. They are coiled tubular glands lying deep inside the dermis. Their ducts pass through the epidermis on the surface of the skin as pores through which they empty their secretions, i.e., sweat. The glands are lined by secretory cells and are surrounded by myoepithelial cells.
  - *Apocrine glands:* These glands are located only in a few areas: in the axillae, in the anogenital region, in the external ear as modified glands called ceruminous glands, in the eyelid as Moll's glands, and in the breast as mammary glands. Apocrine glands are also tubular glands but have larger lumina. Apocrine glands have a single layer of secretory cells that contain acidophilic, PAS-positive, prominent granular cytoplasm. The type of secretion in the apocrine glands (*apo*=off) is called the decapitation secretion, as if the cytoplasm of the secretory cells is pinched off.
- *Sebaceous (holocrine) glands:* Sebaceous glands are found everywhere on the skin except on the palms and soles. They are often found in association with hair but can be seen in a few areas devoid of hair as modified sebaceous glands, such as in the external auditory meatus, nipple, and areola of male and female breast; labia minora; prepuce; and meibomian glands of the eyelids. Sebaceous glands are composed of lobules of sebaceous cells containing small, round nuclei and abundant fatty, network-like cytoplasm.
- *Hair:* The hair grows from the bottom of the follicle. It therefore has an intracutaneous portion present in the hair follicle and the shaft. The hair follicles consist of epithelial and connective tissue components. The hair shaft is made up of an outer sheath, pigmented cortex, and inner medulla.
- *Arrectores pilorum:* These small bundles of smooth muscles are attached to each hair follicle. When the muscle contracts, the hair becomes more erect, and the follicle is dragged upward so as to become prominent on the surface of the skin, producing what is known as "goose skin" or "goose bumps."
- *Nails:* The nails are thickenings of the deeper part of the stratum corneum that develop at a specially modified portion of the skin called the nail bed. The nail is composed of clear horny cells, resembling stratum lucidum, but are much more keratinized [21].

11.3.2 Integrity of the Barrier

The stratum corneum layer of epidermis is a major barrier of percutaneous absorption. Anything that alters the structure or function of the stratum corneum will affect epidermal absorption. The integrity of this barrier is reduced by inflammation of the skin, such as any form of dermatitis or psoriasis, which may result in increased percutaneous absorption. Similarly, removal of the stratum corneum by stripping or damage by alkalis, etc., will increase absorption.

11.3.3 Factors Influencing Dermal Absorption

Percutaneous absorption is influenced by many physicochemical and biological factors that are necessary to be considered for safe and effective topical medication [22].

- Skin-related factors
  - Occluded or diseased
  - Area and site of application
  - Differences in races and sex
  - Age of the patient
  - Temperature and moisture
- Physicochemical properties of the drug
  - Concentration of drug at the site of action
  - Molecular weight
  - Partition coefficient
  - Molecular volume
  - Metabolism
  - Melting point
- Vehicle used for the formulation of substances (formulation factors)
  - Partition coefficient
  - Degree of hydration
  - Viscosity of vehicle

11.3.4 Condition of the Skin

The diffusion of some semisolids may be increased more than 10% because of skin occlusion due to profound change in temperature, surface area, blood flow, DNA, microbial flora, and water content in the stratum corneum [23]. Occlusion usually means the skin is covered directly or indirectly by impermeable films or substances such as diapers, tape, chambers, gloves, textile garments, wound dressings, or transdermal devices, but certain topical vehicles that contain fats and/or polymer oils (petrolatum, paraffin, etc.) may also generate occlusive effects [24]. Permeability of topical hydrocortisone may be increased by more than 10-fold after occlusion when applied on the forearm [25]. Occlusion not only increases the permeability but also decreases the mean residence time and alters the first-pass metabolism through the skin [26].

Permeability of skin varies from one part to another part, and it largely depends on the thickness of the stratum corneum. According to the findings of one study, the highest total absorption of hydrocortisone is that from the scrotum, followed (in decreasing order) from forehead, scalp, back, forearms, palm, and plantar surface [27]. Another study reports that ketoprofen 3% absorption is similar in all body parts except the knee [28]. Topical application of hydrocortisone in a vehicle containing ethanol would penetrate faster through leg skin from the lower leg when compared with the thorax or groin, which, depending on cutaneous blood flow, may result in higher systemic drug concentrations or greater efficiency in treating local inflamed tissue [29].

The greatest toxicological response to topical administration has been seen in infants. Preterm infants do not have an intact barrier function and are susceptible to systemic toxicity from topically applied drugs. Normal full-term infants probably have a fully developed stratum corneum barrier with a complete barrier function. However, topical application of the same amount of compound to both adults and newborns reveals greater systemic availability in newborns.

An increase in skin temperature enhances the rate of permeation. This may be attributed to increased blood flow associated with increased skin temperature. It has been observed that temperature has a significant effect on *in vitro* drug diffusivity [30].

Skin contains Phase-1 and Phase-2 enzymes and is capable of metabolizing a wide range of xenobiotics, although the specific activities of these enzymes found in skin are relatively low when compared to their equivalent hepatic forms. The skin also has metabolic potential and can alter chemicals to their more reactive metabolites [31].

11.3.5 Physicochemical Properties of the Penetrant

Absorption is affected by the relative water/lipid solubility of a drug and relative solubility of the drug in a vehicle compared with its solubility in the stratum corneum. In order for a chemical to penetrate through the skin into systemic circulation, it requires both a degree of lipophilicity (to facilitate its entry into the stratum corneum) and hydrophilicity (to aid its passage through the viable epidermis and dermis). Percutaneous absorption of the penetrant depends on the lipid content, appendageal density, and imperfection (pores and correction). Other factors such as molecular weight, molecular volume, and melting point also affect diffusion across the skin [32].

It has been observed that the stratum corneum is a major diffusional barrier, and large molecules hardly penetrate through the skin. Additionally, the diffusion coefficients of the compounds across viable skin are dependent on the molecular weight, size, and shape of the penetrant. Drug permeation through viable skin without the stratum corneum is more than 100 times greater than through intact skin [33].

Melting point also has an important effect on drug permeability. Permeability is inversely proportional to the melting point. It has been reported that the lower the melting point, the higher the solubility and free energy, and the greater is the absorption through the stratum corneum [34].

The partition coefficient of drugs also affects their permeation through skin. A balance between lipophilicity and hydrophilicity is a prerequisite for drug absorption through the skin. The amount and concentration of a drug in a vehicle also affect the solubility and flux of the drug due to increased thermodynamic activity. It has been observed that a higher partition coefficient favors permeation through skin.

11.3.6 Vehicle Used in Formulation

Selection of a vehicle is an important parameter in the formulation of a new dosage form, especially in a dermatological product, due to its unique structure [35]. When one is designing a formulation, the physicochemical properties of the vehicle are also important parameters to produce effective and safe delivery. Some vehicles, such as polyethylene glycol, produce occlusions on the stratum corneum and increase skin permeability of the drug. These vehicles increase the penetration of hydrophilic drugs to a certain extent but are not applicable for all drugs.

The partition coefficient of a vehicle is also an important factor in percutaneous absorption. A lipophilic drug easily enters into the stratum corneum due to its high lipid content, but a viable epidermis restricts the entry of a highly lipophilic drug. Ointments can enhance percutaneous absorption of a topical product by providing an occlusive barrier. Creams, lotions, and gels have lower oil content and therefore are less absorptive. Certain vehicles can also cause more irritation, altering the skin's permeability and resulting in enhanced absorption.

Volatility of a vehicle also plays an important role in the topical absorption of a drug. Permeation of hydrocortisone improves in the presence of ethanol in the vehicle. Significant regional differences (i.e., among the thorax, neck, and groin areas) have also been observed in the transdermal penetration and skin retention of hydrocortisone [36].

From the equation of diffusion coefficient, it is clear that the diffusion coefficient is inversely proportional to the viscosity of a vehicle. The more viscous the vehicle, the less dermatological absorption of the drug. Contradictory results were obtained in a study where a viscous substance was applied in "in use" (i.e., finite amount) doses. In this study, thickening agents promoted penetration, probably through greater stratum corneum diffusivity due to an enhanced hydration caused by the thicker formulations [99]. In another study, there was no effect of a vehicle's viscosity on drug absorption through the skin [100].

In another study, the permeation rates of a homologous series of primary alcohols (C_1-C_{10}) through skin were measured. On the basis of our understanding of physicochemical properties of drugs and knowledge of the solubility character of the vehicles, we can qualitatively predict the permeation of different substances [100].

11.3.7 Mechanism of Absorption through Skin

The penetration of a drug through the stratum corneum involves partition phenomena of applied molecules between lipophilic and hydrophilic compartments. For many substances, the penetration takes place through an intercellular way, more than transcellular, diffusing around the keratinocytes. The functions of different parts of skin are shown in Table 11.1. The rate of diffusion in creams, ointments, gels, and other semisolids may be determined by the following:

- Transdermal permeation, through the stratum corneum
- Intercellular permeation, through the stratum corneum
- Transappendaged permeation, via hair follicles and sebaceous and sweat glands

A drug readily diffuses from the stratum corneum into the epidermis and then into the dermis, where it enters the capillary microcirculation of the skin and thus the systemic circulation. There may be a degree of presystemic metabolism in the epidermis and dermis, a desirable feature to the extent that it limits the systemic effects.

Transcellular movement: Intracellular components of the stratum corneum lack a functional lipid matrix around keratin and keratohyalin, resulting in low permeability of corneocytes [38]. Degradation of the corneodesmosomes causes the formation of a continuous lacunar dominio ("aqueous pore"), allowing intercellular penetration; the lacunae formed are scattered and form as a result of occlusion, ionophoresis, and ultrasound waves. They may become larger and connect, thus forming a net ("pore-way"). Various methods can induce such an increase in permeability [39].

Intercellular movement: The lipid lamellae of the intercellular spaces (each one including two or three bilayers and made mainly of ceramides, cholesterol, and free fatty acids) are the intercellular structure of the horny layer, having the main role in barrier function. Most solute substances, nonpolar or polar, penetrate across intercellular lipid avenues. The permeability of very polar solutes is constant and

TABLE 11.1 Function of Skin [37]

Function	Structure/Cell Involved
Protect against:	Stratum corneum
Chemical, particle, dessication	Melanin produced by melanocytes and transferred to keratinocytes
UV radiation	Langerhans cells, lymphocytes, mast cells, and mononuclear phagocytes
Antigen, haptens	Stratum corneum, Langerhans cells, mast cells, and mononuclear phagocytes
Microbes	
Preserve balanced internal environment	Stratum corneum
Prevent loss of water, electrolytes, and macromolecules	
Shock absorber	Dermis and subcutaneous fat
Strong yet elastic and compliant covering	
Sensation	Specialist nerve-ending pain, leading to withdrawal; itch leading to scratch; and hence removal of parasite
Vitamin D synthesis	Keratinocytes
Temperature regulation	Eccrine sweat gland and blood vessel
Protection and fine manipulation of small objects	Nails
Hormonal	Hair follicle and sebaceous gland
Testosterone synthesis and conversion to other anderogenic steroids	

similar to the transport of ions (e.g., potassium ions). Lipophilic solute permeability increases according to specific lipophilic properties.

Transfollicular movement: Such movement through hair follicles, pilosebaceous units, and eccrine glands is limited. The orifices of the pilosebaceous units represent about 10% in areas where their density is high (face and scalp) and only 0.1% in areas where their density is low. This is a possible selective way for some drugs. Follicular penetration may be influenced by sebaceous secretion, which favors the absorption of substances soluble in lipids. The penetration through the pilosebaceous units is dependent on the property of the substance and the type of preparation.

11.4. THEORY OF SEMISOLID DOSAGE FORMS

11.4.1 Hydrophilic Properties

The water-absorbing capacity of oleaginous and water-in-oil bases may be expressed in terms of the water number, which is defined as the maximum quantity of water that is held (partly emulsified) by 100 g of a base at 20°C. The test consists of adding increments of water to the melted base and triturating until the mixture has cooled. When no more water is absorbed, the product is placed in a refrigerator for several hours, removed, and allowed to come to room temperature. The material is then rubbed on a slab until water does not exude, and finally, the amount of water remaining in the base is determined.

11.4.2 Rheological Properties

Different semisolid dosage forms exhibit different rheological properties. Semisolids do not flow at low shear stresses but undergo reversible deformation like elastic solids. When a characteristic shear stress, called the yield value or yield stress, is exceeded, these forms flow like liquids. Yield stresses usually are caused by structural networks extending throughout an entire system. To break such a network requires stress that produces no flow, but only elastic deformation. When the yield stress is exceeded, the network is partly ruptured and flow occurs.

Gels or jellies are characterized by a comparatively high degree of elasticity. They undergo rather large elastic deformation at shear stresses below the yield value, from which they recover their shape when the stresses are removed. Recoverable deformations of 10%–30% are not unusual, especially for polymer gels. Clay gels are less elastic, and their rheological properties resemble paste.

Pastes possess little elasticity and cannot recover their shape except from very small deformations. At stresses above their yield values, pastes behave like free-flowing liquids. This type of rheological behavior is called plasticity. Brownian motion builds up the networks in gels and pastes and restores them when they have been ruptured by stress higher than the yield value. Examples of plastic materials are ointments and pastes, creams, butter and margarine, dough, putties, and modeling clay.

Semisolids with high yield values are described as "hard." When their plastic viscosity is high, they are described as "stiff." For example, in Figure 11.4 hydrophilic petrolatum has a higher yield value as compared to hydrophilic petrolatum containing water and may be termed hard petrolatum. The best instrument for determining the rheologic properties of pharmaceutical semisolids is some form of a rotational viscometer. The cone-plate viscometer is particularly well adapted for the analysis of semisolid emulsions and suspensions. The Stormer viscometer, consisting of a stationary cup and rotating bob, is also satisfactory for semisolids.

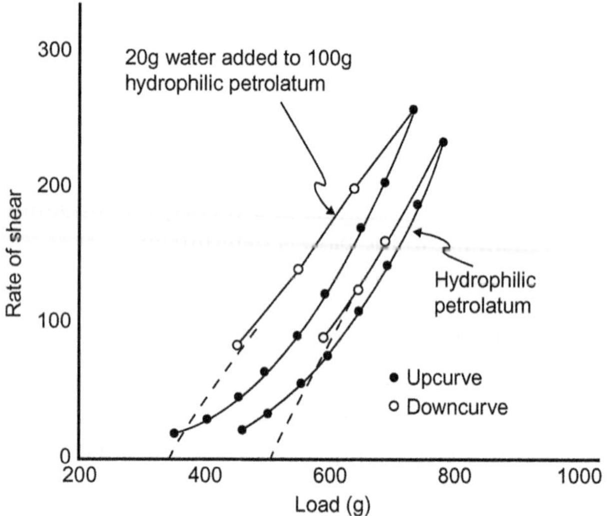

FIGURE 11.4 Flow curves obtained for hydrophilic petrolatum and hydrophilic petrolatum containing water [40].

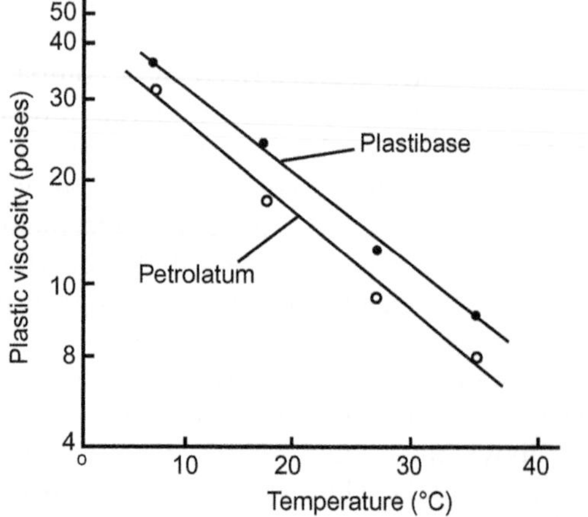

FIGURE 11.5 Plastic viscosity of petrolatum and plastibase as a function of temperature [41].

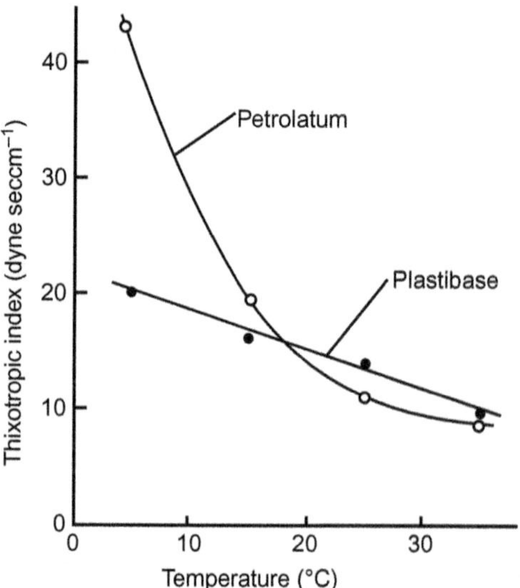

FIGURE 11.6 Thixotropic behavior of petrolatum and plastibase as a function of temperature [41].

Consistency curves for the emulsifiable bases, hydrophilic petrolatum, and hydrophilic petrolatum in which water has been incorporated are shown in Figure 11.4. The addition of water to hydrophilic petrolatum lowers the yield-point (the intersection of the x-axis and extrapolated downcurve). The plastic viscosity (the reciprocal of the slope of the downcurve) and the thixotropy (the area between the upcurve and downcurve generally termed the hysteresis loop) are increased by the addition of water to hydrophilic petrolatum.

Figure 11.5 shows the change in plastic viscosity, and Figure 11.6 shows the thixotropic behavior of petrolatum and plastibase as a function of temperature. The modified Stormer viscometer was used to obtain such curves. As observed in Figure 11.5, both of the bases show about the same temperature coefficient of plastic viscosity. These results account for the fact that the bases have about the same degree of softness.

The mechanical properties of gels are characterized by two separate parameters, rigidity and viscosity, which are affected by temperature. The rigidity index, f, of a gel is the force required for depressing its surface to a fixed distance. To measure rigidity, one subjects a sample of gel mass to penetrative compression using a flat-ended cylindrical plunger that operates at a constant speed when the strain (rate of deformation of gel) is constant and independent of stress (force applied). The thermal degradation of a gel with respect to rigidity follows second-order kinetics, as shown in Eq. 11.2:

$$-\frac{df}{dt} = k_f f^2 \tag{11.2}$$

The preceding equation can be integrated into Eq. 11.3:

$$\frac{1}{f} - \frac{1}{f_0} = k_f t \tag{11.3}$$

where f is the rigidity index of the gel at time t, f_0 is the rigidity index at time zero, k_f is the rate constant (g^{-1} hr^{-1}), and t is the heating time in hours. Eq. 11.3 conforms to a straight-line equation; therefore, f_0 and k_f can be calculated from its intercept and slope, respectively, at a given temperature.

The effect of temperature on the rate constant, k_f, can be expressed using the Arrhenius equation (Eq. 11.4):

$$k_f = Ae^{-E_a/RT} \tag{11.4}$$

The preceding equation can be represented also by Eq. 11.5:

$$ln\ k_f = In\ A - \frac{E_a}{RT} \tag{11.5}$$

Equation 11.5 conforms to a straight-line equation. Thus, a plot of $ln\ k_f$ versus 1/T would result in a straight line with slope and intercept equal to $-\frac{E_a}{R}$ and $ln\ A$, respectively, which in turn can be used to measure the Arrhenius constant A and the energy of activation E_a.

11.4.3 Rheological Changes

Homogenization frequently increases the consistency of a semisolid emulsion because it increases the number of emulsified particles. Homogenization can also have the opposite effect, that of decreasing the viscosity of the product owing to the electrolyte effect. Some creams are sensitive to agitation and stress. The continuous rotation of an auger in the hopper of the filling machine may cause cream to liquefy. Such creams may be made more resistant to agitation through a formula change.

11.5. METHODS OF ENHANCEMENT OF PERCUTANEOUS ABSORPTION

Due to the composition of the stratum corneum, this is the main barrier in the absorption of drugs through the skin. Various methods that have been adopted to increase the percutaneous absorption of drugs are discussed in the following sections.

11.5.1 Chemical Method

A permeation enhancer enters through the stratum corneum, interferes with the lipid content, and disrupts the barrier of the skin. Some examples of penetration enhancers are water, sulfoxides (e.g., dimethylsulfoxide, or DMSO), azones [98] (e.g., laurocapram), pyrrolidones (e.g., 2-pyrrolidone, 2P), alcohols and alkanols (ethanol or decanol), glycols (e.g., propylene glycol, PG), surfactants (also common in dosage forms), fatty acids, and terpenes [42].

A penetration enhancer should have the following properties:

- It should be nontoxic to the skin.
- It should be inert and not show any pharmacological activity.
- It should be effective at a very low concentration.
- It does not have any incompatibility with other substances (active ingredients or excipients).
- It should have a rapid and reversible onset of action.

11.5.1.1 Water

Water is a well-recognized solvent used in many pharmaceutical preparations. This is innocuous physiologically but reactive chemically. Due to its innocuous nature, water is also used in the dermatological field as a penetration enhancer to promote the permeation of a number of drugs (especially steroids). This causes the occlusion or hydration of the stratum corneum but has no effect on the lipid bilayer. A problem involved with this solvent is the presence of numerous inorganic ions that interfere with the action of surfactants and slow down the effects of surfactants. Another drawback is the possibility of the presence of a microorganism as a contaminant, which may degrade the formulation.

11.5.1.2 Sulfoxides

Dimethyl sulfoxide (DMSO) has been the most frequently used penetration enhancer in the past few years. DMSO is a clear, colorless to yellowish liquid with a characteristic bitter odor and taste. It is a highly polar, stable compound that can easily absorb moisture and dissolve polar, nonpolar, and lipoidal drugs. DMSO has very good absorption in skin and oral mucosa. When DMSO is applied topically, a taste of this solvent comes into the mouth within 5 minutes and creates lethargy in people. Many adverse effects have been observed with continuous topical administration of the drug. DMSO at a concentration of 5%–10% is suitable for the enhancement of percutaneous absorption [43]. It alters the protein structure and lipid content of the stratum corneum. Moreover, it also alters the partition coefficient of the drug. DMSO also possesses mild anti-inflammatory activity at low concentrations [44]. The most frequent adverse effect associated with DMSO is dry skin [45].

An experiment was performed to evaluate the neurotoxic effects of DMSO, but no toxic effects on the neural and arterial tissues of rats were observed when it was slowly infused into the carotid artery [46]. DMSO, an aprotic solvent, has been found to be useful as a topical agent with antioxidant effects in treatment of chronic wounds. It prevents TNF-α-induced proteolytic activity in cutaneous inflammatory reactions [47]. Despite its many beneficiary effects, it should be used with caution.

11.5.1.3 Azone

Azone, or 1-Dodecylazacyloheptan-2-one (laurocapram, Azone; Nelson Research and Development, Irvine, CA), is a smooth, oily, hydrophobic liquid that has been reported to be nonirritating to human skin and is capable of enhancing the percutaneous penetration of a variety of compounds.

Topical formulations of the antiviral compound trifluorothymidine (TFT) were prepared with different proportions of azone, propylene glycol (PG), polyethylene glycol (PEG-300), and/or water and evaluated by measuring *in vitro* diffusion of TFT through excised guinea pig skin. Azone dramatically increases drug flux. Azone and PG may enhance membrane permeability relative to water and act synergistically on the penetration of the active ingredient. The concentration of azone, which maximally enhances penetration, varies with different compounds and also with the nature of the formulation.

Azone is a good candidate for the enhancement of dermatological absorption, but the vehicle in ophthalmic formulation that contains azone showed ocular toxicity when applied on rat eyes. The toxicity signs were elucidated by the conjunctivae and iris, discharge, and corneal edema. This toxicity can occur due to the direct penetration of azone in the stratum corneum or the increased permeation of benzalkonium chloride in the formulation. The capacity of azone as a penetration enhancer was evaluated from dermatological absorption of metronidazole on human skin. Azone in a 1% concentration was found to be more effective as compared to other concentrations in the enhancement of metronidazole transport in comparison to other drugs and it remains on the skin for several days (Walton et al., 1985).

11.5.1.4 Pyrrolidone

Pyrrolidone is a colorless liquid used in industrial settings as a high-boiling noncorrosive polar solvent for a wide variety of applications. It is miscible with a wide variety of other solvents, including water, ethanol, diethyl ether, chloroform, benzene, ethyl acetate, and carbon disulfide. It has been reported that pyrrolidone increases the penetration of various drugs such as sulfaguanidine, aminopyrine, flurbiprofen, and Sudan III. A derivative of pyrrolidine and pyrrolidone interacts with skin lipids and penetrates through it.

From different studies, it has been suggested that pyrrolidone is a very good penetration enhancer, but it also shows a hypersensitive reaction on rabbit skin. So, there should always be a balance between the penetration-enhancing effects and other adverse effects. Methyl pyrrolidone and azone have been observed to be good penetration enhancers for the improvement of dermatological absorption of heparin sodium salt through human skin [48].

11.5.1.5 Alkanol

In alkanol, ethanol has been an attractive candidate for the enhancement of penetration for the past few decades. Ethanol is a semipolar solvent that is miscible with water and other organic solvents. Ethanol shows less irritation as compared to other penetration enhancers. In addition, it leaves a cooling sensation upon evaporation. Migration of 1-alkanol in the lipid bilayer is very rapid. A bond is assembled between the hydroxyl group of 1-alkanol and the carbonyl group of the lipid, and a hydrocarbon chain is formed, which resides in the hydrophobic core of the lipid bilayer. Ethanol diffuses easily in the lipid bilayer as compared to other long-chain alkanols [49].

11.5.1.6 Propylene Glycol

Propylene glycol is a water-miscible, colorless, highly flammable liquid substance. It is a type of alcohol made from fermented yeast and carbohydrates, and is commonly used in a wide variety of products. Even though there are warnings against skin contact with propylene glycol, it is still used in skin-care products. Propylene glycol has been used in many formulations as humectants, antibacterial agents, and antifungal agents in semisolid dosage forms. Propylene glycol interferes with the lamellar lipid in corneocytes and improves the partition of the drug and acts as a penetration enhancer. For the delivery of drugs from topical formulations of 5-fluorouracil and haloperidol, having an appropriate propylene glycol content in the vehicle is useful [50]. Despite its various uses in semisolid dosage forms, propylene glycol at higher doses may result in reversible acute renal failure caused by proximal renal tubular cell injury [51].

11.5.1.7 Surfactants

Surfactants are multipurpose excipients used in many industries, such as the pharmaceutical, cosmetics, and food industries. Surfactants reduce the interfacial tension between two phases and stabilize a formulation. They can act as solubilizers, soaps, detergents, wetting agents, adhesives, emulsifiers, foaming agents, and suspending agents. They have a lipophilic alkyl or aryl chain, together with a hydrophilic potion in their structure. According to the number and nature of a group, surfactants may be classified as predominantly hydrophilic or predominantly lipophilic.

Solubilizing agents, detergents, and o/w emulsifying agents come under the hydrophilic category due to its value of hydrophilic lipophilic balance (HLB), whereas wetting agents, antifoaming agents, and w/o emulsifying agents come under the second category. Surfactants such as Span are lipophilic and have low HLB (1.8–8.6), whereas Tween is hydrophilic and has a higher HLB value. These substances are absorbed at the interface and exhibit a self-association at a specific concentration. Nonionic surfactants like Polyoxyethylene-2-oleyl ether (Poloxamer, a nonionic surfactant) show higher percutaneous transportation of drugs as compared to other nonionic surfactants. Thermal analysis suggests that the stratum corneum is fluidized to form a loosely layered stratum corneum, and thus, the intercellular space becomes broad in the presence of poloxamer. Sodium lauryl sulphate causes transepidermal water loss and should be avoided in daily-applied cosmetics [52]. It has been observed that glyceryl monocaprylate/caprate increased 5-FU flux up to 10-fold because it is the least lipophilic, and being amphiphilic, it has the optimum alkyl chain length for surfactants [53].

11.5.1.8 Fatty Acids

Natural oil is obtained directly from plant and vegetable sources. These are the main sources of fatty acids containing the carbon-carbon double bond and hydroxyl bond. Viscosity depends on the molecular weight and hydroxyl content. Natural vegetable oil is safe and less irritating but goes rancid easily. Dermatological absorption of drugs is enhanced with an increase in the carbon chain length of fatty acids [54]. Corn oil is considered to be a naturally safe and effective penetration enhancer. Various fatty acids are considered to be safe and inert ingredients and are used in formulations. The fatty acids enhance the partitioning of drugs into the lipid core in the stratum corneum [55]. The unsaturated fatty acid portion of cod liver oil, for example, makes it an effective permeation enhancer. Greater piroxicam flux through the skin was observed when administered in the form of a gel containing oleic acid, which doubles the percutaneous absorption of piroxicam [56].

11.5.1.9 Terpenes

Terpenes are natural penetration enhancers that are classified as generally regarded as safe (GRAS) and less irritating, as recognized by the Food and Drug Administration [57]. Terpenes interfere with lipid bilayers in the keratinocytes from the stratum corneum and have no effect on the highly ordered structure of keratins [50]. Terpenes increase the penetration of hydrophilic drugs by partitioning the drugs from aqueous solutions to the stratum corneum. Terpenes showed significant synergistic effect when used with other penetration enhancers. For example, the flux of 5-Fluorouracil increases when propylene glycol is used along with terpene. The change in entropy causes disruption of the lipid of the stratum corneum and causes phase separation of the lipid in the stratum corneum [58].

11.5.2 Physical Penetration Enhancers

Dermatological penetration can be enhanced through physical means, such as with the help of microneedles, jet propulsion, electric current, ultrasonic or photomechanical waves, etc.

11.5.2.1 Electrically Based

11.5.2.1.1 ELECTROPORATION

Electroporation is a very effective technique used in the enhancement of penetration through skin. This technique utilizes a controlled electric field of high voltage for milliseconds to a few seconds to disturb the lipid bilayer of a cell membrane for a temporary period to allow the entry of aqueous substances. When molecules enter into the cell membrane, pores are closed readily and regain their highly ordered structure. The stratum corneum also contains the same structure as other cell membranes with the hydrophobic core encapsulated in a hydrophilic layer that permits entry of lipophilic substances only. This technique involves many applications, including the transfer of DNA, large-molecular-weight drugs, and also lipophilic as well as hydrophilic molecules. This technique reduces the pain or discomfort of injection and quickly passes the drug through the skin barrier. The rate of diffusion of a drug depends on the electrical and physical properties. The application of electroporation has many advantages but may cause cell death and muscle contraction due to improper pulse [59].

11.5.2.1.2 IONTOPHORESIS

Iontophoresis is a technique used to enhance dermatological absorption of drugs in topical and transdermal drug delivery through the application of a constant electric current. Many diseases can be cured through the use of this technique, especially hyperhidrosis. This technique is based on the general concept of coulombic force in which two anions experience a mutual repulsive force, as do two cations. When a positively charged molecule is transported through the barrier, it is placed under the anode electrode, which repels the ion toward skin that behaves like a cathode (human skin and rat skin both are negatively charged at a pH more than 4) and attracts a positive-charged ion to it by removing other positive ions from its inner surface. In this technique, a constant electric current nearly $0.5\,mA/cm^2$ is applied to increase the diffusion of drug through the stratum corneum, a lipoidal barrier. This is based on the principle of electro-osmosis and electromigration, which push the ionic or nonionic molecule through the cell membrane and provide a programmed and controlled drug delivery for those drugs in which hydrophilicity, lipophilicity, and molecular weight are issues [60]. Ions with a high-density current show an increase in skin permeability although it may damage skin. Iontophoresis bypasses the first-pass metabolism in liver; in addition, it can deliver drugs having a short biological half-life, high molecular weight, as well as lipophilic and ionic substances. It provides sustained drug delivery, increased patient compliance, and ease in termination of therapy at any stage; it also reduces inter- and intrasubject variability because this therapy is based directly on applied current.

A variety of drugs can be delivered through this drug delivery system, including small molecules such as apomorphine [61], sumatriptan [62], 5-fluorouracil [63], rotigotine [64], and buspirone hydrochloride [65]; and large molecules having high molecular weight (heparin and hormones), insulin, etc. [66].

11.5.2.1.3 SONOPHORESIS

Sonophoresis is a process that utilizes the microwaves or ultra sound waves of frequency (20 kHz to 3 MHz), which enhance the absorption of drugs through skin by formation of cavitation, streaming, and heating. Acoustic streaming occurs at low-intensity waves, whereas heating and acoustic cavitations will predominate on a high level. Low-frequency sonophoresis is said to be more significant than the high-frequency waves [67]. The highly ordered structure of the stratum corneum is disrupted by low-frequency waves and enhances percutaneous absorption. The examination of the permeation pathway of lanthanum nitrate tracer suggests that microwaves interfere with the diffusion of stratum granulosum (SG) or the upper SG layer. Additionally, lanthanum nitrate also diffuses into the viable epidermis through the intercellular pathway. It shows a synergistic effect with other chemical penetration enhancers such as oleic acid [68]. This technique can be applied to a number of therapeutic agents that can be delivered through the skin.

11.5.2.1.4 PHOTOMECHANICAL WAVES

Compressed photomechanical waves contain high-amplitude pressure waves of 100 atmospheres for a few seconds; they interact with cells and tissues. This interaction depends on the pressure, duration, and time. Photomechanical waves can be high-power pulse or low-power pulse used for medical purposes, but the low-power waves have more advantages in drug delivery, such as gene therapy. Stress or compressed waves can enhance the diffusion of macromolecules (40 kDa dextran and 20 nm latex particles) by increasing the permeability of cell membranes of the stratum corneum by forming a cavity, increasing permeability, and increasing the diffusion rate of drug molecules into the viable epidermis and dermis. This delivery system diffuses the drug in the depth of the tissue and produces a systemic effect, as in insulin, which reduces the blood sugar level for many hours when delivered through stress waves. These waves reduce the pain and discomfort from other delivery systems, and the occluded barriers regain their structure easily [69].

11.5.2.2 Structure-Based Physical Approach

11.5.2.2.1 MICRONEEDLE

Many patients panic when they learn that they are going to be injected with a needle, although the treatment is meant for their benefit. One advanced technique uses microneedles that do not induce any pain; these needles vary in size. This alternative method to deliver drugs does not affect the blood vessels and nerve endings in the hypodermis layer. There also is less risk of infection and contamination from the device used for drug administration. Shape and size also affect the magnitude of pain and discomfort. Pyramidal wet-etch microneedles can cause less pain and discomfort because the microchannel created by these needles is quickly repaired. Enhanced skin permeability has been observed with microneedles that have a size greater than 600 μm. As a result, flux of a drug in the epidermis is increased as compared to the use of other size microneedles [70].

Researchers have developed biodegradable microneedles made from polymer poly-N-isopropylacrylamide (PNIPAAm) and poly-lactic-co-glycolic acid (PLGA). The hydrogel swells on contact with body fluid and absorbs water quickly. The swollen hydrogel causes microneedles to swell, and structural breakdown of biodegradable needles releases drugs from the matrix. Many drugs can be successfully delivered from these biodegradable polymers [71]. Applications with microneedles include delivery of cosmetics, vaccines of oligonucleotides, reduction of blood glucose level by insulin, induction of immune responses from protein, and DNA vaccine delivery through transcutaneous routes.

11.5.2.3 *Velocity-Based Physical Approach*

11.5.2.3.1 JET PROPULSION

The jet propulsion technique is a needle-free injection that uses a high-velocity stream of drugs to penetrate the blood circulation system through the skin. Jet diameter and velocity are the two main parameters for the penetration of drugs into the skin. Jet streams that flow through a gauge diameter of 152 microns have a threshold velocity in the range of 80–100 m/s. Jet propulsion is not very popular in the market due to pain induced on injection. The drug is delivered from a traditional jet injector, which penetrates near the pain receptors located in the deep layers of skin. Recently, conventional jet injectors were replaced with micro jet injectors, which deliver the drug on the superficial layer or above the pain receptors. A number of factors affect the depth of penetration of a drug into the skin.

11.5.3 Biochemical Enhancers

11.5.3.1 *Liposomes*

Liposomes are composed of artificial microscopic vesicles in which the aqueous compartment is encapsulated between a membranous lipid bilayer composed of natural and synthetic phospholipids. The release rate of a drug depends on the composition and morphology of the lipid vesicle. Liposomes (lipid vesicles) are formed when thin lipid layers of phospholipids are hydrated and stacks of liquid crystalline become fluid and swell. The hydrated fatty acid chain separates itself during agitation and forms a large vesicle that prevents an interface between water and the hydrocarbon bilayer at the edges.

Generally, phospholipids are amphiphilic molecules containing a polar head and hydrophilic (phosphoric acid bound to water-soluble molecules) and hydrophobic tail, composed of two fatty acid chains containing 10–24 carbon atoms and 0–6 double bonds in each chain.

The structure of intracellular lipids in skin resembles the composition of liposomes; hence, liposomes have been tested for better skin penetration with faster diffusion. Many investigations have been performed using reconstructed human skin to determine the exact mechanism of permeation of drugs through topical liposomes. Two distinctive mechanisms are responsible for enhanced topical localization: the transepidermal pathway and the transfollicular pathway.

Liposomes have proved to be useful carriers for a number of drugs, including peptides, proteins, plasmid DNA, antisense oligonucleotides, and ribozymes, for pharmaceutical, cosmetic, and biochemical purposes [72].

The enormous versatility in particle size and in the physical parameters of the lipids affords an attractive potential for constructing tailor-made vehicles for a wide range of applications, including drug targeting. One proprietary product currently being marketed is Celadrin® Topical Liposome Lotion, although it is not approved by the FDA.

11.5.3.2 *Niosomes*

Niosomes are also a carrier-type vesicular drug delivery system like liposomes. In niosomes, the lipid bilayer of liposomes is replaced with a nonionic surfactant. They are used as an alternative to liposomes due to their stable character and cost-effectiveness in formulation [73]. Nonionic surfactant vesicles follow the same procedure of synthesis as in liposomes, i.e., hydration of nonionic surfactants. A wide variety of nonionic surfactants have been found to be useful in the fabrication of niosomes. However, vesicles may also be prepared using ionic amphiphiles such as negatively charged diacetyl phosphate and positively charged stearyl amine. Niosomes appear to have applications in topical and transdermal dosage forms containing hydrophilic and hydrophobic drugs; they also can be used to encapsulate biotechnological products including vaccines [74].

11.5.3.3 *Nanoparticles*

Nanoparticles are solid colloidal drug carriers ranging from 10–1,000 nm in diameter and are composed of synthetic, natural, or semisynthetic polymers encapsulating the drug molecule [75]. Many hydrophilic (gelatin, albumin, casein, polysaccharide lectin, etc.) and hydrophobic polymers (polycaprolactone, polyesters, polyanhydrides, polycyanoacrylate) are used in the formation of nanoparticles. Recent biomedical applications include efficient and controlled drug delivery targeting skin and skin appendages, transcutaneous vaccination, and transdermal gene therapy. The nanoformulations have modernized conventional transdermal drug delivery for the treatment of various skin diseases. Nanoparticles are being used in the field of cosmetics, but there must be a safety assurance and toxicity check mechanism before application on skin [76].

Solid lipid nanoparticles (SLNs) are composed of a solid and lipid particle matrix that proves to be an alternative carrier system to liposomes and emulsions. SLNs exhibit a wide application in the field of cosmeceuticals and pharmaceuticals due to an increase in the rate of permeation, occlusion, and hydration of skin. Lipid nanoparticles are formed from biodegradable lipids, which are used as safe carriers with excellent tolerability. Cosmetic companies rank high among nanotechnology patent holders in the United States;

L'Oreal, which devotes about $600 million of its annual $17 billion revenues to research, is the industry leader on nanopatents [77].

11.5.3.4 *Transferosomes*

Transferosomes are elastic and deformable vesicles applied to the skin. The vesicles contain soya phosphatidylcholine encapsulating sodium cholate; ethanol is added in small concentrations as an accelerant. The drug can penetrate through the skin into the systemic circulation by hydration and osmotic force without affecting the occlusion process. Recent investigation demonstrates the potential use of small molecules, peptides, steroids, proteins, and vaccines, both *in vitro* and *in vivo*. Transferosomes are also used in gene therapy on skin and achieve drug delivery through transfection [78].

11.6. CHARACTERIZATION AND EVALUATION OF SEMISOLID DOSAGE FORMS

Many significant factors such as particle size and shape, texture, rheological properties, mucoadhesive properties, and surface pH can influence the complex structure of semisolid dosage forms. These properties directly affect the dermatological absorption and therapeutic efficacy of drugs.

11.6.1 Particle Size

Particle size is an important property for the pharmaceutical and cosmeceutical industry because it directly affects drug bioavailability; a decrease in particle size results in increased surface area, leading to enhanced dissolution and finally the absorption of the drug. Particle size and size distribution in dispersion play important roles in the safety and efficacy of dosage forms. Content uniformity, dose uniformity, rheological properties, grittiness, and irritability are directly related to the size and shape of particles [79]. One study on porcine skin suggested that nanoparticles with a smaller particle size favor follicular localization [102]. Particle size significantly affects the penetration of drugs. Drugs with a particle size less than 3 nm may penetrate both in the stratum corneum and hair follicle, whereas drugs with a particle size greater than 10 nm usually do not cross the epidermal layer. Drugs with a particle size between 3 and 10 nm may get concentrated on the hair follicle.

Because particle size is a critical parameter in the performance of topical dosage forms, it must be carefully controlled. A number of techniques have been explored to determine the particle size of drugs, including laser diffraction, dynamic light scattering (DLS), disc centrifugation, and light microscopy.

11.6.1.1 *Laser Diffraction*

Any particle that passes through a laser beam scatters light in proportion to its size depending on the angle through which it travels. The intensity of scattered light depends on particle size and its volume. The wider the angle, the higher the particle scattering intensity and vice versa. A laser diffraction technique currently is being used for the determination of particle size and as a quality assurance tool in large-scale production lines in industry. Laser diffraction can determine particle size during manufacturing of the semisolid dosage form so that sedimentation can be determined and formulations can be optimized at the initial stage. The laser diffraction equipment can measure the particles in the size range of 0.5–3,500 μm. This technique shows good reproducibility in its results[103].[161]

11.6.1.2 *Dynamic Light Scattering*

The dynamic light scattering technique involves an optical procedure that measures the fluctuation of scattered light intensities as defined through Brownian motion of particles in the submicron range (5 nm–5 μm). The upper limit of the range is decided by the weight of the scattered particles. Dynamic light scattering can be used as an analytical technique to determine particle size, polydispersity and the size distribution of highly complex samples of proteins, nanoparticles, and cosmetics [80].

11.6.1.3 *Disc Centrifuge*

A disc centrifuge works on the principle of centrifugal sedimentation in a liquid medium where centrifugal force is generated by a rotating disc. The sedimentation is stabilized by a slight density gradient within the liquid. This procedure is used for particle size determination where sedimentation of particles depends on the viscosity of the solution, the density gradient, and the centrifugal force generated by the disc centrifuge.

11.6.1.4 *Optical Microscopy*

The optical microscopy method uses a large number of photomicrographs to capture particle size distribution through a technology-intensive method that automatically analyzes particle size through an optical microscope that is fitted with a dedicated digital camera that can handle the collective analysis of images. This analysis helps in measuring the length, width, area, and circle diameter and in studying surface properties of particles under observation. The upper limits of the particles under observation can be enhanced up to several millimeters at low magnification, while the lower limits can be enhanced close to a micrometer through the use of white light illumination [81].

11.6.1.5 Raman Chemical Imaging

The Raman chemical imaging technique is a combination of optical microscopy and Raman spectroscopy used to generate hyper-spectral images that contain a high-resolution power that separates the individual spectrum. It can detect droplets of different chemical agents and is used to analyze the morphology, composition, and spatial distribution of particles in semisolid preparations. It yields better results as compared to conventional microscopy in terms of speed, image clarity, droplet size distribution of oil and emulsion, and simultaneous detection of droplets of different compositions. Raman chemical imaging has been utilized successfully to determine the particle size, chemical identity, and particle size distribution of corticosteroids in nasal spray suspension. This technique can be used for differentiation between the excipient and active pharmaceutical ingredient, total number, shape, and size of particles [82].

11.6.2 Rheological Properties

Semisolid dosage forms represent a wide class of dosage forms containing creams, ointments, gels, pastes, suppositories, etc. They are dispersions containing flow properties of both solids and liquids. A deformation of structure occurs on application of external force or extrusion from a bottle. Higher shear stress in viscometers is useful to determine the viscosity during manufacturing, but it can change the structure of semisolid dosage forms. Therefore, application of low shear stress should be preferred wherever possible, as it does not cause any change in the structure and can be performed on the ground state. Viscosity has a considerable effect on the percutaneous absorption of the drug. It is generally considered that the higher the viscosity of the dosage form, the lesser is the rate of diffusion of medicament, although sometimes a drug product having a higher concentration of a drug exhibits a greater rate of drug diffusion. Evaluation of rheological parameters is important not only for assessing the rate of diffusion but also for evaluating the consistency of dosage, which has a significant effect on spreadability and duration of action of a topical dosage form. Batch-to-batch uniformity in consistency is required for a quality product during manufacturing to maintain reproducibility in the production process, because most semisolid dosage forms, when sheared, exhibit non-Newtonian behavior. The rheological behavior of semisolids is attributable to properties like shear thinning viscosity, thixotropy, and irreversible shear stress [83]. A large number of factors affect the viscosity of semisolid dosage forms, such as inherent physical structure of the product, product sampling technique, sample temperature for viscosity testing, container size, and shape. Temperature has a significant effect on the rheology of semisolid dosage forms. As the temperature is raised, semisolid products show a decrease in viscosity, thixotropy, and yield value. For many of the semisolids, there appears to be a straight-line relationship between thixotropic area and temperature. Hydroxypropyl cellulose gels can be formed with water, ethanol, and propylene glycol, whose viscosity does not exhibit hysteresis in their rheograms. The viscosity increases and the gel shows non-Newtonian behavior with an increase in the molecular weight and concentration of the polymer. Concentration of propylene glycol in ternary solvent mixtures with water and ethanol increases the elasticity of gel and hence makes it highly viscoelastic in nature. Spreading capacity, stickiness, and fluidity of the formulation after application depend on rheological characteristics and significantly affect patient acceptability of semisolid dosage forms [84].

11.6.2.1 Measurement of Rheological Property

11.6.2.1.1 VISCOMETER/ RHEOMETER

A number of viscometers and rheometers are used to characterize the shear rate and viscoelastic properties of solids, semisolids, and liquids. A rheometer can be classified in the following categories based on the geometry: concentric cylinder, cone and plate, parallel plate, and rectangular torsion, as shown in Figure 11.7. The small-angle cone and plate and small-gap concentric

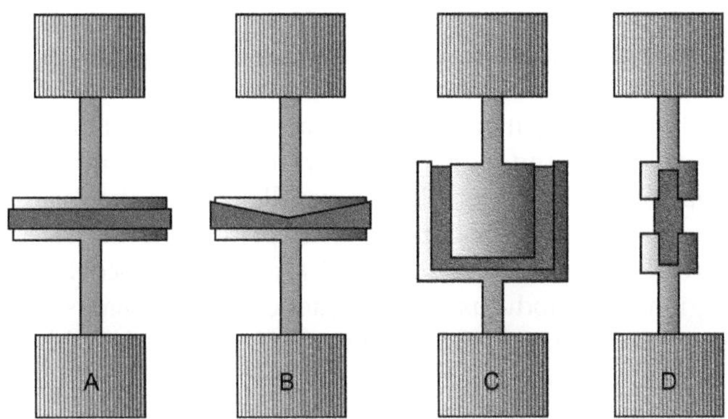

FIGURE 11.7 Schematic diagrams for dynamic rheometers: (A) parallel plates, (B) cone and plate, (C) concentric cylinder (couette), and (D) solid or torsion rectangular. The appropriate geometry is dictated primarily by the properties of sample material, but may also be dictated by the desire to simulate a process or in situ application. *(Adapted from http://www.ceramicindustry.com/articles/print/using-rheology-to-improve-manufacturing).*

cylinder have the same shear rate and shear stress at each portion of liquid/semisolid to be tested [85].

11.6.2.1.2 CONCENTRIC CYLINDER VISCOMETER

The concentric cylinder viscometer functions on a moderate shear rate, making this a good choice for measurement of rheological properties in different fields of pharmacy and engineering. This type of instrument consists of two coaxial cylinders: the outer cylinder forms the cup, and the inner cylinder forms a bob. Two types of instruments exist depending on whether the cup or bob rotates. One is a couette-type system, in which the cup rotates and the bob is stationary; this type can be used to calculate shear rate of low viscous substances. In another type known as the Searle type, the bob is rotated and the cup is stationary. The Brookfield viscometer, which comes under the second category, is widely used in the viscosity measurement of diverse topical formulations.

11.6.2.1.3 CONE AND PLATE VISCOMETER

When a cup plate viscometer is used to calculate rheological properties, the shear stress and shear rate can be obtained directly. The instrument essentially consists of a flat, circular plate with a wide-angle cone placed centrally above it. It contains a moderate shear rate device that is appropriate for semisolids containing smaller particles because the cone angle is small.

11.6.2.1.4 PARALLEL PLATE AND RECTANGULAR TORSIONAL RHEOMETER

In a parallel plate and rectangular torsional rheometer, shear stress is determined from the torque response of the instrument, which is evaluated by constructing a force-balance equation on disk and integrating over the radius. With a cone plate viscometer, the shear stress is constant and can be easily evaluated, whereas in a parallel plate system, shear stress is a function of the radius of the semisolid between the plates, making it more complicated. It shows nonuniform strain and adjustable gap height. Samples are applied on the lower plate in parallel and to the inside of the stator in the concentric plate. The stress is directly proportional to the strain in the viscoelastic region and modulus. The frequency sweep analysis is performed in a frequency range of 0.1–10 Hz with a constant stress and is used to calculate the modulus and dynamic viscosity [86].

11.6.3 Consistency

Batch-to-batch uniform consistency (i.e., thickness or firmness) of semisolid dosage forms is important for quality control. A cone penetration test is used to measure the consistency of various substances, such as petroleum products, food, cosmetics, and other semisolid materials. A penetrometer is used to measure the consistency and penetration properties of semisolid substances [97]. This is based on the principle that a standard penetrant such as a cone or a needle penetrates into the depth of the semisolid substance under defined conditions of sample size, penetrant weight, geometry, and time, and a higher penetration of the penetrant indicates an increase in softness of the sample.

11.6.4 Surface pH

Semisolid dosage forms contain very limited quantities of a liquid or aqueous phase. Surface pH of semisolids should be tested during manufacturing and for monitoring batch-to-batch uniformity and for quality control of dosage forms. Surface pH can be measured by using a simple pH meter or by using a probe-type pH meter. If the formulation is thick, the pH can be measured by diluting with distilled water. Because the skin has a neutral pH, the formulation should also have nearly the same pH; otherwise, it may cause local irritation.

11.6.5 Content Uniformity

Uniformity of content may be ensured by using suitable analytical procedures in accordance with official methods or by using suitable validated analytical procedures. Uniformity of content of cyclosporine in the formulation containing poly (lactide-co-glycolide), for example, can be determined by radio immune assay (RIA). Conformational stability can be predicted from other spectroscopy such as FTIR and circular dichroism (CD) spectroscopy [87]. In a study of controlled-release insulin gel, the content of insulin in formulation was evaluated by enzyme-linked immunosorbent assay (ELISA), and conformational stability was confirmed by electrophoresis, FTIR, and circular dichroism spectroscopy [88].

11.6.6 Spreadability

Spreadability depends on the rheological properties of dosage forms. When an external force is applied to the wall of a gel container, it forms a puddle that provides a pharmacological effect on spreading the dosage form at the application site. Therefore, spreading is an important property in the effectiveness of a dosage form to the target site, extrusion from the container, ease of application, and consumer preference. Drug release characteristics, consistency, spreadability, penetrometer readings, extrudability of container, viscosity, and physical and chemical stability are the properties used to select an ointment base.

A number of methods such as the parallel plate method, subject assessment (use of human volunteers), master curve (summation of subject assessment and the instrumental method), and *in vivo* studies on animals and humans are used to measure the spreading of dosage forms. A master curve derived from rheological concepts was plotted to measure the spreadability of creams and ointments using a Ferranti–Shirley cone and plate viscometer at 25°C and 34°C. Creams show better spreading properties than the ointment dosage forms. It was observed that spreadability of formulations depends on the rate of shear, which varies from 400 to 2,500 sec^{-1}. A rheological master curve was plotted between the rate of shear and consistency of spreading. The spreadability parameter was found to be similar with all types of scaling (ordinal, preference, and ratio scaling), and it was observed that such screening tests are useful in dosage form development [89].

11.6.7 Texture Analysis

Texture is the feel of a substance, which can be quantified through properties such as silkiness, roughness, and stiffness. All the mechanical properties including texture, hardness, compressibility, adhesiveness, and cohesiveness of a vaginal gel containing clomiphene citrate, for example, can be analyzed using the TA-XT Plus Texture analyzer (Stable Micro Systems, UK) containing controlled penetrometer software at a temperature of 37 ± 0.5°C. The assembly contains a universal bottle at a fixed height of 8 cm, which is kept in an ultrasonic water bath to remove air bubbles. It also contains a Perspex probe with a 10 mm diameter that is twice compressed into each formulation at a particular depth and time, and the compression property is evaluated with the help of software in the instrument [90].

11.6.8 Mucoadhesive Properties

Mucoadhesive strength is the force required to detach a hydrated formulation from the mucous membrane. In semisolid dosage forms, mucoadhesive formulations include ointments, pastes, gels, etc, which may contain bioadhesive polymers incorporated into the hydrophobic base. The mechanism of mucoadhesion gives an idea about the retention time of formulation on the mucosa, which depends on the surface energy, along with viscoelastic properties of liquid [91].

The mucoadhesive properties of a formulation may be evaluated by using a texture analyser in which mucin discs are attached horizontally with double-sided adhesive tape to the lower end of a probe. Samples of each formulation are packed into a shallow cylindrical vessel. The mucin disc in the analytical probe is lowered to the surface of each formulation with a particular force and time in order to ensure intimate contact between the mucin disc and sample; then the probe is moved upward at a constant speed. The force required to detach the mucin disc from the surface of the formulation can be measured from a force-time plot. At least four readings should be taken for accuracy of result [86]. However, a modified physical balance can also be used to measure the mucoadhesive strength of formulations, where force required to detach the film is measured [92].

11.6.9 Drug Content

Drug content in topical dosage forms can be evaluated by adding a fixed quantity of a formulation containing the drug to a solvent in sealed ampoules. The mixture is stirred in a constant temperature bath at 37°C for a defined time, and the samples are withdrawn at the time of separation of the aqueous and oily phases. The samples are then analyzed using a suitable analytical technique such as spectrophotometry or chromatographic technique such as HPLC.

11.6.10 Evaluation of Drug Release and Permeation

In semisolid dosage forms, the stratum corneum of skin acts as a barrier for most drugs. A lipophilic drug, however, can more easily cross through this barrier. Therefore, an *in vitro* and/or *in vivo* evaluation of dosage form is required to determine the route of penetration and the amount of drug permeated through the skin so that an effective formulation can be developed that can easily cross the skin barrier and provide a safe and efficacious drug delivery.

11.7. PROCEDURE AND APPARATUS FOR DIFFUSION EXPERIMENT

Diffusion is a process by which a mass transfer of molecules is brought about by random molecular motion due to a concentration gradient across a barrier, which is the region that offers resistance to the diffusant. Generally, a membrane consisting of a sheet of solid or semisolid material is used as a barrier to separate the phases and materials passing through it.

The driving force for diffusion is the concentration gradient (or more correctly, the gradient of chemical potential).

Examples:

Transport of drugs through a polymeric membrane
Percutaneous absorption of drugs
Passive diffusion of drugs in the GI tract

11.7.1 Mathematics of Diffusion

Diffusion can be schematically represented as shown in Figure 11.8, where S is the cross-sectional area, h is the thickness, C_1 is the concentration in the membrane on the donor side, C_2 is concentration in the membrane on the receptor side, C_d is concentration in the donor side, C_r is the concentration in the receptor side.

From Fick's first law:

$$J = \frac{dM}{Sdt} = -D\frac{dc}{dx} = -D\left(\frac{(c_2 - c_1)}{h}\right) \quad (11.6)$$

$$J = D\left(\frac{c_1 - c_2}{h}\right) \quad (11.7)$$

Assumptions:

1. A quasi–steady state exists.
2. No aqueous boundary layer exists.

Since C_1 and C_2 are difficult to measure, C_d and C_r are generally monitored.

If the partition coefficient = K, as follows:

$$K = \frac{C_1}{C_d} = \frac{C_2}{C_r} \quad (11.8)$$

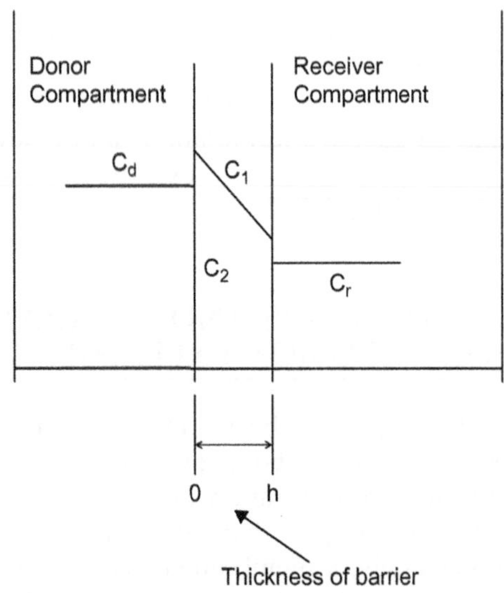

FIGURE 11.8 Diffusion through the isotropic membrane.

Then $C_1 = K\,C_d$ and $C_2 = K\,C_r$.
Substituting these values in Eq. 11.6, we get

$$\frac{dM}{dt} = \frac{DSK(c_d - c_r)}{h} \quad (11.9)$$

If the sink condition prevails in the receptor compartment (when the drug concentration in the receptor compartment is less than 15%–20% of the solubility of the drug in the medium of interest), then $C_r \approx 0$ such that

$$\frac{dM}{dt} = \frac{DSK(c_d)}{h} = PSc_d \quad (11.10)$$

where

$$\frac{Dk}{h} = P = \text{Permeability coefficient (cm/sec)} \quad (11.11)$$

Then

$$\mathrm{M} = PSc_d t \quad (11.12)$$

The amount of material (M) flowing through a unit cross-section (S) of a barrier in unit time (t) is defined as flux:

$$J = \frac{dM}{Sdt} \quad (11.13)$$

According to Fick's first law, the flux is proportional to the concentration gradient, as shown in Eqs. 11.14 and 11.15:

$$J \propto \frac{dC}{dx} \quad (11.14)$$

$$J = -D\frac{dc}{dx} \quad (11.15)$$

where D is the diffusion coefficient of the substance that is diffusing through a barrier, in cm^2/sec, and x is the distance in centimeters of movement perpendicular to the barrier. The mass, M, is usually given in grams and moles; the barrier surface in cm^2; and the time, t, in seconds. The diffusion constant, D, is treated as a constant in Eq. 11.15. This may not always be the case, and D may be affected by the temperature, pressure, concentration, solvent properties, and the chemical nature of the diffusant.

Fick's second law allows us to determine the rate of change of concentration relative to the position in a system. According to Fick's second law, the rate of change in concentration in a volume element within the diffusional field is proportional to the rate of change in concentration gradient at the point in the field, as shown in both Eqs. 11.16 and 11.17:

$$\frac{\delta c}{\delta t} = -\frac{\delta J}{\delta x} = \frac{\delta\left[-D\left(\frac{\delta c}{\delta x}\right)\right]}{\delta x} \quad (11.16)$$

$$\frac{\partial c}{\partial t} = D\frac{\partial^2 C}{\partial x^2} \qquad (11.17)$$

Fick's laws are very important in pharmacy, and numerous equations that account for drug release from delivery systems and drug absorption in biological systems have been derived from these laws.

11.7.2 Diffusion Apparatus

The apparatus used for measuring diffusion coefficients of substances are called diffusion cells. These cells basically consist of two chambers (donor and receiver chambers) separated by a membrane, and they differ widely in shape and size. Figure 11.9 shows a schematic representation of a horizontal side-by-side diffusion cells.

To measure the diffusion coefficients of substances, one adds the drug to the donor chamber, and the amount of drug that penetrates into the receiver chamber is measured as a function of time. The result of this experiment is usually a curve, as shown in Figure 11.10.

Flux can be determined from the slope of the steady-state portion of the plot, and lag time is equal to its intercept on abscissa. The diffusion coefficient of the drug can be readily determined from the lag time, using Eq. 11.18:

$$t_L = \frac{h^2}{6D} \qquad (11.18)$$

where h is the thickness of the membrane used.

The release of drugs suspended in ointment bases can be calculated by using the Higuchi equation, Eq. 11.19 [93]:

$$Q = 2Co\,(Dt/\pi)^{1/2} \qquad (11.19)$$

where Q is the amount of drug released into the receptor phase per unit area (mg/cm^2), Co is the initial drug concentration in the dosage form (mg/mL), D is the apparent diffusion coefficient of the drug (cm^2/s), t is the time after application (s), and π is a constant.

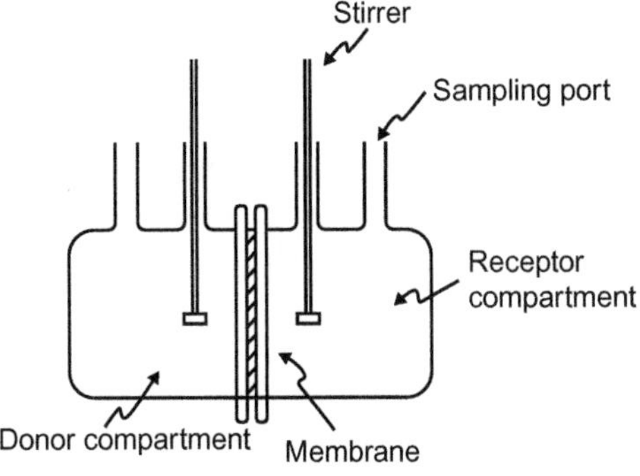

FIGURE 11.9 Schematic representation of a horizontal diffusion cell.

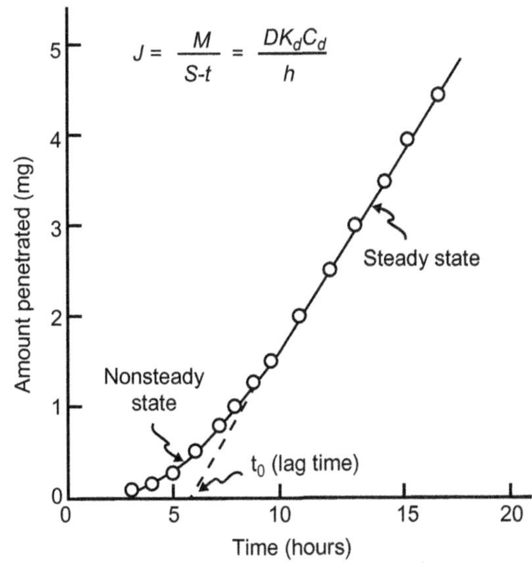

FIGURE 11.10 Graphical plot of a typical diffusion data.

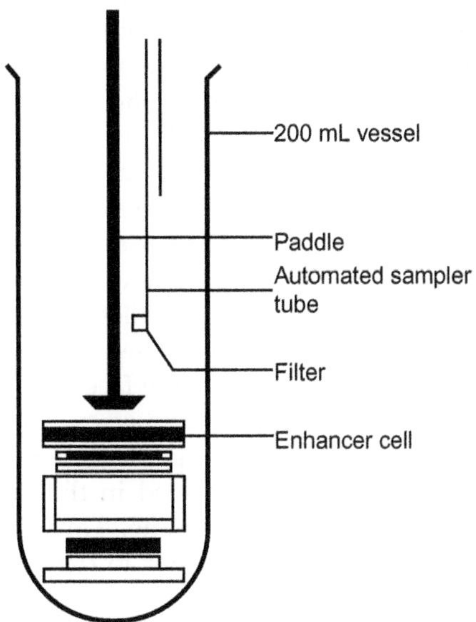

FIGURE 11.11 The Enhancer Cell™ assembly.

A number of apparatus and diffusion cells have been used to determine the flux or diffusion coefficient of drugs. The following sections provide details on diffusion cells described in the USP.

11.7.3 Modified USP Apparatus with Enhancer Cell

The Enhancer Cell assembly contains an enhancer cell placed in a USP apparatus (see Figure 11.11). The Enhancer Cell™ (VanKel, NJ), made of Teflon, consisting of a cap, an o-ring, a washer, and a drug reservoira

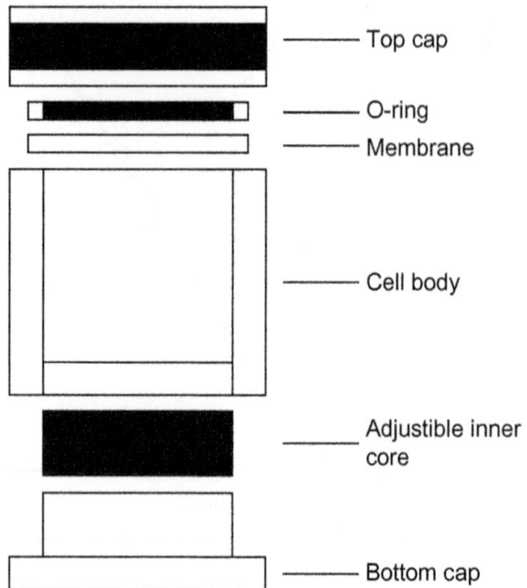

FIGURE 11.12 Modified USP apparatus with enhancer cell.

is used for *in vitro* release studies of semisolid dosage forms, placing a membrane on the top of the reservoir. The diameter of the body, cap and solid ring are kept identical, which helps in keeping the membrane in its position while tightening the cell. The cell is placed in a USP dissolution tester that is a modified form of a USP apparatus 2 with 200 mL capacity flask instead of a 900 mL flask. Also part of this equipment are an adapter plate to prevent evaporation from the receptor phase, a small size shaft, and collets, along with a small receptor cell for analysis. The sample is placed on the membrane mounting, on the face of the receptor medium in the reservoir, and the screw cap is tightened on the membrane. During the experiment, one must ensure that no air is trapped in the interface of the formulation and the membrane. Thus, the equipment is degassed using a sonicator to remove air bubbles. The Enhancer Cell is then placed in a modified USP apparatus (see Figure 11.12). The receptor medium is stirred constantly with a magnetic stirrer. Further samples are collected by means of an automatic sampler and are replaced with fresh samples. This simple method ensures batch-to-batch consistency of semisolid dosage forms and can detect products of different strengths. It reduces costs by requiring fewer accessories and apparatus that give reliable and reproducible results as compared to data obtained from other diffusion cells used as screening devices in preformulation and product development [94].

11.7.4 USP Apparatus 4 with Dialysis Adapter

In 1957, a flow-through cell was developed by the FDA to evaluate the release rate of dosage forms. Bhardwaj et al. later modified the USP apparatus 4 with a dialysis adapter (see Figure 11.13). The dialysis adapter is made of a hollow cylinder containing a circular Teflon fabricated base and top, supported by metallic wire to provide a framework for the adapter. A dialysis membrane is placed over the Teflon top and sealed with an o-ring at the top and bottom. The whole assembly is then placed in the USP apparatus in an upright position. The base of a sample cell is filled with ruby beads or glass beads at the bottom of the cell. The dosage form is applied on the adapter and sealed with a screw on the top. The sample is withdrawn from the media reservoir container of the apparatus and replaced with a fresh solvent to maintain the sink condition during the experiment. This method can provide better simulations for *in vivo* conditions. Additionally, it can provide biorelevant conditions such as the addition of serum or enzymes, change in temperature or pH, and addition of a surfactant to trigger release and does not alter the mechanism of drug release. It is used mainly for liposome, microemulsion, suspension, etc., but now it can be used to study semisolid dosage forms where microdialysis is recommended.

A number of *in vitro* release methods can be used to evaluate semisolid dosage forms. These methods can provide simple, reproducible quality control tests that can be used to test the quality and stability of semisolid dosage forms containing hydrophilic and lipophilic drugs but not applied for bioequivalence studies of dosage forms. None of these methods can be used as official methods in the Pharmacopoeia. Regulatory agencies are continuously trying to search for more stringent methods comparable to dissolution testing of oral dosage forms.

11.7.5 Method of Preparation of Semisolid Dosage Form

As mentioned previously, semisolid dosage forms include ointments, creams, gels, pastes, and suppositories. Mixing of semisolids depends on the type of dosage form, the quantity of product, and the types of bases used in formulation of the product (see Tables 11.2 and 11.3). The ointments, pastes, and gels can be prepared from two methods: trituration and fusion. The trituration method, which is performed on a laboratory scale, involves mixing the drug with a base and other excipients using a metal spatula. The fusion method, used for large-scale manufacturing, involves heating waxes and solids according to the descending order of melting points with continuous mixing in a mixer or in homogenizers in order to produce the desired homogeneity of products. One problem involved in the process of mixing of semisolids is dead-spot formation, which can be prevented if the

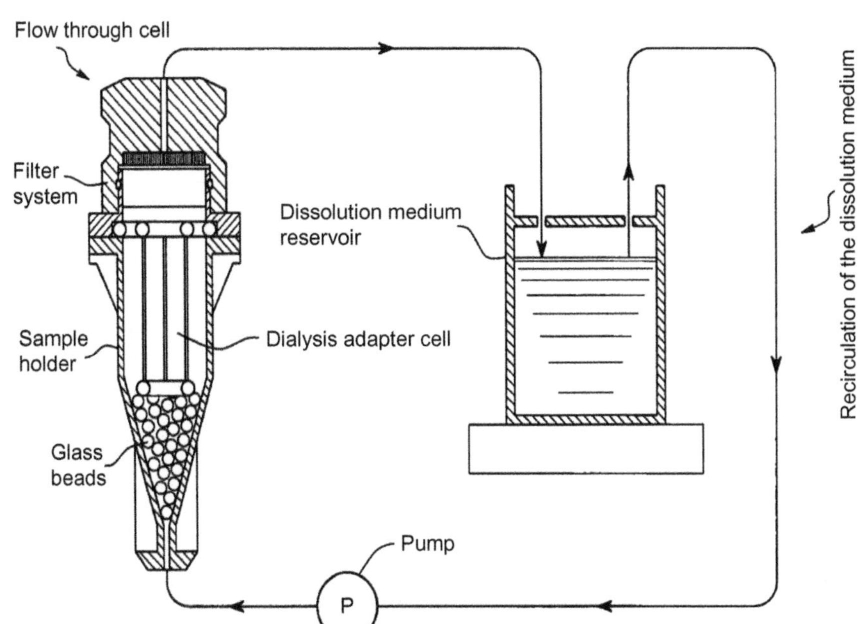

FIGURE 11.13 USP Apparatus 4 with dialysis adapter.

proper shape blade is used. The mixing process includes low-speed shear, smearing, wiping, folding, stretching, and compressing. Low-speed shear is required due to changes in rheological properties with the changes in shear stress of semisolids.

Two types of mixers are used for mixing semisolids: double-kneading machines and Banbury mixers. For very stiff masses, the kneading machine is commonly used. It consists of an open trough with an approximately semi-cylindrical bottom. Within this trough, two horizontal knives in a roughly Z-shaped outline rotate. This construction is usually known as a sigma blade. These knives are placed and shaped so that the material turned up by one knife is immediately turned under by the adjacent one. These machines are built in large sizes and may be designed to consume a very large amount of power. They may be jacketed for heating or cooling, and they may be closed to retain volatile solvents. They always operate on the batch principle and are therefore mounted so that they can be dumped by power-operated jacks. The Banbury mixer is an exceedingly heavy machine with two pear-shaped knives or blades, each rotating in a cylindrical shell, but these cylinders partly intersect each other. The projection is spiral along the axis, and the two spirals interlock. Because heat may be produced during mixing in the cylinder, the walls are cooled by a water spray.

Creams can be prepared by simultaneously heating both the aqueous phase and oily phase at the same temperature, 70°C, and the two phases mixed. After mixing, the congealed mass is cooled, and volatile ingredients are added after cooling to 25–30°C. In order to avoid grittiness, particle size reduction can be achieved by using a colloidal mill or triple-roller mill. According to the USP, dilution should not be preferred in creams and ointments until and unless it is required, because excessive dilution can affect the stability of the formulation. The dilution should be performed in hygienic conditions in order to avoid any microbial contamination. Any unsuitable diluents, excessive dilution, or heating during mixing can cause incompatibility or instability. The preparations should be used within 2 weeks after the dilution.

11.7.6 Packaging, Storage, and Labeling

Packaging for semisolid preparations is often dictated by the nature of the medicament and the base. It is also dependent on the manner in which the semisolid is applied or the shipment of the product is done, depending on the quantity involved in the packaging. Stainless steel, tin plate drums, and collapsible aluminum tubes [96] are used where the semisolids are devoid of reactive ingredients with the metals; i.e., they do not cause any corrosion or rusting. Glass packaging is used mostly in products that are not affected by light and mainly used for medium bulk quantities up to 2 kg in weight. Most bulk packaging is done in high-density polyethylene containers because they are light, moldable, and they regain their original shape, causing no wastage. They therefore are more suitable for semisolids in which sensitive applications are involved, such as eye ointments and ointments used for oral treatments. The most extensively used

TABLE 11.2 Summary Chart: Properties of Ointment Bases

	Oleaginous Ointment Bases	Absorption Ointment Bases	Water/Oil Emulsion Ointment Bases	Oil/Water Emulsion Ointment Bases	Water-miscible Ointment Bases
Composition	oleaginous compounds	oleaginous base + w/o surfactant	oleaginous base + water (<45% w/w) + w/o surfactant (HLB <8)	oleaginous base + water (>45% w/w) + o/w surfactant (HLB >9)	Polyethylene Glycols (PEGs)
Water Content	anhydrous	anhydrous	hydrous	hydrous	anhydrous, hydrous
Affinity for Water	hydrophobic	hydrophilic	hydrophilic	hydrophilic	hydrophilic
Spreadability	difficult	difficult	moderate to easy	easy	moderate to easy
Washability	nonwashable	nonwashable	non- or poorly washable	washable	washable
Stability	oils poor; hydrocarbons better	oils poor; hydrocarbons better	unstable, especially alkali soaps and natural colloids	unstable, especially alkali soaps and natural colloids; nonionics better	stable
Drug Incorporation Potential	solids or oils (oil solubles only)	solids, oils, and aqueous solutions (small amounts)	solids, oils, and aqueous solutions (small amounts)	solid and aqueous solutions (small amounts)	solid and aqueous solutions
Drug Release Potential	poor	poor, but > oleaginous	fair to good	fair to good	good
Occlusiveness	yes	yes	sometimes	no	no
Uses	protectants, emollients (+/−), vehicles for hydrolyzable drugs	protectants, emollients (+/−), vehicles for aqueous solutions, solids, and non-hydrolyzable drugs	emollients, cleansing creams, vehicles for solid, liquid, or non-hydrolyzable drugs	emollients, vehicles for solid, liquid, or non-hydrolyzable drugs	drug vehicles
Examples	White Petrolatum, White Ointment	Hydrophilic Petrolatum, Anhydrous Lanolin, Aquabase™, Aquaphor®, Polysorb®	Cold Cream type, Hydrous Lanolin, Rose Water Ointment, Hydrocream™, Eucerin®, Nivea®	Hydrophilic Ointment, Dermabase™, Velvachol®, Unibase®	PEG Ointment, P

packing material for pharmaceuticals these days is collapsible plastic tubes, but they do have the disadvantage of possibly causing oxidation. Metal tubes provide good protection from oxidation and do not let aqueous solutions dry out because they retain the volatile ingredients of the medicaments; however, these tubes may not be cost effective [95].

Semisolids must be stored very carefully at a suitable temperature for a given period of time depending on the nature of products to be stored. Aluminium-collapsible tubes containing an epoxy-resin coating are used for products that must be stored for a longer period of time because they are known for their good mechanical properties and chemical resistance [96]. These tubes are good for semisolid dosages that are sterile in nature and are stored in air-tight, tamper-proof containers at less than 25°C.

11.7.7 Packaging, Storage, and Labeling of Suppositories

The preferred storage for suppositories is glass and plastic screw-top jars due to their hygroscopic nature. Suppositories are packed and stored at low temperatures. The label must contain the "use for" instructions, i.e., "for rectal use only," "for vaginal use only." It also should mention the temperature at which they are to be stored, such as "store in a cool place."

The next step before launching a drug requires marketing surveillance, ensuring the labeling of the drug in accordance with drug regulatory authority and pharmacopeial guidelines. The label on the container should state "For external/internal use"; the strength of active ingredient as a percentage or volume; the "best before" date/date of expiry/manufacturing date; name and

TABLE 11.3 Formulation and Component of Semisolid Dosage Form

Component	Properties	Example
BASES		
Ointment Bases		
Oleaginous bases	Occlusive, hydrophobic, greasy, nonwashable	White petrolatum, white ointment
Absorption bases	Occlusive, water absorbent, anhydrous, greasy	Anhydrous lanolin, hydrophilic petrolatum
W/O type emulsion bases	Occlusive, hydrous, greasy, hydrophilic, nonwashable	Lanolin, cold cream
O/W type emulsion bases	Washable, nongreasy, can be diluted with water, non occlusive	Hydrophilic ointment
Water-soluble bases	Water-soluble and washable, nongreasy, nonocclusive, lipid free	Polyethylene glycol ointment
Suppository Bases		
Oily bases	Low absorption of water, hydrophobic, immiscible with mucus	Theobroma oil, hydrogenated oil
Water-soluble/Water-miscible	Hydrophilic, some are hygroscopic	Glycero gelatin, polyethylene glycol
Emulsifying bases	Water-dispersible, contain nonionic surfactant with oils or waxy solids	Witespol, massupol, massa esterinum
Vehicle		
Aqueous vehicle	Hydrophilic, nonreactant and nontoxic	Ethanol and water
Nonaqueous vehicle	Hydrophobic, oily	Mineral oil and volatile oil
Emulsifying Agents		
Anionic	Contain a negative charge, produce o/w emulsions, high pH	Soaps, sulphated alcohols, dioctyl sodium sulpho succinate
Cationic	Bear a positive charge, used in creams and lotions	Benzalkonium chloride, cetrimide
Nonionic	Stable, used in both o/w and w/o emulsion	Sorbitan monostearate, macrogol ethers
Gelling Agents/ Thickening Agents	Form gel by increasing viscosity, may be natural, semisynthetic and synthetic	Silicates, bentonites, carbomers, cellulose derivatives, gelatins
Antioxidants	Prevent or reduce rate of oxidation, chelating agent acts as catalyst for oxidation process	BHA, BHT, ascorbic acid, citric acid, tartaric acid,
Buffers	Control pH and provide stability by preventing drug ionization	Citrate, phosphate, and acetate buffer
Humectants	Minimize water loss and prevent drying out	Glycerol, propylene glycol, sorbitol
Preservatives	Kill or inhibit the growth of micro-organisms	Benzoic acid, hydroxyl benzoates, benzalkonium compounds

amount of added antimicrobial preservatives; storage condition; batch number; dilution required, if any; and/or sterility of preparation, as the case may be.

11.8. CONCLUSIONS

Semisolid dosage forms constitute a significant type of treatment and hold a lot of potential; it is up to us to effectively utilize these dosage forms to effectively harness their potential in effective therapy and healthcare management. There is a rising demand for dermatological products in the world market today, and this trend will continue in the future. The treatment subareas of dermatology that will see the highest boost in the future include infectious skin disease, psoriasis, dermatitis, acne, and skin protection. Novel and innovative drug delivery approaches to deliver therapeutic agents via skin have seen some dramatic improvements over the past decade and will be explored much more in the future.

CASE STUDIES

Case 11.1

Mrs. Turner needs to purchase a prescription of 0.25% (w/w) steroid cream to treat eczema on her infant son's cheeks. She asks the pharmacist about a prescription she got from her doctor two weeks ago for the same steroid but at a higher concentration (1%). Since the cost of this topical formulation is very high, she wants to know why she needs to purchase the 0.25% cream for her son when she could use the left-over 1% ointment instead. How should the pharmacist respond to Mrs. Turner?

Approach: This is an interesting case because it deals with multiple factors:

1. The cream formulation is not the same as an ointment.
2. An infant's skin is very different from that of an adult, with different barrier properties. One has to consider the percutaneous absorption properties of the topical formulation, which is quite different from that for adult.
3. The strength of the ointment is four times more concentrated than the prescription for the cream. Therefore, caution should be taken not to substitute the ointment for the cream.

Case 11.2

A family of three is planning a long trip to Europe. Both parents and their teenage son suffer from travel sickness during long-term air travel. Unfortunately, the trip was so quickly arranged that the teenage son does not have a scopolamine patch to use during this travel. His mother calls the pharmacist for a consultation, explaining that her son's age is exactly half of her age. She wants to know why she cannot cut one of her transdermal patches in half and use a half patch for her son. What should you, as an attending pharmacist, respond to the mother?

Approach: You should explicitly say no to this query. Explain to the mother that by cutting her patch into two, she will destroy the rate-controlling membrane and the patch will lose its controlled mechanism of release; therefore, there may be a possibility of a dumping effect for the drug.

References

[1] Eros I, Ehab JA, Cserne A, Csoka I, Csanyi E. Factors influencing liberation of drug from semisolid dosage forms. Acta Pharm Hung 2000;70:29–34.
[2] Chalupova Z, Masteikova R, Savickas A. Pharmaceutical hydrophilic gels. Ceska Slov Farm 2005;54:55–9.
[3] Durgin JM, Hanan ZI. Pharmaceutical dosage forms. In: Bellegarde M, editor. Pharmacy practice for technicians. 4th ed. New York, USA: Cengage Learning; 2010.
[4] Niazi S. Handbook of pharmaceutical manufacturing formulations: semisolid products. Boca Raton, Florida, USA: CRC Press; 2004.
[5] Petró E, Balogh A, Blazsó G, Erös I, Csóka I. *In vitro* and *in vivo* evaluation of drug release from semisolid dosage forms. Eighth central european symposium on pharmaceutical technology, vol. 78. Graz, Austria: Scientia Pharmaceutica; 2010. p. 597.
[6] Buhse L, Kolinski R, Westenberger B, Wokovich A, Spencer J, Chen CW, et al. Topical drug classification. Int J Pharm 2005;295:101–12.
[7] Vintiloiu A, Leroux JC. Organogels and their use in drug delivery. A review. J Control Rel 2008;125:179–92.
[8] Juch RD, Rufli T, Surber C. Pastes: what do they contain? How do they work? Dermatology 1994;189:373–7.
[9] Carneiro RL, Poppi RJ. Homogeneity study of ointment dosage forms by infrared imaging spectroscopy. J Pharm Biomed Anal 2012;58:42–8.
[10] Ezzedeen FW, Shihab FA, Stohs SJ. Release of sorbic acid from ointment bases. Int J Pharm 1986;28:113–7.
[11] Velissaratou AS, Papaioannou G. *In vitro* release of chlorpheniramine maleate from ointment bases. Int J Pharm 1989;52:83–6.
[12] Bennett PN, Brown MJ. Clinical pharmacology. 9th ed. UK: Churchill Livingstone/Elsevier; 2008.
[13] Bharat B. Nanotribological and nanomechanical properties of skin with and without cream treatment using atomic force microscopy and nanoindentation. J Coll Interface Sci 2011;367 (1):1–33 2012.
[14] Yahagi R, Onishi H, Machida Y. Preparation and evaluation of double-phased mucoadhesive suppositories of lidocaine utilizing Carbopol and white beeswax. J Control Rel 1999;61:1–8.
[15] Takatori T, Shimono N, Higaki K, Kimura T. Evaluation of sustained release suppositories prepared with fatty base including solid fats with high melting points. Int J Pharm 2004;278:275–82.
[16] Feingold KR. Thematic review series: skin lipids. The role of epidermal lipids in cutaneous permeability barrier homeostasis. J Lipid Res 2007;48:2531–46.
[17] Tortora GJ, Derrickson B. Principles of anatomy and physiology. 10th ed. New York: John Wiley and Sons; 2008.
[18] Kokate A, Marasanapalle VP, Jasti BR, Li X. Design of controlled release drug delivery systems. In: Li X, Jasti BR, editors. Design of controlled release drug delivery systems. New York: McGraw-Hill; 2006. p. 41–74.
[19] Sembulingam K, Sembulingam P. Structure of skin. In: Sumbulingam K, Sembulingam P, editors. Essentials of medical physiology. 2nd ed. New Delhi: Jaypee Brothers, Medical Publishers; 2004. p. 256.
[20] Mohan H. Textbook of pathology. 4th ed. New Delhi, India: Jaypee Brothers; 2005. p. 754–756.
[21] Waugh A, Grant AW, Chambers G, Ross JS, Wilson KJW. Ross and Wilson anatomy and physiology in health and illness. Churchill Livingstone; 2006.
[22] Newton SJ, Cook JM. Considerations for percutaneous absorption. Int J Pharm Compound 2010;301–4.
[23] Leow YH, Maibach HI. Effect of occlusion on skin. J Dermatol Treat 1997;8:139–42.
[24] Zhai H, Maibach HI. Effects of occlusion (II): wound healing. Cosmetics Toiletries 2004;36–9 April 2004.
[25] Millikan LE. Drug therapy in dermatology. In: Angela N, Anigbogu HIM, editors. Drug therapy in dermatology, vol. 18. New York: Dekker; 2000. p. 18–20.
[26] Qiao GL, Riviere JE. Significant effects of application site and occlusion on the pharmacokinetics of cutaneous penetration and biotransformation of parathion *in vivo* in swine. J Pharm Sci 1995;84:425–32.
[27] Wester RC, Maibach HI. Regional variation in percutaneous absorption. In: Wester RC, Maibach HI, editors. Percutaneous absorption: mechanism methodology. New York: Marcel Dekker; 1989. p. 111–20.
[28] Shah AK, Wei G, Lanman RC, Bhargava VO, Weir SJ. Percutaneous absorption of ketoprofen from different anatomical sites in man. Pharm Res 1996;13:168–72.

[29] Mills PC, Cross SE. Regional differences in the *in vitro* penetration of hydrocortisone through equine skin. J Vet Pharmacol Ther 2006;29:25–30.
[30] Akomeah F, Nazir T, Martin GP, Brown MB. Effect of heat on the percutaneous absorption and skin retention of three model penetrants. Eur J Pharm Sci 2004;21:337–45.
[31] Hewitt P, Maibach HI. Systemic toxicity. In: Kanerva L, editor. Handbook of occupational dermatology. New York: Springer; 2000. p. 44–54.
[32] Akomeah FK, Martin GP, Brown MB. Variability in human skin permeability *in vitro:* comparing penetrants with different physicochemical properties. J Pharm Sci 2007;96:824–34.
[33] Miyagi T, Hikima T, Tojo K. Effect of molecular weight of penetrants on iontophoretic transdermal delivery *in vitro*. J Chem Eng Japan 2006;39:360–5.
[34] Mackay KM, Williams AC, Barry BW. Effect of melting point of chiral terpenes on human stratum corneum uptake. Int J Pharm 2001;228:89–97.
[35] Williams A. Pharmaceutical solvents as vehicles for topical dosage forms. In: Augustijns P, Brewster M, editors. Solvent systems and their selection in pharmaceutics and biopharmaceutics. Springer; 2007. p. 403–26.
[36] Mills PC, Magnusson BM, Cross SE. Effects of vehicle and region of application on absorption of hydrocortisone through canine skin. Am J Vet Res 2005;66:43–7.
[37] Schofield OMV, Rees JL. Skin disease. In: Boon NA, Davidson S, editors. Davidson's Principles and Practice of Medicine. Edinburgh: Elsevier/Churchill Livingstone; 2006. p. 1257–316.
[38] Roberts MS, Cross SE, Pellett MA. Skin transport. Dermatological and transdermal formulations, vol. 119. New York: Marcel Dekker, Inc.; 2002. p. 89–195.
[39] Menon GK, Elias PM. Morphologic basis for a pore-pathway in mammalian stratum corneum. Skin Pharmacol 1997;10:235–46.
[40] Kostenbauder HB, Martin AN. A rheological study of some pharmaceutical semisolids. J Am Pharm Assoc Am Pharm Assoc (Baltim) 1954;43(7):401–7.
[41] Chun, AHC. The measurement of hydrophile-lipophile balance of surface Active agents. MS Thesis, Purdue University, 1959.
[42] Williams AC, Barry BW. Penetration enhancers. Adv Drug Deliv Rev 2004;56:603–18.
[43] Zafar S, Ali A, Aqil M, Ahad A. Transdermal drug delivery of labetalol hydrochloride: feasibility and effect of penetration enhancers. J Pharm Bioallied Sci 2010;2:321–4.
[44] Hollebeeck S, Raas T, Piront N, Schneider YJ, Toussaint O, Larondelle Y, et al. Dimethyl sulfoxide (DMSO) attenuates the inflammatory response in the *in vitro* intestinal Caco-2 cell model. Toxicol Lett 2011;206:268–75.
[45] Fuller P, Roth S. Diclofenac sodium topical solution with dimethyl sulfoxide, a viable alternative to oral nonsteroidal anti-inflammatories in osteoarthritis: review of current evidence. J Multidiscip Health 2011;4:223–31.
[46] Bakar B, Kose EA, Sonal S, Alhan A, Kilinc K, Keskil IS. Evaluation of the neurotoxicity of DMSO infused into the carotid artery of rat. Injury 2012;43(3):315–22.
[47] Majtan J, Majtan V. Dimethyl sulfoxide attenuates TNF-alpha-induced production of MMP-9 in human keratinocytes. J Toxicol Environ Health A 2011;74:1319–22.
[48] Bonina FP, Montenegro L. Penetration enhancer effects on *in vitro* percutaneous absorption of heparin sodium salt. Int J Pharm 1992;82:171–7.
[49] Griepernau B, Leis S, Schneider MF, Sikor M, Steppich D, Bockmann RA. 1-Alkanols and membranes: a story of attraction. Biochim Biophys Acta 2007;1768:2899–913.
[50] Vaddi HK, Ho PC, Chan SY. Terpenes in propylene glycol as skin-penetration enhancers: permeation and partition of haloperidol, Fourier transform infrared spectroscopy, and differential scanning calorimetry. J Pharm Sci 2002;91:1639–51.
[51] Yorgin PD, Theodorou AA, Al-Uzri A, Davenport K, Boyer-Hassen LV, Johnson MI. Propylene glycol-induced proximal renal tubular cell injury. Am J Kidney Dis 1997;30:134–9.
[52] Tupker RA, Pinnagoda J, Nater JP. The transient and cumulative effect of sodium lauryl sulphate on the epidermal barrier assessed by transepidermal water loss: inter-individual variation. Acta Derm Venereol 1990;70:1–5.
[53] Cornwell PA, Tubek J, van Gompel HAHP, Little CJ, Wiechers JW. Glyceryl monocaprylate/caprate as a moderate skin penetration enhancer. Int J Pharm 1998;171:243–55.
[54] Choi J, Choi M-K, Chong S, Chung S-J, Shim C-K, Kim D-D. Effect of fatty acids on the transdermal delivery of donepezil: *in vitro* and *in vivo* evaluation. Int J Pharm 2012;422 (1–2):83–90.
[55] Ibrahim SA, Li SK. Efficiency of fatty acids as chemical penetration enhancers: mechanisms and structure enhancement relationship. Pharm Res 2010;27:115–25.
[56] Santoyo S, Arellano A, Ygartua P, Martin C. Penetration enhancer effects on the *in vitro* percutaneous absorption of piroxicam through rat skin. Int J Pharm 1995;117:219–24.
[57] Aqil M, Ahad A, Sultana Y, Ali A. Status of terpenes as skin penetration enhancers. Drug Discov Today 2007;12:1061–7.
[58] Qian L, Ma Z, Zhang W, Wang Q. Influence of penetration enhancers on *in vitro* transdermal permeation of L-tethrahydropalmatine. Zhongguo Zhong Yao Za Zhi 2011;36:1729–32.
[59] Escobar-Chavez JJ, Bonilla-Martinez D, Villegas-Gonzalez MA, Revilla-Vazquez AL. Electroporation as an efficient physical enhancer for skin drug delivery. J Clin Pharmacol 2009;49:1262–83.
[60] Batheja P, Thakur R, Michniak B. Transdermal iontophoresis. Expert Opin Drug Deliv 2006;3:127–38.
[61] Li GL, de Vries JJ, van Steeg TJ, van den Bussche H, Maas HJ, Reeuwijk HJ, et al. Transdermal iontophoretic delivery of apomorphine in patients improved by surfactant formulation pretreatment. J Control Release 2005;101:199–208.
[62] Pierce MW. Transdermal delivery of sumatriptan for the treatment of acute migraine. Neurotherapeutics 2010;7:159–63.
[63] Fang JY, Hung CF, Fang YP, Chan TF. Transdermal iontophoresis of 5-fluorouracil combined with electroporation and laser treatment. Int J Pharm 2004;270:241–9.
[64] Nugroho AK, Li G, Grossklaus A, Danhof M, Bouwstra JA. Transdermal iontophoresis of rotigotine: influence of concentration, temperature and current density in human skin *in vitro*. J Control Rel 2004;96:159–67.
[65] Meidan VM, Al-Khalili M, Michniak BB. Enhanced iontophoretic delivery of buspirone hydrochloride across human skin using chemical enhancers. Int J Pharm 2003;264:73–83.
[66] Pillai O, Kumar N, Dey CS, Borkute, Sivaprasad N, Panchagnula R. Transdermal iontophoresis of insulin: III. Influence of electronic parameters. Methods Find Exp Clin Pharmacol 2004;26:399–408.
[67] Mitragotri S, Kost J. Low-frequency sonophoresis: a review. Adv Drug Deliv Rev 2004;56:589–601.
[68] Lee SE, Choi KJ, Menon GK, Kim HJ, Choi EH, Ahn SK, et al. Penetration pathways induced by low-frequency sonophoresis with physical and chemical enhancers: iron oxide nanoparticles versus lanthanum nitrates. J Invest Dermatol 2010;130:1063–72.
[69] Doukas AG, Kollias N. Transdermal drug delivery with a pressure wave. Adv Drug Deliv Rev 2004;56:559–79.
[70] Yan G, Warner KS, Zhang J, Sharma S, Gale BK. Evaluation needle length and density of microneedle arrays in the

pretreatment of skin for transdermal drug delivery. Int J Pharm 2010;391:7–12.

[71] Kim M, Jung B, Park J-H. Hydrogel swelling as a trigger to release biodegradable polymer microneedles in skin. Biomaterials 2012;33:668–78.

[72] Ulrich AS. Biophysical aspects of using liposomes as delivery vehicle. Biosci Rep 2002;22:129–50.

[73] Rajera R, Nagpal K, Singh SK, Mishra DN. Niosomes: a controlled and novel drug delivery system. Biol Pharm Bull 2011;34:945–53.

[74] Azeem A, Anwer MK, Talegaonkar S. Niosomes in sustained and targeted drug delivery: some recent advances. J Drug Target 2009;17:671–89.

[75] Nagpal K, Singh SK, Mishra DN. Chitosan nanoparticles: a promising system in novel drug delivery. Chem Pharm Bull (Tokyo) 2010;58:1423–30.

[76] Papakostas D, Rancan F, Sterry W, Blume-Peytavi U, Vogt A. Nanoparticles in dermatology. Arch Dermatol Res 2011;303:533–50.

[77] Kaur IP, Agrawal R. Nanotechnology: a new paradigm in cosmeceuticals. Recent Pat Drug Deliv Formul 2007;1:171–82.

[78] Rai K, Gupta Y, Jain A, Jain SK. Transferosomes: self-optimizing carriers for bioactives. PDA J Pharm Sci Technol 2008;62:362–79.

[79] Shekunov BY, Chattopadhyay P, Tong HH, Chow AH. Particle size analysis in pharmaceutics: principles, methods and applications. Pharm Res 2007;24:203–27.

[80] Moore J, Cerasoli E. Particle light scattering methods and applications. In: John L, editor. Encyclopedia of spectroscopy and spectrometry. 2nd ed. Oxford: Academic Press; 2010. p. 2077–88.

[81] Philo Morse AL. Light microscopic determination of particle size distribution in an aqueous gel. Drug Delivery Technology, vol. 9, 2009. Available from: <http://www.particlesciences.com/docs/DDT-Particle_Size_Dist-May_09.pdf>

[82] Doub WH, Adams WP, Spencer JA, Buhse LF, Nelson MP, Treado PJ. Raman chemical imaging for ingredient-specific particle size characterization of aqueous suspension nasal spray formulations: a progress report. Pharm Res 2007;24:934–45.

[83] Ueda CT, Kris Derdzinski VPS, Ewing G, Flynn G, Maibach H, Marques M, et al. Topical and transdermal drug products. Pharmacopeial Forum 2009;35:750–64.

[84] Marty JP, Lafforgue C, Grossiord JL, Soto P. Rheological properties of three different vitamin D ointments and their clinical perception by patients with mild to moderate psoriasis. J Eur Acad Dermatol Venereol 2005;19(Suppl. 3):7–10.

[85] Barnes HA, Maia JM. Rheometry. In: Gallegos C, editor. Rheology, encyclopedia of life support systems, vol. 1. Oxford: EOLSS Publishers UK; 2010. p. 331–63.

[86] Jones DS, Bruschi ML, de Freitas O, Gremião MP, Lara EH, Andrews GP. Rheological, mechanical and mucoadhesive properties of thermoresponsive, bioadhesive binary mixtures composed of poloxamer 407 and carbopol 974P designed as platforms for implantable drug delivery systems for use in the oral cavity. Int J Pharm 2009;372:49–58.

[87] Dhawan S, Kapil R, Kapoor DN, Kumar M. Development and evaluation of *in situ* gel forming system for sustained delivery of cyclosporine. Curr Drug Deliv 2009;6:495–504.

[88] Dhawan S, Kapil R, Kapoor DN. Development and evaluation of *in situ* gel-forming system for sustained delivery of insulin. J Biomater Appl 2011;25:699–720.

[89] Barry BW, Grace AJ. Sensory testing of spreadability: investigation of rheological conditions operative during application of topical preparations. J Pharm Sci 1972;61:335–41.

[90] Cevher E, Sensoy D, Taha M, Araman A. Effect of thiolated polymers to textural and mucoadhesive properties of vaginal gel formulations prepared with polycarbophil and chitosan. AAPS Pharm Sci Tech 2008;9:953–65.

[91] Smart JD. The basics and underlying mechanisms of mucoadhesion. Adv Drug Deliv Rev 2005;57:1556–68.

[92] Bansal K, Rawat MK, Jain A, Rajput A, Chaturvedi TP, Singh S. Development of satranidazole mucoadhesive gel for the treatment of periodontitis. AAPS Pharm Sci Tech 2009;10:716–23.

[93] Franz TJ. Percutaneous absorption on the relevance of *in vitro* data. J Invest Dermatol 1975;64:190–5.

[94] Rege PR, Vilivalam VD, Collins CC. Development in release testing of topical dosage forms: use of the Enhancer Cell™ with automated sampling. J Pharm Biomed Anal 1998;17:1225–33.

[95] Lockhart H, Paine FA. Packaging of pharmaceuticals and healthcare products. 1st ed. Madras, India: Blackie Academic and Professional; 1996.

[96] Haverkamp JB, Lipke U, Zapf T, Galensa R, Lipperheide C. Contamination of semisolid dosage forms by leachables from aluminium tubes. Eur J Pharm Biopharm 2008;70:921–8.

[97] Goldenberg WS, Shah R. A useful tool for the determination of consistency in semi-solid substances. Available from: <http://www.koehlerinstruments.com/literature/applications/Penetration-Paper.pdf>, accessed August 13, 2013.

[98] Wotton PK, Møllgaard B, Hadgraft J, Hoelgaard A. Vehicle effect on topical drug delivery. III. Effect of azone on the cutaneous permeation of metronidazole and propylene glycol. Int J Pharms 1985;24:19–26.

[99] Cross SE, Jiang R, Benson HA, Roberts MS. Can increasing the viscosity of formulations be used to reduce the human skin penetration of the sunscreen oxybenzone? J Invest Dermatol 2001;117:147–50.

[100] Ashley JJ, Levy G. Effect of vehicle viscosity and an anticholinergic agent on bioavailability of a poorly absorbed drug (phenolsulfonphthalein) in man. J Pharm Sci 1973;62:688–90.

[101] Scheuplein RJ, Blank IH. Mechanism of percutaneous absorption. IV. Penetration of nonelectrolytes (alcohols) from aqueous solutions and from pure liquids. J Invest Dermatol 1973;60:286–96.

[102] Shim J, Seok Kang H, Park WS, Han SH, Kim J, Chang IS. Transdermal delivery of mixnoxidil with block copolymer nanoparticles. J Control Release 2004;97:477–84.

[103] Malvern Instruments. Laser diffraction. Available from: <http://www.malvern.com/labeng/technology/laser_diffraction/laser_diffraction.htm> [accessed 13.08.2013].

CHAPTER

12

Special Dosage Forms and Drug Delivery Systems

Sarat K. Mohapatra and Alekha K. Dash

Department of Pharmacy Sciences, School of Pharmacy and Health Professions, Creighton University, Omaha, NE, USA

CHAPTER OBJECTIVES

- Distinguish the difference between a drug, a conventional dosage form, and a specialized dosage form.
- Recognize innovations in technology and their impact on special dosage forms of the future.
- Understand the various parenteral technologies in practice.
- Appraise the various osmotic drug delivery systems.
- Recognize the growing field of nanotechnology in drug delivery.
- Understand the use of liposomes as special dosage forms.
- Understand the application of magnetic drug delivery and its challenges.
- Describe the various implantable dosage forms in pharmacy practice and their future prospects.
- Recognize the application of prodrugs as special dosage forms.

Keywords

- Conventional dosage form
- Implantable drug delivery
- Liposomal delivery
- Magnetic delivery
- Nanodelivery
- Osmotic delivery
- Parenteral delivery
- Prodrug
- Specialized dosage form

12.1. INTRODUCTION

A dosage form is a combination of both active and inactive drug ingredients, also known as excipients, in any of the three physical forms of matter. The addition of excipients is essential to deliver sometimes a very small quantity of the drug that will have therapeutic value without causing toxicity. For example, a therapeutically significant dose of 10 mg of Clotrimazole, an antifungal drug, or even 0.05 mg of Ethinyl Estradiol, an estrogen drug, is too small to weigh and dispense to patients. Excipients are needed in such instances as inactive fillers to create a safe and accurate bulk dose that can be easily weighed and administered to patients more reliably. Conventional dosage forms are available in different categories depending on the route of delivery. Pills, tablets, capsules, thin films (e.g., Listerine pocketpaks®), liquid solutions (e.g., syrup), suspension powder, and solid crystals enable drug delivery through the oral route. Aerosol, inhaler, and nebulizer forms are used for inhalational drug delivery. Intradermal, intramuscular, intraperitoneal, intravenous, subcutaneous, and intrathecal injections are examples of parenteral drug delivery methods. Creams, gels, balms, lotions, ointments, ear drops, eye drops, and skin patches are delivered topically. Suppositories are used for rectal and vaginal routes. Even today, these conventional dosage forms are the primary pharmaceutical products available.

Note that dosage forms are designed for specific routes based on their chemical stability and pharmacokinetic properties. For example, insulin cannot be delivered orally because it will be metabolized in the gastrointestinal (GI) tract before entering the

Pharmaceutics. DOI: http://dx.doi.org/10.1016/B978-0-12-386890-9.00012-1

bloodstream. Similarly, if we need to avoid first-pass metabolism in the liver, intravenous or intramuscular drug delivery may be among the preferred choices. Details on various conventional dosage forms are covered in a number of chapters in this book. The objective of this chapter is to make readers aware of a number of special dosage forms and drug delivery approaches either currently in practice or on the horizon. Numerous tables provide various dosage forms currently on the market.

An ideal drug delivery system has two prerequisites [1]. First, it should be a single dosage form to last the duration of the treatment. Second, it should be directed to the site of interest. This is not possible with conventional dosage forms. In fact, conventional dosage forms have a number of drawbacks:

- Drugs may be released rapidly, requiring frequent administration of the drugs.
- Such forms are difficult to monitor.
- Careful calculation may be necessary to prevent overdosing.
- There is an increased chance of missing a dose.
- Fluctuations in the plasma concentration lead to overshooting or undershooting the therapeutic window. This fluctuation causes adverse effect for drugs with a small therapeutic index.
- Drugs can go to nontarget cells and therefore be ineffective.
- Such forms can be expensive because of the need to use more drugs than may be necessary.

In the past three decades, many new techniques and drug delivery systems that were not realized through conventional dosage forms have been developed to improve the drug delivery process. These techniques can be divided into three main categories:

- Controlled-release drug delivery
- Sustained-release drug delivery
- Site-specific or targeted drug delivery

The aforementioned techniques are capable of controlling the rate of drug delivery, extending the duration of drug delivery, or delivering the drug at the appropriate location in the human body. Figure 12.1 shows a hypothetical plasma concentration profile of the drug versus time for conventional, controlled, and sustained drug delivery techniques. Note that the conventional dosage form requires frequent delivery of doses. It can overshoot or undershoot the therapeutic window, reducing not only the effectiveness of the drug but also easily creating a toxic effect. An ideal sustained drug delivery system should be able to maintain plasma concentration of the drug over an extended period of time. Sustained-release systems developed so far mimic zero-order release through a

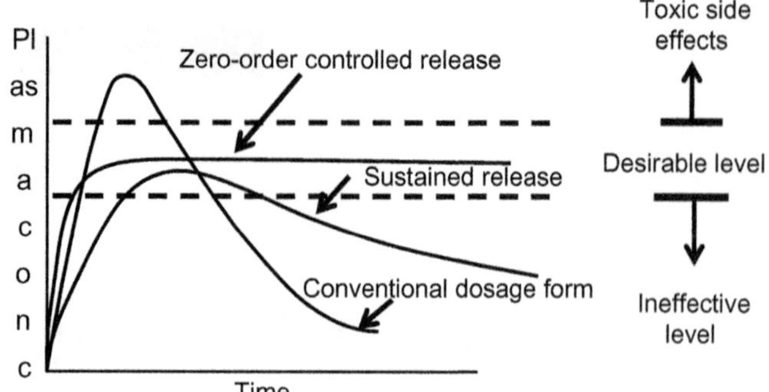

FIGURE 12.1 Plasma drug concentration versus time for zero-order controlled release, sustained-release and release from conventional dosage forms.

slow first release. On the other hand, a controlled-release system delivers an agent at a controlled rate for an extended period of time. Properly designed, it will provide steady-state drug delivery within the therapeutic window. Normally, it follows zero-order kinetics. It may also target drug action by spatially targeting the drug at the site. Thus, controlled-release drug delivery has the following advantages:

- The rate is reproducible, resulting in prolonged delivery.
- Zero-order kinetics is feasible.
- Less frequent administration is necessary, which results in increased convenience and better patient compliance.
- Site-specific targeting is possible, which eliminates damage to nonspecific organs.
- Less drug is used, resulting in reduced cost.
- Repatenting is possible without the need for new drug development.

In the following sections, we discuss numerous special dosage forms and drug delivery systems, their operating principles, and their current status.

12.2. SPECIAL DOSAGE FORMS

Five primary areas are covered in this chapter: (1) parenteral drug delivery, (2) osmotic drug delivery, (3) nanotechnology, (4) implantable drug delivery, and (5) prodrug approaches. These areas were chosen because of current marketed products. The nanotechnology area is fairly extensive. We briefly cover different nanotechnology areas with the exception of liposomes and super paramagnetic iron oxide nanoparticles (SPIONs). Marketable products using SPIONS are very limited at this time. It is expected that they will have a large impact in different facets of medicine in the future.

12.3. PARENTERAL DRUG DELIVERY

The term "parenteral" is derived from two Greek words: *para* (besides) and *nteron* (the gut). This means administration of drugs other than the gastrointestinal tract. A parenteral drug is defined as a sterile product that is suitable for administration by injection, internal irrigation, or for use in dialysis procedures.

12.3.1 Routes of Parenteral Administration

Parenterals are administered through various routes. Common parenteral routes of administration, as shown in Figure 12.2, include intravenous (IV), intramuscular (IM), subcutaneous (SQ/SC), and intradermal (ID). Each parenteral route of administration is described in detail in Chapter 13.

12.3.1.1 *Intravenous*

Intravenous (IV) injections are introduced directly into the bloodstream. The IV route is used when immediate systemic response is desired. These solutions are generally administered slowly so that they are diluted by the blood flowing past the needle point. The intravenous route is indicated when a drug is poorly absorbed via the oral route or is destroyed by digestive enzymes. This route is helpful when the patient is uncooperative, unconscious, and therefore unable to take medications by the oral route. Much greater volumes of the drug can be administered via this route. Adverse effects of this mode of administration include thrombosis, phlebitis, embolism, particulate material, and infection.

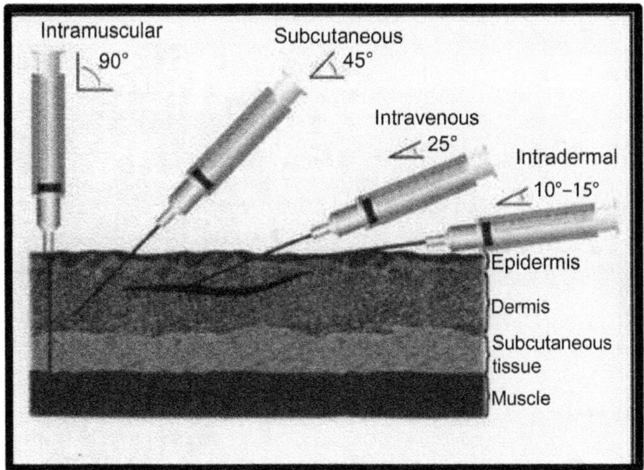

FIGURE 12.2 Various common routes for parenteral drug delivery.

12.3.1.2 *Intramuscular*

Intramuscular (IM) injections are administered into the striated muscle fibers under the subcutaneous skin layer. Limited sites are available for administration, such as the deltoid, gluteus medius, and vastus lateralis muscles. The usual needle length is from 1 to $1^1/_2$ inches. Volume limitations are 2 mL deltoid and thigh and 5 mL for gluteus medius. The IM route is less hazardous and easier to use than IV. However, the IM route is more painful than IV, and the onset of action is longer than that of IV but shorter than that of SQ.

12.3.1.3 *Subcutaneous*

Subcutaneous (SQ/SC) injections are introduced into the loose interstitial tissues under the skin surface. A drug may be injected directly into the SQ space or released into SQ tissues via an implanted device. This route of administration is useful for short-term and long-term therapies. There are many sites available, such as the upper arm, anterior thigh, lower abdomen, and upper back. Usual needle length is 3/8 to 1 inch. Volume limitation is about 2 mL. SQ absorption is slower than that of IM but faster and more predictable than the oral route. Solutions, suspensions, and emulsions are appropriate for this route. Commonly used medications include heparin, enoxaparin, insulin, and some vaccines. Drugs that are irritating or highly viscous can produce induration, tissue sloughing, abscess formation, or can be painful to the patient.

12.3.1.4 *Intradermal*

The intradermal (ID) route is otherwise known as intracutaneous (IC). Injection is introduced directly into the more vascular layers of the skin just under the epidermis. Usual sites are the volar surface (inside) of the forearm, upper chest, and back. Usual needle length is 3/8 inch. Volume limitation is about 0.1 mL. This route of administration is used for diagnosis, desensitization, and immunization. Solutions, suspensions, and emulsions are appropriate for this route.

A few special administration sites for parenteral injections are given in Table 12.1.

12.3.2 Advantages and Limitations of Parenteral Administration

12.3.2.1 *Advantages*

- Drug action is quick.
- The whole drug is administered, and bioavailability can be fast if the drug is given by the IV route.
- Administration of intravenous fluids in case of dehydration or shock will save the life of the patient.

TABLE 12.1 Special Administration Sites for Parenteral Injections

Sites	Description
Intrathecal	Solution is injected directly into the subarachnoid space. Volumes of 1–2 mL are usually administered.
Intra-articular	Therapeutic agents are injected into the joint spaces.
Intracardial	Solutions are directly injected into the heart.
Intraperitoneal	The solutions are injected directly into the peritoneal cavity (for example, the rabies vaccine).
Intravesical	Solution is injected into the bladder.
Intraosseous	Solution is injected into the bone marrow. It's, in effect, an indirect IV access route because bone marrow drains directly into the venous system.

- Some drugs such as insulin and heparin are destroyed if given orally. However, they can be effective when given by parenteral routes.

12.3.2.2 *Limitations*

- The dosage form must be administered by trained personnel.
- The effect of overdose or hypersensitive reaction to the drug is difficult to reverse.
- There is a need for strict adherence to aseptic procedures.
- Contamination of dosage form prior to injection is possible.
- Due to strict requirements in manufacturing and packaging, the dosage form is more expensive than preparations given by other routes.

12.3.3 Drug Containers

12.3.3.1 *Small Volume Parenteral*

Small volume parenteral (SVP) solutions are usually 100 mL or less and are packaged in different ways depending on the intended use. If the SVP is a liquid that is used primarily to deliver medications, it is packaged in a small plastic bag called a minibag of 50–100 mL. SVPs can also be packaged as ampules, vials, and prefilled syringes. Liquid drugs are supplied in prefilled syringes, heat-sealed ampules, or in vials sealed with a rubber closure. Powdered drugs supplied in vials must be reconstituted (dissolved in a suitable liquid).

12.3.3.2 *Large Volume Parenteral*

Large volume parenteral (LVP) solutions are single-dose injections intended for intravenous use and packaged in containers labeled as containing more than 100 mL. LVPs are packaged in glass bottles or in large-volume flexible containers. LVPs may contain greater than 100 mL to greater than 1–2 L of solution, and have to be sterile, pyrogen-free, and essentially free of particulate matter. LVPs should not have any antimicrobial agents and should be isotonic. LVPs can consist of electrolytes, carbohydrates, nutritional solutions (proteins and lipid emulsions), peritoneal dialysis, and irrigating solutions.

12.3.4 Drug Administration

Parenteral administration is done through syringes and needles.

12.3.4.1 *Syringes and Needles*

The word "syringe" is derived from the Greek word *syrinx*, meaning "tube." A syringe is a simple pump consisting of a plunger that fits inside a tube. The pump can be pulled and pushed inside the pump to intake or expel a liquid or gas through an orifice at the open end of the tube. The open end of the syringe can be fitted with a hypodermic needle, a nozzle, or tubing.

The barrel of the syringe is made of plastic or glass and usually has graduated marks indicating the volume of fluid inside the syringe. The glass syringes can be sterilized in an autoclave. However, most modern syringes are made of plastic with a rubber piston for a better seal inside the tube. These are cheap and can be disposed of after each use.

Various parts of a 10 mL Luer–Lock hypodermic syringe with a needle are shown in Figure 12.3.

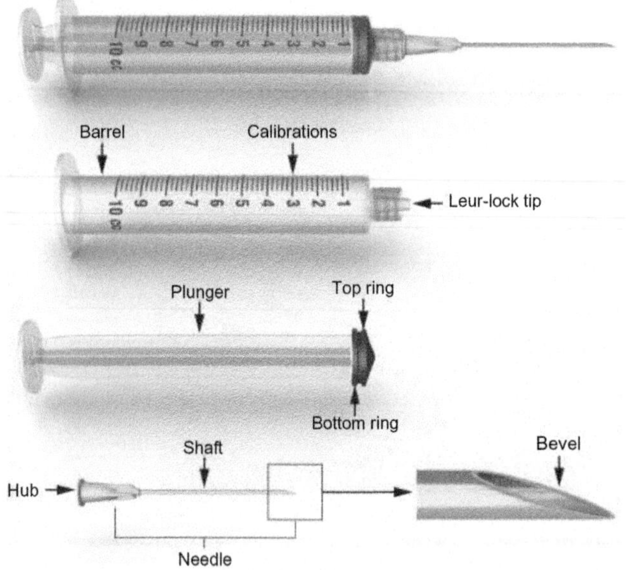

FIGURE 12.3 Parts of a 10 mL Luer–Lock hypodermic syringe.

12.3.4.2 *Types of Syringes*

The two major types of syringes are hypodermic and oral.

12.3.4.2.1 HYPODERMIC SYRINGE

In 1853, Drs. Charles Pravaz and Alexander Wood were the first to develop a syringe with a needle that was fine enough to pierce the skin. This is known as a hypodermic syringe. These syringes are calibrated in cubic centimeters (cc) or milliliters (mL). The smaller capacity syringes (1, 2, 2½, and 3 mL) are used most often for subcutaneous or intramuscular injections of medication. The larger sizes (5, 6, 10, and 12 mL) are commonly used to draw blood or prepare medications for intravenous administration. Syringes 20 mL and larger are used to inject large volumes of sterile solutions. The 1 mL syringe is also known as a tuberculin syringe and is calibrated in a hundredth of a milliliter. Insulin syringes are used for the subcutaneous injection of insulin and calibrated in "units" rather than milliliters. The most commonly prepared concentration of insulin is 100 units per mL, which is referred to as "units 100 insulin." A 50-unit Lo-Dose insulin syringe is shown in Figure 12.4.

12.3.4.2.2 ORAL SYRINGE

An oral syringe is a measuring device used to accurately measure dosage of liquid medicine expressed in milliliters. Oral syringes are available in sizes 1–10 mL and larger. The most commonly used sizes are 1, 2.5, and 5 mL.

12.3.4.3 *Types of Needles*

A needle is composed of two parts: a hub, which locks to the tip of the syringe, and the canula, the pointed hollow tube as shown in Figure 12.3.

Needles have three dimensions:

1. The length of the needle (from the hub to the tip) usually ranges from ¼ in to 1½ in.
2. The outside diameter (gauge) usually ranges from 13 to 27 gauge, according to the English Wire Gauge System. For example, an 18-gauge needle is larger than a 22-gauge needle.
3. Canula wall thickness is either a regular or thin wall.

Various canula designs are shown in Figure 12.5.

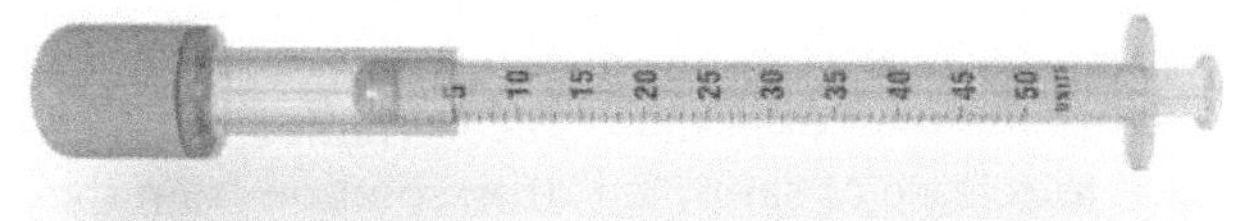

FIGURE 12.4 Insulin syringe with 50-unit capacity.

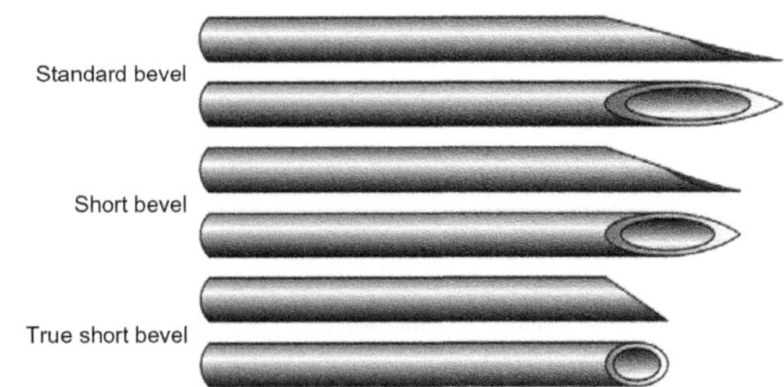

FIGURE 12.5 Various canula designs used in needles.

12.4. OSMOTIC DELIVERY

In the osmotic drug delivery system, the driving force is the osmotic pressure, and the operating principle is osmosis. Osmosis is the passive net movement of solvent molecules through a semipermeable membrane from a region of lower concentration of solute to a region of higher solute concentration.

Abbé Nollet discovered Osmotic effect in 1748. In 1877, Pfeffer used semipermeable membrane to separate sugar solution from pure water and found that osmotic pressure is proportional to the solute concentration and temperature. It was Van't Hoff who identified the proportionality between osmotic pressure, solute concentration and temperature. Van't Hoff osmotic pressure equation is shown in Eq. 12.1:

$$\Pi = iC\,R\,T \tag{12.1}$$

Where Π is the osmotic pressure, i is the Van't Hoff factor (the number of ions produced due to dissociation of one molecule of a solute), C is the concentration in molarity, R is the gas constant, and T is the absolute temperature. Osmotic pressure is the pressure which, if applied, will prevent movement of solvent through the semipermeable membrane to the region of higher solute concentration.

Osmosis has played a very important role in the osmotic pump first pioneered by the Alza Corporation. Note that a constant osmotic pressure implies a constant drug release rate and, therefore, a controlled drug delivery. Significant osmotic pressure can be developed by a number of compounds or mixtures of compounds. They are listed in Table 12.2.

12.4.1 Osmotic Pump

The Alza Corporation pioneered the development of the first osmotic pump for drug delivery. It was called an elementary osmotic pump (EOP) [2,3]. Figure 12.6 shows a cross-section of an elementary osmotic pump. It consists of an osmotic core containing the drug,

TABLE 12.2 Osmotic Pressure of Saturated Solutions of Common Pharmaceutical Solutes

Compound or Mixture	Osmotic Pressure (atm)	Compound or Mixture	Osmotic Pressure (atm)
Lactose-fructose	500	Mannitol-sucrose	170
Dextrose-fructose	450	Sucrose	150
Sucrose-fructose	430	Mannitol-lactose	130
Mannitol-fructose	415	Dextrose	82
Sodium chloride	356	Potassium sulfate	39
Fructose	335	Mannitol	38
Lactose-sucrose	250	Sodium phosphate tribasic · $12H_2O$	36
Potassium chloride	245	Sodium phosphate dibasic · $7H_2O$	31
Lactose-dextrose	225	Sodium phosphate dibasic · $12H_2O$	31
Mannitol-dextrose	225	Sodium phosphate dibasic anhydrous	29
Dextrose-sucrose	190	Sodium phosphate monobasic · H_2O	28

surrounded by a semipermeable membrane and a delivery orifice. When exposed to water, the drug in the core imbibes water osmotically at a controlled rate determined by the permeability of the membrane and osmotic pressure of the core formulation. If the internal volume is constant, the osmotic pump delivers a volume of the saturated solution at a controlled rate. Delivery of the system is constant as long as excess solid is present.

The rate of drug release, dm/dt, can be expressed by Eq. 12.2:

$$dm/dt = (A/h)\, L_p\, (\sigma\Delta\Pi - \Delta P)\, C \qquad (12.2)$$

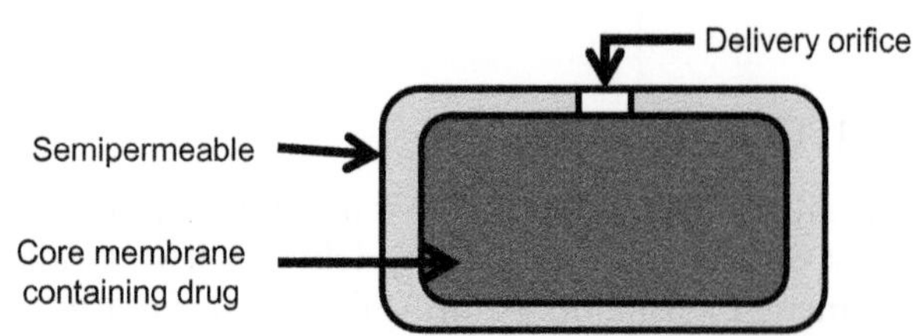

FIGURE 12.6 Cross-section of an elementary osmotic pump.

where $\Delta\Pi$ and ΔP are the osmotic and hydrostatic pressure differences, respectively, between the inside and outside of the system; L_p is the mechanical permeability of the membrane; σ is the reflection coefficient; A is the membrane area; h is the membrane thickness; and C is the concentration of the compound in the dispensed fluid. Normally, $\Delta\Pi \gg \Delta P$ with the appropriate selection of the size of the orifice. Also, when osmotic pressure, Π, of the formulation is large compared to the osmotic pressure of the environment, Eq. 12.2 simplifies to

$$dm/dt = (A/h)\, L_p\, \sigma\, \Pi\, C \qquad (12.3)$$

Equation 12.2 gives zero-order kinetics with a constant value of C. As the formulation gets saturated and no excess solid is present, the release rate follows non-zero order release kinetics. A single chamber osmotic pump such as the EOP just discussed is useful for a moderately soluble active pharmaceutical ingredient (API).

12.4.2 Advantages and Limitations of Osmotic Drug Delivery

12.4.2.1 Advantages of the Osmotic Drug Delivery System

- Zero-order release is achievable.
- Delivery can be designed for delayed or pulsed delivery.
- Drug delivery is independent of pH variations.
- Delivery can be predictable based on mathematical calculations.
- Agitation outside the pump doesn't have any effect on drug delivery.
- Greater latitude in the size of the opening orifice is possible.
- This delivery system is relatively simple to fabricate using conventional pharmaceutical manufacturing equipment.
- Implantable systems can deliver a drug for a very long time (≥6 months).

12.4.2.2 Limitations of the Osmotic Drug Delivery System

- Special equipment is needed to fabricate.
- The manufacturing process is more complicated than that of conventional dosage forms.
- Osmotic pump residence time in the body varies with gastric motility and food intake.
- This delivery system may cause irritation or ulcer due to release of saturated drug solution from the reservoir.
- The drug release rate is fixed by the manufacturer.

12.4.2.3 *Key Parameters Influencing the Design of the Osmotic Pump*

- Solubility of the solute inside the drug delivery system affects the drug release rate. Some general strategies can be employed to increase the solubility of low-solubility compounds such as swellable polymers, use of wicking agents to increase the surface area of the drug with the incoming aqueous fluids (colloidal silicon dioxide, sodium lauryl sulfate, etc.), use of effervescent mixtures (a mixture of citric acid and sodium bicarbonate), use of cyclodextrin derivatives that increase solubility of poorly soluble drugs, etc.
- The osmotic pressure gradient inside the compartment and outer ambient needs to be optimized. The simplest way to control the osmotic pressure is to maintain a saturated solution of appropriate osmotic agent inside the device. Table 12.2 shows osmotic pressure of commonly used solutes in formulations [4].
- Osmotic agents maintain a concentration gradient across the membrane. Osmotic compounds usually are ionic compounds such as the chlorides of Li, Na, K, Mg, sodium or potassium hydrogen phosphate; and water-soluble salts of organic acids such as sodium and potassium acetate, sodium benzoate, citrate, ascorbate, etc. They generate a driving force for the uptake of water through the semipermeable membrane.
- A semipermeable membrane is one of the most important components of the osmotic system. It helps in unidirectional movement of water from the body fluid into the osmotic chamber. It should possess certain performance criteria, such as sufficient wet strength and water permeability and good biocompatibility. It should be rigid and nonswelling and should be thick enough to withstand the pressure in the device. Good permeability to water and impermeability to solute are important. Some examples are cellulose esters such as cellulose acetate, cellulose acetate butyrate, cellulose triacetate, ethyl cellulose, and eudragits.
- Plasticizers change viscoelastic behavior of polymers, and these changes may affect the permeability of the polymeric films. Some of the plasticizers used include polyethylene glycols, ethylene glycol monoacetate and diacetate, triethyl citrate, diethyl tartrate, or diacetin for more permeable films.
- The size of the orifice is critical to obtain zero-order kinetics in osmotic drug delivery. It must be smaller than the maximum size to minimize drug delivery by diffusion. The orifice area should be larger than the minimum to minimize hydrodynamic pressure build-up in the system. Typical orifice size in osmotic pumps is between 600 micron and 1 mm. Although the orifice can be mechanically drilled, it is normally laser-drilled by a CO_2 laser for volume manufacturing.

12.4.3 Variations in Osmotic Pumps

Since the arrival of the EOP, a number of variations of osmotic pumps have been designed and developed. Some important variations are described in the following sections.

12.4.3.1 *Push-Pull Osmotic Pump*

The push-pull osmotic pump (PPOP) is used for the delivery of APIs having extremes of water solubility (poorly water-soluble to highly water-soluble drugs). This consists of two separate chambers: one containing the drug and the other containing the osmotic agents that are surrounded by a semipermeable membrane. Water can enter into both chambers. The osmotic agent swells after water absorption through the semipermeable membrane and pushes the drug through the orifice. A cross-section of the POP before and during operation is shown in Figure 12.7.

12.4.3.2 *Osmotic Controlled Drug Delivery in the Colon*

Osmotic controlled drug delivery in the colon (OROS-CT) was developed by Alza Corporation to target the delivery of the drug locally to the colon for the treatment of colon-specific diseases or for systemic absorption that is otherwise unattainable. This can consist of a single osmotic unit or multiple units (5–6 push-pull units), each 4 mm in diameter. Each unit is surrounded by an enteric coating to prevent fluid entry in the high acidic environment of the stomach. Note that enteric polymer coatings are primarily weak acids containing acidic functional groups, which are capable of ionization at elevated pH. Therefore, in low

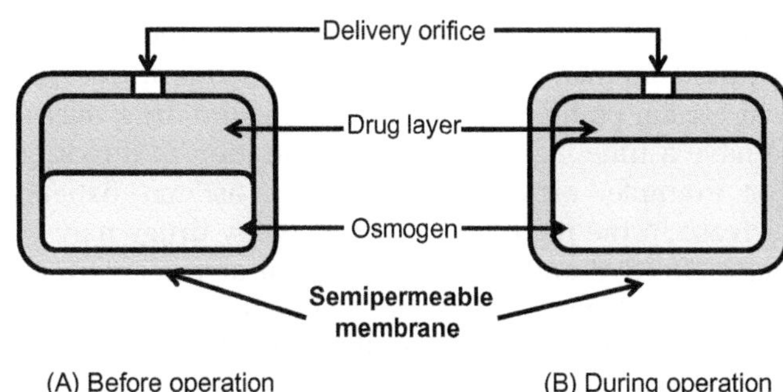

FIGURE 12.7 Schematic of a push-pull osmotic pump (A) before and (B) during operation.

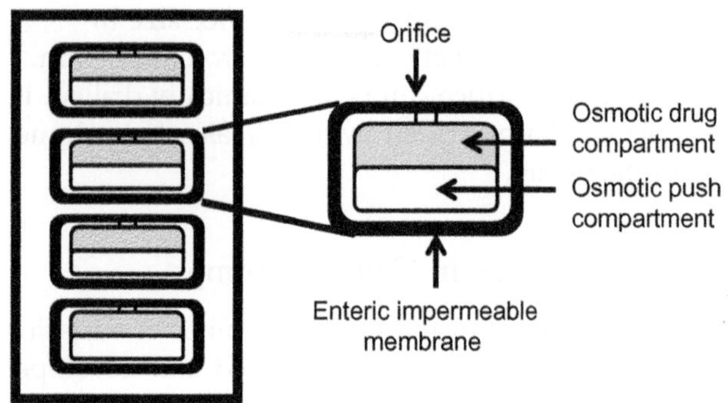

FIGURE 12.8 Schematic of an OROS-CT osmotic pump.

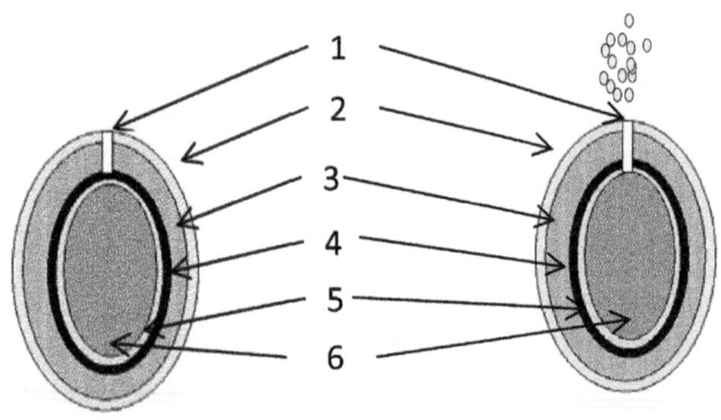

FIGURE 12.9 Schematic cross-sectional view of the L-OROS drug delivery system before and after drug release. 1 = Delivery orifice, 2 = Semipermeable membrane, 3 = Osmotic layer, 4 = Inner layer, 5 = Gelatin layer, and 6 = Liquid drug formulation.

stomach pH, these are protonized and are insoluble. The entire capsule is surrounded by a gelatin layer. Immediately after the capsule is swallowed, the gelatin layer dissolves. These individual POP units escape the stomach because of the enteric coating. The enteric coating dissolves in the high pH of the small intestine. Each push-pull unit is designed with a 3–4-hour gastric delay to prevent drug release in the small intestine. Drug release starts in the colon. A schematic cross-section of OROS-CT is shown in Figure 12.8.

OROS-CT is also used as one of the approaches for the pulsatile drug delivery system (PDDS) in which a delay time from the administration of the drug is required for maximum benefit. This is due to the fact that certain pathological conditions require drug release to have a time lag after the administration of the drug. For example, airway restrictions in asthma patients increase in the nighttime. Chemotherapy drugs may be more effective and less toxic if given at proper tumor cell cycles. Pain in rheumatoid arthritis patients peaks in the morning and decreases throughout the day.

12.4.3.3 *Liquid Oral Osmotic System Pump*

The Liquid Oral Osmotic System, abbreviated L-OROS, is targeted to deliver liquid drug formulations. A schematic cross-sectional view of the L-OROS system is shown in Figure 12.9 before ingestion and during release. The liquid drug formulation is surrounded consecutively by a soft gelatin layer, an osmotic layer, and a rate-controlling membrane, the semipermeable membrane. The delivery orifice is formed through the three outer layers but not through the gelatin layer. As the osmotic engine expands, hydrostatic pressure inside the system increases, thereby breaking the gelatin layer at the orifice, and starts releasing the drug. The inner barrier layer isolates the gelatin wall of the drug solution chamber from hydration.

The L-OROS system comes in soft cap, hard cap, and delayed liquid bolus configurations. The delayed liquid bolus configuration has an additional placebo delay layer. The acetaminophen soft gelatin capsule is an over-the-counter product by Leiner Health Products, Inc.

There are numerous proposed configurations of osmotic drug delivery systems. They have been covered in numerous papers [4–6]. In addition to the osmotic pump tablets for oral drug delivery, there are numerous implantable osmotic pumps such as ALZET® and DUROS® implantable systems currently available. They are manufactured by the Alza Corporation. The implantable osmotic pumps are discussed in detail in Section 12.6 on implantable drug delivery.

Numerous osmotic pump systems are currently available in the market. Table 12.3 provides a summary of many of these systems.

12.5. NANOTECHNOLOGY FOR DRUG DELIVERY

Nanotechnology deals with submicron particles and systems. "Nano" is a Greek word meaning "dwarf." One nanometer is the same as one billionth of a meter (10^{-9} meter). There are various size definitions of nanoparticles. It suffices to say that nanoparticles range in size from 1 nm to 1,000 nm. For more practical applications in biology, we deal with nanoparticles in the 3–300 nm range. Table 12.4 shows the scale of some biological species.

Liposomes, polymer conjugates, polymeric micelles, nanospheres, nanocapsules, dendrimers, etc., can be prepared as nanoparticulate (NP) systems. A number of these nanoparticle systems that have potential uses in pharmacy and medicine are schematically shown in Figure 12.10. Polymer conjugates, polymer micelles, dendrimers, liposomes, nanospheres, nanocapsules, and nanosuspensions (not shown in the Figure 12.10) belong to polymer therapeutics. Solid lipid nanoparticles (SLNs) and variants thereof, such as

TABLE 12.3 Osmotically Controlled Drug Delivery Systems in the Market [7]

Product Name	Drug	Formulation	Dose(mg)	Use	Manufacturer
Acutrim	Phenylpropanolamine	EM	75	Congestion associated with allergies, hay fever, sinus infection	Alza/Heritage
Alpress LP	Prazosin	PP	2.5, 5	Hypertension	Alza/Pfizer
Cardura XL	Doxazosin	PP	4, 8	Hypertension	Alza/Pfizer
Concerta	Methyl phenidate	Imp	18, 27, 36, 54	Psychostimulant drug approved for ADHD	Alza
Coverta HS	Verapamil	PP	180, 240	Hypertension, angina	Alza/GD Searle
Ditropan XL	Oxybutynin chloride	PP	5,10	Overactive bladder	Alza/UCB Pharma
Dynacirc CR	Isradipine	PP	5,10	Hypertension	Alza/Novatris
Sudafed 24	Pseudoephedrine	EP	240	Stuffy nose and sinus pressure	Alza/Novatris
Efidac 24	Chlorpheniramine maleate	EP	4,12	Sneezing, runny nose	Alza/Novatris
Glucotrol XL	Glipizide	PP	5,10	Hyperglycemia	Alza/Pfizer
Minipress XL	Prazosin	EP	2.5,5	Antihypertensive agent	Alza/Pfizer
Procardia XL	Nifedipine	PP	30,60,90	Calcium channel blocker	Alza/Pfizer
Teczem	Enalapril maleate and diltiazem maleate	EP	280 & 5	Hypertension	Merck/ Aventis
Tiamate	Diltiazem HCl	PP	120, 240	Cardiovascular disorder	Merck/ Aventis
Volmax	Albuterol	EP	4,8	Bronchospasm	Alza/Muro Pharma
Tegretol XR	Carbamazepine	EP	100, 200, 400	Anticonvulsant drug	Alza/Novatris
Viadur	Leuprolide acetate	Imp	18, 27, 37 & 54		
Chronogesic	Sufentanil	Imp		Anesthetics, IV narcotics	

EP, Elementary pump; PP, Push-pull pump; Imp, Implantable pump

TABLE 12.4 Examples of Particle Size from Atoms to Protozoa

Specie	Size (nm)
Protozoa	100,000
Cells	10,000
Bacteria	1,000
Viruses	100
Macromolecules	10
Width of DNA	2.5
Atoms	0.1

nanostructured lipid carriers (NLCs) and lipid drug conjugates (LDCs), belong to the lipidic systems. Super paramagnetic iron oxide NPs can be categorized as ceramic systems. Another area not represented in Figure 12.10 is nanoemulsion, which may act as a precursor for the preparation of some of the nanoparticulate systems described here.

12.5.1 Advantages of Nanotechnology

Nanotechnology offers some unique advantages for drug delivery applications. Some of them are as follows:

- Nanoparticles can encapsulate both hydrophobic and hydrophilic agents and thereby protect the encapsulated drug from harmful external conditions.
- Because of small size of the nanoparticles, they provide high dissolution rate, improve aqueous solubility, and thereby improve bioavailability. Note that roughly 40% of all investigational compounds

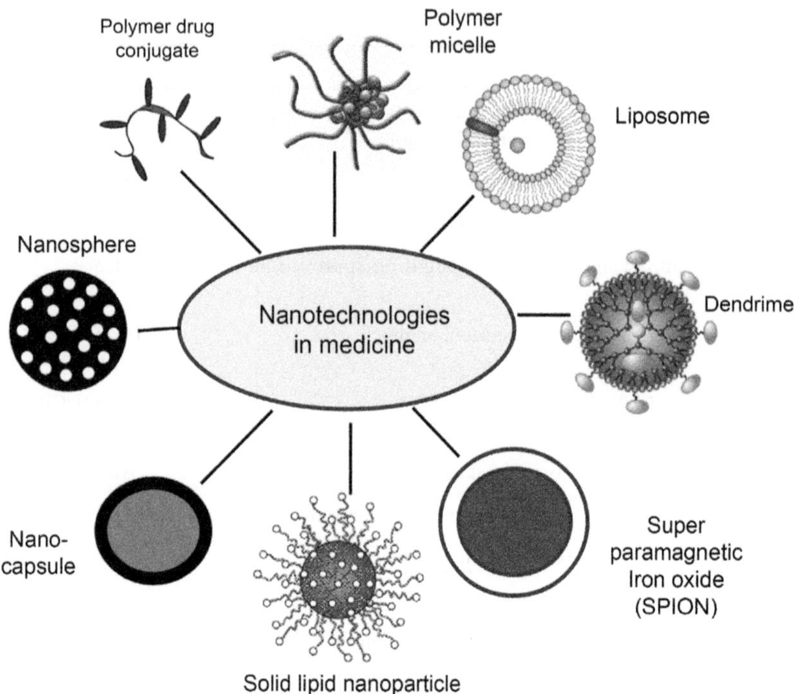

FIGURE 12.10 Schematic representation of various nanotechnologies in medicine.

fail at the developmental stage because of their poor bioavailability often associated with their poor aqueous solubility [8].

- Because of their small size, nanoparticles can be passively targeted at the leaky vasculature of a tumor. Active targeting is possible by attaching ligands/antibodies to the nanoparticles, which helps in preferential anchoring of the drug-loaded nanoparticles at the tumor site. Targeted nano-drug carriers reduce drug toxicity and provide more efficient drug distribution.
- Nanoparticles are taken up by cells more efficiently than the large-sized microparticles [9].
- The system can be used for various routes of administration, such as oral, nasal, parenteral, intraocular.

12.5.2 Nanoparticle Systems

12.5.2.1 Dendrimers

Dendrimers are three-dimensional highly branched macromolecules. They consist of an initiator core and multiple layers of repeating groups. Each layer is called a generation, with the core denoted as generation zero. Precise control over size can be achieved by the extent of polymerization. Dendrimers are made up of different types of polymers such as polyamidoamine (PAMAM), poly(L-glutamic acid), polyethylene imine, polypropylene imine, and polyethylene glycol (PEG). Drugs can be loaded into the dendrimers using cavities in their cores through hydrophobic interaction, hydrogen bonds, or chemical linkage. Drugs can also be adsorbed or attached to surface groups. An excellent review on dendrimers was published by Sonke and Tomalia [10].

VivaGel® contains an innovative antimicrobial agent that is being applied to a range of sexual health products in development by Star Pharma and its partners. VivaGel is a platform product approved by the U.S. FDA and is going through a number of clinical trials for a number of applications such as prevention of bacterial vaginosis and prevention of sexually transmitted infections. The active ingredient of VivaGel is the proprietary dendrimer SPL7013, which has been shown in scientific studies to inhibit viral infections from HIV and the genital herpes virus. Other dendrimer products in the market include Stratus® CS from Dade Behring as a cardiac marker and SuperFect® by Qiagen for gene transfection.

12.5.2.2 Nanospheres and Nanocapsules

Nanospheres are nano-sized spherical objects consisting of synthetic or natural polymers such as collagen and albumin. The drug of interest is dissolved/dispersed or entrapped inside the polymer matrix. These matrices range in size from 100 to 200 nm. Depending on the nature of preparation and the polymer matrix, the release characteristics can be tailored. The surface of these particles are hydrophobic and are more susceptible to opsonization. Therefore, their surfaces need to be modified with hydrophilic materials to avoid opsonization.

Polymeric nanocapsules are colloidal-sized vesicular systems in which the active drug is confined within a cavity surrounded by a membrane or coating. The outer shell prevents direct interaction of the drug. The core is usually an oily liquid with the surrounding shell as a single polymer layer. Polymers typically used in nanocapsule preparation are biodegradable, such as polylactic acid (PLA), polylacticglycolic acid (PLGA), and polycaprolactone (PCL). Polyethylene glycol (PEG) and PLA prevent opsonization and help in long plasma circulation time. Nanocapsules have a higher drug-loading efficiency compared to nanospheres. In physically loaded nanocapsules, the drug-to-polymer ratio can be as high as 5:1 when the core consists of pure drug. This ratio is about 1:10 for nanospheres [11].

12.5.2.3 *Polymeric Micelles*

Amphiphilic molecules have both hydrophobic and hydrophilic ends. When put in an aqueous solution, the hydrophilic tail orients toward water, and the hydrophobic block is removed from the aqueous environment to assume a minimum free energy. At a certain critical amphiphilic concentration (termed critical micellar concentration or CMC), several amphiphiles will self-assemble to create colloidal-size particles called micelles. These are 10–100 nm in size. These micellar colloids form a cargo space for lipophilic drugs. The core of the micelles can entrap hydrophobic drugs. Above the CMC, the micelles will be thermally stabilized against disassembly. The core region of these micelles is surrounded by a corona of the hydrophilic portion of the amphiphilic polymer. The corona provides steric stabilization of the micelles, resists phagocytosis by macrophases, and increases the plasma circulation time of the micelles. Estrasorb™ by Novavax is a polymeric micellar product approved by the FDA. A number of other products are at different stages of clinical trial; they are listed in Table 12.5.

TABLE 12.5 Polymer Micellar Products in the Market or in Clinical Trial

Product	Application	Company
Genexol PM	Non-small cell lung cancer, breast cancer	Samyang
Estrasorb	Topical estrogen therapy	Novavax
NK 105 (Paclitaxel micelle)	Stomach and breast cancer	NanoCarrier
Flucide	Anti-influenza	NanoViricides
Basulin	Long-acting insulin	Flamel Technologies
DO/NDR/02	Paclitaxel delivery	Dabur Research Foundation

12.5.2.4 *Solid-Lipid Nanoparticles*

Lipids are known to improve oral absorption of drugs [12]. Vitamins such as A and E and antifungal agent Griseofulvin are better absorbed orally in the presence of fats. An excellent model drug such as Cyclosporin A in the form of microemulsion reduces the bioavailability variation of the drug. In the early 1960s, the first parenteral administration (Intralipid) began the administration of lipophilic drugs. In the early 1990s, various groups focused attention on solid lipid nanoparticles. As the name suggests, these nanocarriers contain solid lipids. They have the advantages of physical stability, controlled release, and low toxicity; they also help in protecting labile drugs from degradation from the external environment. They are generally prepared with physiological lipids or molecules that have a history of safe use and are better tolerated than the polymeric carriers. Additionally, avoidance of organic solvents makes them better candidates compared to many of the polymeric systems. There are three important variations of lipid nanoparticles tested in the pharmaceutical literature: solid lipid nanoparticles (SLNs), nanostructured lipid carriers (NLCs), and lipid–drug conjugates (LDCs).

12.5.2.4.1 SLNs

SLNs are nanoparticles that are solid at room temperature and also at body temperature. The starting material is solid lipid such as triglycerides (e.g., Triacaprin), partial glycerides (e.g., glyceryl monostearate), fatty acids (e.g., stearic acid), steroids (e.g., cholesterol), and waxes (e.g., cetyl palmitate). Additionally, emulsifiers or mixtures of emulsifiers are used to stabilize the lipid emulsion [13]. The choice of the emulsifier depends on the administration route. High-pressure homogenization [14], breaking of (o/w) microemulsion [15], solvent emulsification-evaporation [16], and high-shear homogenization [15] are some of the techniques used in the manufacturing of these nanocarriers. In spite of a number of advantages of the SLNs, the drug-loading capacity of conventional SLNs is limited by the solubility of the drug in the lipid matrix. Drugs are normally incorporated between the fatty acid chains of the lipids. Highly purified lipids crystallize in a more ordered state and leave little room for drug incorporation and thereby reduce the drug-loading capacity of the SLNs.

Drug expulsion during storage is another factor in reducing the drug-loading capacity of the SLNs. After production, drugs crystallize in a highly ordered state. During storage, the lipids show a slow transition to a low energy and stable ordered state. This contributes to drug expulsion.

12.5.2.4.2 NLCs

NLCs were developed to improve the drug payload or drug-loading capacity of SLNs. Three different approaches are followed in the manufacturing process. (1) NLC I is produced by mixing spatially different lipids, i.e., glycerides composed of different fatty acids, to create more space in the fatty acid chains. This creates imperfect lipid nanoparticle structure to create more space for drug molecules. (2) When liquid lipid (oil) is added to the lipid (e.g., isopropyl myristate with hydroxyoctacosanylhydroxystearate), the lipid solidifies in the amorphous state. Increased disorder of the lipid increases drug loading and reduces drug expulsion. This is known as NLC II structure. (3) NLC III is produced by increasing the amount of oil such that there is a phase separation of oil droplets. More of the drug is partitioned in the liquid droplets than the solid lipid. For example, when Compritol is mixed with Miglyol 812 (> 30%) and the mixture is subjected to hot homogenization, Miglyol droplets are formed inside the Compritol lipid matrix after cooling [17,18].

12.5.2.4.3 LDCs

SLNs and NLCs are useful for the incorporation of lipophilic drugs. Lipid drug conjugates, or LDCs, help in the incorporation of hydrophilic drugs. In this process, an insoluble drug-lipid conjugate is formed either through salt formation (e.g., conjugation through fatty acid) or through covalent linking of the drug with the lipid [19].

12.5.3 Nanoemulsions

Emulsion is a heterogeneous system consisting of two immiscible liquid phases dispersed in one another in the presence of a surface active agent. In emulsion, one liquid (the dispersed phase) is dispersed in the other liquid (the continuous phase). Milk and vinaigrettes are some examples of emulsions. Nanoemulsions are submicron-sized droplets in the continuous phase with approximate droplet size of 100–500 nm. The droplets can be oil (oil-in-water or o/w) or water (water-in-oil or w/o). Variations such as o/w/o or w/o/w exist. These nanoemulsions act as carriers for hydrophobic (o/w) or hydrophilic (w/o) drugs.

Some advantages of nanoemulsions include the following:

- Very small particles are less susceptible to gravitational settling. Brownian motion can negate the gravitational settling.
- The rate of absorption can be increased.
- They provide an aqueous dosage form for water-insoluble drugs.
- The drug is protected from hydrolysis and oxidation because it is in the oil phase (o/w emulsion).
- They can be formulated into a variety of dosage forms such as foams, creams, liquids, and sprays.
- The ingredients are safe and therefore are nontoxic and nonirritating and can be easily applied to skin and mucous membranes.
- They provide better uptake of oil-soluble supplements (o/w emulsion) for cell culture technologies.

Nanoemulsions or emulsions in general don't form spontaneously. If oil is added to water, it will separate immediately. However, when a surface active agent, i.e., surfactant, is added to this mixture with high mechanical agitation, a stable emulsion may form. Small droplets can be formed by applying extra energy or shear force to the two-layer system. This is schematically shown in Figure 12.11.

Application of high shear can be achieved through high-pressure homogenization, microfluidization, ultrasonication, and high-shear stirring techniques [20,21]. The fundamental relationship governing the rupture of an isolated liquid droplet in another immiscible and

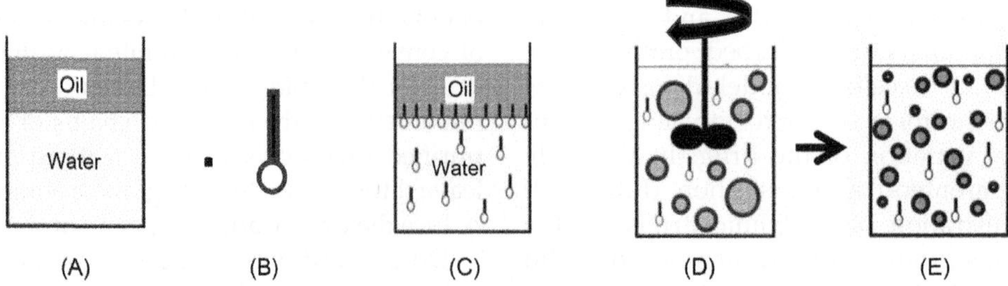

FIGURE 12.11 Steps in the formation of nanoemulsion. (A) Oil added to water; (B) surfactant added; (C) surfactant primarily at the oil-water interface; (D) high shear applied; (E) nanoemulsion formed.

continuous liquid phase was developed by Taylor [22]. This can be expressed as shown in Eq. 12.4:

$$a \sim (\sigma)/(\eta_c \gamma') \quad (12.4)$$

where a is the size of the liquid droplet, σ is the interfacial tension, η_c is the viscosity of the continuous phase, and γ' is the shear rate applied. Using the preceding expression, we are able to get an estimate of the shear rate needed to create a 100 nm droplet. Using a surface tension value of 10 dyn/cm and viscosity of 10^{-2} poise (o/w emulsion with water as the continuous phase), we need a shear rate of 10^8 sec^{-1}. These shear rates are feasible with high-frequency ultrasonic devices and microfluidic systems.

12.5.3.1 *Components of Nanoemulsion*

The four main components of a nanoemulsion are oil, surfactants and cosurfactants, an aqueous phase, and other additives. Some examples of excipients used for o/w emulsion of various excipients are given in Table 12.6. Oils should be appropriately chosen for enhanced solubility and stability of the lipophilic drug. Sometimes, a mixture of oils may be employed to improve solubility. Additionally, oils should be compatible with other excipients. Since oils are triglycerides, care should be taken to prevent oxidation by adding antioxidants such as α-Tocopherol. Sometimes, components such as lecithin and oils with high caloric potential may promote microbial growth. Preservatives such as parabens and EDTA are used to prevent microbial growth. Glycerol, sorbitol, and xylitol are used as tonicity modifiers, and NaOH and HCl can be used for adjusting the pH.

12.5.3.2 *Stability of Nanoemulsions*

Nanoemulsions are thermodynamically unstable, exhibiting flocculation, creaming, and coalescence. Instability comes from the positive free energy change in the process where the generally higher interfacial term combined with the large surface area of the small particles dominate over the entropy term. Flocculation is a process by which the dispersed phase comes out of the formulation in flakes. Coalescence is a process in which small droplets bump into each other and combine to make bigger droplets. Emulsions can also undergo creaming such that one of the phases rises to the top or sedimentation settles to the bottom depending on the relative densities of the two phases (oil or water). Degradation can also be due to Ostwald ripening, wherein small particles can slowly dissolve and migrate toward larger particles and thereby promote growth of larger particles. Note that this process doesn't require proximity of the small particle with the larger particles, as in coalescence.

TABLE 12.6 Formulation Additives for Nanoemulsion

Oil	Surfactant	Other Additives
Sesame oil	Natural lecithins	α-Tocopherol
Castor oil	Phospholipids	Glycerol
Soya oil	Polysorbate 80	Xylitol
Paraffin oil	Poloxamer 407	Sorbitol
Lanolin	Poloxamer 188	EDTA
Glyceryl monostearate	Miranol C2M	Methy and propyl paraben
Linseed oil	Tyloxapol	NaOH, HCl

Thermodynamic instability of a nanoemulsion can be minimized through the appropriate additions of surfactants into the formulation. Surfactants reduce the interfacial tension between oil and water and help in the formation of the nanoemulsion. At the same time, they help in the stability of the nanoemulsion against flocculation, coalescence, and creaming. Van der Waals–London attractive forces induce particle flocculation or agglomeration. In order to overcome the attractive forces, one can put electric charges on the surface of the nanoparticles or provide steric hindrance between particles. Based on the surfactant or combination of surfactants to produce submicron droplets, anionic surfactants produce a negative charge on the surface. Cationic surfactants yield a positive surface charge, and nonionic surfactants such as poloxamers like Tyloxapol stabilize emulsion through steric hindrance.

There have been attempts to rationalize surfactant behavior in terms of hydrophilic-lipophilic balance (HLB). The HLB takes into account the relative magnitudes of the hydrophilic and lipophilic fragments of the molecules. The approach is highly empirical but provides a guide to surfactant selection. It is generally accepted that a low HLB value (3–6) is more suitable for w/o emulsions, whereas surfactants with a high HLB value (8–18) are suitable for o/w emulsions. A required HLB value can be obtained through the appropriate combination of surfactants.

12.5.3.3 *Applications of Nanoemulsions*

Nanoemulsions have been used in numerous pharmaceutical applications in cosmetics, prophylactics, bioterrorism attacks, mucosal vaccines, nontoxic disinfectant cleaners, oral delivery of poorly soluble drugs, vehicles for transdermal drug delivery, cancer therapy and targeted drug delivery, and parenteral and pulmonary drug delivery [21,23]. Some nanoemulsion products available in the market are listed in Table 12.7 [23].

TABLE 12.7 Commercial Therapeutic Nanoemulsion Products

Drug	Brand Name	Manufacturer	Indications
Propofol	Diprivan	AstraZeneca	Anesthetic
Propofol	Troypofol	Troikaa	Anesthetic
Dexamethasone	Limehason	Mitsubishi Pharmaceutical	Steroidal anti-inflammatory
Alprostadil palmitate	Liple	Mitsubishi Pharmaceutical	Vasodilator platelet inhibitor
Flurbiprofen axetil	Ropion	Kaken Pharmaceuticals	Nonsteroidal analgesic
Vitamin A, D, E, K	Vitalipid	Fresenius Kabi	Parenteral nutrition

TABLE 12.8 Nanosuspension Drug Products in the Market [24–26]

Product	Drug	Indication	Manufacturer	Route of Administration
Abraxane	Paclitaxel	Anticancer	American Pharmaceutical Partners/American Bioscience	Intravenous
Rapamune	Sirolimus	Immunosuppressant	Wyeth/Elan Nanosystems	Oral
EMEND	Aprepitant	Anti-emetic	Merck/Elan Nanosystems	Oral
Triglide	Fenofibrate	Lipid lowering	First Horizon Pharma/ SkyPharma	Oral
MEGACEES	Megestrol Acetate	Steroid hormone	Par Pharma/Elan Nanosystems	Oral
Tricor	Fenofibrate	Lipid lowering	Abbott/Elan Nanosystems	Oral

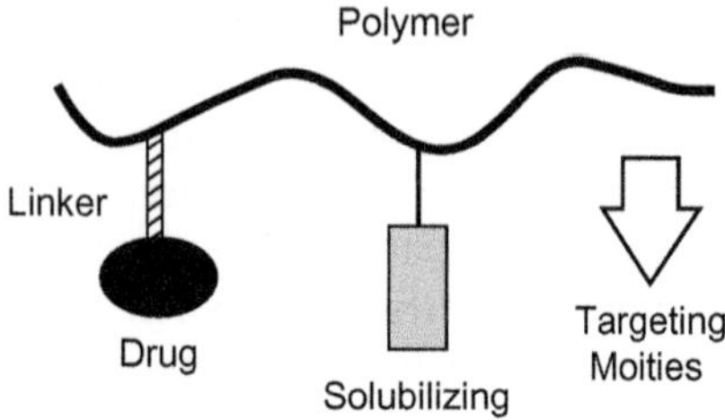

FIGURE 12.12 Schematic of drug-polymer conjugate model proposed by Ringdorf [30].

12.5.4 Nanosuspensions

In nanosuspensions, the particle sizes of the dispersed particles in the suspensions are in the nano range. These systems have an advantage of higher mass-to-volume loading. Therefore, nanosuspensions are useful when there is a higher dosing requirement. For intramuscular or ophthalmic delivery in which there is a need for low administration volume, a nanosuspension is a better choice because of high drug loading in the nanosuspension. In many conventional approaches, excessive amounts of co-solvents are used to solubilize the drug, i.e., Cremophore EL in paclitaxel delivery. However, high dosages of co-solvents have toxic side effects.

A number of drugs using the nanosuspension technique are in the market as well as in clinical trials. The drugs marketed as nanosuspension dosage forms are summarized in Table 12.8.

12.5.5 Polymer Conjugates

Polymer conjugates are a rapidly growing drug delivery area. Today, the vast majority of clinically approved drugs have a low molecular weight (typically under 500 $gmol^{-1}$) [27]. They typically have a short half-life in the blood plasma and a high overall clearance rate. An important requirement for drug delivery is to improve the pharmacological and pharmacokinetic profiles of therapeutic molecules. Two possible routes to improve drug delivery are through chemical conjugation and physical encapsulation. The encapsulation approach originated from the seminal work by Folkman and Long [28] and later by Langer and Folkman [29]. In these systems, drugs are physically incorporated in the nanoparticulate systems such as emulsions, liposomes, polymeric micelles, and lipid nanoparticles, described earlier.

The covalent conjugation approach was first introduced by Ringdorf in 1975 [30]. A schematic of this approach is shown in Figure 12.12.

It's important to know the mechanism of drug action, i.e., whether the conjugated drug is the active moiety or the released free drug. In most cases the covalent bond between the drug and the linker or spacer breaks and makes the drug active. A covalent link formed between the hydrophilic polymer to protein to form polymer-protein conjugates has been the preferred strategy. Targeting moieties to the polymer backbone can help in the active targeting of the

TABLE 12.9 Polymer Conjugate Products in the Market [31]

Compound and Name	Year to Market	Indication	Manufacturer
SMANCS (Zinostatin Stimalmer)	1993	Hepatocellular carcinoma	Yamanouchi Pharmaceuticals
Oncaspar (PEG-asparaginase)	1994	Acute lymphoblastic leukemia	Enzon
Adagen (PEG-adenosine deaminase)	1990	SCID syndrome	Enzon
PEG-Intron (Linear PEG-interferon α 2b)	2000	Hepatitis C, clinical evaluation on cancer, multiple sclerosis, and HIV/AIDS	Schering–Plough/ Enzon
Pegasys (Branched PEG-interferon α 2a)	2002	Hepatitis C	Roche
Pegvisomant (PEG-growth hormone receptor antagonist)	2002	Acromegaly	Pfizer
Neulasta (PEG-G-CSF)	2002	Prevention of neutropenia associated with cancer chemotherapy	Amgen
Macugen (Branched PEG-anti-VEGF aptamer	2004	Age-related macular degeneration	OSI Pharmaceuticals/ Pfizer
CD870 (PEG-anti-TNF Fab)	2008	Rheumatoid arthritis and Crohn's disease	UCB

conjugated drug. Significant progress in the protein-polymer conjugate was possible after the introduction of polyethylene glycol (PEG) or PEGylation of the protein. PEG is a linear chain polymer that is flexible, highly water soluble, nondegradable, nontoxic, and nonimmunogenic. Conjugation increases hydrodynamic volume of the macromolecular carrier, decreasing renal filtration. Additionally, PEGylation helps in shielding the protein from the reticuloendothelial system, thereby improving stability, increasing half-life, and improving the enhanced permeability and retention (EPR) effect. Protein PEGylation has been responsible for the introduction of numerous drugs, which are listed in Table 12.9. A large number of polymer-drug conjugates are in various clinical trials. Xytotax™ [Polyglutamic acid (PGA)-Paclitaxel] by Cell Therapeutics, which is undergoing a Phase III clinical trial, may be the first polymer-drug conjugate to be available in the market.

12.5.6 Liposomes

Liposomes were discovered in the early 1960s by British scientist Alec Bangham during electron microscopic observation of lecithin suspensions [32]. He observed that hydration of dry lipids would form closed-shell structures encapsulating part of the liquid medium core. The closed-shell structure has a lipid bilayer similar to a biological membrane. Since this discovery by Bangham, significant progress has been made by scientists in utilizing these closed structures for drug delivery applications. The first liposomal drug delivery system to be marketed was a formulation of Amphotericin B (AmBisome®, NeXstar Pharmaceuticals Inc, San Dimas, CA, USA). This formulation received approval for sale in Ireland in late 1990, followed by other European countries. Other Amphotericin B formulations (Amphotec®) in 1994 and Abelcet® in 1995 followed.

12.5.6.1 Constituents and Configurations

The primary constituents of a liposome are phospholipids. Some of the phospholipids used in the preparation of liposomes are Dimyristoyl Phosphatidylcholine (DMPC), Dipalmitoyl Phosphatidylcholine (DPPC), Distearoyl Phosphatidylcholine, Dioleyl Phosphatidylcholine (DOPC), Dimyristoyl Phosphatidyl Ethanolamine (DMPE), Distearoyl Phosphatidyl Ethanolamine (DSPE), Dilauryl Phosphatidylcholine (DLPC), Dilauryl Phosphatidyl Ethanolamine (DLPE), Dioleoyl Phosphatidyl Ethanolamine (DOPE), and Distearoyl Phosphatidyl Serine (DSPS). Cholesterol can be added to the bilayer mixtures to act as a fluidity buffer and as an intercalator with the phospholipid molecules. All these lipids have a hydrophilic head group and a hydrophobic tail group. In general, a hydrophobic tail with a single chain (tail) forms micelles and a double chain forms a bilayer. The hydrophobic tails are composed of 10–24 carbon atoms. The hydrophilic head group will point toward water in the core and outside the membrane. The transformation of the lipid to the bilayer structure is shown in Figure 12.13.

A liposome bilayer can have a surface charge. It can be associated with an antibody for active targeted delivery. Hydrophilic polymers such as polyethylene glycol can be attached to the bilayer membrane surface

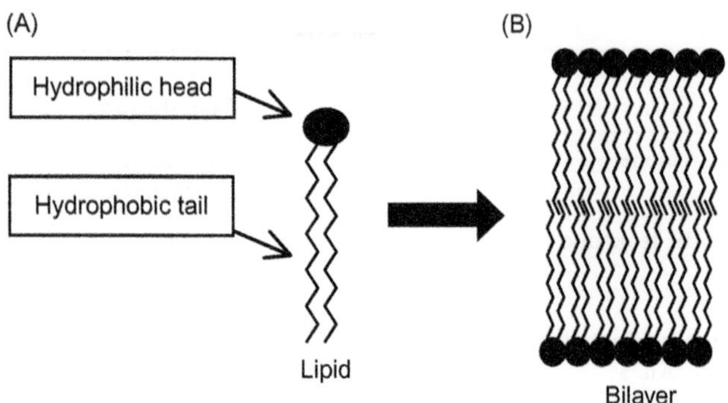

FIGURE 12.13 (A) An amphiphilic lipid molecule showing a double chain hydrophobic tail and a hydrophilic head. (B) Formation of a bilayer membrane from the amphiphilic lipid film under hydration.

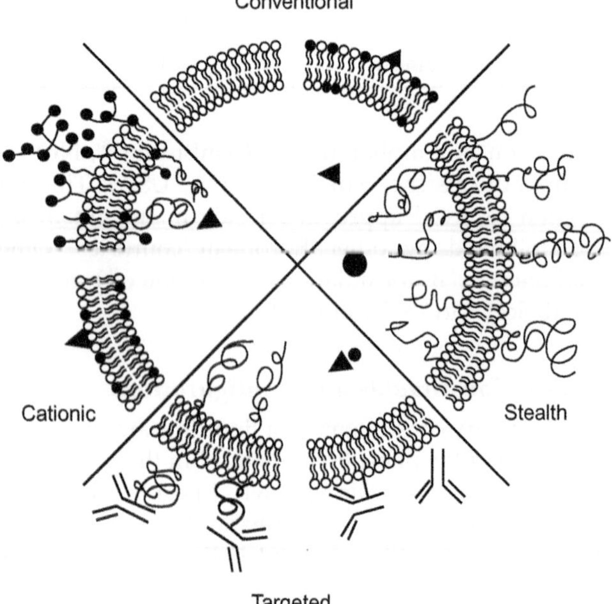

FIGURE 12.14 Schematic representation of different configurations of Liposome. Conventional liposomes are either neutral or negatively charged. Stealth liposomes carry polymer coatings such as polyethylene glycol to improve circulation. Immunoliposomes or targeted liposomes carry antibody for selective targeting. Cationic liposomes carry a net positive charge through mono or multivalent cations. Hydrophobic drug molecules are shown embedded (Triangles) in the bilayer and hydrophilic drug molecules (triangle or circle) are shown inside the liposome core [33].

to improve the systemic circulation time. This is schematically shown in Figure 12.14.

The vesicular structure of liposomes can have different configurations. They can be unilamellar, or a single bilayer enclosure; multilamellar with many layers separated by a water layer in between; or multivesicular, where a large vesicle encapsulates a number of small vesicles. Table 12.10 shows these configurations along with their approximate size ranges.

TABLE 12.10 Liposome Structures [34]

Liposome Structure	Size (μm)	Structure (Schematic)
Unilamellar vesicles (UVs)	~ 0.02–0.2	
Large unilamellar vesicles (LUVs)	~ 0.2–1.0	
Giant unilamellar vesicles (GUVs)	>1.0	
Oligolamellar vesicles (OLVs)	~ 0.1–1.0	
Multilamellar vesicles (MLVs)	>0.5	
Multivesicular vesicles (MVVs)	>1.0	

Unilamellar vesicles are used in research applications because of their well-characterized membrane properties. Oligolamellar vesicles cannot be reproducibly prepared and are rarely used. Multilamellar vesicles are frequently used in drug delivery and cosmetic applications. Multivesicular vesicles are used in nanoreactor assemblies and drug delivery tools.

12.5.6.2 *Advantages and Challenges of Liposomes*

12.5.6.2.1 ADVANTAGES OF LIPOSOMES

- Liposomes are biocompatible, biodegradable, and nontoxic because they are composed of natural lipids.
- They can encapsulate both hydrophilic (in the core) and hydrophobic drugs (in the bilayer membrane).
- By encapsulating the drugs, liposomes can protect the drugs from the external environment and help in the extended release of the drugs.
- By encapsulating the drugs, liposomes reduce the drug toxicity to the tissues.
- Through passive and active targeting, site-specific drug delivery can be achieved.
- Size, charge, and surface properties can be modified by appropriate addition of chemicals to the lipid mixture before or after liposome preparation.
- Liposomes can be formulated to various dosage forms such as aerosol and to semisolid forms such as gel, creams, and lotions. These forms can be lyophilized for subsequent reconstitution and administration through various routes, such as intravenous, ocular, nasal, subcutaneous, and intramuscular.

TABLE 12.11 Liposome Preparation Techniques

MLV	UV	LUV	GUV
Thin film hydration of lipids prepared by evaporation, spray drying or lyophilization process	• Bath or probe sonication • Extrusion • High pressure homogenization • Ink-Jet injection into an aqueous phase	• Freeze-thaw cycling • Swelling in non-electrolytes • Dehydration/Rehydration • Extrusion • Detergent dialysis • Reverse evaporation	• Dehydration/Rehydration • Electroformation • Solid film hydration • Detergent dialysis

12.5.6.2.2 CHALLENGES OF LIPOSOMES

- Production costs are high.
- Hydrophobic drug solubility needs to be increased.
- Liposomes suffer from leakage and fusion of encapsulated drug molecules.
- An effective sterilization process is needed for parenteral application.

12.5.6.3 Liposome Preparation

Thin film hydration is widely used in the preparation of MLVs. In this approach, lipid solution is dried by evaporation, spray drying, or lyophilization. The dried film is hydrolyzed in the presence of a buffer and agitated to form multilamellar vesicles. Liposomes of different sizes require different preparation techniques. An abbreviated description of various techniques is given in Table 12.11. Details of the techniques can be found in numerous references [33–40].

12.5.6.4 Factors Affecting Liposome Performance

A number of factors responsible for liposome stability in storage as well as during *in vivo* performance are given here [41].

12.5.6.4.1 SURFACE CHARGE

Based on the head group of the lipid and the pH, the surface charge of the liposome can be positive, negative or neutral. The nature of the surface charge can affect stability, site-specific drug delivery and biodistribution. Neutral surface charge will have lower suspension stability. These also have a lower tendency to be cleared by reticuloendothelial system (RES). Liposomes with negative surface charge can be endocytosed faster than the neutral liposomes. Positively charged liposomes can have an enhanced uptake by the RES. Positively charged liposomes are often used for intracellular gene delivery.

12.5.6.4.2 SURFACE HYDRATION AND STERIC EFFECT

The surface of the liposome can be modified to reduce aggregation and with appropriate attachment of hydrophilic polymers to be recognized by RES. This is often achieved by conjugating polyethylene glycol to the terminal amine of the phospholipid material. The resulting liposomes can't be recognized by macrophages and RES as foreign particles. The optimum PEG molecular weight is 1–2000, and the PEG should be 5%–10% of the total lipid composition.

12.5.6.4.3 FLUIDITY OF THE LIPID BILAYER

Liposomes and the lipid bilayer exhibit a well-ordered gel phase below a critical transition temperature (T_c). At and above this critical temperature, liposomes show leaky behavior. This will give rise to enhanced permeability, protein binding, aggregation, and fusion. Addition of cholesterol ($>$30 mol%) can eliminate phase transition and reduce permeability.

12.5.6.4.4 LIPOSOME SIZE

Increase in the liposome size can enhance the uptake by RES. Unilamellar vesicles 50–100 nm in size help in drug delivery by increasing systemic circulation time. This small size also applies to PEG-treated liposomes. Note that antifungal medication such as Ambisome® is formulated to the size specification of 45–80 nm to reduce RES uptake.

12.5.6.4.5 LIPOSOME APPLICATIONS

Over the past three decades, liposomal drug delivery has made a lot of progress. Based on the information from multiple sources, we have come across 20 clinically approved products in the United States and a number of products at various stages of clinical trials. The clinically approved products are shown in Table 12.12. Note that these products operate in wide-ranging applications as shown in the table.

12.5.7 Magnetic Nanoparticle Delivery

Magnetic nanoparticles offer some attractive possibilities both in the areas of therapeutics and diagnostics in biomedicine. Because of their small size (few nanometers to tens of nanometers), they are smaller than or comparable to cells (10–100 microns), viruses (20–50 nm), proteins (5–50 nm), or a gene (2 nm wide to 20–450 nm long) and can bind to a biological entity of interest [42].

12.5.7.1 Magnetic Nanoparticles

Magnetic nanoparticles can be formed from various metals such as iron, cobalt, or nickel. Bimetallic nanoparticles such as Fe_xCo_{1-x} and FePt have demonstrated

TABLE 12.12 Liposome Products Currently Available in the Market

Product Name	Active Drug	Routes of Administration	Indications
Daunoxome	Daunorubicin	IV	Antineoplastic
Myocet	Doxorubicin	IV	Breast cancer
Doxil/Caelyx	Doxorubicin in PEG Liposome	IM	Antineoplastic
AmBisome	Amphotericin B	IV	Antifungal
Abelcet	Amphotericin B	IV	Antifungal
Funzizone	Amphotericin B	IV	Fungal infections
Amphotec	Amphotericin B	IV	Fungal infections
Alec	Dry protein free powder of DPPC-PG	Aerosol	Expanding lung diseases in babies
DepoCyt	Cytarabine	IT	Lymphomatous meningitis
Onco-TCS	Vincristine	IV	Non-Hodgkin's lymphoma
NX211	Lurtotecan	IV	Ovarian cancer
Nyotran	Nystatin	IV	Topical antifungal agent
Lipoplatin	Cisplatin	IV	Solid tumors
Evacet	Doxorubicin	IV	Ovarian cancer, AIDS
Allovectin-7	DNA Plasmid encoding HLA-B7 and a2-microglobulin	IV	Metastatic melanoma
Epaxal	IRIV vaccine	IM	Hepatitis-A
Inflexal V	IRIV vaccine	IM	Influenza
DepoDur	Morphine	Epidural	Post-surgical analgesia
Visudyne	Verteporfin	IV	Macular degeneration
Estrasorb	Micellular estradiol	Topical	Menopausal therapy

IV, Intravenous; IM, Intramuscular; IT, Intrathecal.

good magnetic saturation and superparamagnetic (SPM) behavior and are useful for magnetic targeting. Many of these nanoparticles have been coated with graphitic carbon, gold, or other polymeric materials to prevent oxidation [43]. A significant amount of research and development has gone into magnetic iron oxide (Fe_3O_4 and γ-Fe_2O_3) since these materials have high magnetic moments, exhibit superparamagnetic behavior, and more importantly, are biocompatible [44].

There are many different approaches in synthesizing magnetic nanoparticles. The most commonly used approach is through coprecipitation of bivalent and trivalent iron chlorides [46]. In the aqueous media, iron oxide nanoparticles have a tendency to aggregate and precipitate without appropriate surface coatings. For *in vivo* applications, these nanoparticles need to be coated with a variety of moieties to prevent aggregation and attack by macrophages. Amphiphilic polymeric surfactants such as poloxamers, poloxamines, and polyethylene glycol are generally used. Antibody attachment to these moieties can improve active targeting of these nanoparticles.

Magnetization behavior (change in magnetization with magnetic field) of these materials dictates the range of applications of these materials. Magnetization characteristics of superparamagnetic, paramagnetic, and ferromagnetic particles are shown in Figure 12.15.

12.5.7.2 *Applications of Superparamagnetic Iron Oxide Nanoparticles*

Because of their magnetic properties, superparamagnetic particles can be used for a number of important applications:

- Magnetic contrast agents in MRI imaging.
- Hyperthermia agents in which the magnetic particles are heated by the application of a high-frequency magnetic field.
- Targeted drug delivery by an external magnetic field gradient. This is otherwise known as magnetic targeting.
- Cell labeling and magnetic separation.

Of these applications, magnetic drug delivery through magnetic targeting and magnetic hyperthermia are important therapeutic applications.

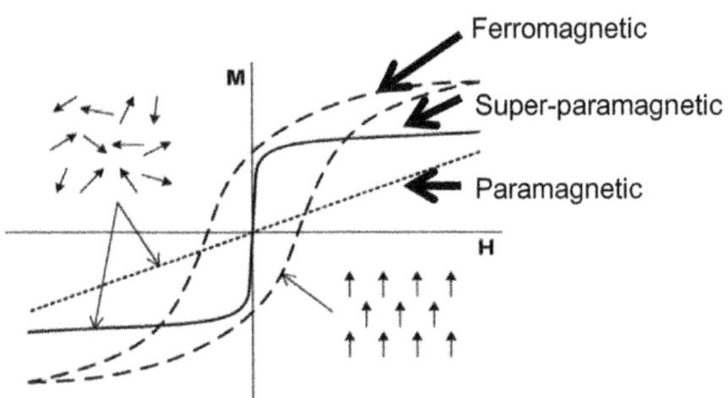

FIGURE 12.15 Magnetization characteristics of ferromagnetic, paramagnetic, and superparamagnetic nanoparticles.

12.5.7.3 Hyperthermia

Hyperthermia is a promising approach for cancer therapy aside from the traditional approach to surgery. There are two different regimens of hyperthermia. A temperature change between 41°C and 46°C stimulates the immune response in cancer cells. This is considered as mild hyperthermia. A temperature increase from 46°C to 56°C is a region of thermoablation. This causes tumor destruction by cell necrosis, coagulation, and carbonization.

Ferromagnetic particles (FM) possess hysteretic properties between magnetization (M) and magnetic field (H), as shown in Figure 12.15. In general, these are multimagnetic domain particles. Alternating magnetic fields induce heating of these particles. The amount of heat generated per unit volume is given by the frequency multiplied by the area of the hysteretic loop, as shown in Eq. 12.5:

$$P_{FM} = \mu_0 f \int H\, dM \qquad (12.5)$$

where μ_0 is the permeability of free space and f is the frequency. Since frequency is not part of the integral in the preceding equation, P_{FM} can be evaluated from quasistatic measurements. Even though substantial hysteretic heating can be achieved by the FM particles, the amplitude of H required will be high. Also, when the field is turned off, there will be some remnant magnetization.

Magnetic particle hyperthermia has been revitalized by the advent of magnetic fluid hyperthermia (MFH), in which the magnetic particles are superparamagnetic. These are single-domain nanoparticles with a diameter of 10–50 nm. Superparamagnetism in drug delivery is necessary because once the external magnetic field is removed, magnetization disappears (negligible remanence and coercivity), and therefore, these particles don't have hysteretic M-H loop behavior as shown in Figure 12.15. Lack of remanence also helps in reducing agglomeration and possible embolization of capillary vessels.

Another key requirement is the biodegradability of the nanoparticles. Superparamagnetic iron oxide nanoparticles (SPIONs) are considered to be biodegradable.

SPION is heated through several relaxation mechanisms, such as Brownian motion relaxation or Néel relaxation or both. Brownian motion is due to the rotation of the magnetic nanoparticle in a fluid such as ferrofluid. Néel relaxation occurs when the magnetic domain reorients in the magnetic field. If the nanoparticle is fixed in place and is not able to rotate, Néel relaxation will dominate. For particles in a fluid, both Brownian motion relaxation and Néel relaxation will dominate. For superparamagnetic nanoparticles, the magnetization response to the AC field can be described by the complex susceptibility, $\chi = \chi' + i\,\chi''$. Both the susceptibility components are frequency dependent, unlike the case of ferromagnetic particles. The out-of-phase component of the susceptibility χ'' results in heat generation, as given by Eq. 12.6:

$$P_{SPM} = \mu_0 \pi\, f\, \chi''\, H^2 \qquad (12.6)$$

This equation suggests that if M lags behind H, there is a positive contribution of magnetic energy into internal energy, which results in heating.

Measurements of heat generation from magnetic particles are usually expressed in terms of specific absorption rate (SAR) in units of W g^{-1}. SAR is measured as shown in Eq. 12.7:

$$SAR = C\, \Delta T/\Delta t \qquad (12.7)$$

where C is the specific heat of the sample (J g^{-1} K^{-1}) and $\Delta T/\Delta t$ is the initial rate of rise in temperature. Multiplying SAR by the density of the particles gives P_{FM} and P_{SM}. Magnetic saturation in FM particles requires a much higher magnetic field compared to SPM nanoparticles, for example, SPION. The best of ferrofluids reported by Hergt et al. [45] has an SAR of 45 Wg^{-1} at 6.5 kAm^{-1} and 300 kHz, which extrapolates to 209 Wg^{-1} for 14 kAm^{-1}. This compares with 75 Wg^{-1} at 14 kA m^{-1} for the best FM magnetic sample. This suggests superiority of SPION over FM particles.

There are two modes of delivering magnetic nanoparticles to a tumor. Intratumoral delivery injects the particles directly into the tumor. The intratumoral injection may be appealing at first sight, but efficiency of particle delivery isn't well known. An intravenous injection route through antibody targeting is a possible alternative route. The efficiency of magnetic particle delivery to the tumor site is unknown.

12.5.7.4 Magnetic Targeting Drug Delivery

Chemotherapeutic drugs are mostly nonspecific, and when administered intravenously, they are

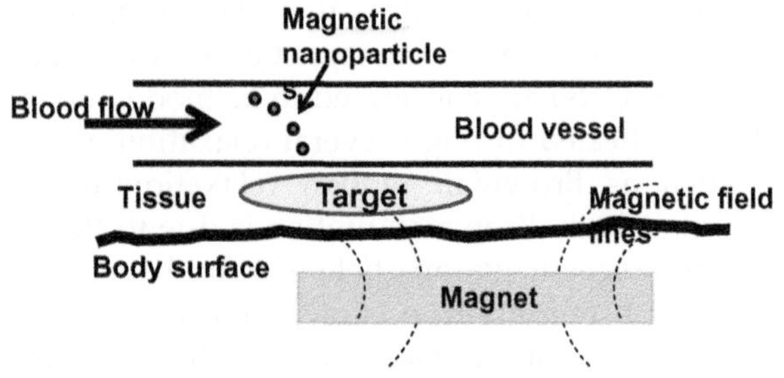

FIGURE 12.16 Schematic representation of magnetic nanoparticle targeting with external magnetic field.

available for general systemic distribution and cannot distinguish healthy cells from tumor cells. Therefore, specific targeting is a real delivery challenge. However, a number of approaches are being developed to have site-specific delivery. Some of these approaches use drug-loaded solid lipid nanoparticles, liposomes, magnetic micro- and nanoparticle carrier systems, etc. The idea of using magnetic particles for therapeutic drug delivery goes back to the 1970s [47]. Application of a magnetic field attracts the magnetic nanoparticles to the target site. This is known as magnetic targeting, which is shown schematically in Figure 12.16.

The geometry of the magnetic field is very important to direct the drug-loaded magnetic nanoparticles to the tumor and not to the peripheral tissues. Since the magnetic gradient decreases with distance, for effective tumor treatment, the tumor location should be within 10–15 cm from the surface of the body.

Targeted drug delivery through magnetic nanoparticles holds a lot of promise but has to overcome a number of challenges for clinical practice. A number of companies currently manufacture and supply coated and uncoated magnetic nanoparticles for drug delivery research and magnetic particle hyperthermia application. A list of these companies is given in Table 12.13.

12.6. IMPLANTABLE DRUG DELIVERY

Oral delivery is a preferred approach to drug delivery. However, the bioavailability of many therapeutic drugs dictates alternative approaches such as parenteral dosage forms, polymer depots, osmotic pumps, and implantable drug delivery. In 1861, Lafarge pioneered the concept of the implantable drug delivery system (IDDS) [48] for long-term continuous administration of crystalline hormone in the form of a solid steroidal pellet. In the late 1930s, Danckwerts et al. [49] began research on sustained-release implantable drug delivery systems administered through subcutaneous routes. Research and product commercialization have steadily increased, and IDDS has grown to a market size greater than $6 billion annually.

The implantable therapeutic systems are used for long-term, continuous, and sustained-release application of drugs. The IDDS systems are surgically placed below the skin or cornea (for intraocular drug delivery). Ideal requirements of an IDDS system are environmental stability, biocompatibility, sterility, improvement in patient compliance by reducing the frequency of drug administration through the entire cycle of drug administration, controlled drug release, easy termination, and manufacturability. It is also important that the implanted system should be readily recoverable (surgical removal) by trained personnel or should be biodegradable. There are three classes of implantable drug delivery systems in use today: drug implants, drug-coated implants, and implantable pumps containing the drug. The first uses various types of polymers and polymeric membranes to control the release kinetics of drug delivery. Polymeric systems are further classified as nondegradable and biodegradable systems [50].

12.6.1 Nondegradable Systems

Two types of nondegradable implants are shown in Figure 12.17. In the reservoir type system, a central compact core contains the drug, surrounded by a permeable nondegradable outer membrane. Drug release is governed by diffusion through the polymer outer membrane. A potential complication may come from a rupture of the outer membrane. This will result in "drug dumping." Depending on the nature of the drug, this will cause potential toxic side effects. The "drug dumping" has made the system less popular. The most widely used reservoir system is Norplant. This was a set of six small (2.4 mm × 34 mm) silicone capsules each filled with 36 mg of Levonorgestrel, a progesterone implant for birth control. It was implanted intradermally on the inside of the upper arm and effective for 5 years. Norplant was approved by the FDA in 1990 and was phased out in 2002. Norplant II (Jadelle) is a two-capsule system approved by the FDA in 1996.

In the past, anticancer drugs such as doxorubicin were studied as nondegradable microcapsule-based reservoir systems. However, the biodegradable matrix system containing doxorubicin had fewer toxic side effects compared to the nondegradable reservoir system.

Matrix systems are also used as nondegradable implants. Note that it's generally easier to fabricate a matrix-type implant than a reservoir-based system. Matrix systems consist of uniformly distributed drug

TABLE 12.13 Companies Involved in the Development and Production of Magnetic Particles for Drug Delivery

Company	Application	Website
Micromod Partikeltechnologie GmbH	Drug delivery, biomagnetic separation, nucleic acid purification	www.micromod.de
Advanced Magnetics, Inc.	Treatment of anemia, MRI contrast agents	www.amagpharma.com
MagForce Nanotechnologies AG	Hyperthermia	www.magforce.com
Sirtex Medical, LTD	Radiation therapy	www.sirtex.com
Biophan Technologies, Inc.	Drug delivery	www.biophan.com
Magnamedics GmbH	Drug delivery, *in vitro* diagnostics	www.magnamedics.com
Chemicell GmbH	Drug delivery (FluidMag), bioseparation, gene transfection and detection	www.chemicell.com

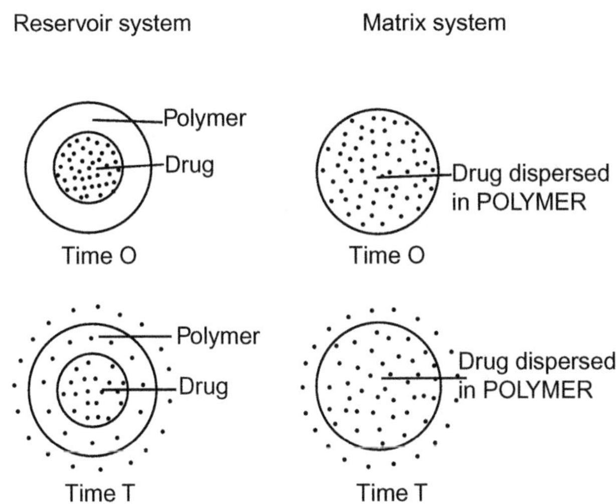

FIGURE 12.17 Cross-sectional view of idealized nonerodible reservoir and matrix systems, showing diffusion of the drug across the polymer.

throughout a solid nondegradable polymer (Figure 12.17). Similar to reservoir systems, these systems also rely on the diffusion of drug particles through the polymer matrix network. Kinetics of drug release from the matrix system isn't constant and depends on the volume fraction of the drug in the polymer.

The major drawback of the nondegradable polymer implant system is the surgical removal of the implant after the completion of the intended drug delivery cycle. One of the major uses of nondegradable polymer matrix systems is the sustained release of hormones in animals. Compudose is a matrix-type implant in which microcrystalline estradiol is dispersed in a silicone rubber matrix, which is then used to coat a biocompatible inert core of silicone rubber without any drug particles. Depending on the structure of the implant, estradiol in Compudose gets released in 200–400 days.

Another nondegradable carrier system that has found wide use in the treatment of osteomyelitis is polymethyl methacrylate (PMMA). Gentamicin (as a sulphate salt) incorporated into PMMA beads is commercially available under the trade name Septopal. It is implanted close to the site of surgery to prevent infection. Other antibiotics incorporated into PMMA are Tobramycin, Kanamycin, and Ceftriaxone.

A reservoir/matrix hybrid approach has also been approved for a number of nondegradable implants. One such implant is Implanon, which is fabricated by dispersing the drug, 3-ketodesogestrel, in an ethylene vinyl acetate (EVA) copolymer matrix. This polymer matrix is then coated with another layer of EVA copolymer without the drug. Diffusion through the membrane is rate limiting. Implanon, made by Organon International, is a single-rod long-acting hormonal contraceptive implanted under the skin of a woman's upper arm. It lasts for 3 years. The reasoning behind the hybrid approach is to improve the drug release kinetics from a $t^{0.5}$ dependence (square root of time release) as observed in the matrix-type implant to close to zero-order kinetics.

12.6.2 Biodegradable Systems

Two types of biodegradable implant systems are currently used: solid and injectable. In a solid biodegradable implant, the implant is inserted during surgery. It doesn't require surgical removal, as in the nondegradable implants discussed in the preceding section. This improves patient compliance. Developing biodegradable systems is more complicated compared to developing nondegradable systems because many variables need to be controlled. Drug-release kinetics from a degradable polymeric system depends on both diffusion and polymer erosion. Alteration in body pH or temperature can cause a change in the degradation rate of the polymer. The surface area of the polymer also changes with polymer erosion. In order to obtain a more uniform and constant release, one needs to use geometric shapes whose surface area doesn't change as a function of time.

TABLE 12.14 Synthetic Polymers Used in the Fabrication of Biodegradable Implants [50]

Water-Soluble Polymers	Degradable Polymers
Poly(acrylic acid), or PAC	Poly(hydroxyl butyrate), or PHB
Poly(ethylene glycol), or PEG	Poly(lactide-co-glycolide), or PLG
Poly(vinyl pyrrolidone), or PVP	Polyanhydrides, or PA

Polymers used in biodegradable implants must be water soluble and/or degradable in water. Some examples of synthetic polymers used in the fabrication of biodegradable implants are given in Table 12.14.

Lupron Depot (Tap Pharmaceuticals, USA) is used for the treatment of prostate cancer in male patients and treatment of endometriosis and anemia in female patients. It is composed of a PLA/PLG microsphere delivery system with leuprolide. It is supplied in a single-dose vial containing lyophilized microspheres and an ampule containing a diluent. Prior to the intramuscular injection, the diluent is mixed with the lyophilized microspheres. Depending on the polymer ratio (PLA/PLG), the release rate can last from 1 to 4 months.

Gliadel is a biodegradable polyanhydride implant composed of poly[bis(p-carboxyphenoxy) propane: sebacic acid] in a 20:80 monomer ratio for the delivery of carmustine. The implant is indicated in the treatment of recurrent glioblastoma multiforme, a common and fatal type of brain cancer. Up to eight Gliadel wafers are implanted in the cavity formed after the removal of the brain tumor, providing a highly localized dosage of anticancer agent for a long time.

Atrigel (Atrix Laboratories) is an injectable implant. It can be used for parenteral and site-specific drug delivery. It consists of biodegradable polymers in a biocompatible carrier. When injected, it solidifies in the body at body temperature and releases the active drug over a prolonged time.

The FDA has approved a few products using Atrigel technology; they include Atridox, for periodontal treatment; Atrisorb, a free-flow polymer that, when injected at a bone graft site, helps in cell regeneration; and Atrisorb D, which provides a controlled release of Doxycycline for a period of 7 days and prevents bacterial colonization at the barrier.

Regel is a proprietary drug delivery system from MacroMed. It employs 23% (w/w) copolymer of PLGA−PEG-PLGA in phosphate buffer saline. It's a thermally reversible polymer developed for parenteral delivery. The thermal characteristics of Regel can be modified as a function of molecular weight, hydrophobicity, and polymer concentration to help in programmed delivery of the active agent.

The synthetic process involves additions of Poly (ethylene glycol), lactide, and glycolide monomers along with stannous octoate catalyst, which results in 95% yield and 99% purity. Sterilization of the product is done by filtration and gas sterilization. Prior to injection, the product is reconstituted, yielding aqueous Regel as a free-flowing liquid with a viscosity of less than 1 poise. After injection, the polymer undergoes a phase change and becomes a water-insoluble biodegradable implant.

MacroMed's first product, OncoGel, is supplied as a frozen formulation of Paclitaxel in Regel in clinical trials. This unique drug therapy delivers a highly concentrated dose of the chemotherapy gel injected directly onto hard-to-reach tumors in the esophagus nonsurgically.

The Alazamer Depot technology (Alza Corporation, Mountain View, CA, USA) was designed to offer sustained delivery of therapeutic agents, including proteins, other biomolecules and small-molecular-weight compounds. The technology consists of a biodegradable polymer, suitable solvent, and formulated drug particles. The formulation is injected subcutaneously, with the drug released by diffusion from the system, while water and other biological fluids diffuse in. At later stages, the polymer degrades and further contributes to drug release.

Delivering proteins is often a challenging task because of their large size, stability issues, and fragile three-dimensional structure, which must be maintained for their therapeutic activity. The development of an effective system would require overcoming some key obstacles such as: (i) iprotein's fragile conformation, which is maintained in the processing and formulation process, (ii) controlling the release to maintain the therapeutic levels for the required time and (iii) developing a sterile product to produce quantities of materials for clinical trial and commercialization.

Alkermes, a global company headquartered in Dublin, Ireland, developed a microencapsulation process to achieve high encapsulation efficiency while maintaining protein integrity. The process involves preparing freeze-dried proteins by atomization into liquid nitrogen. The lyophilized protein powder is added to the polymer solution and dispersed through sonication or high-pressure homogenization to reduce the drug particle size. Frozen drug/polymer microspheres are produced by atomization into liquid nitrogen. Filtration and vacuum drying are done to produce the final protein product inside the polymer microspheres. The polymer most commonly used is poly(lactide-co-glycolide), or PLG.

The microsphere may be administered by subcutaneous or intramuscular injection after dispersion in viscous aqueous diluents and delivery through a

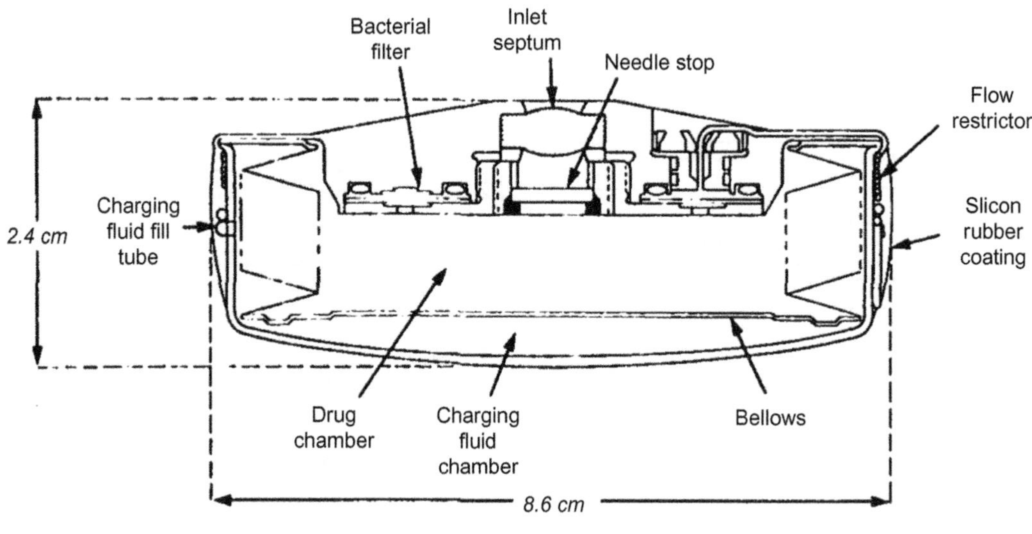

FIGURE 12.18 Schematic diagram of diaphragm pump.

hypodermic needle. The first approved long-acting formulation of a therapeutic protein, Neutropin Depot (Genetech Inc., San Francisco, CA, USA), a human growth hormone (hGH) product, is manufactured by the ProLease process.

12.6.3 Pump Systems

12.6.3.1 Diaphragm Pumps

Many different drugs require external control of delivery rate and volume over a prolonged period of time. Such control isn't achievable by nondegradable or biodegradable delivery. Pump systems provide the required control needed in such situations. The first such implantable infusion pump was invented at the University of Minnesota [52,53] and developed in a combined effort with the Metal Bellows Corporation of Sharon, Massachusetts, USA, which was spun out to form Infusaid Corporation; the implantable pump was called the Infusaid pump. A schematic of the pump is shown in Figure 12.18.

Briefly, the pump is a hollow titanium disc divided into two chambers by a flexible titanium bellows. A volatile charging fluid is sealed in the outer chamber, and the inner chamber is filled with the appropriate drug. Vapor pressure from the volatile fluid at the physiological temperature displaces the bellows, causing the drug to be pushed out through a bacterial filter. The flow is controlled by a capillary flow control mechanism. The inner chamber of the pump can be filled by a needle injection through a self-sealing septum, simultaneously compressing and condensing the vapor in the outer chamber. This first pump had a single flow rate. The pump was placed in the peritoneal cavity through surgery.

Since the invention of the Infusaid implantable pump, there have been numerous developments on the design, controlled drug delivery, and remote programmability of implantable pumps. A cross-sectional view of Medtronic's programmable, implantable MiniMed pump is shown in Figure 12.19. This type of pump is used for delivering insulin to Type 1 diabetic patients.

The pump in Figure 12.19 is completely encased in a biocompatible titanium case. It operates in an open-loop configuration. A closed-loop configuration for insulin delivery is now available. This has a two-chamber configuration like the Infusaid pump. The pumping mechanism is a solenoid operated in a hermetically sealed pulsatile pump (Peristaltic pump). The pump electronics has a microprocessor designed to receive telemetry signals, store programming information, control the pulsing of the pump, and send information from stored memory. The battery life is 3–5 years. The future of insulin delivery is in closed-loop control where the blood glucose is continuously measured and fed back to the electronic module of the pump for controlling insulin delivery. The Medtronic MiniMed uses a needle-type glucose sensor that has been approved by FDA. The sensor is implanted in the subcutaneous tissue using a specifically designed indwelling tool to prevent tissue trauma. It is connected by wire to a portable page-size external monitoring unit that monitors the glucose level in the patient and sends appropriate signals to the implanted pump in the peritoneal cavity. Frequent calibration and inter-sensor variability are some of the issues in

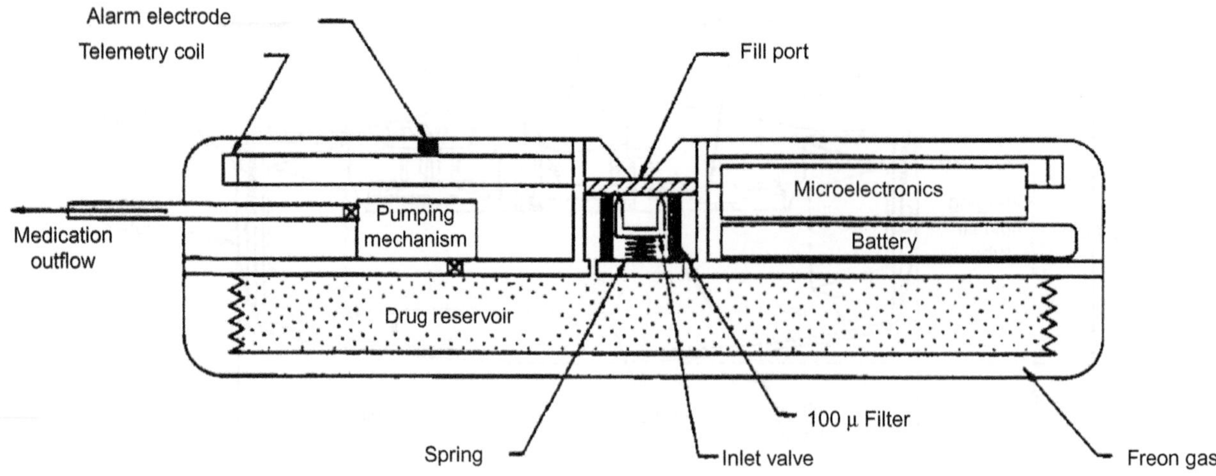

FIGURE 12.19 Schematic of a programmable implanted pump.

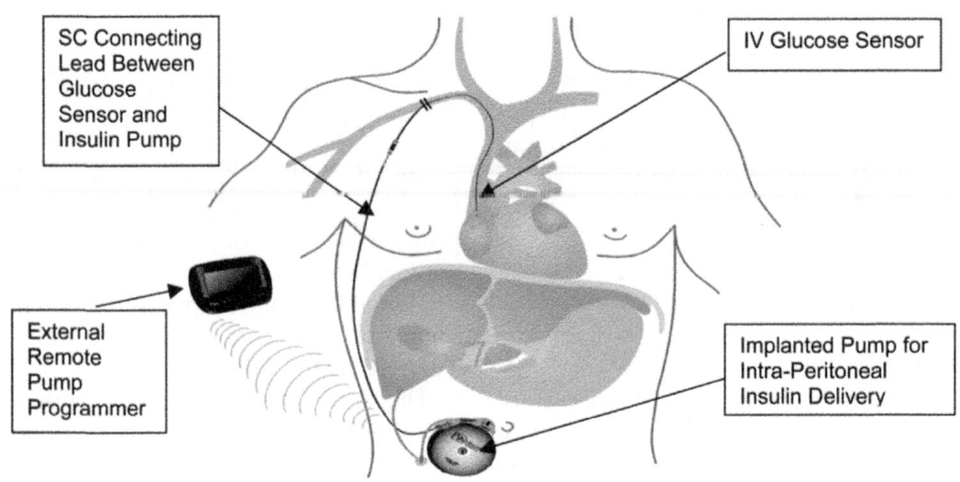

FIGURE 12.20 An artistic rendering of the closed-loop glucose control system.

this approach. Additionally, stopping the glucose infusion shows a persistently lower sensor signal. In the near future, it may be possible to use closed-loop glucose sensing by IV glucose sensor. Such an effort is currently in clinical trials. An artistic rendering of such a system is shown in Figure 12.20 [54].

12.6.3.2 Micro-Electromechanical Pumps

There has been a surge of interest in miniaturizing implanted drug delivery systems, reducing cost, improving performance, and integrating features. Micro- and nano-electromechanical systems (MEMS and NEMS) for drug delivery will provide some unique opportunities in the future for advanced drug delivery techniques. Some additional benefits of these techniques are that they are fast acting; deliver drugs in a pulsatile or continuous mode; deliver multiple drugs at their optimum therapeutic level; are stable; provide hermetic storage of therapeutic drugs in solid, liquid, or gel form; and provide wireless communication with an external controller for device monitoring and therapy modification. Some but not all of these benefits are met in the implantable pumps discussed earlier. MEMS and NEMS are based on well-established technologies in microelectronic industries.

Micro-electromechanical systems, or MEMS, is a technology that in its most general form can be defined as miniaturized mechanical, electrical elements (i.e., devices and structures) that are made using the techniques of microfabrication. The critical physical dimension can vary from less than a micron to several millimeters. Also, MEMS can have simple structures with no moving parts to more complex electromechanical systems with multiple moving parts with integrated microelectronics. MEMS technology borrows a lot of microfabrication technologies from the silicon microelectronic industries and therefore has seen rapid growth in many areas, including biology and drug delivery devices.

When the devices get small, the usual question is whether they will be practical. Let's consider a few examples [55]. Fentanyl, a powerful narcotic drug widely used for anesthesia and analgesia, has a dosage regimen of $\sim$25 μg for a typical 50 kg adult. Adult dosages for antibiotics, such as penicillin and amoxicillin, are typically 1 g/day. If we scale down the size as in MEMS, we reduce available volume. Let's consider a drug reservoir size of 10 micron × 10 micron × 1 mm. Volume of this drug reservoir is around 100 pL. A Synchromed 8637-20 pump comes with a volume of 20 mL. This is some eight orders of magnitude greater than the small MEMS reservoir. This volume can be circumvented by using these small structures in conjunction with a large reservoir attached to it or using an array of small reservoirs. Also, note that many of the drugs come with a large number of excipients. These may be unnecessary for the MEMS drug delivery systems.

Currently, no MEMS micropumps are available for implanted drug delivery. Many of the technologies are in clinical or preclinical trials or under development. If we look at the time horizon, they may take 5–15 years before FDA approval. Let us consider a few examples that have undergone a number of clinical trials. Figure 12.21 shows a device with cross-sections of several drug reservoirs. Some of the early prototypes were made with a 10 × 10 matrix array of drug reservoirs. Each of these can be individually addressed. Each microchip was $15 \times 15 \times 1\ mm^3$ with a reservoir capacity of 300 nL [56]. Application of a voltage between the gold cathode and anode causes electrochemical dissolution of the gold thin film protecting the drug based on the following chemical reactions:

$$Au + 4\,Cl^- \rightarrow [AuCl_4]^- + 3\,e^-$$

$$Au + m\,H_2O \rightarrow [Au(H_2O)m]3^+ + 3\,e^-$$

$$2\,Au + 3\,H_2O \rightarrow Au_2O_3 + 6\,H^+ + 3\,e^-$$

$$2\,Cl^- \rightarrow Cl_2 + 2\,e^-$$

$$Au_2O_3 + 8\,Cl^- + 6\,H^+ \rightarrow 2\,[AuCl_4]^- + 3\,H_2O$$

The body naturally contains an aqueous solution containing sodium (Na^+) and chloride (Cl^-) ions, which help in the gold dissolution process under the application of a voltage between the gold cathode and anode. This device by Microchips Inc. is undergoing clinical trial.

Intraocular diseases such as retinitis pigmentosa, age-related macular degeneration, diabetic retinopathy, and glaucoma are presently incurable and affect a large number of people worldwide. Innovative drug therapy is the most effective way of treating these diseases. Oral and topical drugs require large doses to reach therapeutic levels in the intraocular space. Implantable pumps haven't been successful because of their large size. A small, active MEMS device has been designed, fabricated, and tested in porcine eyes. The intraocular device and surgical implantation are shown in Figure 12.22 (A) and (B), respectively.

The drug delivery device consists of an electrolysis pump, drug reservoir, and a transscleral cannula. The electrolysis pump consists of an interdigitated platinum electrode immersed in an electrolyte. Application of a current gives rise to electrolysis of water. The gas bubbles thus formed applies the pressure to inject the drug into the eye through the cannula.

12.6.4 Osmotic Pumps

12.6.4.1 ALZET® Osmotic Pumps

Similar to the other osmotic pumps, the ALZET osmotic pump operates because of an osmotic pressure difference between the osmotic agent chamber or the salt chamber and the drug chamber. The basic principle of this drug delivery is outlined in Section 12.4 on osmotic drug delivery.

The ALZET osmotic pump consists of three concentric cylinders. The outermost layer is a semipermeable membrane constructed from cellulose materials. A supersaturated salt solution is kept in this layer. This outer cylinder surrounds the impermeable drug reservoir. A 25- or 27-gauge filling tube is used to fill the drug in this cylinder. A schematic of the ALZET pump is shown in Figure 12.23.

When this pump is implanted, the interstitial fluid enters the semipermeable membrane and creates an osmotic pressure in the salt chamber. This compresses the drug reservoir and forces the drug solution out of the delivery portal.

These pumps can be implanted subcutaneously or intraperitoneally or used with a catheter to infuse a vein or artery or target tissues such as the brain. Implanting the pump subcutaneously is much quicker and less stressful than using intravenous catheterization.

Three sizes of ALZET pumps are available. These pumps can deliver drugs from 3 days to 6 weeks depending on the size of the pump. The drug delivery rates can vary from 0.11 μL/hr to 10 μL/hr. The delivery profiles of these pumps are independent of the drug formulation to be dispensed. Note that each pump configuration is fixed at the factory for one delivery rate. The drug delivery follows zero-order kinetics. These pumps have been used successfully with a wide range of drugs, largely for animal studies.

(A)

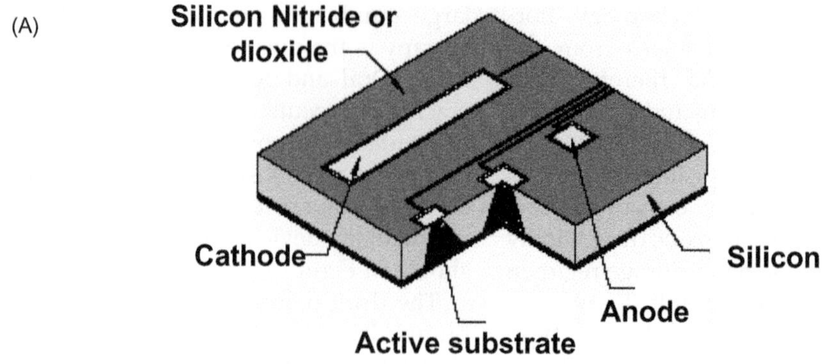

(B)

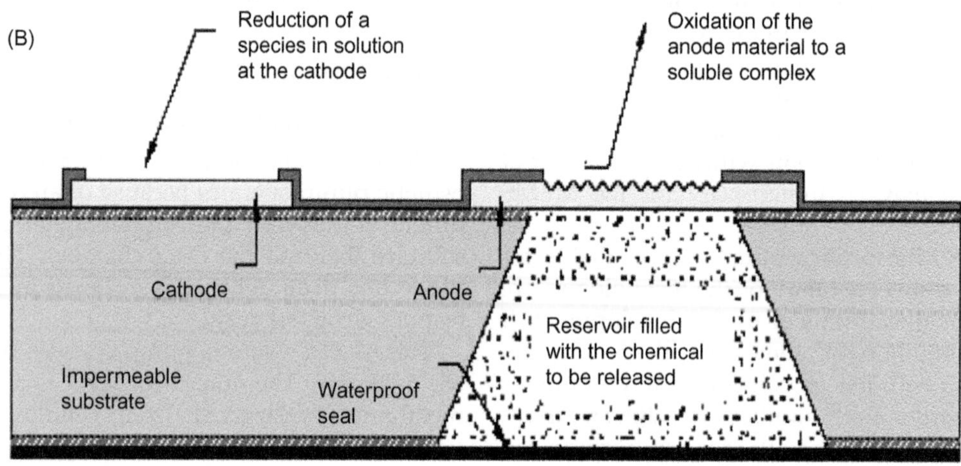

(C)

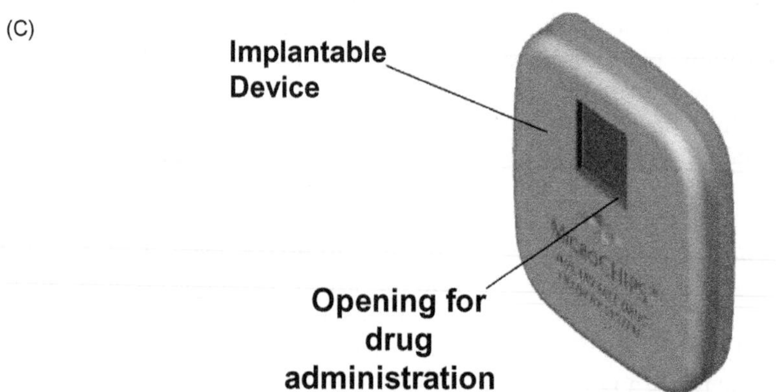

FIGURE 12.21 An implantable MEMS structure on silicon substrate. (A) Fabricated device with micro-reservoir and the electrode structure; (B) cross-section of the device showing a single reservoir with cathode, anode, drug, and partial oxidation of the anode material; and (C) a completed device with enclosure.

12.6.4.2 *DUROS® Osmotic Pumps*

The success of the ALZET osmotic pump showed the breadth of applicability of osmosis for parenteral drug delivery by the osmotic process. This gave rise to the DUROS platform technology. A schematic of the implant is shown in Figure 12.24.

The DUROS device consists of a cylindrical titanium alloy reservoir capped at one end by a semipermeable membrane made of polyurethane polymer and capped

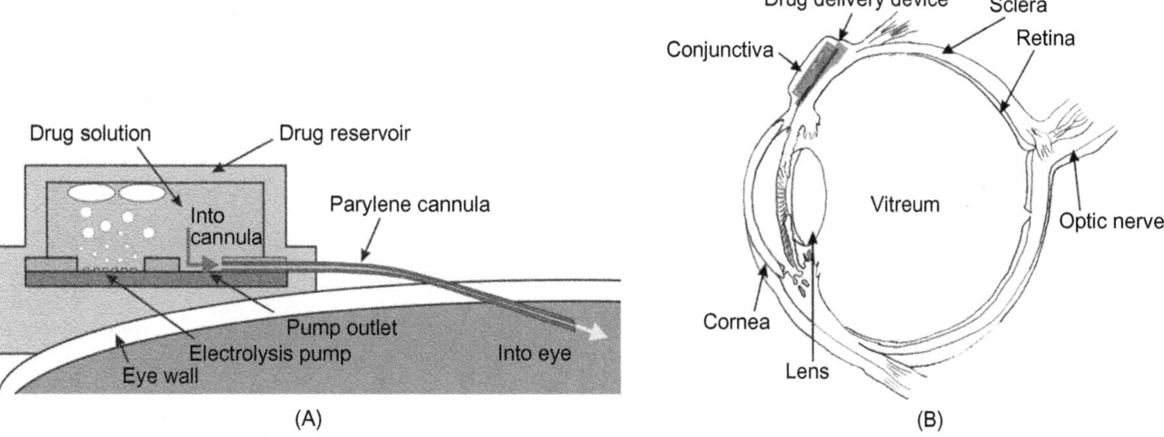

FIGURE 12.22 (A) Cross-section of the ocular drug delivery device showing the electrochemical pumping of the drug into the eye; (B) conceptual illustration of the implanted ocular drug delivery device [57].

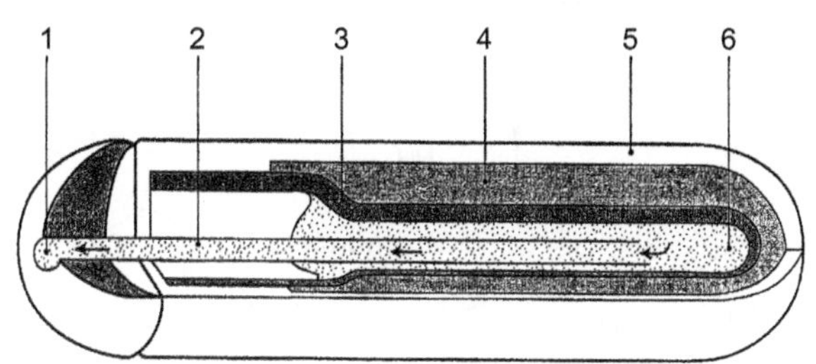

FIGURE 12.23 Schematic of the implantable ALZET osmotic pump showing (1) delivery portal, (2) flow moderator, (3) impermeable reservoir wall, (4) osmotic agent, (5) semipermeable membrane, and (6) drug reservoir [3].

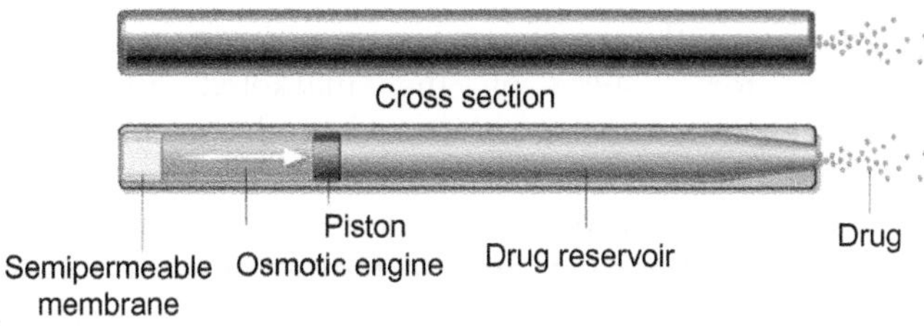

FIGURE 12.24 A schematic of the DUROS osmotic pump.

at the other end by a diffusion moderator. Positioned next to the membrane is the osmotic engine, which contains primarily NaCl along with other pharmaceutical excipients in tablet form. Next to the osmotic engine is a piston made from elastomeric materials; it serves to separate the osmotic engine from the drug reservoir.

All DUROS components are biocompatible. Radiation (gamma radiation) sterilization of the device may be used to sterilize the final drug product. If the drug formulation can't withstand the sterilizing radiation, the device is radiation sterilized with the drug sterilized by appropriate aseptic techniques.

The device comes in two different sizes (4 mm OD × 44 mm length or 10 mm OD × 44 mm length) and can last from 3 months to a year. For many applications, the preferred site for implantation is subcutaneous placement in the inside of the upper arm. An implanter is used in the implantation process. Targeted delivery of the drug is possible through a catheter integrated at the exit port. The catheter can give rise to more effective drug delivery at targeted sites.

Viadur® by Alza Corporation using the DUROS technology platform was the first such product approved by the FDA in 2000. Viadur (leuprolide acetate implant) is a sterile, nonbiodegradable, osmotically driven miniaturized implant designed to deliver leuprolide acetate for 12 months at a controlled rate. To address the needs of chronic pain sufferers, the DUROS technology platform has been applied to the delivery of the drug Sufentanil. This DUROS system has the trade name Chronogesic® and is designed to deliver the drug for 3 months. Because Sufentanil is 500x more potent than morphine, a 1-month therapy can be contained in a 155 μL drug reservoir. Chronogesic is undergoing clinical trials.

The Viadur delivery platform has been licensed to Bayer Pharmaceuticals, Inc. DUROS has been licensed to Intarcia Therapeutics, Inc. Intarcia is using the DUROS platform to deliver Exenatide (Intarcia for Type 2 diabetes); this is in Phase 3 clinical trials.

12.7. PRODRUGS

Almost all drugs have some undesirable characteristics in their physicochemical and biological properties. These undesirable characteristics and therapeutic efficiency can be improved by suitable modification through biological, physical, or chemical means. The biological approach is to alter the route of administration. The physical approach is to modify the dosage form. The third approach is to enhance drug selectivity while minimizing toxicity [58]. This third approach leads to the design of prodrugs. The concept of prodrugs isn't new. Adrian Albert [59] was the first to introduce the concept of prodrugs and suggested that the technique can be used to temporarily alter and therefore optimize the physicochemical properties and thus the pharmacological and toxicological profiles of an agent.

According to International Union of Pure and Applied Chemistry (IUPAC), a prodrug is defined as any compound that undergoes biotransformation before exhibiting pharmacological effects. Prodrugs are considered to be inactive or at least less significantly active than the released drugs. Once inside the body, these prodrugs undergo enzymatic or chemical reaction to show drug-like properties (i.e., absorption, distribution, metabolism, and excretion). The transformation of a prodrug to actual drug behavior is schematically shown in Figure 12.25.

Note the "barrier" shown in Figure 12.25. Prodrugs provide possibilities to overcome various barriers to drug formulation and delivery, such as aqueous solubility, chemical instability, insufficient oral absorption, rapid presystemic metabolism, insufficient penetration into the brain, toxicity, local irritation, and patient compliance such as odor and taste [60].

The design of the prodrug structure is considered in the early phase of clinical development. This will include the appropriate functional groups (promoiety) for derivatization. Promoiety should be safe and rapidly excreted from the body. The choice of promoiety should be appropriate for the disease state. Some of the common functional groups used in prodrug design are carboxylic, hydroxyl, amine, phosphates, and carbonyl groups. They are shown in Table 12.15.

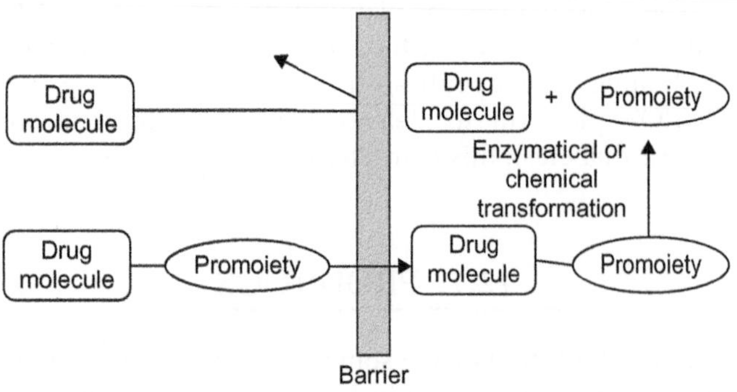

FIGURE 12.25 A simplified representation of the prodrug concept.

TABLE 12.15 Functional Groups and Their Derivatives Used in the Design and Synthesis of Prodrugs

Functional Group	Derivative
–COOH Carboxylic Acid	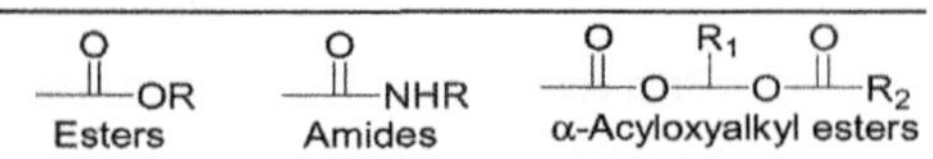 Esters; Amides; α-Acyloxyalkyl esters
–OH Alcohol	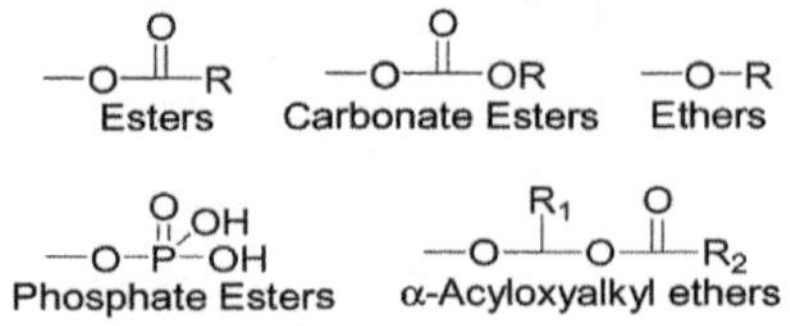 Esters; Carbonate Esters; Ethers; Phosphate Esters; α-Acyloxyalkyl ethers
$-NH_2$ Amine	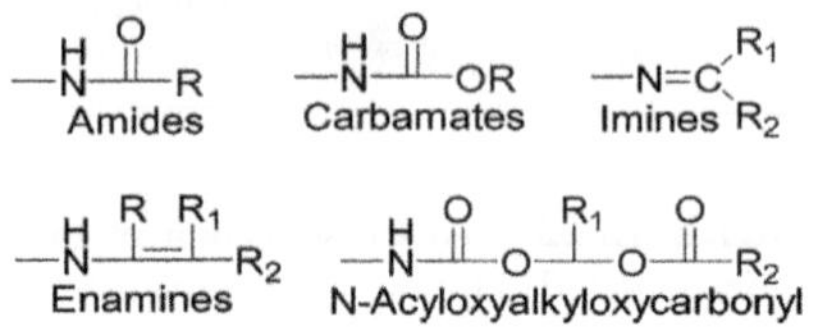 Amides; Carbamates; Imines; Enamines; N-Acyloxyalkyloxycarbonyl

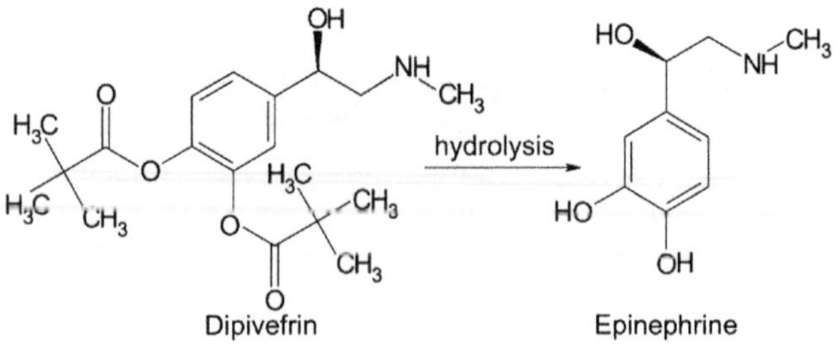

FIGURE 12.26 Hydrolysis of the prodrug dipivefrin to functional epinephrine inside the anterior chamber of the eye.

Esters are the most common prodrugs used and account for ~49% of the marketed products. Following are some examples of prodrugs and their principles of action.

Dipivefrin is a prodrug that gives rise to epinephrine used as an intraocular drug to reduce pressure in the eye (see Figure 12.26). The addition of pivaloyl groups to the epinephrine molecule improves the lipophilic character of the drug and thereby increases penetration into the anterior chamber of the eye. Once inside the anterior chamber, Dipivefrin is converted to epinephrine through hydrolysis. Epinephrine reduces the intraocular pressure by reducing humor production.

Parkinson's disease is known to be due to a deficiency in dopamine. Because of its polar characteristic, dopamine can't cross the blood-brain barrier. Levodopa (L-3,4-dihydroxy-phenylalanine), an amino acid, is recognized by the amino acid carrier proteins and is carried across the cell membrane (see Figure 12.27). It is a prodrug for dopamine. When Levodopa is inside the cell, the enzyme decarboxylase removes the acid group to produce dopamine.

Most drugs administered orally or intravenously go through the bloodstream to the site where they are required. During this process of transport, they can cause other toxic effects. Anticancer chemotherapeutic drugs are cytotoxic because they also affect normal growing cells. A site-specific prodrug can alleviate the toxicity to normal cells. Diethylstilbestrol diphosphate is a prodrug designed for breast cancer; this prodrug can be activated through an enzyme in the breast tissue as shown in Figure 12.28.

Fosphenytoin sodium salt is a prodrug for phenytoin used as an anti-epileptic agent (see Figure 12.29). This prodrug is used to reduce drug precipitation and consequent local irritation by phenytoin at the injection site. The prodrug has an aqueous solubility more than 7,000 times greater than phenytoin. The prodrug has a short half-life (<15 minutes) in blood and is rapidly converted to phenytoin in blood. The enzymatic action initially releases an unstable intermediate, which is rapidly converted to phenytoin.

Prodrugs currently available in the market are shown in Table 12.16.

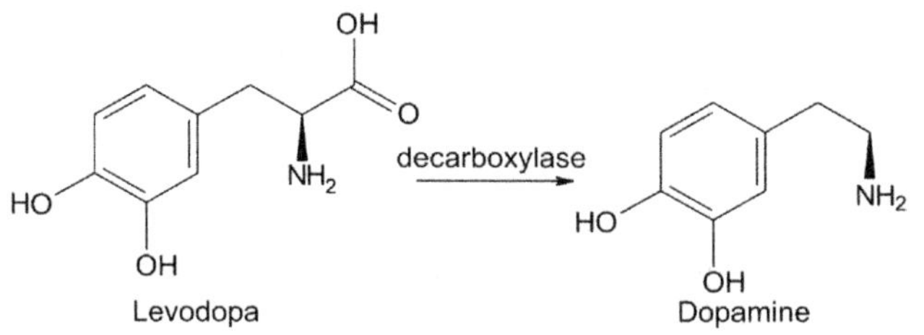

FIGURE 12.27 Enzymatic conversion of the prodrug levodopa to functional dopamine inside the cell.

12.8. CONCLUSIONS

Development of new chemical entities (NCEs) is expensive. Additionally, more than 60% of the NCEs in the pipeline have poor aqueous solubility, and most of them have some bioavailability issues. This chapter describes some of the special dosage forms and drug delivery systems that have emerged over the past few decades to address some of the deficiencies of the conventional dosage forms. For example, osmotic drug delivery provides a means of controlled and site-specific drug delivery without significant effect of pH variation in the gastrointestinal tract. Liposomes are

TABLE 12.16 Produgs Currently Available in the Market

Therapeutic Area	Prodrug Name (Trade Name)
Proton pump inhibitors	Esomeprazole (Nexium)
	Lansoprazole (Prevacid)
	Pantoprazole (Protonix)
	Rabeprazole (Sciphex)
Antiplatelet agent	Clopidogrel (Plavix)
Antiviral agent	Valacyclovir (Valtrex)
Hypercholesterolemia	Fenofibrate (Tricor)
Antiviral agent	Tenofovir disoproxil (Atripla)
Psychostimulant	Lisdexamfetamine (Vyvanse)
Influenza	Oseltamivir (Tamiflu)
Hypertension	Olmesartan medoxomil (Benicar)
Immunosuppressant	Mycophenolate mofetil (CellCept)
Glaucoma	Latanoprost (Xalatan)

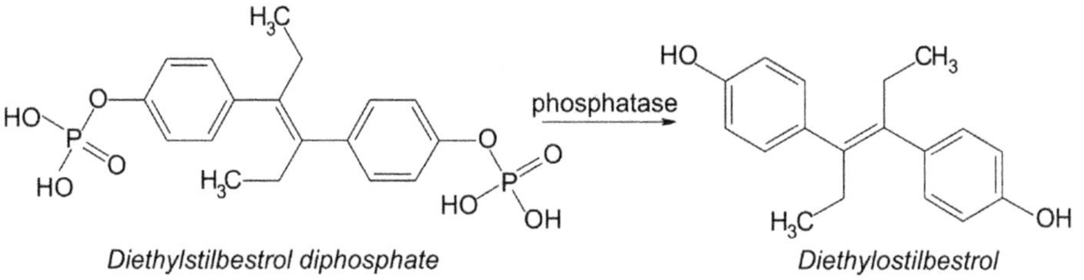

FIGURE 12.28 Breast cancer prodrug diethylstilbestrol diphosphate converts to diethylstilbestrol in the breast tissue in the presence of an enzyme phosphatase.

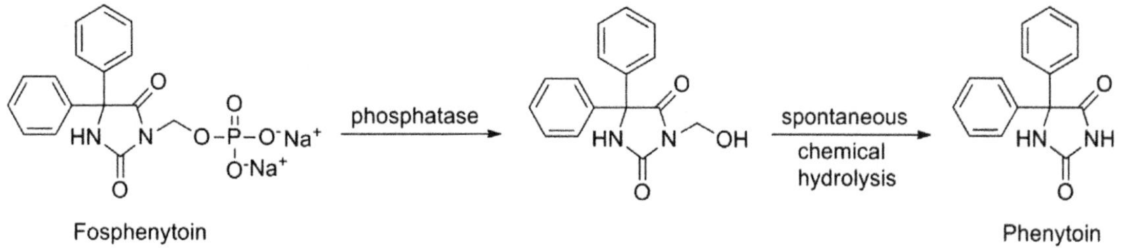

FIGURE 12.29 A two step conversion of the prodrug fosphenytoin sodium to phenytoin in the blood.

biocompatible and can deliver both hydrophilic and hydrophobic drugs. Liposomes provide versatility in the formulation of various dosage forms such as aerosols, gels, creams, and lotions and deliver the drugs through various routes such as intravenous, ocular, nasal, and subcutaneous. Dosage forms incorporating solid lipid nanoparticles, nanoemulsions, and nanosuspensions improve the apparent solubility of the drugs. Parenteral formulations using nanotechnologies can result in long systemic circulation as well as site-specific drug delivery. Magnetic nanoparticles can provide a multifunctional approach with site-specific drug delivery at the tumor site with the added benefit of hyperthermia, leading to tumor cell death. Implantable drug delivery is an approach used to prolong the delivery of a drug from weeks to months to years, resulting in improved patient compliance. Pharmacological effectiveness of a drug can be improved by the formulation of prodrugs.

This chapter also lists many of the products currently available in the market using the special dosage forms. Amorphous solid dispersions, co-crystals, etc., are some of the emerging technologies that are not described in this chapter. All these technologies will harness the benefits of the existing drugs and enhance the therapeutic effects of the new ones.

CASE STUDIES

Case 12.1

Mr. Smith, a cardiac patient, recently visited his physician and was put on Procardia XL® 60 mg tablet per day. His physician advised him to reduce the nifedipine dose from 60 mg to 30 mg/day. He still had 24 tablets left from his previous prescription, so he decided to cut the 60 mg tablet in half to meet his dosage need. When he brought this decision to the attention of his pharmacist, the pharmacist immediately called Mr. Smith and wanted to talk to him before he used the remaining 60 mg tablets. Is there any concern with the approach to cut tablets in half? If so, what type of counseling to the patient is needed for this case?

Approach: One should first understand the specialized dosage form of Procardia XL®. This is not a conventional oral tablet. Even though, this extended release tablet is similar in appearance to a conventional tablet, it consists of a semipermeable membrane surrounding an osmotically active drug core. The core itself is divided into two layers: an "active" layer containing the drug nifedipine and a "push" layer containing pharmacologically inert (but osmotically active) components. As water from the gastrointestinal tract enters into the tablet via the semipermeable membrane, pressure increases in the osmotic layer and "pushes" against the drug layer, releasing drug through the precision laser-drilled tablet orifice in the active layer in a zero-order manner. The Procardia XL® extended release tablet is designed to provide nifedipine at an approximately constant rate over 24 hours as long as the osmotic gradient remains constant, and then it gradually falls to zero. When the patient swallows the tablet, the biologically inert components of the tablet remain intact during gastrointestinal transit and are eliminated in the feces as an insoluble shell. This controlled rate of drug delivery into the gastrointestinal lumen is independent of pH or gastrointestinal motility. Procardia XL depends on the existence of an osmotic gradient between the contents of the bilayer core and fluid in the gastrointestinal tract for its action. Cutting this tablet into two halves will destroy the membrane and will dump the entire drug content at one time, and no constant release will be achieved.

Therefore, the pharmacist's advice is not to use the 60 mg tablet any more. Instead, the patient should use 30 mg Procardia XL extended release tablets.

Case 12.2

A healthy man is admitted to an emergency room for a hernia repair due to a suspected obstruction. The patient's medical history reveals an uneventful anesthesia for an orthopedic surgery in the past year. It is decided to use a modified rapid sequence induction with rocuronium (40 mg) and thiopental sodium (375 mg) through a 20 G cannula connected to a 1000 mL Hartmann's solution. It is noted that the patient, upon intubation, is not fully relaxed despite an appropriate dose of relaxant. It is noticed that the Hartmann's infusion stopped, and there is a 10 cm long column of fluid containing a flaky precipitate in the IV line, which was unsuccessfully flushed with 10 mL of saline through the injection port. Explain the possible cause of this problem to the attending surgeon and the nursing staff based on your knowledge of pharmaceutics.

Approach: This problem was possibly caused by drug incompatibility due to acid base properties, pH, and solubility. Rocuronium given through a poorly flowing cannula may have led to crystallize thiopental and subsequent obstruction of the cannula. Literature data [61] reveal the pH of thiopentone is 11–12, and for the muscle relaxant, rocuronium, is 4.0. In a highly acidic pH, the basic drug will precipitate to thiopentone acid, which has a very low solubility <0.1 mg/mL as compared to the sodium salt (700 mg/mL). A combination of a free-flowing drip as well as fluids running through the drip can minimize this precipitation. Another alternative is to change the drugs. Use of propofol or any of the muscle relaxants instead may be an alternative and better choice.

References

[1] Jantzen GM, Robinson JR. Sustained and controlled release drug delivery systems. 3rd ed. Modern pharmaceutics, vol. 575. New York: Marcel Dekker; 1995.

[2] Theeuwes F. The elementary osmotic pump. J Pharm Sci 1975;64(12):1987–91.

[3] Theeuwes F, Yum SI. Principles of the design and operation of generic osmotic pumps for the delivery of semisolid or liquid drug formulations. Ann Biomed Eng 1976;4:343–53.

[4] Zentner, GM, Rork, GS, Himmelstein, KJ. Controlled porosity osmotic pump, U.S. Patent 4968507 1990.

[5] Verma RK, Krishna DM, Garg S. Formulation aspects in the development of osmotically controlled oral drug delivery systems. J Control Release 2002;79:7–27.

[6] Santus G, Baker P. Osmotic drug delivery: a review of the patent literature. J Control Release 1995;35:1–21.

[7] Gupta BP, Thakur N, Jain NP. Osmotically controlled drug delivery system with associated drugs. J Pharm Pharm Sci 2010;13:571–88.

[8] Prentis RA, Lis Y, Walker SR. Pharmaceutical innovation by the seven UK owned pharmaceutical companies (1964–1984). Brit J Clin Pharmacol 1998;25:387–96.

[9] Panyam J, Labhasetwar V. Biodegradable nanoparticles for drug and gene delivery to cells and tissues. Adv Drug Deliv Rev 2003;55:329–47.

[10] Sonke S, Tomalia DA. Dendrimers in biomedical applications—reflections on the field. Adv Drug Deliv Rev 2005;57:2106–29.

[11] Courveur P, Couarrazze G, Devissaguet JP, Puisieux F. Nanoparticles: preparation and characterization. In: Benita S, editor. Microencapsulation methods and industrial applications. New York: Marcel Dekker; 1996. p. 183–211.

[12] Charman WN. Lipids, lipophilic drugs and oral drug delivery—some emerging concepts. J Pharm Sci 2000;89:967–78.

[13] Mehnert W, Mader K. Solid lipid nanoparticles: production, characterization and applications. Adv Drug Deliv Rev 2001;47:165–96.

[14] Muller RH, Runge. Solid lipid nanoparticles for controlled drug delivery. In: Benita S, editor. Submicron emulsion in drug targeting and delivery. Netherlands: Harwood Academic Publishers; 1998. p. P219–34.

[15] Gasco, MR. Method of producing solid lipid microspheres having a narrow size distribution, U.S. Patent 5250236.

[16] Sjostrom B, Bergenstahl B. Preparation of submicron drug particles in lecithin-stabilized O/W emulsions I. Model studies of the precipitation of cholesterylacetate. Int J Pharm 1992;88:53–62.

[17] Wissing SA, Kayser O, Muller RH. Solid lipid nanoparticles for potential drug delivery. Adv Drug Deliver Rev 2004;56:1257–72.

[18] Muller RH, Radtke M, Wissing SA. Nanostructured lipid matrices for improved microencapsulation of drugs. Int J Pharm 2002;242:121–8.

[19] Olbrich C, Gessner A, Kayser O, Muller RH. Lipid-Drug-Conjugate (LDC) nanoparticles as novel carrier system for the hydrophilic antitrypanosomal drug diminazediaceturate. J Drug Target 2002;10(5):387–96.

[20] Koroleva MY, Yurtov EV. Nanoemulsions: the properties, methods of preparation and promising applications. Russ Chem Rev 2012;81:21–43.

[21] Lovelyn C, Attama AA. Current state of nanoemulsions in drug delivery. J Biomater Nanobiotechnol 2011;2:626–39.

[22] Taylor G. The formation of emulsions in definable fields of flow. Proc Royal Soc A 1934;146:501.

[23] Abolmaali SS, Tamaddon AM, Farvadi FS, Daneshamuz S, Moghimi H. Pharmaceutical nanoemulsions and their potential topical and transdermal applications. Iran J Pharm Sci 2011;7:139–50.

[24] Rabinow BE. Nanosuspensions in drug delivery. Nat Rev/Drug Discov 2004;3:785–96.

[25] Pu X, Sun J, Li M, He Z. Formulation of nanosuspensions as a new approach for the delivery of poorly soluble drugs. Curr Nanosci 2009;5:417–27.

[26] Chingunpituk J. Nanosuspension technology for drug delivery, Walailak. J Sci Tech 2007;4:139–53.

[27] Haag R, Kratz F. Polymer therapeutics: concepts and applications. Angew Chem Int Ed 2006;45:1198–215.

[28] Folkman J, Long DM. The use of silicone rubber as a carrier for prolonged drug delivery. J Surg Res 1964;4:139–42.

[29] Langer R, Folkman J. Polymers for sustained release of proteins and other macromolecules. Nature 1976;263:797–800.

[30] Ringdorf H. Structure and properties of pharmacologically active polymers. J Polym Sci Polym Symp 1975;:135–53.

[31] Pasut G, Veronese FM. Polymer-drug conjugation, recent achievements and general strategies. Prog Poly Sci 2007;32:933–67.

[32] Bangham AD, Stondish MM, Watkins JC. Diffusion of univalent ions across the lamellae of swollen phospholipids. J Mol Biol 1965;13:238–52.

[33] Storm G, Crommelin DJA. Liposomes: quo vadis? PSTT 1998;1:29–31.

[34] Jesorka A, Owe Orwar O. Liposomes: technologies and analytical applications. Annu Rev Anal Chem 2008;1:801–32.

[35] Szoka F, Papahadjopoulos D. Procedure for preparation of liposomes with large internal aqueous space and high capture by reverse-phase evaporation. Proc Natl Acad Sci 1978;75:4194–8.

[36] Woodbury DJ, Richardson ES, Grigg AW, Welling RD, Knudson BH. Reducing liposome size with ultrasound: biomedical size distribution. J Liposome Res 2006;16:57–80.

[37] Hauschild S, Lipprandt U, Rumplecker A, Borchert U, Rank A, Schubert R, et al. Direct preparation and loading of lipid and polymer vesicles using inkjets. Small 2005;1:1170–80.

[38] Estes DJ, Mayer. Giant liposomes in physiological buffer using electroformation in a flow chamber. Biochim Biophys Acta 2005;1712:152–60.

[39] Lasic DD. Liposomes. Sci Med 1996;May/June:34–43.

[40] Mozafari, MR, Khosravi-Darani, K. An overview of liposome-derived nanocarrier technologies. In: Mozafari, MR, editor. Nanomaterials and nanosystems for biomedical applications. 2005. p.113–23.

[41] Lian T, Ho RJY. Trends and developments in liposome drug delivery systems. J Pharm Sci 2000;90(6):667–80.

[42] Pankhurst QA, Connolly J, Jones SK, Dobson J. Applications of magnetic nanoparticles in biomedicine. J Phys D, Appl Phys 2003;36:R167–81.

[43] Sun CC, Lee JSH, Zhang MM. Magnetic nanoparticles in MR imaging and drug delivery. Adv Drug Deliv Rev 2008;60:1252–65.

[44] Corchero JL, Villaverde A. Biomedical applications of distally controlled magnetic nanoparticles. Trends Biotechnol 2009;27:468–76.

[45] Hergt R, Andra W, d'Amby CG, Hilger I, Kaiser WA, Richter U, et al. Physical limits of hyperthermia using magnetite fine particles. IEEE Trans Magnetics 1998;34(5):3745–54.

[46] Jain TK, Torres MM, Sahoo SK, Leslie-Pelecky D, Labhasetwar V. Iron oxide nanoparticles for sustained delivery of anticancer agents. Mol Pharm 2005;2:194–205.

[47] Widder KJ, Senei AE, Scarpelli DG. Magnetic microspheres: a model system for site specific drug delivery *in vivo*. Proc Soc Exp Biol Med 1978;58:141–6.

[48] Bharodiya PK, Solanski AB. Approaches to the development of implantable drug delivery system, <http://www.slideshare.net/pareshbharodiya/implantable-drug-delivery-system>; 2010.

[49] Danckenwerts M, Fassini A. Implantable controlled release drug delivery systems: a review. Drug Dev Ind Pharm 1991;17:1465–502.

[50] Dash AK, Cudworth II GC. Therapeutic applications of implantable drug delivery systems. J Pharmacol Toxicol Methods 1998;40:1–12.

[51] Sah H, Chien YW. Rate control in drug delivery and targeting: fundamentals and applications to implantable systems. In: Hilery AM, Lloyd AW, Swarbrick A, editors. *Drug delivery and targeting for pharmacists and pharmaceutical scientists*. Taylor Francis; 2001. p. 73–103.

[52] Blackshear PJ, Dorman FD, Blackshear Jr PL, Varco RL, Buchwald H. A permanently implantable self-recycling low flow constant rate multipurpose infusion pump of simple design. Surg Forum 1970;21:136.

[53] Blackshear PJ, Dorman FD, Blackshear Jr PL, Varco RL, Buchwald, HA. Implantable Infusion Pump, U.S. Patent 3,731,681 1973.

[54] Renard E. Implantable closed-loop glucose-sensing and insulin delivery: the future of insulin pump therapy. Curr Opin Pharmacol 2002;2:708–16.

[55] LaVan DA, McGuire T, Langer R. Small scale systems for *in vivo* drug delivery. Nat Biotechnol 2003;21:1184–91.

[56] Prescott JH, Lipka S, Baldwin S, Sheppard NF, Maloney JM, Coppeta J, et al. Chronic programmed polypeptide delivery from an implanted, multireservoir microchip device. Nat Biotechnol 2006;24:437–8.

[57] Li PY, Shih J, Lo R, Saati S, Agrawal R, Humayun MS, et al. An electrochemical intraocular drug delivery device. Sens Actuators A 2008;143:41–8.

[58] Verma A, Verma B, Prajapati SK, Tripathi K. Prodrugs as a chemical delivery system: a review. Asian J Res Chem 2009;2:100–3.

[59] Albert A. Chemical aspects of selective toxicity. Nature 1958;182:421–3.

[60] Rautio J, Kumpulainen H, Heimbach T, Oliyai R, Oh D, Jarvinen T, et al. Prodrugs: design and clinical applications. Nat Rev/Drug Discov 2008;7:255–70.

[61] Khan S, Stannard N, Greign J. Precipitation of thiopental with muscle relaxant: a potential hazard. J R Soc MedSh Rep 2011;2:58.

PART III

BIOLOGICAL APPLICATIONS OF PHARMACEUTICS

CHAPTER

13

Membrane Transport and Permeation

Justin A. Tolman[1] *and Maria P. Lambros*[2]

[1]Creighton University School of Pharmacy and Health Professions, Omaha, NE, USA [2]Department of Pharmaceutical Sciences, College of Pharmacy, Western University of Health Sciences, Pomona, CA, USA

CHAPTER OBJECTIVES

- Describe the composition of biological membranes.
- Explain the fluid mosaic model of membranes.
- Compare and contrast the membrane transport processes of diffusion, carrier-mediated, and vesicular transport.
- Develop and evaluate clinically relevant scenarios that involve medications that target or interact with membrane transport processes.

Keywords

- Active transport
- Carrier-mediated transport
- Diffusion
- Drug transport
- Efflux transport
- Lipid bilayer
- Passive transport
- Phospholipid
- Vesicle-medicated transport

13.1. INTRODUCTION

Drug movement in biological systems is usually governed by interactions between the drug molecule and cellular membranes. These interactions principally describe drug permeation, or movement, from one side of a membrane to the other. That is, permeation is the ability of a drug molecule to pass through biological membranes and can include both passive and active transport phenomena. Often, drug transport can be predominantly affected by one type of membrane permeation and then be affected by perturbations to these systems. This chapter briefly reviews the composition of cell membranes and then describes membrane transport processes.

13.2. CELL MEMBRANES

All the cells in our body are surrounded by plasma membranes [13]. The plasma membrane is a semipermeable barrier that functions as a protective shield from the external environment. Although substantial variability exists in cell membrane composition throughout the body, most cell membranes consist of amphiphilic lipids arranged in a lipid bilayer with proteins imbedded in or through this bilayer (Figure 13.1).

13.2.1 Membrane Composition

Most membrane lipids are glycerol molecules that contain an esterified phosphate and two fatty acid chains (Figure 13.2). These fatty acid chains can be of varying lengths and can be saturated or unsaturated to affect membrane properties. Other membrane lipids can have substituted hydrophilic functional groups in place of the phosphate or might lack fatty acid groups. The resulting amphiphilic lipid molecules have a hydrophilic head group attached to two lipophilic fatty acid tails. Some examples of common cell membrane lipids include phosphatidylcholine, phosphatidylserine, phosphatidylinositol, sphingomyelin, glycolipids, and cholesterol.

In physiologic conditions, these lipids orient into a bilayer with hydrophilic head groups toward the external aqueous environment and hydrophobic fatty acid

Pharmaceutics. DOI: http://dx.doi.org/10.1016/B978-0-12-386890-9.00013-3

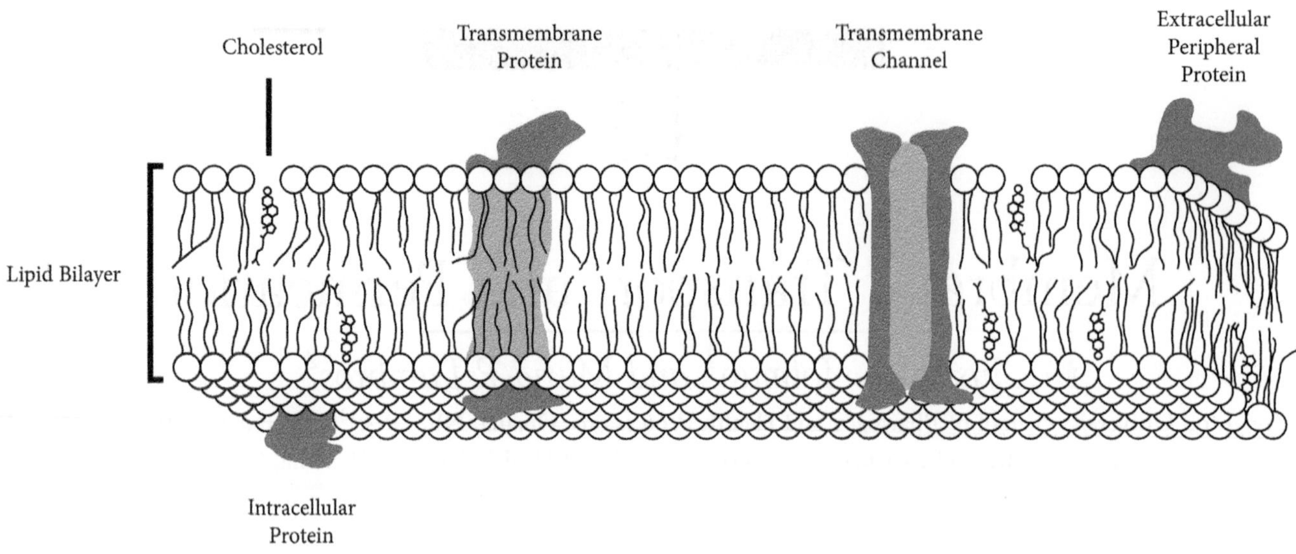

FIGURE 13.1 A schematic representation of a cell membrane. It consists of a lipid bilayer and embedded protein structures.

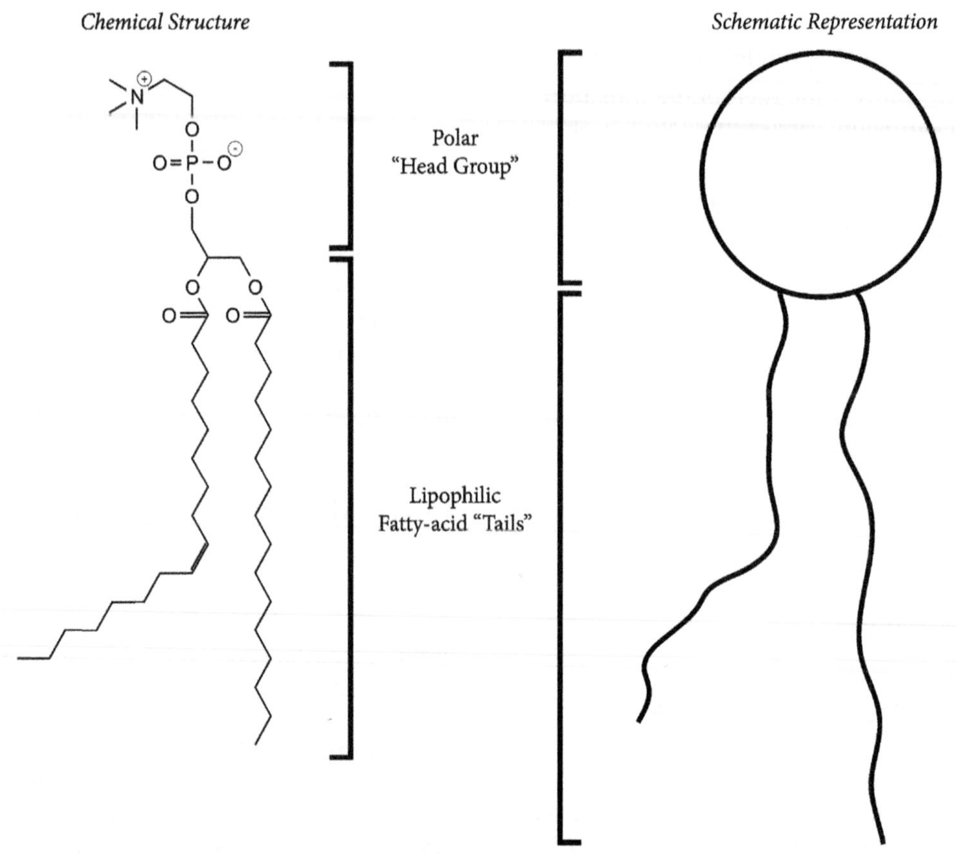

FIGURE 13.2 Chemical structure of phospholipids.

chains pointed into a lipophilic core region. These membrane bilayers are often stable under normal physiologic conditions to minimize aqueous exposure of lipophilic membrane lipid portions. Despite relative membrane integrity, there is a great deal of flexibility and "fluidity" due to the fatty acid chains in the lipophilic membrane core [9]. The majority of lipid movement in intact membranes is lateral (sideways) within

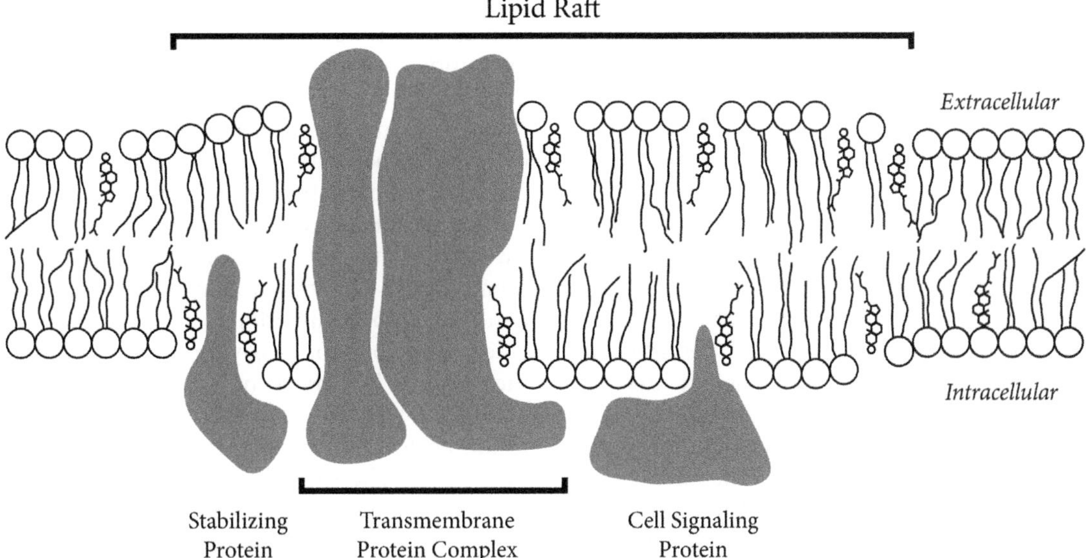

FIGURE 13.3 Schematic representation of a lipid raft.

one layer of the membrane. Rarely, a lipid in one layer of the bilayer may exchange position with another lipid in the other monolayer. Lipid movement and distribution within biological membranes can be substantially affected by normal cellular functions and changes to the cellular shape [9].

Lipid composition is an important factor in the properties of biological membranes. Long-chain fatty acids tend to thicken the cell membrane and create a more substantial lipophilic core. The presence of double bonds in the fatty acid chains also prevents close association of lipophilic tails and induces more membrane fluidity. In contrast, cholesterol can intercalate between fatty acids to induce more close association of lipophilic tails and induce membrane rigidity.

13.2.2 Fluid Mosaic Model for Membranes

In 1972, Singer and Nicolson originally proposed a "fluid mosaic" model from which our current view of biological membranes has evolved [14]. The fluid portion of this model is derived from the flexible and fluid lipid bilayer as previously described. The mosaic portion of this molecule describes heterogeneous globular protein structures either partially or fully embedded in the lipid bilayer (Figure 13.1). The lipid and protein constituents of the bilayer float freely in the plane of the bilayer and form a mosaic pattern.

The scientific understanding of the fluid-mosaic model has evolved with recent advances. Specifically, cell membranes are not freely fluid but have regions of increased order imposed by large-scale structures and complexes (Figure 13.3). Lipid rafts are heterogeneous membrane domains with clusters of lipids and associated protein complexes in ordered spatial relationships [1]. These organized regions have varied structures and temporal stabilities but exist for proper functioning of cellular processes. One example of a lipid raft includes a membrane domain that contains a cell surface receptor and intracellular machinery for the communication of extracellular signals to intracellular second messenger systems and functions. Another type of lipid raft includes membrane domains that stabilize protein-mediated transport systems for the physical transfer of substances into or out of the cell.

13.3. MEMBRANE TRANSPORT

The semi-permeable nature of biological membranes is due to the fluid mosaic nature of membranes. The composition of both lipid bilayers and embedded protein structures can affect the permeation of substances through membranes. That is, a substance must then be able to pass directly through the membrane, be transported through the membrane with the assistance of a protein structure, or be transported through membranes through vesicles that merge with, or are formed from, the cell membrane. These three broad categories of permeation are described as diffusion, carrier-mediated transport, or vesicular transport. Within these categories, some substances are able to be transported passively without cellular expenditure of energy, whereas other transport systems require energy to move substances. Most substances are predominantly transported through biological membranes by limited permeation mechanisms based on substance physicochemical properties such as molecular size, polarity, ionization state, aqueous solubility, hydrophilicity/lipophilicity balance, and mimicry of endogenous compounds [5].

13.3.1 Diffusion

Diffusion is the movement of substances from a region of high concentration to a region of low concentration. The process of diffusion can be described by Fick's First Law of Diffusion. When used to describe diffusion through a semipermeable biological membrane, the flux (J) of a substance through the membrane is inversely proportional to the membrane thickness (X) and proportional to the diffusion coefficient (D) of the drug through the membrane and the concentration gradient ($C_1 - C_2$) across the membrane:

$$J = DK(C_1 - C_2)/X \quad (13.1)$$

where K is the partition coefficient of the diffusing molecule in the membrane (K = Concentration of the drug in the membrane/Concentration of the drug in the donor, C_D or receiver compartment, C_R). In equation 13.1 the units for D are in cm^2/sec; the thickness, X, in cm; the concentration, C, in g/cm^3, and the flux, J, in $g\ cm^{-2}\ sec^{-1}$.

The driving force then for diffusion is the concentration gradient while the resistive force for diffusion is the thickness of the membrane (Figure 13.4). As a result, diffusion is a passive phenomenon that does not directly require energy for the movement of substances. This passive process will continue with net substance movement occurring from a region of high concentration to low concentration (with a concentration gradient) until an equilibrium is established such that there is no difference in drug concentrations across the membrane. During this equilibrium, drug movement will continue to occur but with no net change in drug concentrations across the membrane.

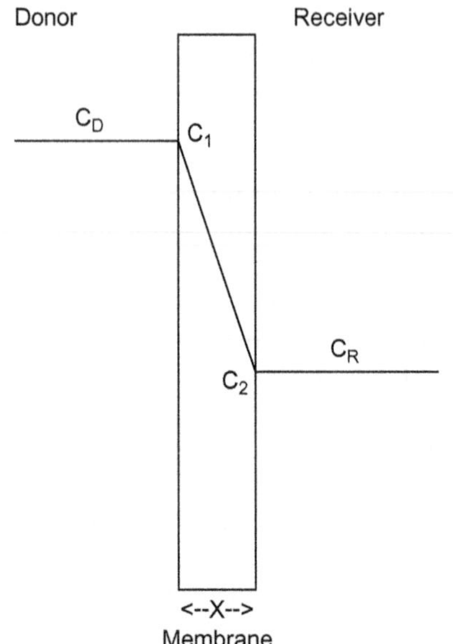

FIGURE 13.4 Steady-state diffusion through a thin membrane.

Not all substances are able to diffuse across biological membranes. Water is able to diffuse through cell membranes. Many nonpolar substances such as oxygen and carbon dioxide, as well as many drug molecules, are able to passively diffuse directly through membranes. The drug molecule must also be lipophilic enough to pass through the membrane but not so lipophilic as to be retained within the lipid bilayer lipophilic core. The rate of diffusion is then limited by the surface area across which diffusion can take place. If a substance is unable to pass directly through the lipid bilayer, protein-mediated phenomena can potentially cause transport across biological membranes.

13.3.2 Carrier-Mediated Transport

Many biologically relevant substances are able to pass through membranes through specialized pores and channels or protein structures. Many small charged species (e.g., Na^+, K^+, Ca^{2+}, and Cl^- ions) pass via specific channels that allow dissolved ion movement through membranes in response to electrical or chemical stimuli. It is important to note that these pores or channels principally allow passive ion movement with a concentration gradient. Other protein transporters can facilitate the passive diffusion of small polar molecules (e.g., glucose) into cells with transport described as facilitated diffusion.

In contrast, other embedded protein structures promote direct substance movement against concentration gradients and are termed primary active transport systems. Some of these systems are specialized protein structures that move ions or small polar molecules against concentration gradients for maintenance of electrochemical gradients and transport of important biological substances. Separate protein systems are referred to as efflux pumps or transporters and cause substance movement out of cells for protective purposes. Many primary active systems allow substances to permeate through membranes based on distinct chemical or molecular properties, whereas others are promiscuous and might transport substances based on a broad range of properties such as molecular size, polarity, ionization state (including cations and anions), lipophilicity, and functional groups.

Protein-mediated systems that cause substance movement against gradients but do so through co-transport of other ions with a gradient are designated as secondary active transport systems. These systems simultaneously transport a small polar molecule or ion against an established concentration gradient while a separate ion or molecule is transported with an established ion gradient. Secondary active transport systems then do not directly require energy for movement of substances but instead rely on ion gradients established by primary active transport systems. Most secondary active transport systems are highly specialized for the movement of specific molecules or ions.

Despite numerous differences in protein function, all carrier mediated transport systems are dependent on specialized protein structures embedded in biological membranes (Figure 13.5). Carrier-mediated systems require some degree of protein conformational change to effect substance permeation through membranes. Due to the physical reliance on a distinct protein structure, these carrier-mediated systems can become saturated to demonstrate transport maxima. The rate of substance transport is then limited by the number of transport proteins available for substance movement.

The rate, V, of active transport can be described by the Michaelis-Menten equation:

$$V = V_{max}C/(K_m + C)$$

where C is the concentration of the solute, V_{max} is the maximum transport rate that can be attained and K_m is the Michaelis-Menten constant.

13.3.3 Vesicular Transport

Vesicular transport is a cellular mechanism to allow the permeation of large polar substances or of large volumes of substances through biological membranes by the formation or fusion of membrane-enclosed vesicles with the cellular membrane (Figure 13.6) [2]. Endocytosis is the process in which a substance enters the cell because the cell engulfs. Exocytosis is the process in which a substance inside an intracellular vesicle exits the cell after fusion of the intracellular vesicle with the cell membrane. The rates of endocytosis and exocytosis are regulated processes to maintain constant cellular membrane surface area and cell volume. Endocytosis and exocytosis are also mechanisms by which lipid bilayer components and embedded protein structures can be regulated on the cell surface. Both endocytosis and exocytosis require energy for the formation and movement of vesicles within cells.

13.4. PHARMACOLOGICALLY RELEVANT MEMBRANE TRANSPORT PROCESSES

Most drug molecules must be transported through various biological membranes to exert pharmacologic effects. Numerous potential transport phenomena could affect a single dose the patient receives (Figure 13.5) [11]. For example, following the delivery of a dose, a given drug molecule could first encounter a biological membrane on the apical surface of an

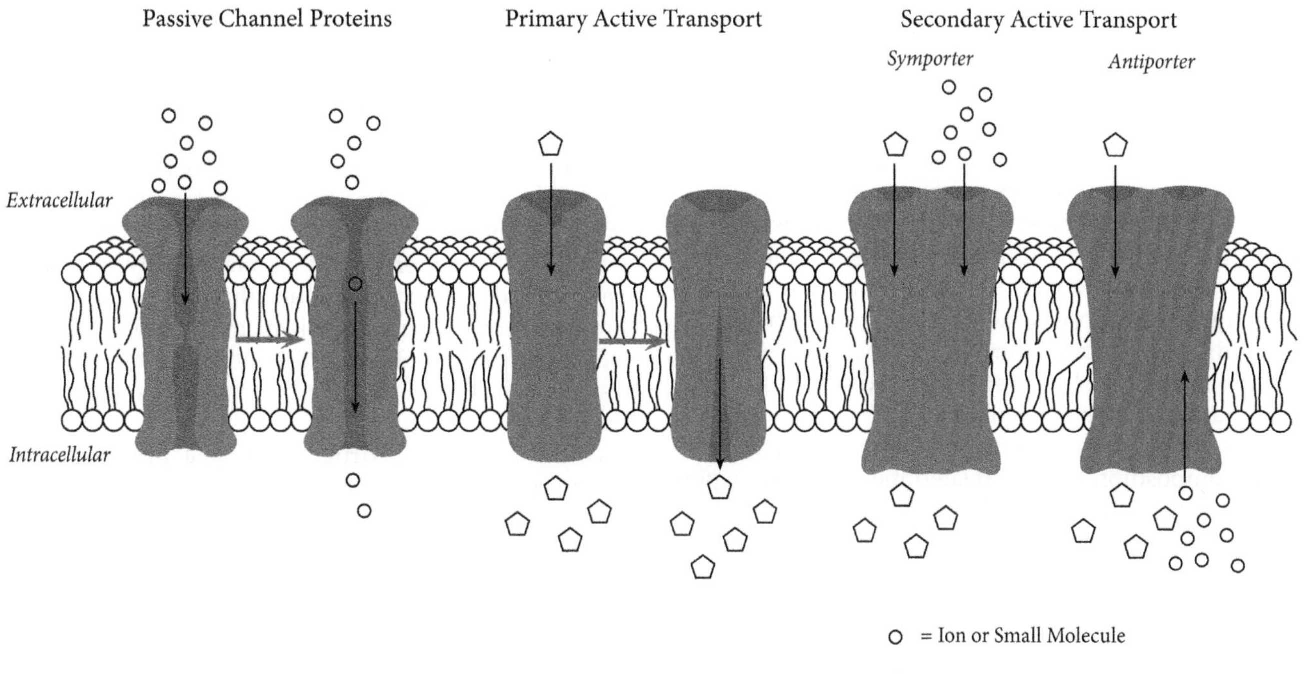

FIGURE 13.5 Schematic representations of various protein structures embedded in biological membranes involved in membrane transport.

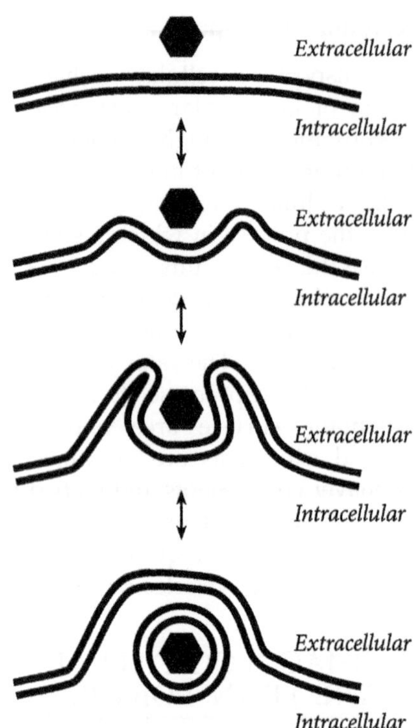

FIGURE 13.6 Schematic representation of vesicular transport.

epithelial site of administration. There could then be a second membrane on the basolateral epithelial surface for the drug molecule to leave the site of administration. The drug molecule could then encounter a capillary membrane before the drug can enter the systemic circulation. Following drug movement through the systemic circulation and transport out through a capillary cell membrane, numerous cell membranes are potentially encountered throughout the body. Following this membrane encounter and movement into an organ or tissue, there could even be a subsequent subcellular organelle or nuclear membrane encounter.

These diverse membranes could have varied permeability to the drug molecule. In fact, substantial variability exists in cell surface composition and membrane transport systems throughout the body. These differences can contribute to pharmacologic variability as reflected by diverse gene expressions of protein transport system components due to genetic differences between patients. Additionally, each membrane composition and the related membrane transport mechanisms introduce differences in potential drug targets and drug-interactions.

13.4.1 Select Membrane Transport Systems as Drug Targets

Many drugs affect membrane transport systems to exert their pharmacologic action. A very large number of currently marketed therapeutic agents as well as environmental or chemical agents exert effects through disruptions of the lipid bilayer, protein-mediated transport systems, and vesicular formation and transport.

13.4.1.1 Diffusion

Amphotericin B is a large macrocyclic polyene antifungal agent (Figure 13.7) that is formulated in a variety of commercially available preparations (Amphotec®, Abelcet®, and AmBisome®) [10]. The amphilic faces of this large molecule are thought to intercalate into the lipid bilayer of fungal cell membranes through association with prevalent lipid sterols in fungal membranes. Clusters of amphotericin B molecules then associate into loose lipid raft structures and form indiscriminate holes [18] or gaps in the fungal cell membrane integrity. The disruption of membrane integrity or alteration of diffusion parameters then has catastrophic effects on fungal cell viability and contributes to cell death. Amphotericin B also can cause nephrotoxicity that is thought to be due in part to association with sterols present in renal cell lipid bilayers. Other drugs that affect cell membranes are often cytotoxic and used for cell-killing pharmacologic effects as antibacterial or antifungal agents.

13.4.1.2 Carrier-Mediated Transport

Numerous drugs and agents exert pharmacologic action on protein-mediated membrane transport systems. Many drugs affect the regulation of ion gradients across cell membranes through inhibition of ion transporters. These ion-regulating drugs are therapeutically used in a variety of disease states including hypertension, cardiac arrhythmias, seizures, and nerve signal transduction. Nontherapeutic insecticides, chemical warfare agents, and chemical toxins can also affect ion gradients and ion transport systems [3,12]. Other therapeutic and nontherapeutic agents directly affect primary active transport systems that are used for the movement of endogenous biochemical substances and exogenous drug molecules. Secondary active transport systems can also be directly and indirectly affected by drugs.

One example of a drug affecting a primary active transport system is omeprazole (Prilosec®) [10]. It is a small molecule in a drug class that targets a specific ion transporter in the gut (Figure 13.8). This class is referred to as proton-pump inhibitors (PPIs) and irreversibly inhibits the H^+/K^+ ATPase co-transporter present on the apical surface of gastric parietal cells of the stomach. This primary active co-transport system pumps protons against the pH gradient to concentrate acid in the gastric lumen while also scavenging a

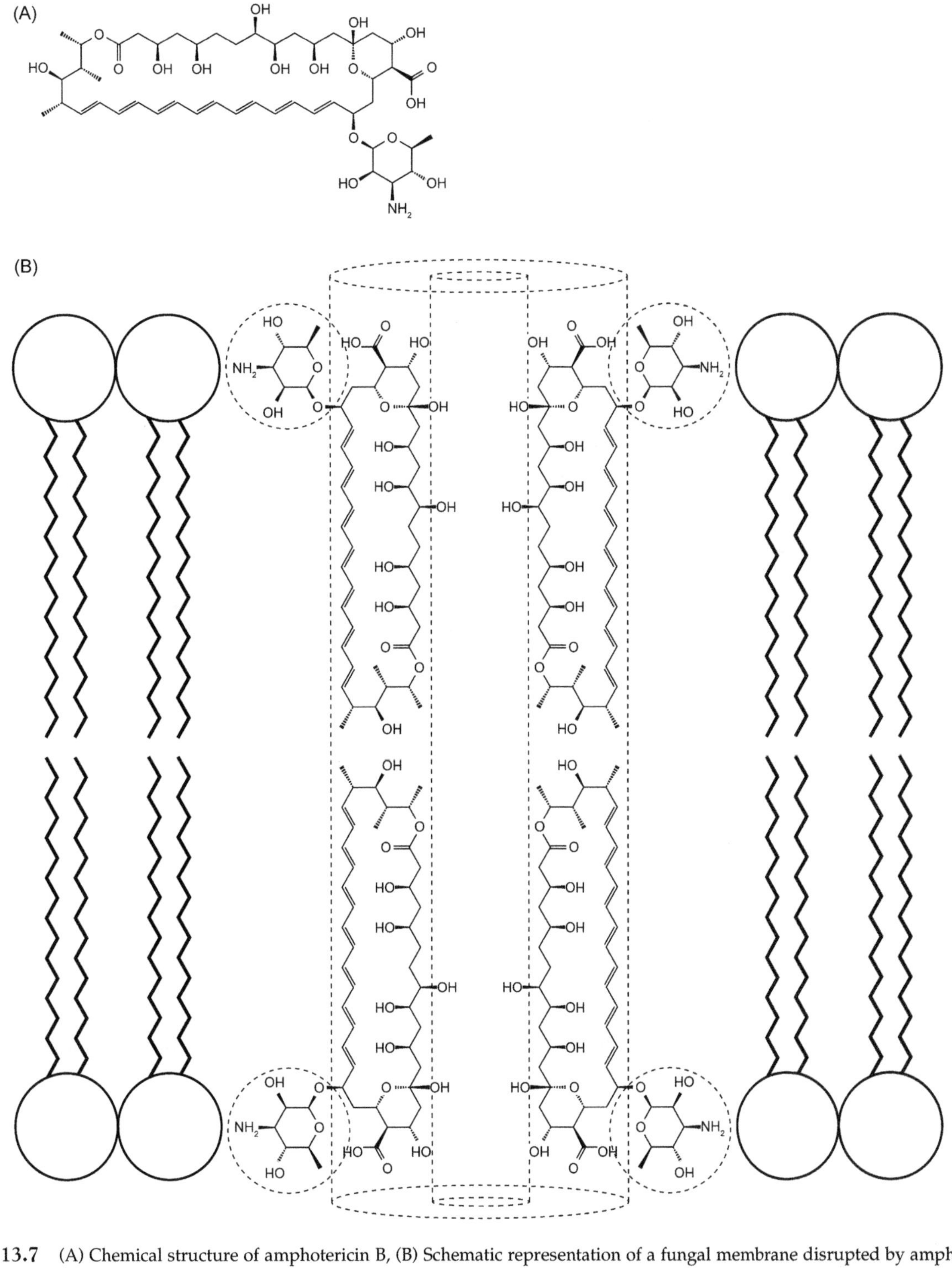

FIGURE 13.7 (A) Chemical structure of amphotericin B, (B) Schematic representation of a fungal membrane disrupted by amphotericin B.

potassium ion from the gastric lumen and transporting it against the potassium gradient into the cell. Omeprazole and other PPIs covalently bind to cysteine residues in hydrogen-potassium pumps to irreversibly inhibit their function and result in inhibition of the gastric acid secretion [17].

13.4.1.3 Vesicular Transport

The gastrointestinal epithelium contains specialized M-cells for the vesicular transport of macromolecules and microorganisms [6]. M-cells function to internalize antigenic pathogens or particles by engulfing them in vesicles on the apical side of the cell and transporting

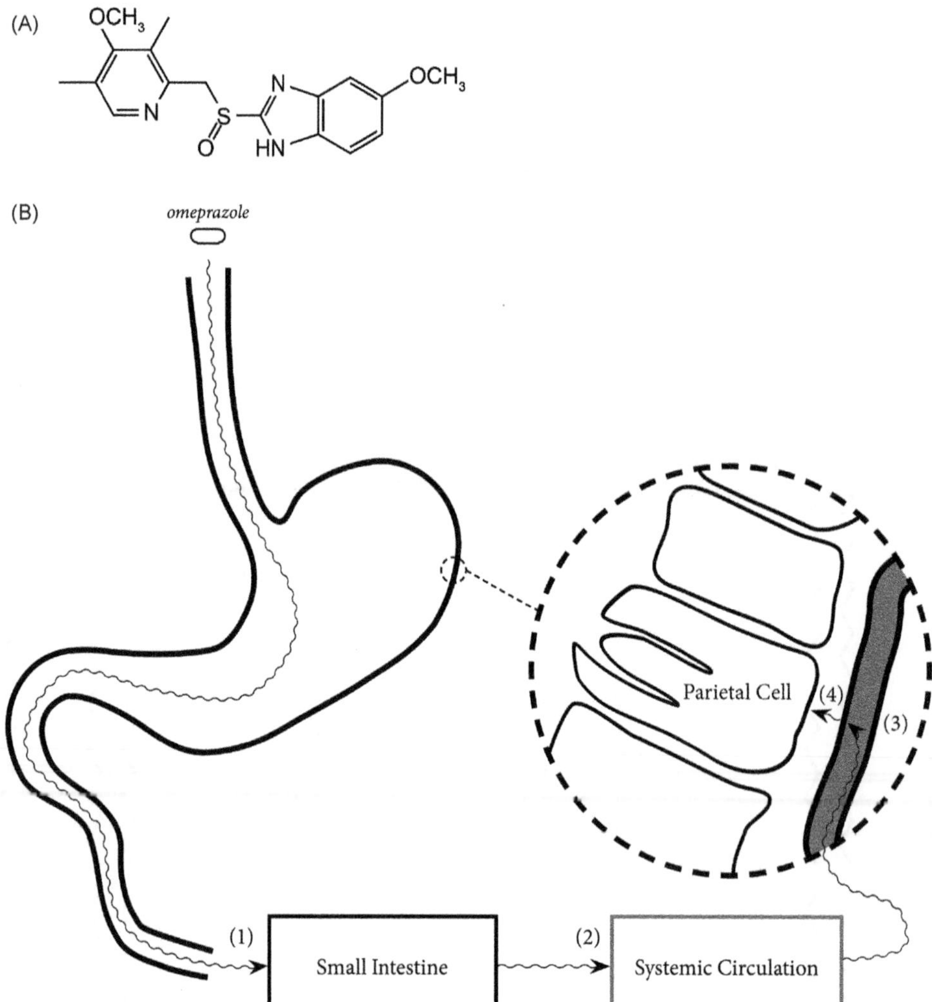

FIGURE 13.8 (A) The chemical structure of omeprazole, B) Representative membrane transport processes for omeprazole. (1) Dissolution of omeprazole in the small intestine and absorption of the drug across the apical membrane of the intestinal epithelium, (2) Transport of omeprazole through the basolateral membrane of the intestinal epithelium through the capillary epithelium and into the systemic circulation, (3) Transport of omeprazole through the capillary epithelium and to the parietal cell, (4) Transport of omeprazole through the parietal cell membrane to exert pharmacologic action on proton pumps located in the apical membrane of parietal cells.

them to the basolateral through transcytosis. In this way, appropriate immune responses can be generated against ingested antigens. However, the normally nonspecific vesicle formation can be attuned to provide mucosal vaccination against specific ingested antigens through oral vaccination strategies. The live, attenuated oral polio vaccine (OPV) takes advantage of M-cell vesicular transport to promote vesicle formation [4]. Specifically, the OPV causes epithelial M-cells to be primed for increased vesicular formation and transport of ingested polio virus particles to provide polio immunity [7].

13.4.2 Select Membrane Transport Systems as Drug Interactions

Many drugs utilize carrier-mediated transport systems through facilitated, primary, or secondary systems for drug permeation through membranes. This increases the likelihood that some drug/substance combinations could utilize or affect the same protein system for drug movement processes. These interactions could be competitive or beneficial for therapeutic drug effects but must be considered for appropriate drug therapy evaluation.

One example of membrane transport–based drug interactions involves a promiscuous efflux pump referred to as P-glycoprotein (Pgp) [16]. Pgp belongs to the ATP-binding cassette transporter (ABC) protein superfamily. ABC transporters involved in translocation of substances through biological membranes are a very diverse group and include numerous protein structures that impart multi-drug resistance (MDR) [15]. Pgp is a well-characterized protein that is widely distributed and expressed throughout the body [8].

It actively inhibits net drug permeation across biological membranes. Pgp is a protective efflux pump that can cause the expulsion of exogenous substances that have permeated through a membrane back into the lumen of various organs or tissues. Many hydrophobic drugs are affected by Pgp efflux under normal physiologic conditions, whereas some pathogenic conditions, including cancer, can cause overexpression of Pgp. Pgp primary active transport expression can be a significant cause of MDR for many pathologic conditions.

13.5. CONCLUSIONS

Drug permeation through biological membranes is a nontrivial barrier to pharmacologic action. Thankfully, permeation is potentially possible through the semipermeable nature of biological membranes. A large diversity of substances is able to pass through membranes based on a surplus of transport mechanisms. These transport mechanisms include passive drug diffusion and facilitated diffusion as well as active transport phenomena of primary and secondary active transport as well as vesicular-mediated transport. In the next chapter, the process of drug absorption and disposition in biological systems will expand on this understanding of the membrane transport process and drug permeation.

CASE STUDIES

Case 13.1

Loperamide is an over-the-counter antidiarrheal drug taken orally. *In vitro* studies have shown that it is a very potent μ-opioid receptor agonist. The expected activity would include analgesia, sedation, drowsiness, constipation, respiratory depression, etc. However, *in vivo*, it exhibits only antidiarrheal activity. Can you suggest why such central nervous system (CNS) activity is not seen in the case of oral loperamide use? If the drug will be co-administered with quinidine, do you expect any drug-drug interaction problem? Hints: *Quinidine is a potent Pgp inhibitor.*

Approach: We did not see any central nervous activity due to abundant P-gp activity at the blood-brain barrier (BBB). Therefore, transport of this molecule to the brain is restricted. When Pgp inhibitors such as quinidine are co-administered, things change and we expect a drug-drug interaction. We see elevated antidiarrheal activity along with CNS side effects.

Case 13.2

Targeted delivery to a tumor by nanoparticles has gained tremendous attention because of their extra permeability and retention (EPR) effect. Explain how it works in the case of a solid tumor.

Approach: Nanoparticles in particle sizes at approximately 100 nm can pass through leaky vasculature. Therefore, their tumor uptake is very high. Because of their particle size range, they are not cleared by reticuloendothelial systems (RES) and can be circulated in the blood for a long time. Finally, because solid tumors are devoid of lymphatic drainage, once nanoparticles are taken into tumors, they stay for a longer time in the tumors. This combined phenomenon is called the EPR effect.

References

[1] Catalá A. Lipid peroxidation modifies the picture of membranes from the "Fluid Mosaic Model" to the "Lipid Whisker Model". Biochimie 2012;94(1):101–9.
[2] Doherty GJ, McMahon HT. Mechanisms of endocytosis. Annu Rev Biochem 2009;78:857–902.
[3] Doherty JD. Insecticides affecting ion transport. Pharmacol Ther 1979;7(1):123–51.
[4] Gebert A, et al. Antigen transport into Peyer's patches: increased uptake by constant numbers of M cells. Am J Pathol 2004;164(1):65–72.
[5] Golan DE, editor. Principles of pharmacology: the pathophysiologic basis of drug therapy. 3rd ed. Philadelphia, PA: Lippincott Williams & Wilkins; 2011.
[6] Hathaway LJ, Kraehenbuhl JP. The role of M cells in mucosal immunity. Cell Mol Life Sci 2000;57(2):323–32.
[7] Knox C, et al. DrugBank 3.0: a comprehensive resource for 'omics' research on drugs. Nucleic Acids Res 2011;39(Database issue):D1035–41.
[8] Lum BL, Gosland MP. MDR expression in normal tissues. Pharmacologic implications for the clinical use of P-glycoprotein inhibitors. Hematol/Oncol Clin North Am 1995;9 (2):319–36.
[9] Marguet D, et al. Dynamics in the plasma membrane: how to combine fluidity and order. EMBO J 2006;25(15):3446–57.
[10] McEvoy GK. AHFS drug information. American hospital formulary service. American Society of Health-System Pharmacists; 2013. Available from: http://www.ahfsdruginformation.com/.
[11] Mizuno N, et al. Impact of drug transporter studies on drug discovery and development. Pharmacol Rev 2003;55 (3):425–61.
[12] Schiavo G, Matteoli M, Montecucco C. Neurotoxins affecting neuroexocytosis. Physiol Rev 2000;80(2):717–66.
[13] Sherwood L. The plasma membrane and membrane potential (Ch 3.) In: Sherwood, L. Human physiology: from cells to systems. Belmont, CA: Brooks/Cole; 2013.
[14] Singer SJ, Nicolson GL. The fluid mosaic model of the structure of cell membranes. Science (New York, N.Y.) 1972;175 (4023):720–31.
[15] Sun J, et al. Multidrug resistance P-glycoprotein: crucial significance in drug disposition and interaction. Med Sci Monitor: Int Med J Exp Clin Res 2004;10(1):RA5–14.
[16] Yu DK. The contribution of P-glycoprotein to pharmacokinetic drug-drug interactions. J Clin Pharmacol 1999;39(12):1203–11.
[17] Shin JM. Pharmacology of proton pump inhibitors. Curr Gastroenterol Rep 2008;10(6):528–34.
[18] Gray KC, Palacios DS, Dailey I, et al. Amphotericin primarily kills yeast by simply binding ergosterol. Proc Natl Acad Sci USA 2012;109(7):2234–9.

CHAPTER

14

Factors Affecting Drug Absorption and Disposition

Chong-Hui Gu[1], Anuj Kuldipkumar[1] and Harsh Chauhan[2]

[1]Vertex Pharmaceuticals, Inc., Cambridge, MA, USA [2]College of Pharmacy, Creighton University, Omaha, NE, USA

CHAPTER OBJECTIVES

- Describe the process of drug absorption from a drug product into the systemic circulation.
- Relate the processes that govern drug dissolution, permeation, and first-pass metabolism to overall drug absorption from the gastrointestinal tract.
- Compare and contrast the factors affecting drug absorption from the gastrointestinal tract.
- Describe the factors that affect drug disposition following absorption.
- Understand the concept of volume of distribution to describe the extent of distribution of drugs in patients.
- Understand the various processes of drug elimination pathways.

Keywords

- Absorption
- Disposition
- Distribution
- Elimination
- Food effects
- Oral absorption
- Permeation

14.1. INTRODUCTION

To treat a disease with a drug therapy, a sufficient amount of drug should be delivered to the site of action to achieve desirable therapeutic effects with minimal undesirable side effects. As the drug concentration in the action site is influenced by absorption and disposition processes in the body, it is therefore important to study the factors affecting how these processes affect drug action and to select optimal drug products.

After drug administration, except for local treatment, a drug molecule must first enter the systemic circulation to reach the site of action and exert pharmacologic effects. The processes of drug transfer from the extravascular site of administration to systemic circulation are defined as absorption [1]. This chapter describes the general process of absorption and then focuses on the process of oral absorption and the factors affecting oral absorption. Although a drug is absorbed from numerous routes of administration, the specific factors that affect drug absorption from those sites do not necessarily correlate with those that affect oral absorption [2].

The term "drug disposition" is used in this chapter to describe distribution (the processes of drug movement within a patient) and elimination (the removal of a drug from a patient) [1]. Detailed descriptions of drug disposition lie in the field of pharmacokinetics (PK), which is beyond the scope of this textbook. However, this chapter introduces the basic concepts of drug disposition and factors affecting drug disposition.

14.2. DRUG ABSORPTION

Drug absorption is a heterogeneous process by which a drug travels into a patient. For many drugs, absorption into the patient is preceded by several steps

Pharmaceutics. DOI: http://dx.doi.org/10.1016/B978-0-12-386890-9.00014-5

and followed by several others before pharmacologic effects can be seen (Figure 14.1). First, the drug is incorporated into a formulation of some type for the preparation of a drug product. Second, that drug product is administered to the patient. Third, the drug is released from the drug product and becomes potentially available for absorption. Fourth, the drug is absorbed into the systemic circulation. Fifth, the drug travels to the site of action via the systemic circulation.

Not all drug products experience these steps for pharmacologic action. For example, there is no absorption process for drugs that are administered directly into the systemic blood circulation by injection or infusion. All other routes of drug administration will have some absorption potential. However, the route of administration is not the only factor influencing drug absorption in patients. The physicochemical properties of the drug molecule, the dosage form, membrane permeation, and physiologic and pathologic processes in the patient are some factors that can affect absorption.

Although the complexities of drug absorption are substantial in the various organs and tissues involved in drug administration, oral absorption provides clear and common explanations and illustrations of these factors. Following this discussion of oral drug absorption, the pharmaceutical expert should be able to synthesize anatomical and physiological understandings of organs and tissues with the pharmaceutics principles for a basic understanding of drug absorption in various organs and tissues. Chapter 15 also provides brief overviews for absorptive processes in common sites of drug administration.

14.3. ORAL DRUG ABSORPTION PROCESSES

Oral drug absorption involves the release of drugs in a solubilized form in the gastrointestinal (GI) tract (dissolution), permeation through the GI membrane, and entrance into systemic circulation after passing though the portal vein and liver. The absorbed drug molecules must survive gut metabolism and first-pass extraction by the liver before reaching systemic circulation [3]. Figure 14.2 illustrates the oral absorption processes.

14.3.1 Dissolution

The first step of oral absorption after administration of a solid dosage form is the dissolution of the drug in the GI lumen. The process of drug dissolution is explained in detail in Chapters 5 and 8. In review, drug dissolution consists of two steps: (1) the formation of a loose drug molecule at the solid-liquid interface, similar to a surface reaction, and (2) the diffusion

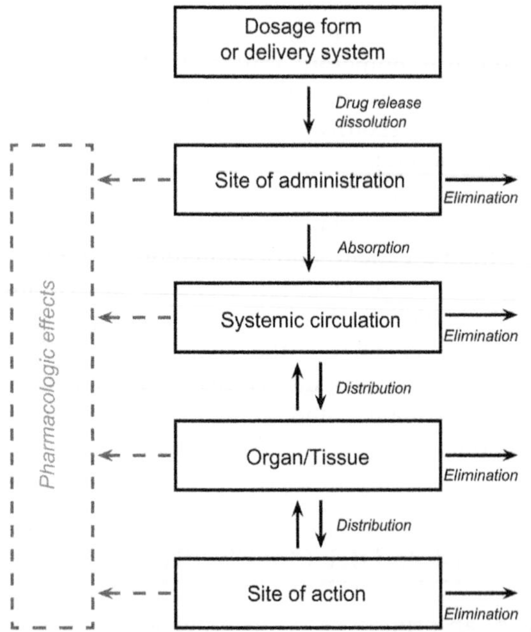

FIGURE 14.1 Schematic diagram illustrating the processes of drug movement preceding pharmacologic effects.

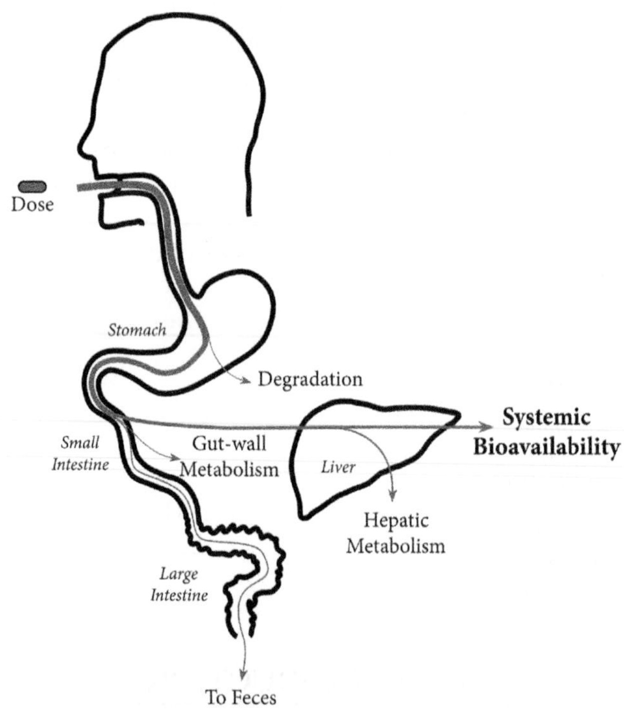

FIGURE 14.2 Oral drug absorption processes. A drug, given as a solid orally, must overcome dissolution, permeation, and metabolism barriers to reach systemic circulation. Incomplete dissolution, incomplete permeation, and removal of drugs by metabolism in the gut and liver are often the causes of poor oral absorption.

of the loose drug molecule through the solid-liquid interface into the bulk of the solution. Many dissolution profiles can be described by the diffusion rate limited process in the form of the Noyes–Whitney equation, as shown in Eq. 14.1 [4]:

$$\frac{dM}{dt} = \frac{DA(S-c)}{h} \tag{14.1}$$

where M is the amount dissolved, t is time, D is a diffusion rate constant of the drug molecule, h is the diffusion layer thickness, A is the surface area, c is the concentration of drug in the dissolution medium at time t, and S is the solubility of the drug in the dissolution medium. For spherical particles under the sink condition when c is much smaller than S, the Noyes–Whitney equation can be expressed as shown in Eq. 14.2:

$$M_0^{1/3} - M^{1/3} = kt, \quad k = \frac{DS}{h}\left(\frac{4\pi\rho}{3}\right)^{1/3} \tag{14.2}$$

where M_0 is the initial drug mass, M is the remaining undissolved drug mass at time t, and k is the dissolution rate constant determined by the diffusion coefficient, diffusion layer thickness, solubility, and density of the material (ρ) [5]. Equation 14.2 is well known as Hixson–Crowell's cubic root law of dissolution. However, under different conditions, it is also possible that the dissolution rate is controlled by the formation of loose drug molecules at the solid-liquid interface. For the surface reaction–controlled dissolution, the dissolution rate can be described similar to the equation used to describe chemical reactions [6].

It is clear from the Noyes–Whitney equation that the dissolution rate of diffusion-controlled dissolution is influenced by diffusivity, diffusion layer thickness, surface area, and solubility. These factors are determined by the physicochemical properties of the drug molecule and its formulation as well as the physiological conditions of the GI tract. Among these factors, solubility not only directly influences the dissolution rate, which can then control the absorption rate if the permeation rate is fast enough, but also determines the maximum amount of drug dissolved, which may control the extent of absorption.

The dissolution step as the first step of oral absorption presents both a challenge and an opportunity for drug delivery. Recently, many drugs in development have very poor aqueous solubility, as discussed in Chapters 5 and 8 [7]. The challenge of delivering these drugs is to improve the solubility and dissolution rate to ensure that enough drugs are absorbed to provide a therapeutic effect. New technologies have been developed to improve the oral bioavailability of these drugs. For example, by reducing the drug particle size through micronizing or nano sizing, the surface area of the drug can be increased to improve the dissolution rate [8]. Using either salt or cocrystal forms of a drug substance or by developing amorphous or lipid formulations, one can achieve higher apparent solubility to improve both the rate and extent of dissolution and absorption [7,8]. On the other hand, by altering the dissolution rate to control the absorption rate and the site of absorption in the GI tract, the modified release formulation technology is able to deliver an optimal plasma drug concentration-time profile. Figure 14.3 shows the dissolution and plasma drug concentration-time profiles of orally administered isosorbide mononitrate immediate- and sustained-release formulations [9]. By decreasing the rate of drug dissolution in the GI tract, the sustained-release formulation was able to maintain drug concentrations above the therapeutic effective concentration for a longer duration of time.

The physiological factors that influence dissolution of drugs in the GI tract include GI anatomy, volume, pH and composition of fluid in the GI, and GI motility. These factors are further influenced by other variables such as age, genetics, disease state, co-medication, and food consumption. It is therefore not surprising that significant inter- and intra-individual variability of factors important for absorption (e.g., solubility) are observed in a population and can contribute to variability in oral drug absorption rates [10]. For weakly acidic or basic drugs with pH-dependent solubility, the gastric pH can significantly affect the dissolution rate and solubility. For example, itraconazole is a poorly soluble weak base that is more soluble under low pH. When 200 mg of itraconazole (Sporanox® Capsules) were administered after ranitidine pretreatment, which raised gastric pH to 6, itraconazole was absorbed to a lesser extent than when Sporanox® Capsules were administered alone, with decreases in the total amount of drug absorbed and the maximal drug concentrations [11]. Interestingly, the reduced amount absorbed was mitigated when Sporanox® Capsules were administered with a cola beverage, which is acidic, after ranitidine pretreatment [11]. To avoid reduced absorption due to elevated gastric pH, patients are advised on the prescription label of Sporanox® that antacids be administered at least 1 hour before or 2 hours after the administration of Sporanox®.

14.3.2 Permeation

After dissolution, the next step in oral absorption is for the drug molecule to permeate through the gastrointestinal membrane. It is generally believed that the vast majority of drug molecules can permeate through the GI barrier only as a single molecule or as small aggregates of molecules. Therefore, drug dissolution

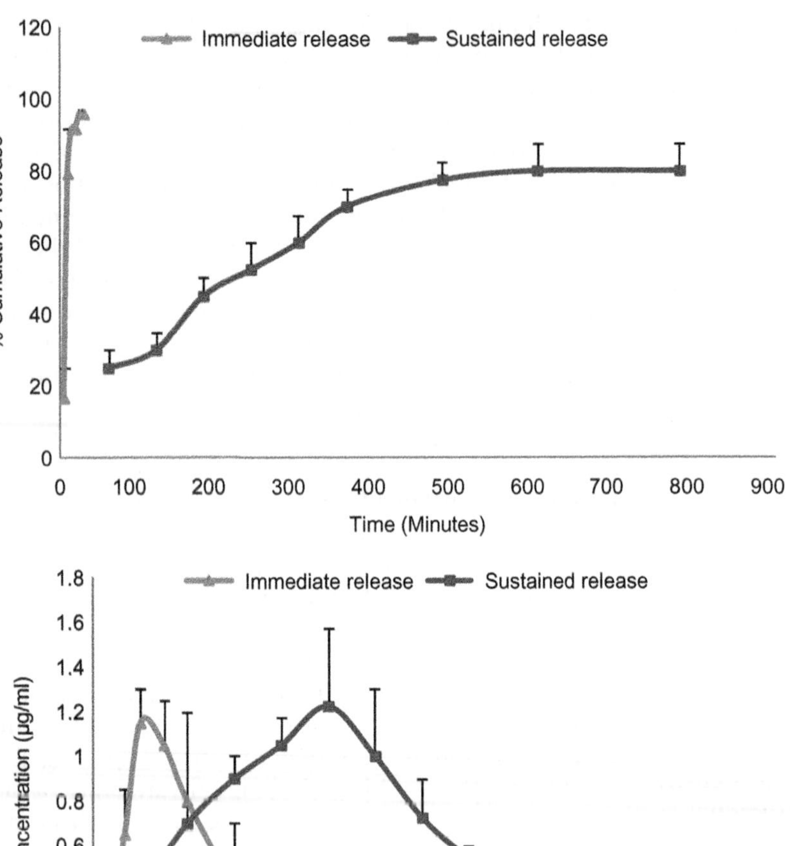

FIGURE 14.3 (A) *In vitro* dissolution profile of immediate-release and sustained-release profile of isomorbide nitrate. (B) *In vivo* plasma concentration-time profile of the same immediate-release and sustained-release formulation of isomorbide nitrate. *(Adapted from reference [9].)*

must occur before absorption when administering a nondissolved drug dosage form. The GI tract maintains a barrier between the luminal environment and the internal environment of the body through a continuous sheet of polarized columnar epithelial cells, often called an epithelial barrier [12]. When a drug is administered orally, the drug molecules must pass through the epithelial barrier to be absorbed into the gastric vasculature and subsequently into the systemic circulation. Two routes are available for the drug to permeate through this barrier: either transcellularly (through cells) or paracellularly (through spaces between cells). A series of intercellular junctions connects the individual cells, among which the tight junction is the most important for the paracellular barrier. The tight junction is perforated by aqueous pores, with a wide size range of 4–40 Å radius [13]. For the transcellular pathway, a drug can permeate either through passive transcellular diffusion or carrier-mediated uptake or endocytosis. Enterocytes also contain efflux transporters, such as p-glycoprotein, which can pump drugs to the outside of cells [14]. Recent studies have found that transporters are often involved in permeation of most drugs [15]. Figure 14.4A provides a list of transporters in the enterocytes [15].

As discussed in Chapter 13, the effective drug permeability is the net result of passive diffusion, active transport mechanisms, and vesicular transport. For each process, the permeation rate is influenced by different relationships to the drug concentration at the site of drug transport. For passive diffusion, the rate is proportional to the concentration, whereas carrier-mediated uptake follows a sigmoidal relationship with the concentration as protein and vesicular mediated transport systems become saturated.

Practically, the overall effective permeability is often used to characterize the rate of drug permeation. Permeability of drugs across human epithelial colorectal adenocarcinoma (Caco-2) cells or Mardin–Darby canine kidney (MDCK) cells grown on a membrane is

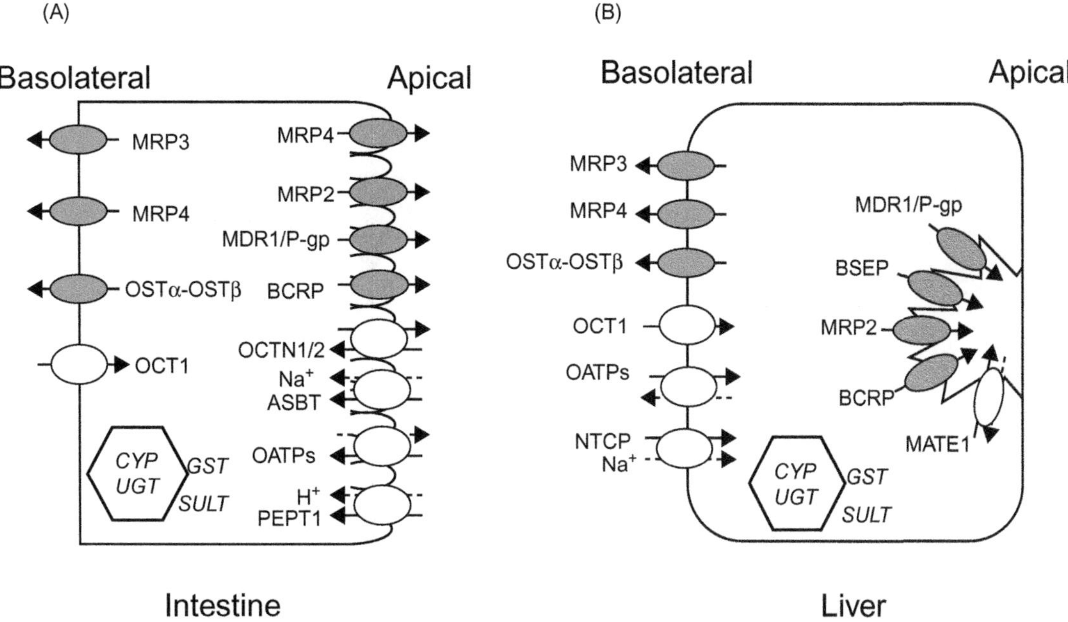

FIGURE 14.4 Schematic diagram of transporters and enzymes in the enterocyte (A) and hepatocyte (B). ASBT = Apical Sodium dependent Bile acid Transporter, BCRP = Breast Cancer Resistant Protein, BSEP = Bile Salt Export Pump, MATE = Multidrug and Toxin Extrusion, MRP = Multidrug-Resistance Protein, MDR = Multidrug-Resistance, NTCP = Sodium-taurocholate Cotransporting Polypeptide, OATP = Organic Anion-Transporting Protein, OCT = Organic Vation, OCTN = Organic zwitterions/Cation, OST = Organic Solute, PEPT = Peptide Transporter, SULT = Sulfotransferases *(Reproduced from reference [27] with permission.)*

often studied to characterize *in vitro* drug permeability [16]. Permeability of drugs in the human jejunum has also been measured using *in situ* intestinal perfusion. A perfusion tube is placed in the human jejunum to allow passage of a drug through a 10-cm segment. By measuring the drug concentration at the inlet and outlet of the perfusion tube, one determines drug permeability [17]. A correlation between caco-2 permeability and human jejunum permeability has been established using statistical [18] and mechanistic [19] approaches. Attempts have been made to predict drug intestinal permeability based on molecular structure. However, a reliable model is still evasive, partially due to a lack of reliable prediction of the role of membrane transporters in permeability [20].

Absorption of most orally administered compounds occurs in the small intestine. This can be attributed to the significantly larger surface area available for absorption in the small intestine as compared to other parts of GI tract. The absorptive surface area of jejunum and ileum is approximately 120 m^2 in humans as compared to 0.25 m^2 in the colon [21]. The uneven presence of transporters in various segments of the GI tract also contributes to the different absorption rate in different GI segments. Expression levels of the major transporters (uptake and efflux) have been shown to vary depending on the region of the GI tract (Table 14.1) [22]. However, there are conflicting reports regarding the distribution of transporters. For instance, P-glycoprotein (P-gp, an efflux transporter) expression was found to be the highest in jejunum in one study [22] but was reported to progressively increase from proximal to distal regions of the intestine in another study [23]. The activity of transporters is unlikely to be important for highly permeable drugs but will play a dominant role for drugs with low passive permeability [24]. Depending on the passive permeability and propensity for active transport of any drug, absorption may occur along the entire GI tract or may be limited to the proximal GI tract. The absorption of lefradafiban (a highly permeable compound) has been shown to occur along the entire GI tract, whereas danoprevir is preferentially absorbed from the upper small intestine and has very low bioavailability upon colonic administration [25,26].

TABLE 14.1 Distribution of ATP-Binding Cassette (ABC) Transporters P-gp, MRP1, MRP2, and Cytochrome P450 3A4 (CYP3A4) in Different Segments of the Gastrointestinal Tract [22]

	Based on mRNA Level	Based on Protein Level
P-gp	Jejunum ~ ileum > colon	Jejunum ~ colon > ileum
MRP1	Jejunum ~ ileum ~ colon	Jejunum ~ ileum ~ colon
MRP2	Jejunum > ileum > colon	Jejunum > ileum > colon
CYP3A4	Jejunum > ileum > colon	Jejunum > ileum ~ colon

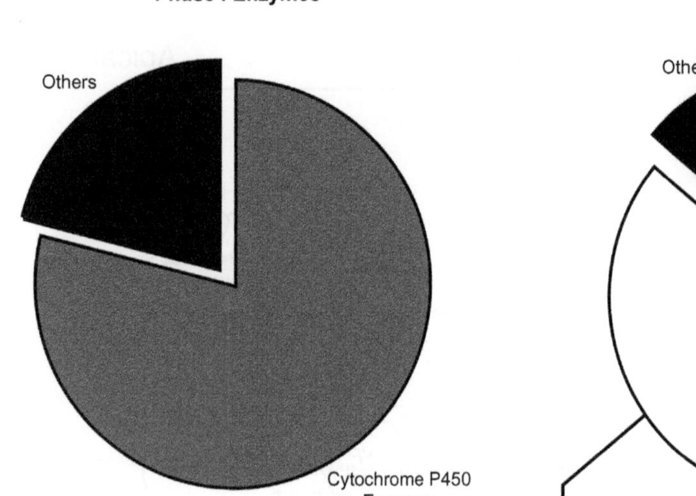

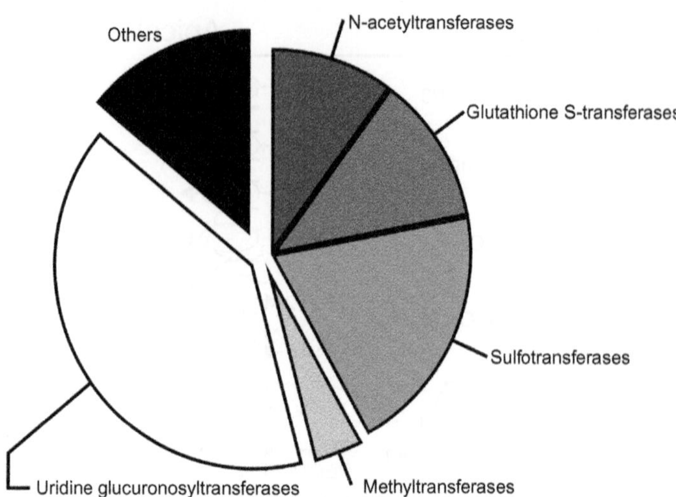

FIGURE 14.5 A chart representing the Phase I and Phase II drug metabolizing enzymes. The relative size of each pie section represents the prevalence of that enzyme in overall drug metabolism. ADH, alcohol dehydrogenase; ALDH, aldehyde dehydrogenase; CYP, cytochrome P450; DPD, dihydropyrimidine dehydrogenase; NQO1, NADPH:quinone oxidoreductase or DT diaphorase; COMT, catechol O-methyltransferase; GST, glutathione S-transferase; HMT, histamine methyltransferase; NAT, N-acetyltransferase; STs, sulfotransferases; TPMT, thiopurine methyltransferase; UGTs, uridine 59-triphosphate glucuronosyltransferases. *(Reproduced from reference [28] with permission.)*

TABLE 14.2 Distribution of Metabolic Enzymes in the Liver and Small Intestine [22]

	*Phase I Enzymes	*Phase II Enzymes	Enzyme P450s	**SULT
Liver	Cytochrome P450, Flavin monooxygenases, Monoamine oxidase, Carbonyl reductase, Sulfatase, Glucuronidases, Carboxylesterases	SULT, UGT, GST, Methyltransferase, N-cetyltransferase, Amino acid Nacetyltransferase	CYP3A (>40%), CYP2C (25%), CYP1A2 (18%) CYP2E1 (9%), CYP2A6 (6%), CYP2D6 (2%)	SULT1A1 (>50%) SULT2A1, SULT1B1, and SULT1E1 are also present in the liver.
Small Intestine			CYP3A (82%), CYP2C9 (14%), CYP2C19 (2%), CYP2D6 (0.7%)	SULT1B1 (36%), SULT1A3 (31%), SULT1A1 (19%), SULT1E1 (8%), SULT2A1 (6%)

Liver contains much higher amounts of Phase I and Phase II enzymes than the small intestine.
**The small intestine contains the largest overall amount of SULT of any of the tissues.*

14.3.3 Gut Metabolism and First-Pass Extraction by Liver

A drug molecule that permeates into the enterocytes must then survive gut metabolism (also referred to as intestinal first-pass extraction) and first-pass metabolism by the liver before it reaches the systemic circulation [27]. Intestinal epithelial cells and hepatocytes contain a variety of enzymes involved in phase I and II metabolism (Figure 14.5) [28]. Phase I metabolism reactions typically affect the drug molecular structure and include oxidation, reduction, and hydrolysis reactions. Phase I drug metabolism is conducted by a variety of enzymes, with Cytochrome P450 enzymes (CYP) being the most prominent class (Figure 14.5) [29]. Phase II metabolism includes conjugation reactions such as glucuronidation, glycosidation, sulfation, methylation, acetylation, glutathione conjugation, amino acid conjugation, fatty acid conjugation, and condensation. Phase II metabolism enzymes, such as glucuronidating UDP-Glucuronosyltransferases (UGT) [30], sulfotransferases, and glutathione S-transferases, are present in both the small intestine and liver (Figure 14.5) [31]. Table 14.2 summarizes the relative abundances of enzymes in the intestine and liver as well as the distribution of CYP enzyme types in different segments of the GI tract [22].

It is estimated that the CYP3A enzyme subfamily is involved in the metabolism of a large portion of currently marketed drugs [32]. Both CYP3A4 and CYP3A5 are present in all regions of the GI tract [33]. Among them, CYP3A4 is the most common CYP enzyme found in the human intestine and liver. The level of CYP3A4 expression is lower in the duodenum before rising in the jejunum and subsequently decreasing toward the ileum and colon [33]. Although the liver contains substantially more drug metabolizing enzymes than the intestine, intestinal first-pass metabolism has been shown to be significant for many drugs. For example, cyclosporine [34], midazolam [35], tacrolimus [36], nifedipine [37], felodipine [38], and verapamil [39] have been identified to undergo substantial intestinal Phase I metabolism, whereas raloxifene undergoes intestinal Phase II metabolism [40].

After the drug molecule permeates the GI membrane, it enters the mesenteric vessels surrounding the intestine. These vessels then drain into the hepatic portal vein system and carry the drug to the liver. In the liver, the blood from the hepatic portal vein system (approximately 75% of total hepatic blood flow) is mixed with those from hepatic arteries [41]. The blood then flows through liver sinusoids and leaves the liver through the central vein. The liver is a major site for the metabolism of many drugs due to prevalent metabolizing enzymes and transporters (Figure 14.4B) [27]. Some drug molecules entering the liver will not be able to reach the systemic circulation due to hepatic metabolism. This phenomenon is called first-pass metabolism or the first-pass effect. First-pass extraction happens when a drug permeates into hepatocytes and is either metabolized by enzymes or secreted into bile. The portion that is secreted into the bile will drain into the small intestine and can either be reabsorbed through enterohepatic recirculation or eliminated into the feces.

It has been recognized that the interplay between membrane transporters and enzymes in both the intestine and liver plays an important role in the first-pass effect. To explain the significant intestinal metabolism of some drugs, it was proposed that the existence of efflux transporters, such as P-gp, play an important role in increasing the exposure of susceptible drugs to metabolizing enzymes in the intestine through repeated cycling of drug into and out of the gut enterocytes via passive diffusion and active efflux, i.e., secretion by P-gp. This process is thought to result in reduced drug concentration in the enterocyte and thereby a reduced saturation of the metabolizing enzymes in terms of concentration and duration above saturated level, a higher exposure of drug to enzymes and an increased mean residence time of the drug in the intestine [42]. In the liver, the degree of first-pass metabolism is also influenced by the rate and extent of uptake mediated through the uptake transporters and excretion mediated through biliary transporters relative to the metabolic rate by liver enzymes [43].

Because first-pass metabolism is influenced by blood flow rate and activity of transporters and enzymes in the intestine and liver, food uptake and comedication can significantly affect the extent of first-pass extraction. The increase of splenic blood flow rate postprandially leads to a significant decrease in the first-pass metabolism of propranolol and a bioavailability increase of up to 250% [44,45]. The involvement of a drug with membrane transporters and metabolizing enzymes in both the intestine and liver is a major underlying cause of drug-drug interactions that must be evaluated for inappropriate drug utilization reviews. For example, ketoconazole, an antifungal medication, is a known CYP inhibitor that will inhibit the metabolism of many co-administered medications. When ketoconazole was co-dosed with cyclodextrin, the oral bioavailability of cyclodextrin was more than doubled, with approximately one-third of the increase attributed to the decreased liver first-pass effect and the rest attributed to the decreased gut metabolism by ketoconazole [34].

14.4. FOOD EFFECTS ON ORAL DRUG ABSORPTION

Food intake causes physiological changes in the gastrointestinal tract and exerts complicated effects on the oral absorption of drugs. Postprandial changes in GI physiology include delayed gastric emptying, changes in gastric pH, increased bile flow, and increased splanchnic blood flow [46]. Additionally, food components may change gut metabolism or have a physicochemical interaction with the drug molecule, thereby interfering with its absorption [46]. These changes can alter the drug product GI transit time, drug dissolution, permeability, and first-pass extraction ratio, leading to changes in the rate and extent of drug absorption and subsequently systemic drug concentrations.

The effect of food on drug absorption is generally influenced by drug solubility, membrane permeability, and metabolism. Many drugs with low aqueous solubility and either high membrane permeability or extensive metabolism have increased absorption with food intake, referred to as a "positive food effect." In contrast, many drugs with high aqueous solubility and either low membrane permeability or poor metabolism have reduced absorption with food intake, referred to as a "negative food effect" [47]. No trends in drug absorption with food intake are observed for drugs with high solubility and permeability or for drugs that have low solubility and low permeability [46]. However, drug-specific exceptions to these general relationships can exist for compounds with very high first-pass effects (e.g., the propranolol example earlier in this chapter), extensive drug adsorption or binding to substances, complexation, or chemical instability of the drug substance in the GI tract.

More detailed and drug-specific analyses of food effects are often reported in the pharmaceutical literature. Some studies have revealed that a positive food effect is most likely due to an improved solubility of the poorly soluble drug under fed conditions, whereas a negative food effect is often due to the negative interference on permeation of poorly permeable drugs in the presence of food [48]. Due to a significant effect of food intake on the absorption of some drugs, the prescription label of these drugs often specifies when to administer the drugs with regard to food intake. For example, Mepron® (atovaquone) showed a three-fold increase in its bioavailability when taken with a meal, and subsequently, patients are instructed to take Mepron with meals to improve its oral absorption [49,50]. Grapefruit or orange juice was found to reduce the bioavailability of Allegra® (fexofenadine HCl) by 36%, likely due to the inhibition of uptake transporters responsible for the permeation of fexofenadine [51]. It is therefore recommended to take Allegra with water only [50].

14.5. EVALUATION OF ORAL ABSORPTION

It is desirable to understand the influence of these multiple factors on the oral absorption and subsequent systemic drug concentrations for a drug in order to design a drug product accordingly for optimal efficacy with low propensity for adverse effects. When drug dissolution is the rate-limiting step for oral absorption, it is often possible to correlate the *in vitro* dissolution profile of a drug product with *in vivo* systemic drug concentrations. This correlation is often referred as the *in vitro–in vivo* correlation (IVIVC) [52]. A more broad definition of IVIVC may also include correlating other *in vitro* data with *in vivo* parameters [53]. A proper discussion of IVIVC requires an understanding of basic pharmacokinetic principles and is beyond the scope of the present work. However, this chapter provides a brief discussion of IVIVC as it applies to the principles of oral drug absorption.

Generally, IVIVC studies relate data through statistically validated mathematical models. The strongest relationships correlate the entire *in vitro* dissolution profile to the entire *in vivo* drug concentration profile. A slightly less robust correlation can be established using mean *in vitro* dissolution times to either the mean *in vivo* residence time for a drug molecule within the systemic circulation or the mean *in vivo* dissolution time. The least robust IVIVC methods correlate one dissolution time point ($t_{50\%}$, $t_{90\%}$, etc.) to one mean *in vivo* pharmacokinetic parameter. The correlation does not reflect all drug concentrations but selects one datum for comparison.

In order to build a successful IVIVC, drug dissolution must be the rate-limiting step for oral absorption, and the *in vitro* dissolution method needs to be biorelevant by simulating physiological conditions to the best ability possible. As discussed in Chapter 8, a dissolution test has historically been used as a quality control (QC) tool to release a dosage form for commercial use [54]. The focus of dissolution testing in quality control is to ensure batch-to-batch consistency and to detect manufacturing deviations. A dissolution method developed for quality control may or may not be indicative of *in vivo* dissolution performance. New dissolution devices, such as the TIM-1 system [55] and a dynamic dissolution setup [56], as well as new dissolution media, such as simulated intestinal fluid [57], have been proposed to more closely mimic the *in vivo* GI condition. It has been shown in the literature that these newer dissolution tests provide a more realistic prediction of the *in vivo* drug absorption from drug products [58,59].

In general, the IVIVC methods discussed previously use a statistical approach to establish a correlation. Recently, physiology based oral absorption modeling software has been developed to enable mechanism-based IVIVC through direct simulation of *in vivo* systemic drug concentrations based on *in vitro* properties of a drug, including the dissolution profile [60]. The physiology-based oral absorption model describes the steps of oral absorption mechanistically and incorporates physiological parameters of the GI tract into the model. The most widely used model to describe absorption physiology is called the compartment and transition model, which was originally developed at the University of Michigan [61], and has since been adapted by commercial software packages, including GastroPlus (ACAT model) [62], Simcyp (ADAM model) [63], and PKsim [64]. The compartment and transition model divides the GI tract into theoretical sections or compartments (e.g., nine compartments in the case of GastroPlus), and drugs are transferred into the subsequent compartments in a rate defined by first-order kinetic principles and physiological GI residence time. In each compartment, drug dissolution and absorption are modeled using the corresponding rate equations. Because physiology-based oral absorption models take into consideration physicochemical factors, such as p*K*a, solubility, particle size, and permeability, as well as GI physiological factors, such as pH in each GI segment, GI absorption surface area, volume of GI fluid, gastric emptying time, intestinal transit rate, and first-pass, the model enables mechanistic understanding and prediction of oral drug absorption [54]. The effects of membrane transporter systems can also be included in these models for even more accurate IVIVC relationships [46]. Applications of physiology-based oral absorption modeling include simulation of the influence of formulation on oral absorption based on *in vitro* dissolution [65], food effect on oral absorption [66], drug-drug interaction [67], and the effect of changes in GI physiology on absorption [63].

14.6. DRUG DISPOSITION

Following absorption into the systemic circulation, a drug is delivered through the systemic blood flow to all organs and tissues. The drug will eventually leave the body by a process referred to as elimination from a variety of organs, such as the liver, kidney, and lung. Drug concentration can rarely be measured at the site of pharmacologic action. As a result, drug concentrations in the blood or plasma are used to evaluate a drug's bioavailability and are typically evaluated as a function of time after drug administration. The concentration versus time relationship then serves as the basis to understand drug movement in patients and can inform the understanding of pharmacologic or toxicologic effects. Distribution is the process of reversible movement of the drug within the body. Elimination is the irreversible loss of drug from the body and can occur through metabolism as well as excretion. Distribution and elimination are collectively referred to as drug disposition [1]. Pharmacokinetics is the study of drug movement in living systems and uses mathematical models to evaluate the processes of absorption, distribution, metabolism, and excretion [68]. Although a discussion of basic pharmacokinetic concepts is beyond the scope of this textbook, the processes of drug disposition are illustrated to facilitate a conceptual understanding of drug movement following absorption.

14.6.1 Factors Affecting Distribution

Distribution of a drug between blood and various tissues occurs at different rates and to different extents. Numerous factors affect drug distribution including the physicochemical properties of the drug, hydrophilicity and lipophilicity, blood flow rate to the tissue, membrane transport processes, selective organ/tissue permeability, drug binding within the blood or in an organ/tissue, and partitioning into fat [69]. For some drugs, the rate of distribution into organs and tissues is principally affected by blood perfusion or membrane permeability. For example, some drugs stay in a tissue longer when the perfusion rate is slow, whereas others have prolonged perfusion rates when drug affinity to tissue is high.

One key measure of distribution is the volume of distribution (V_d). The V_d represents a theoretical space or volume in which a drug is distributed following administration and is ultimately affected by all those factors mentioned previously. While some V_d values might have a physiological significance (e.g., some highly water soluble drugs have a V_d approximately equal to the total body water volume) or might respond to some pathologic process, the volume of distribution is an imaginary space that has no direct relationship to drug or patient parameters. As a result, the V_d varies widely for different drugs and is a key parameter for the evaluation of drug therapy.

For example, quinacrine, a highly lipophilic compound, has a V_d of 40,000 L. In contrast, the V_d of salicylic acid and warfarin, both of which are highly bound to plasma proteins, is approximately 0.1 L/kg and corresponds to the plasma fluid volume. Erythropoietin, a high molecular weight compound, has a large steric volume and has a V_d of only 0.05 L/kg, which may represent the lower limit of a volume that might correspond to the plasma water [68].

The volume of distribution is governed by partition coefficients that quantify the equilibrium drug concentration ratio between a tissue and plasma. Partition coefficient values describe relative drug affinity to tissues. Many factors affect the tissue affinity of a drug, including lipophilicity (often characterized by logP), ionization state of the drug (characterized by p*K*a and environment pH), binding affinity of the drug to plasma proteins, and membrane transporter systems. Attempts have been made to estimate the tissue affinity based on tissue composition and physicochemical properties of a drug with some success. A study of 18 drugs found that 61% of the drugs had observed V_d values within a two-fold difference of the predicted values [69]. In addition to the properties of a drug, individual subject variability, such as weight, body mass index, disease state, age, etc., can also affect the variability of volume of distribution in a population [70].

14.6.2 Factors Affecting Drug Elimination

A drug is eliminated from the body through two main processes: excretion and metabolism [1]. Excretion is the irreversible loss of chemically unchanged drug while metabolism is the conversion of a drug molecule chemically into its metabolites. Although infrequent, metabolites may be converted back into the original drug through enterohepatic recirculation or other processes [33]. Elimination by metabolism refers, then, to only the portion of metabolism that leads to irreversible drug loss. Although a drug can be eliminated by many organs, most drugs are eliminated by the liver and/or kidneys. Elimination is also typically, but not always, a first-order process where the rate of drug elimination is dependent on the drug concentration in the patient at a given time.

A key pharmacokinetic parameter used to describe the process of elimination is total body clearance (*Cl*). Clearance is defined as the volume that has all drug eliminated from it per unit time (with units of volume/time). Clearance can be used to determine the rate of drug elimination (R_e) from the patient at a given drug concentration (*C*) [68]. The rate of drug elimination is shown in Eq. 14.3:

$$R_e = Cl \times C \tag{14.3}$$

In the absence of metabolic enzyme saturation, intrinsic clearance may be expressed as the sum of V_{max}/K_m values of all the enzymes involved in the metabolism of a particular compound where V_{max} is the maximum rate of enzymatic reaction and K_m is the Michaelis-Menten constant. The value of V_{max}/K_m is often estimated *in vitro* using liver microsome or hepatocytes or recombinantly expressed enzymes [53].

Total body clearance is also equal to the sum total of all organ- or tissue-specific elimination processes that affect a drug, as shown in Eq. 14.4. Specifically,

$$Cl_{total} = \sum Cl_{hepatic} + Cl_{renal} + Cl_{pulmonary} + \ldots \tag{14.4}$$

Clearance can then be evaluated for many drugs if assumptions can be made to simplify the process of drug elimination to one principal eliminating organ. For some drugs, elimination can be assumed to be principally either through hepatic metabolism or renal excretion. The fraction eliminated unchanged in the urine (f_e) is a simple pharmacokinetic parameter used to evaluate the proportion of the total drug dose that is recovered from the urine in an unmetabolized state. Drugs with a low f_e value (<0.1) can be assumed to be hepatically metabolized, whereas drugs with a high f_e value (>0.9) can be assumed to be renally excreted if a clinician can assume no other routes of drug elimination are prevalent. This assumption would then lead to the following equations (Eqs. 14.5 and 14.6):

$$\mathrm{Cl_{renal}} = \mathrm{Cl_{total}} \times \mathrm{f_e} \tag{14.5}$$

$$\mathrm{Cl_{hepatic}} = \mathrm{Cl_{total}} \times (1 - \mathrm{f_e}) \tag{14.6}$$

The rate of hepatic metabolism is influenced by the hepatic blood flow rate, the degree of drug/protein binding in the liver (often represented by measuring plasma protein binding), and the total drug clearance rate. When the liver blood flow is more prevalent than the degree of drug metabolism, hepatic drug clearance will be controlled by the liver blood flow rate and won't change significantly if there is variability in the process of drug metabolism through changes in metabolizing enzyme expression or activity. On the other hand, when the degree of drug metabolism is more prevalent than liver blood flow, the hepatic clearance will be controlled by the metabolizing enzymatic activity and expression, and changes to liver blood flow will not significantly affect drug clearance. Hepatic drug clearance can be influenced by an interplay between both uptake transporters and biliary transporters. It was proposed to include the intrinsic clearance of uptake and efflux across the sinusoidal membrane in the overall description of the intrinsic hepatic clearance [43]. Currently, due to limited knowledge on the abundance of specific transporters in the human liver, it is still difficult to predict the hepatic clearance accurately when the factors involving the transporters need to be considered [53].

The kidney is a major organ for drug excretion [1]. For drugs that are exclusively eliminated by the kidneys and not reabsorbed back into the systemic drug circulation, the rate of renal drug elimination would be equal to the glomerular filtration rate. In typical healthy patients, the glomerular filtration rate is the rate at which plasma water is filtered and has an average value of approximately 120 mL/min [1]. However, most drugs with substantial renal elimination cannot be assumed to have an elimination rate equal to the glomerular filtration rate. The kidneys are designed for reabsorption processes with substantial possibilities for drug diffusion and numerous active membrane transport systems. Drug reabsorption is influenced by the urine pH for ionizable drugs because the urine pH affects the ionization state of the drug and subsequently its permeability. More recently, it is reported that urine pH can also affect transporter activities, such as PEP-T2, which then affects the renal clearance in the case of cephalexin [71].

14.6.3 Pharmacokinetics Models

This discussion on drug distribution and elimination provides a brief introduction to pharmacokinetic processes that affect drug disposition following absorption. A more thorough analysis of basic pharmacokinetic principles is needed to adequately appreciate the processes of absorption, distribution, metabolism, and excretion. In this more thorough analysis, statistically validated modeling systems are used to describe drug movement in patients. The complexity of human anatomy and physiology would make it appear that it is difficult to describe the plasma drug concentration-time profile with a model. Surprisingly, simple compartmental models are predominantly used for clinical

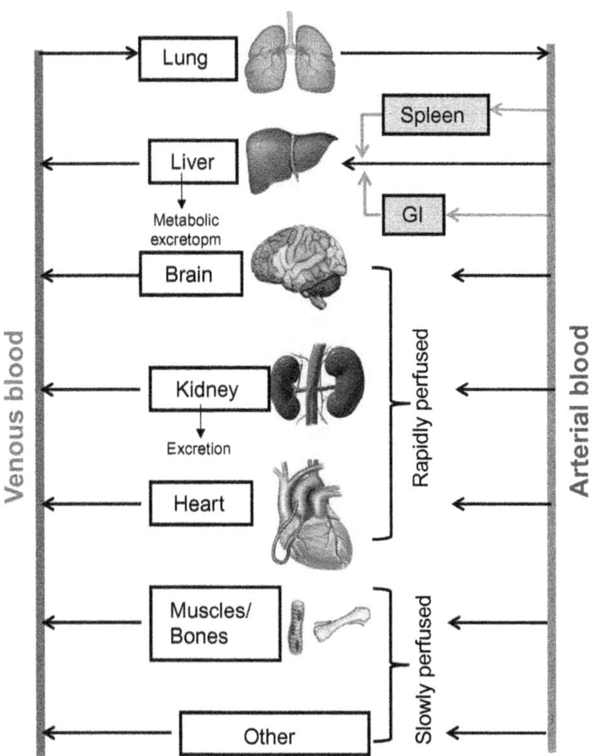

FIGURE 14.6 Illustration of a physiology based pharmacokinetics model. Elimination is depicted as occurring from only the liver and kidneys, whereas it can occur also at other sites for some drugs. Enterohepatic recirculation can be included in the model but is not depicted in the graph. *(Adapted from reference [72].)*

evaluation of drug pharmacokinetic properties and provide an adequate depiction of the concentration versus time profiles for many drugs [68].

Although appropriate and valid pharmacokinetic models are widely used to describe drug movement in patients, these models do not provide detailed mechanistic understandings of the fate of a drug in the body. More complex physiology based pharmacokinetic (PBPK) models attempt to gain mechanistic insight into how a drug is absorbed, distributed, and eliminated in the body. Figure 14.6 depicts a typical PBPK model [72]. The physiology based oral absorption model mentioned previously can be considered a partial PBPK model when simple models are used to depict drug pharmacokinetics post-absorption.

A PBPK model comprises a model structure to describe absorption and disposition processes through utilization of drug physicochemical properties, such as solubility, permeability, and fraction unbound in plasma; and physiological parameters, such as organ/tissue volume, blood flow rates to each organ/tissue, and partition coefficients for each organ/tissue. The PBPK model provides an integrated framework to mechanistically and quantitatively describe the influence of drug properties and physiology parameters on drug absorption and disposition. A unique feature of PBPK models is to understand the influence of individual physiological variables on drug absorption and disposition. PBPK modeling has been used to predict drug absorption [63], human plasma concentration-time profiles based on *in vitro* data [73], as well as influences of drug-drug interaction, age, gender, and disease states on pharmacokinetics [70]. The accuracy of PBPK is expected to be continuously improved as the understanding of drug absorption and disposition processes is enhanced. A major development of PK modeling is likely to connect PBPK with population pharmacokinetics (POPPK) to understand individual variability in PK [72]. PBPK modeling accuracy will further improve with increased understanding of the physiology and more powerful computational technology.

14.7. CONCLUSIONS

Drug absorption and disposition are influenced by both physicochemical properties of a drug and individual physiology conditions. The rate and extent of oral absorption are influenced by the dissolution characteristics of dosage forms, physicochemical and biopharmaceutical properties of the active drug ingredient, physiological condition of the gastrointestinal (GI) tract, and the extent of first-pass extraction at the gut and liver. Both drug distribution and disposition are also influenced by drug properties, individual physiological conditions, and other factors such as co-medication. Figure 14.7 summarizes the factors that influence drug absorption and disposition discussed in this chapter [60,72]. Recent advancement in physiology based absorption and pharmacokinetics modeling offer the opportunity to simulate and predict the influence of multiple factors on absorption and disposition mechanistically. As our knowledge of absorption and disposition processes is enhanced, we will continue to leverage our understanding to provide better pharmaceutical care to patients.

CASE STUDIES

Case 14.1

A doctoral student in pharmacy on a clinical rotation is presented with a plasma chloramphenicol concentration time profile from old pharmaceutical literature, as shown in Figure 14.8, and is asked to explain this graph in the context of the effect of crystal forms of the drug on its bioavailability. What should

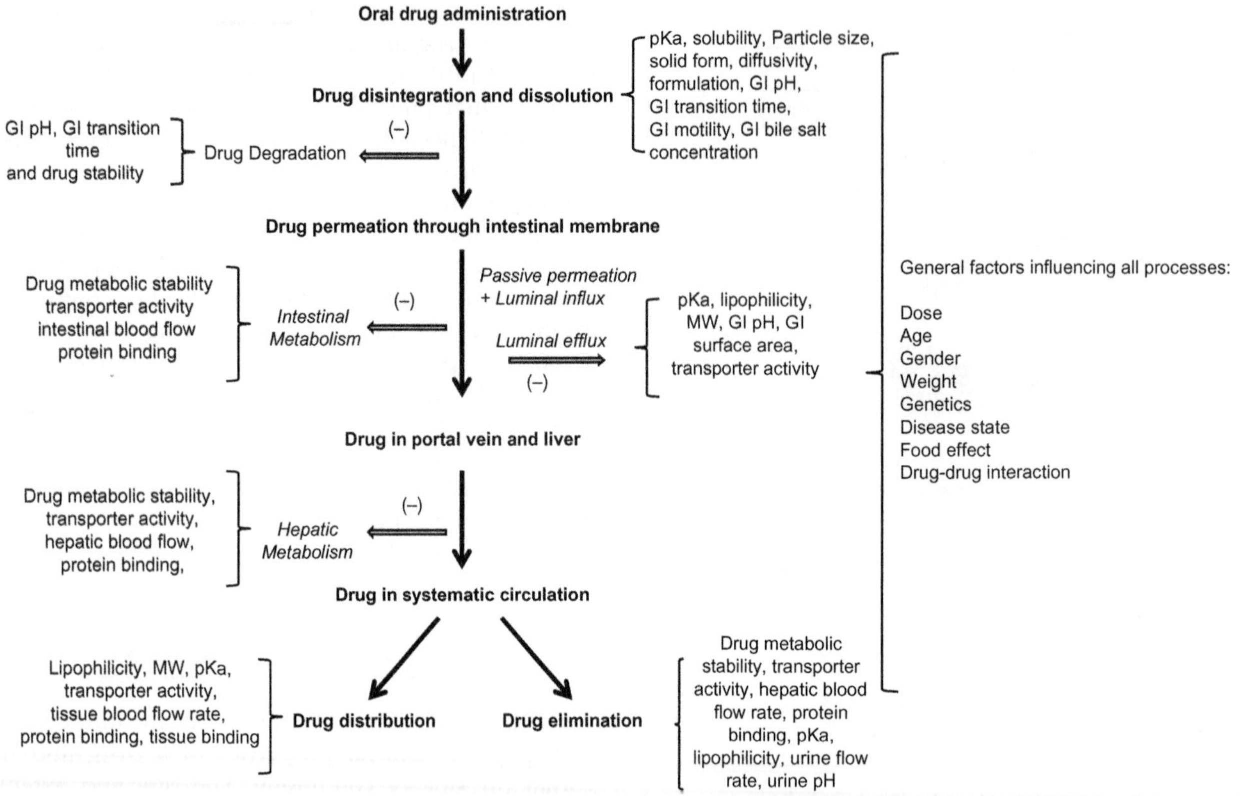

FIGURE 14.7 Scheme of drug oral absorption and disposition processes and major factors that influence the processes. *(Adapted from reference [72].)*

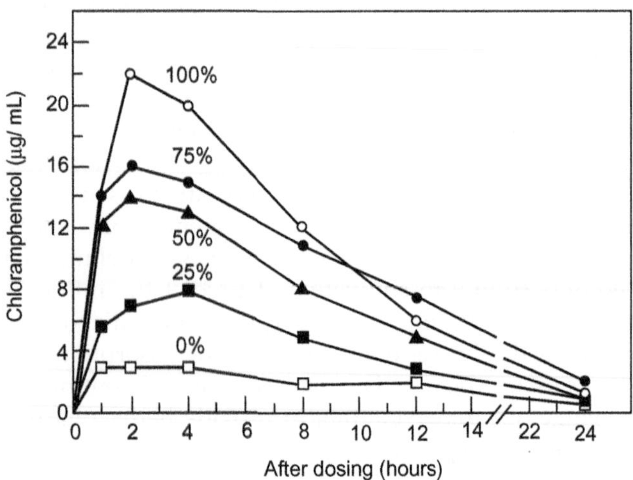

FIGURE 14.8 Comparison of mean blood serum levels obtained with chloramphenicol palmitate suspension containing varying ratios of α and β polymorphs, following single oral dose equivalent to 1.5 g chloramphenicol. Percentage in figure represents percentage of β polymorph in the suspension [74].

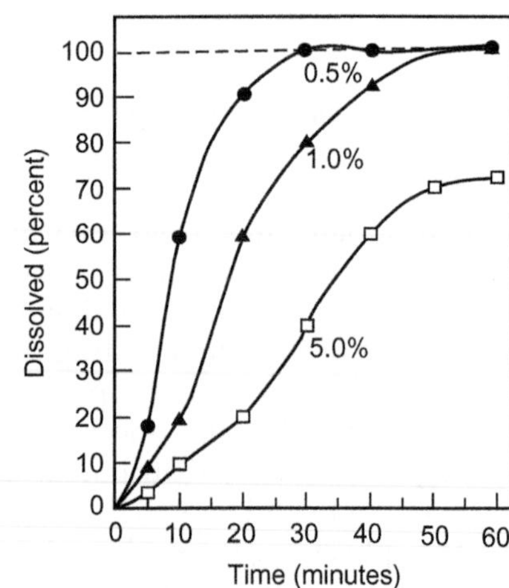

FIGURE 14.9 Effect of lubricant on drug dissolution. The % symbol in the figure represent percentage of magnesium stearate in formulation[75].

be the ideal response of the student to his or her preceptor?

Approach: A crystalline drug can exist in different polymorphic forms. Each polymorph can have distinctly different physical properties that can affect its solubility, dissolution, absorption, and bioavailability. This is a classic example in which chloramphenicol palmitate can exist at least in two forms: α and β. The former has lower absorption and bioavailability as compared to the latter form. This is due to differences in solubility and dissolution of these two different forms of the same drug.

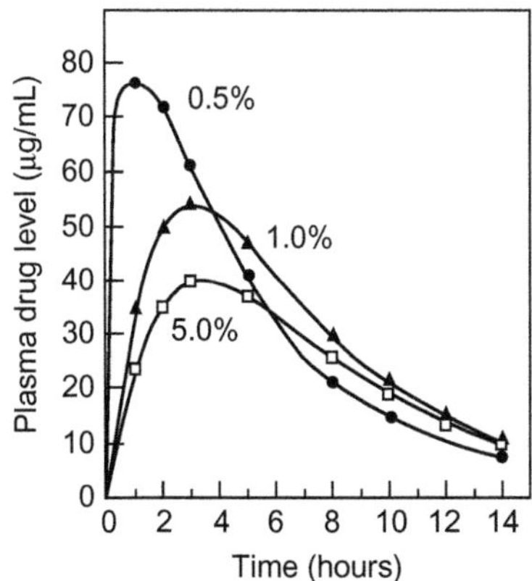

FIGURE 14.10 Effect of lubricant on drug absorption. The % symbol in the figure represent percentage of magnesium stearate in formulation. Incomplete drug absorption occurs for formulation with 5% magnesium stearate [75].

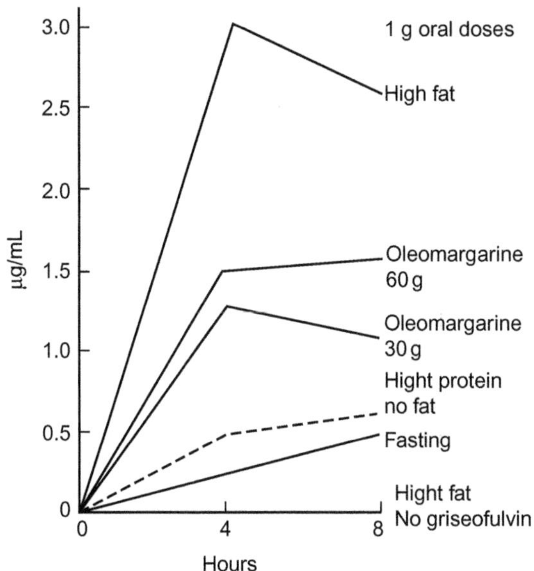

FIGURE 14.11 Comparison of the effects of different types of food intake on the serum griseofulvin levels following the 1.0 gram of oral dose [76].

Case 14.2

An *in vitro–in vivo* correlation study is presented in a midyear pharmacy meeting. The data are presented in Figures 14.9 and 14.10. The preceptor at the rotation site asks you to submit a five-line report on this finding. What is your approach to address this case?

Approach: This *in vitro–in vivo* correlation study compares the effect of lubricant (magnesium stearate) in an oral tablet on dissolution and bioavailability. A good correlation between *in vitro* dissolution and in vivo exposure was observed. An increase in the percentage of magnesium stearate in the tablet reduces its dissolution and thereby slows down oral absorption. In this case, 0.5% magnesium stearate provides better dissolution and AUC compared to 5% of magnesium stearate in the formulation. Hydrophobicity of this excipient is responsible for this difference.

Case 14.3

Literature data suggest the effect of food on the oral absorption of certain specific drugs. One such drug and its absorption data are shown in Figure 14.11. What are your recommendations for a man on griseofulvin for fungal infection of his nails?

Approach: Griseofulvin is a highly hydrophobic drug and has solubility/dissolution limited oral absorption and bioavailability issues. From the graph in Figure 14.11, it is clear that taking the drug with food can increase the oral absorption of this drug. A high fat diet showed the highest absorption compared to any other diets tested. The drug product label should contain guidelines on how to take the drug regarding food intake. The patient should be advised to follow the label carefully regarding the timing of drug administration with food.

References

[1] Rowland M, Tozer TN. Clinical pharmacokinetics concepts and applications. 3rd ed. Philadelphia, PA: Williams & Wilkins; 1995.

[2] Allen LV, Popovich NG, Ansel HC. Ansel's pharmaceutical dosage forms and drug delivery systems. 9th ed. Philadelphia, PA: Lippincott Williams & Wilkins; 2010.

[3] Martinez MN, Amidon GL. A mechanistic approach to understanding the factors affecting drug absorption: a review of fundamentals. J Clin Pharmacol 2002:620–43.

[4] Noyes AA, Whitney WR. The rate of solution of solid substances in their own solutions. J Am Chem Soc 1897;19:930–4.

[5] Hixson A, Crowell J. Dependence of reaction velocity upon surface and agitation (I) theoretical consideration. Ind Eng Chem 1931;23:923–31.

[6] Dokoumetzidis A, Papadopoulou V, Valsami G, Macheras P. Development of a reaction-limited model of dissolution: application to official dissolution tests experiments. Int J Pharm 2008;355(1–2):114–25.

[7] Brouwers J, Brewster ME, Augustijns P. Supersaturating drug delivery systems: the answer to solubility-limited oral bioavailability? J Pharm Sci 2009;98(8):2549–72.

[8] Liu R. Water insoluble drug formulation. 2nd ed. CRC Press; 2008.

[9] Li Z-Q, He X, Gao X, Xu Y-Y, Wang Y-F, Gu H, et al. Study on dissolution and absorption of four dosage forms of isosorbide mononitrate: level A *in vitro–in vivo* correlation. Eur J Pharm Biopharm 2011;79:364–71.

[10] Clarysse S, Psachoulias D, Brouwers J, Tack J, Annaert P, Duchateau G, et al. Postprandial changes in solubilizing capacity of human intestinal fluids for BCS class II drugs. Pharm Res 2009;26:1456–66.

[11] Lange DP, Hardin J, Wu J, Klausner M. Effect of a cola beverage on the bioavailability of itraconazole in the presence of H2 blockers. J Clin Pharmacol 1997;37:535–40.

[12] Ma TY, Anderson JM. Tight junctions and the intestinal barrier. In: Johnson LR, editor. Physiology of gastrointestinal tract. 4th ed. Boca Raton, FL: Elsevier; 2006. p. 1559–94.
[13] Firth JA. Endothelial barriers: from hypothetical pores to membrane proteins. J Anat 2002;200:541–8.
[14] Shugarts SB, Leslie Z. The role of transporters in the pharmacokinetics of orally administered drugs. Pharm Res 2009;26: 2039–54.
[15] Giacomini KMH, Huang S-M, Tweedie DJ, Benet LZ, Brouwer KLR, Chu X, et al. Membrane transporters in drug development. Nat Rev Drug Discov 2010;9:215–36.
[16] Press B. Optimization of the Caco-2 permeability assay to screen drug compounds for intestinal absorption and efflux. In: Turksen, K. (ed) Methods in molecular biology. New York, NY: Springer; 2011. p. 139–154.
[17] Lennernäs H. Human intestinal permeability. J Pharm Sci 1998;87:403–10.
[18] Sun D, Yu LX, Hussain MA, Wall DA, Smith RL, Amidon GL. In vitro testing of drug absorption for drug 'developability' assessment: forming an interface between *in vitro* preclinical data and clinical outcome. Curr Opin Drug Discov Devel 2004;7:75–85.
[19] Avdeef A, Tam KY. How well can the Caco-2/Madin–Darby canine kidney models predict effective human jejunal permeability? J Med Chem 2010;53(9):3566–84.
[20] Geerts TVH, Yvan. In silico predictions of ADME-tox properties: drug absorption. Comb Chem High Throughput Screening 2011;14:339–61.
[21] Kararli TT. Comparison of the gastrointestinal anatomy, physiology, and biochemistry of humans and commonly used laboratory animals. Biopharm Drug Dispos 1995;16:351–80.
[22] Berggren S, Gall C, Wollnitz N, Ekelund M, Karlbom U, Hoogstraate J, et al. Gene and protein expression of P-glycoprotein, MRP1, MRP2, and CYP3A4 in the small and large human intestine. Mol Pharm 2007;4:252–7.
[23] Mouly S, Paine MF. P-glycoprotein increases from proximal to distal regions of human small intestine. Pharm Res 2003;20:1595–9.
[24] Cao XY, Lawrence X, Barbaciru C, Landowski CP, Shin H-C, Gibbs S, et al. Permeability dominates *in vivo* intestinal absorption of P-gp substrate with high solubility and high permeability. Mol Pharm 2005;2:329–40.
[25] Drewe J, Narjes H, Heinzel G, Brickl RS, Rohr A, Begliner C. Absorption of lefradafiban from different sites of the gastrointestinal tract. Br J Clin Pharmacol 2000;50:69–72.
[26] Reddy MB, Connor A, Brennan BJ, Morcos PN, Zhou A, McLawhon P, et al. Physiological modeling and assessments of regional drug bioavailability of danoprevir to determine whether a controlled release formulation is feasible. Biopharm Drug Dispos 2011;32:261–75.
[27] Fan J, Chen S, Chow ECY, Sandy Pang K. PBPK modeling of intestinal and liver enzymes and transporters in drug absorption and sequential metabolism. Curr Drug Metab 2010;11:743–61.
[28] Zhang QY, Dunbar D, Ostrowska A, Zeloft S, Yang J, Kaminsky LS. Characterization of human small intestinal cytochromes P450. Drug Metab Dispos 1999;27:804–9.
[29] Klose TS, Blaisdell J, Goldstein JA. Gene structure of CYP2C8 and extrahepatic distribution of the human CYP2Cs. J Biochem Mol Toxicol 1999;13:280–95.
[30] Doherty MM, Pang KS. First-pass effect: significance of the intestine for absorption and metabolism. Drug Chem Toxicol 1997;20:329–44.
[31] Liu L, Pang KS. The roles of transporters and enzymes in hepatic drug processing. Drug Metab Dispos 2005;33:1–9.
[32] De Waziers I, Cugnenc P, Yang CS, Leroux JP, Beaune PH. Cytochrome P450 isoenzymes, epoxide hydrolase and glutathione transferases in rat and human hepatic and extrahepatic tissues. J Pharmacol Exp Ther 1990;253:387–94.
[33] Paine MF, Khalighi M, Fisher JM, Shen DD, Kunze KL, Marsh CL, et al. Characterization of interintestinal and intraintestinal variations in human CYP3Adependent metabolism. J Pharmacol Exp Ther 1997;283:1552–62.
[34] Gomez DYW, Vincent J, Tomlanovich SJ, Hebert MF, Benet LZ. The effects of ketoconazole on the intestinal metabolism and bioavailability of cyclosporine. Clin Pharmacol Therapeut (St. Louis) 1995;58:15–9.
[35] Paine MF, Shen DD, Kunze KL, Perkins JD, Marsh CL, McVicar JPB, et al. First-pass metabolism of midazolam by the human intestine. Clin Pharmacol Ther 1996;60:14–24.
[36] Lampen A, Christians U, Guengerich FP, Watkins PB, Kolars JC, Bader A, et al. Metabolism of the immunosuppressant tacrolimus in the small intestine: cytochrome P450, drug interactions, and interindividual variability. Drug Metab Dispos 1995;23:1315–24.
[37] Holtbecker N, Fromm MF, Kroemer HK, Ohnhaus EE, Heidemann H. The nifedipine-rifampin interaction. Evidence for induction of gut wall metabolism. Drug Metab Dispos 1996;24:1121–3.
[38] Bailey DG, Arnold JM, Munoz C, Spence JD. Grapefruit juice—felodipine interaction: mechanism, predictability, and effect of naringin. Clin Pharmacol Therapeut (St. Louis) 1993;53:637–42.
[39] Darbar D, Fromm MF, Dell'Orto S, Kim RB, Kroemer HK, Eichelbaum MR. Modulation by dietary salt of verapamil disposition in humans. Circulation 1998;98:2702–8.
[40] Mizuma T. Intestinal glucuronidation metabolism may have a greater impact on oral bioavailability than hepatic glucuronidation metabolism in humans: a study with raloxifene, substrate for UGT1A1, 1A8, 1A9, and 1A10. Int J Pharm 2009;378:140–1.
[41] Brown HS, Halliwell M, Qamar M, Read AE, Evans JM, Wells PN. Measurement of normal portal venous blood flow by Doppler ultrasound. Gut 1989;30:503–9.
[42] Wu CY, Benet LZ, Hebert MF, Gupta SK, Rowland M, Gomez DY, et al. Differentiation of absorption and firstpass gut and hepatic metabolism in humans: studies with cyclosporine. Clin Pharmacol Ther 1995;58:492–7.
[43] Watanabe T, Kusuhara H, Sugiyama Y. Application of physiologically based pharmacokinetic modeling and clearance concept to drugs showing transporter-mediated distribution and clearance in humans. J Pharmacokinet Pharmacodynamics 2010;37(6):575–90.
[44] Power JMM, Denis J, McLean AJ. Effects of sensory (teasing) exposure to food on oral propranolol bioavailability. Biopharm Drug Dispos 1995;16:579–89.
[45] Liedholm H, Wahlin-Boll E, Melander A. Mechanisms and variations in the food effect on propranolol bioavailability. Eur J Clin Pharmacol 1990;38:469–75.
[46] David Fleisher CL, Zhou Y, Pao L-H, Karim A. Drug, meal and formulation interactions influencing drug absorption after oral administration. Clinical implications. Clin Pharmacokinet 1999;36:233–54.
[47] Custodio JM, Wu CY, Benet LZ. Predicting drug disposition, absorption/elimination/transporter interplay and the role of food on drug absorption. Adv Drug Deliv Rev 2008;60: 717–33.
[48] Gu C-H, Hua L, Levons J, Lentz K, Gandhi RB, Raghavan K, et al. Predicting effect of food on extent of drug absorption based on physicochemical properties. Pharm Res 2007;24:1118–30.

[49] Rolan PE, Mercer AJ, Weatherley BC, Holdich T, Meire H, Peck RW, et al. Examination of some factors responsible for a food-induced increase in absorption of atovaquone. Br J Clin Pharmacol 1994;37:13–20.

[50] Reference PDs. Available from http://www.pdr.net/drug-summary/allegra-and-children39s-allerga-allergy-tablets?druglabelid=1459&id=3408. Accessed May 2011.

[51] Stoltz M, Thangam A, Lippert C, Yu D, Bhargava V, Eller M, et al. Effect of food on the bioavailability of fexofenadine hydrochloride. Biopharm Drug Dispos 1997;18:645–8.

[52] U.S. Pharmacopoeia. In Vitro and *In Vivo* Evaluations of Dosage Forms, 27th ed., Revision, Easton, PA: Mack Publishing Co.; 2004.

[53] Rostami-Hodjegan A, Tucker GT. Simulation and prediction of *in vivo* drug metabolism in human populations from *in vitro* data. Nat Rev Drug Discov 2007;6(2):140–8.

[54] Jiang W, Kim S, Zhang X, Lionberger RA, Davit BM, Conner DP, et al. The role of predictive biopharmaceutical modeling and simulation in drug development and regulatory evaluation. Int J Pharm 2011;418(2):151–60.

[55] Blanquet S, Zeijdner E, Beyssac E, Meunier JP, Denis S, Havenaar R, et al. A dynamic artificial gastrointestinal system for studying the behavior of orally administered drug dosage forms under various physiological conditions. Pharm Res 2004;21:585–91.

[56] Gu CH, Rao D, Gandhi RB, Hilden J, Raghavan K. Using a novel multicompartment dissolution system to predict the effect of gastric pH on the oral absorption of weak bases with poor intrinsic solubility. J Pharm Sci 2005;94:199–208.

[57] Jantratid E, Janssen N, Reppas C, Dressman JB. Dissolution media simulating conditions in the proximal human gastrointestinal tract: an update. Pharm Res 2008;25(7):1663–76.

[58] Vertzoni M, Diakidou A, Chatzilias M, Soderlind E, Abrahamsson B, Dressman JB, et al. Biorelevant media to simulate fluids in the ascending colon of humans and their usefulness in predicting intracolonic drug solubility. Pharm Res 2010;27(10):2187–96.

[59] Butler JM, Dressman JB. The developability classification system: application of biopharmaceutics concepts to formulation development. J Pharm Sci 2010;99(12):4940–54.

[60] Huang W, Lee SL, Yu LX. Mechanistic approaches to predicting oral drug absorption. AAPS J 2009;11(2):217–24.

[61] Lawrence X, Yu JRC, Amidon GL. Compartmental transit and dispersion model analysis of small intestinal transit flow in humans. Int J Pharm 1996;140:111–8.

[62] Agoram B, Woltosz WS, Bolger MB. Predicting the impact of physiological and biochemical processes on oral drug bioavailability. Adv Drug Deliv Rev 2001;50(Suppl. 1):S41–67.

[63] Jamei M, Turner D, Yang J, Neuhoff S, Polak S, Rostami-Hodjegan A, et al. Population-based mechanistic prediction of oral drug absorption. AAPS J 2009;11(2):225–37.

[64] Thelen K, Coboeken K, Willmann S, Burghaus R, Dressman JB, Lippert J. Evolution of a detailed physiological model to simulate the gastrointestinal transit and absorption process in humans, part 1: oral solutions. J Pharm Sci 2011;100(12):5324–45.

[65] Okumu A, DiMaso M, Lobenberg R. Dynamic dissolution testing to establish *in vitro/in vivo* correlations for montelukast sodium, a poorly soluble drug. Pharm Res 2008;25(12): 2778–85.

[66] Hannah M, Jones NP, Ohlenbusch G, Lavé T. Predicting pharmacokinetic food effects using biorelevant solubility media and physiologically based modelling. Clin Pharmacokinet 2006;45: 1213–26.

[67] Almond LM, Yang J, Jamei M, Tucker GT, Rostami-Hodjegan A. Towards a quantitative framework for the prediction of DDIs arising from cytochrome P450 induction. Curr Drug Metab 2009; 10:420–32.

[68] Gabrielsson J, Weiner D. Pharmacokinetic and pharmacodynamic data analysis. Stockholm, Sweden: Swedish Pharmaceutical Press; 2006.

[69] Jones RD, Jones HM, Rowland M, Gibson CR, Yates JW, Chien JY, et al. PhRMA CPCDC initiative on predictive models of human pharmacokinetics, part 2: comparative assessment of prediction methods of human volume of distribution. J Pharm Sci 2011. Available from: http://dx.doi.org/10.1002/jps.22553 [Epub ahead of print].

[70] Jamei M, Dickinson GL, Rostami-Hodjegan A. A framework for assessing inter-individual variability in pharmacokinetics using virtual human populations and integrating general knowledge of physical chemistry, biology, anatomy, physiology and genetics: a tale of 'bottom-up' vs 'top-down' recognition of covariates. Drug Metab Pharmacokinet 2009;24:53–75.

[71] Liu R, Tang AM, Tan YL, Limenta LM, Lee EJ. Effects of sodium bicarbonate and ammonium chloride pre-treatments on PEPT2 (SLC15A2) mediated renal clearance of cephalexin healthy subjects. Drug Metab Pharmacokinet 2011;26:87–93.

[72] Rowland M, Peck C, Tucker G. Physiologically-based pharmacokinetics in drug development and regulatory science. Annu Rev Pharmacol Toxicol 2011;51:45–73.

[73] Poulin P, Jones RD, Jones HM, Gibson CR, Rowland M, Chien JY, et al. PHRMA CPCDC initiative on predictive models of human pharmacokinetics, part 5: prediction of plasma concentration-time profiles in human by using the physiologically-based pharmacokinetic modeling approach. J Pharm Sci 2011. Available from: http://dx.doi.org/10.1002/jps.22550 [Epub ahead of print].

[74] Agular AJ, Krc Jr J, Kinkel AW, Samyn JC. Effect of polymorphism on the absorption of chloramphenicol from chloramphenicol palmitate. J Pharm Sci 1967;56(7):847–53.

[75] Shargel L, Wu-Pong S, Yu ABC. Applied biopharmaceutics and pharmacokinetics. 5th ed. New York, USA: McGraw-Hill; 2005.

[76] Crounse RG. Human pharmacology of griseolfulvin: the effect of fat intake on gastrointestional absorption. J Invest Dermatol 1961;37:529–33.

CHAPTER

15

Routes of Drug Administration

Mohsen A. Hedaya[1] *and Justin A. Tolman*[2]

[1]Department of Pharmaceutics, Faculty of Pharmacy, Kuwait University, Safat, Kuwait [2]Creighton University School of Pharmacy and Health Professions, Omaha, NE, USA

CHAPTER OBJECTIVES

- Describe the physiologic make-up of common routes of drug administration.
- Identify acceptable dosage forms based on the route of drug administration.
- Compare the common routes of drug administration based on barriers to systemic drug absorption.
- Evaluate the influence of drug physicochemical and formulation properties on the systemic drug absorption from various routes of drug administration.

Keywords

- Absorption barriers
- Nasal drug administration
- Ocular drug administration
- Oral drug administration
- Parenteral drug administration
- Physiological barriers
- Pulmonary drug administration
- Transdermal drug administration

15.1. INTRODUCTION

Drug administration is the application of a drug on a body surface or introduction of the drug into a body space. Following drug administration, drugs are intended to produce systemic or local effects. Most drugs must be absorbed from the site of drug administration and then distributed throughout the body to exert pharmacologic effects. Locally acting drugs produce their effect at or near the site of administration without the need to be absorbed into the systemic circulation. Whether used for its local or systemic effects, the drug molecule encounters biological barriers that can impede movement from the site of administration to the site of action. The initial barriers include membrane transport across biological membranes through the processes of drug absorption and diffusion. As discussed in Chapters 13 and 14, the characteristics of the biological membranes and cell structures vary substantially throughout the body despite the existence of common structural features. As a result, drug administration by different routes results in varied rates and extents of drug absorption and distribution.

The United States Food and Drug Administration (FDA) has defined approximately 117 terms to describe these various routes of drug administration (Table 15.1). The majority of these terms are very specialized routes of targeted drug administration with only limited clinical utility intended to deliver the drug to a very specific site and minimize systemic exposure. Some commonly used routes of drug administration include intravenous injection or infusion directly to the systemic circulation; intramuscular injections; intradermal or subcutaneous injections; transdermal application to the skin; ophthalmic instillation or injection to the eye; auricular instillation to the ear; nasal application to the nose; respiratory inhalation to the lungs; oral ingestion; rectal application to the rectum; and vaginal application to the vagina. The choice of administration route depends on drug, formulation, and patient factors. For example, the pharmaceutical dosage forms should be prepared with specific characteristics that suit the intended route of administration and optimize the drug availability at its

Pharmaceutics. DOI: http://dx.doi.org/10.1016/B978-0-12-386890-9.00015-7

TABLE 15.1 FDA-Approved Terms for Labeled Routes of Administration

auricular (otic)	intrabiliary	intraepidermal	intrapleural	iontophoresis	subarachnoid
buccal	intrabronchial	intraesophageal	intraprostatic	irrigation	subconjunctival
conjunctival	intrabursal	intragastric	intrapulmonary	laryngeal	subcutaneous
cutaneous	intracardiac	intragingival	intraruminal	nasal	subgingival
dental	intracartilaginous	intrahepatic	intrasinal	nasogastric	sublingual
electro-osmosis	intracaudal	intraileal	intraspinal	not applicable	submucosal
endocervical	intracavernous	intralesional	intrasynovial	occlusive dressing technique	subretinal
endosinusial	intracavitary	intralingual	intratendinous	ophthalmic	topical
endotracheal	intracerebral	intraluminal	intratesticular	oral	transdermal
enteral	intracisternal	intralymphatic	intrathecal	oropharyngeal	transendocardial
epidural	intracorneal	intramammary	intrathoracic	parenteral	transmucosal
extra-amniotic	intracoronal, dental	intramedullary	intratubular	percutaneous	transplacental
extracorporeal	intracoronary	intrameningeal	intratumor	periarticular	transtracheal
hemodialysis	intracorporus cavernosum	intramuscular	intratympanic	peridural	transtympanic
infiltration	intradermal	intranodal	intrauterine	perineural	ureteral
interstitial	intradiscal	intraocular	intravascular	periodontal	urethral
intra-abdominal	intraductal	intraomentum	intravenous	rectal	vaginal
intra-amniotic	intraduodenal	intraovarian	intraventricular	respiratory (inhalation)	
intra-arterial	intradural	intrapericardial	intravesical	retrobulbar	
intra-articular	intraepicardial	intraperitoneal	intravitreal	soft tissue	

site of action. The rate and extent at which the drug becomes available at its site of action depend on the drug properties such as solubility and permeability; dosage form characteristics; and anatomical, physiological, and pathological characteristics of the site of drug administration. This chapter discusses specific characteristics of common routes of drug administration and describes formulation strategies relevant to each route of drug administration.

15.2. PARENTERAL DRUG ADMINISTRATION

Parenteral drug administration refers to drug administration outside the alimentary canal in the broadest sense but is classically used to describe injectable routes of administration. These commonly include intravenous (IV), intramuscular (IM), intradermal (ID), and subcutaneous (SC) injections (Figure 15.1). Other less clinically common parenteral routes could also include intra-arterial, intrathecal, and intra-articular injections. The common feature of parenteral drug administration is that the drug is introduced to the body using a hypodermic needle or catheter. Since parenteral drug administration delivers the drug directly into the body and bypasses the skin and other defense mechanisms for protecting the body from infections, formulations intended for parenteral administration must be sterile, nonimmunogenic, and pyrogen free. IV administered drugs do not undergo an absorption process but are introduced directly to the systemic circulation for subsequent distribution to all parts of the body. However, other parenteral routes necessitate the drug be absorbed from the site of administration to be systemically available. The rate and extent of systemic drug availability following parenteral administration is then influenced by the anatomical and physiological characteristics at the site of injection, drug physicochemical properties, and drug formulation.

15.2.1 Intravenous Injection

Drugs administered into the venous circulation return to the heart, where they are available for distribution to all parts of the body. This route of administration guarantees complete bioavailability, meaning that the entire dose of the drug reaches the systemic circulation (see Chapter 16). In the tissues, the capillary

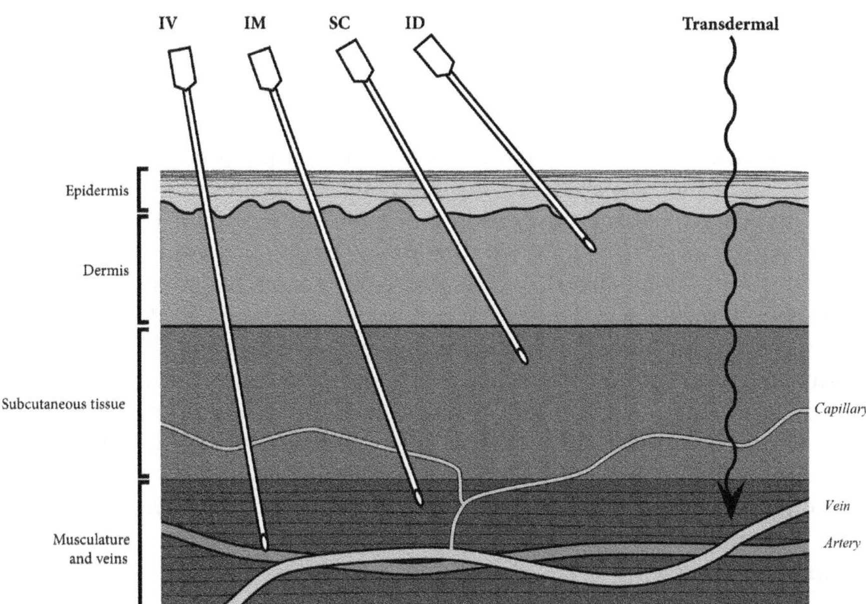

FIGURE 15.1 Schematic representation of parenteral drug delivery routes of drug administration.

endothelium allows passage of small molecules, such as water and low molecular weight drugs and proteins, to the interstitial fluid, which fills the spaces between the cells based on membrane transport processes described in Chapter 13. The movement of fluids between the capillaries and the interstitial fluids is controlled by the balance between the hydrostatic pressure in the capillaries, which favor moving water from the capillaries to the tissues, and the osmotic pressure in the solutes in the capillaries, which favor fluid movement from the tissues to the capillaries. Distribution of drugs from the blood in the capillaries to the tissues occurs through membrane transport processes and usually results in initial net drug transfer from the blood to the tissues. Eventually, a distribution equilibrium is established between the drug in the circulation and the drug in tissues. The extent of drug distribution to tissues depends on the affinity of the drug to different tissues and can be different from one tissue to the other (see Chapter 14) [1].

Drugs are administered via the IV route when rapid drug effect is desired, such as in cases of emergency, when the drug has limited or unpredictable absorption, or in patients who cannot receive the drug administered by other routes. However, IV drug administration must be performed by trained individuals, and special precautions must be considered. IV drug products must be sterile, nonimmunogenic, and pyrogen free. IV drug product formulations should also be solutions free of suspended particles that could obstruct small capillaries, have physiologically compatible pH values near 7.4, be isotonic with the blood, and be formulated in physiologically compatible solvents. Large and small volume intravenous drug products are usually formulated to comply with these requirements. However, some IV drug products cause administration site reactions because the formulations are irritating to the vascular epithelium (often due to high or low pH values; hypertonic or hypotonic solutions; or irritating drug, solvents, or excipients). These irritating formulations can cause phlebitis (inflammation of the vascular epithelium) and potentially severe damage in the tissues surrounding the site of administration after a single injection, during repeated administration, and especially when the injection is inadvertently delivered extravascularly or when extravasation of the dose occurs. However, these formulations should be administered slowly to allow the drug product solution to be diluted in and buffered with the blood to prevent injection-site reactions. For example vancomycin is an IV antibiotic that is associated with inflammatory responses if it is administered too quickly to the patient and must have prolonged rates of IV drug administration to avoid these injection-site reactions.

Drug administration via the IV route can either be by IV bolus administration or by IV infusion. IV bolus administration involves delivery of the entire drug product volume for a short period of time (usually seconds to minutes). IV bolus administration achieves the highest observed drug concentration immediately following the injection. IV infusion is the administration of an intravenous drug product at a constant rate over a period of time. Usually, the rate of drug administration by IV infusions (i.e., the infusion rate) is controlled by a mechanical pump that delivers a set volume per unit time. The period of infusion can be for long (hours to days) or short (minutes to hours) times. Long

IV infusions will cause the drug concentration in the plasma to gradually increase until a constant drug concentration is achieved. These long infusions are typically referred to as continuous infusions and usually involve large fluid volumes. Continuous IV infusions are typically used in hospitalized patients, and the infusion rate can be increased or decreased to achieve a desired drug concentration, desired drug effect, or until the patient condition is stabilized.

Some drugs are administered by repeated short-term infusions of relatively small fluid volumes referred to as intermittent IV infusions. Intermittent IV infusions usually are infused at a constant rate but over a short period of time, usually 30 minutes to 2 hours. Repeated infusions are then administered after a period of time referred to as the dosing interval. Intermittent infusions are used for drugs that might produce injection-site irritation if administered as a bolus dose and allow the drugs to be distributed slowly from the site if injected to the tissues. Drug administration by intermittent IV infusion allows the drug to distribute to the tissues during the infusion, and the maximum drug concentration achieved in blood at the end of the infusion is usually lower than the drug-blood concentration achieved if an equivalent dose were administered by IV bolus.

15.2.2 Intramuscular Injection

Intramuscular (IM) drug administration involves injecting the drug formulation directly into the muscles. Since muscles are usually highly perfused with blood, the drug will be absorbed into the systemic circulation following IM injection. The rate of drug absorption after IM administration is influenced by the formulation properties and the perfusion rate of the site of drug injection. The deltoid muscle is a highly perfused muscle of sufficient size for injection in the shoulder and is preferred when rapid absorption after IM administration is needed. Other large muscle groups can also be considered, such as the Vastus lateralis in the thigh, and may be preferred to avoid possible accidental drug injection into a blood vessel. Regardless of the site of injection, IM drug administration is not a targeted route of drug delivery but will lead to systemic drug concentrations. Therefore, the most important advantage of IM administration as compared to IV injections is the wide variety of formulations that can be administered to the muscles. Formulations such as aqueous solutions and suspensions, emulsions, and oil-based solutions and suspensions can be administered intramuscularly.

The choice of the formulation usually depends on the desired rate of absorption. After IM drug administration, the drug has to leave the injected formulation and dissolve in the interstitial fluid where it can be absorbed to the systemic circulation. Drugs injected in the form of aqueous solutions rapidly mix with interstitial fluids where they become available to be absorbed. In this case, the rate-limiting step for the drug absorption is the perfusion rate of the site of IM injection. On the other hand, IM administration of aqueous or oily solutions or suspensions slows the rate of drug release from the formulation to the interstitial fluid. The rate-limiting step for drug absorption in these formulations is then typically the rate of drug release. IM administration of some oily solutions and suspensions has been used for sustained-release formulations that are absorbed very slowly and provide continuous rates of drug release to the systemic circulation over a prolonged period of time.

15.2.3 Intradermal and Subcutaneous Injection

Intradermal (ID) and subcutaneous (SC) injections deliver drug to specific locations within the skin. The skin consists of multiple layers with differing properties (Figure 15.1). The epidermis is composed of a rapidly dividing inner layer, called the stratum germinativum, which grows upward to renew an outer layer of dead keratinized cells, called the stratum corneum. In this layer, the keratinocytes are surrounded by the lipid matrix that prevents direct contact between these cells and forms continuous lipophilic channels or paths through the stratum corneum. The epidermis protects the body from foreign objects and the outer environment, and also prevents the loss of water and electrolytes from the body. The epidermis is not innervated and does not have a direct blood supply. The thickness of epidermal layers varies significantly in different regions of the body. Underneath the epidermis is the dermis. It is a thick connective tissue layer that is innervated and vascularized. The dermis also contains lymph vessels, hair follicles, and sweat and sebum glands. Underneath the dermis is the subcutaneous tissue that is a loose layer of fat and connective tissue that is also innervated and vascularized. Vascularized muscle tissue can be found underneath the subcutaneous tissue.

ID drug administration is made by injecting a drug product into the dermis or between the dermis and epidermis layers. It is a shallow injection that should not penetrate deep into the skin. SC injections are made by delivering the drug product into the connective tissue underneath the dermis layer. SC injections should not penetrate into the underlying muscle. The volume of the interstitial fluid and the blood perfusion are very limited in the dermis and account for the slower rate of drug absorption after ID administration. ID injections are usually used to administer vaccines or to induce inflammatory responses. In contrast, the SC tissue layer has a larger interstitial fluid volume where the drug can dissolve before it is absorbed. Drug absorption after SC administration usually occurs either by absorption to the blood capillaries or to the lymphatic system, which drains slowly in the systemic circulation, resulting in very slow and unpredictable absorption. This variable absorption then produces unpredictable and erratic systemic drug concentrations after SC drug administration. This problem can be avoided by slowing the rate of drug release from the drug formulation to make it the rate-limiting step for drug absorption. Controlled drug delivery can be achieved in this way for some SC drug products (e.g., some insulin formulations).

15.3. TRANSDERMAL DRUG ADMINISTRATION

While the intradermal and subcutaneous parenteral routes of drug administration inject drug product to specific locations within the skin, the transdermal route of administration is used to deliver drug product through the skin. Transdermal drug delivery requires a drug product be applied topically to the external epidural layer. (Note that the term "topical" refers to a surface or superficial location and does not necessarily imply drug delivery to the skin.) A wide variety of acceptable dosage forms can be used for transdermal drug delivery including solid, semisolid, and liquid formulations. Under most circumstances, topically applied products will have some degree of drug penetration into the skin and potentially be absorbed into the systemic circulation. The rate and extent of drug permeation through the skin are based on numerous factors, including drug physicochemical properties, formulation factors, and pathologic conditions. Some products applied to the skin will have negligible drug absorption and are intended for topical use only. However, pathological conditions or interventional strategies can promote systemic drug absorption even when it does not happen under typical circumstances. Therefore, all topically administered drug products must be clinically evaluated for their potential for intentional and unintentional systemic drug absorption.

Drug absorption through the skin after application of transdermal drug product goes through several steps, which start with the drug release from the dosage form and the drug becoming available to be absorbed. Then the drug must diffuse through the epidural layer, including the keratin/lipid barrier of the stratum corneum, to the dermis, where the drug can be absorbed by the capillary vasculature. The rate of transdermal drug absorption is slow and highly variable. Most of this variability is due to physiological and pathological differences in skin structure, thickness, hydration, and inflammation as well as dose differences and formulation factors. Despite this variability in systemic drug absorption, transdermal drug delivery has several advantages. Transdermal drug delivery bypasses first-pass hepatic metabolism. It is sometimes considered when oral administration is not possible (e.g., veterinary applications), for potent drugs, and for drugs with substantial total body clearance values indicating significant rates of drug elimination from the patient.

The site of drug application can affect the rate of drug absorption across the skin, with thick and keratinized skin providing a more substantial barrier to drug permeation. Transdermal drug products intended for systemic delivery often recommend the drug be applied to the outer upper portions of the arms and shoulders, the upper and lower back, the upper chest, and the lower hips. Pediatric patients and especially neonates have a thinner and more permeable stratum corneum, resulting in faster drug absorption rates compared to adults. Furthermore, skin hydration is influenced by environmental factors and can affect drug permeation. Occlusion at the site of application can substantially increase the permeability of drugs across the skin and might not be clinically advised for products not intended to be occluded. Skin integrity can affect transdermal drug absorption due to disruption at the permeation barrier because the barrier function of the skin is compromised if the skin is damaged or broken.

Transdermal drug delivery requires the drug product be applied to and kept in direct contact with the skin for a certain length of time. There are several mechanisms by which the drug can be absorbed through the skin. Two principal mechanisms involve the lipid channels in the epidermis, through which lipophilic drugs tend to be absorbed, and the hydrophilic keratinized cells, through which hydrophilic drugs are often absorbed. Lipophilic drugs tend to diffuse more slowly through the epidermis and dermis than do hydrophilic drugs. Drugs can also be absorbed through the hair follicles and sebaceous glands. Patients with substantial subcutaneous fat deposits will also have altered rates of transdermal drug absorption, particularly for lipophilic drugs, than typical patients. Skin hydration also increases the moisture content of the lipid channel and the keratinized cells, which increases the possibility of drug dissolution and permeation through the skin. A balance in the hydrophilic and lipophilic drug properties is typically favorable for optimal transdermal administration [2].

The conventional dosage forms for the transdermal route of administration include semisolid preparations of ointments, creams, lotions and gels. Additionally, topically applied powders, aerosols, liquids (aqueous solutions and suspensions as well as oleaginous solutions and suspensions), liniments, collodions, and pastes are used on the skin. Many of these dosage forms are often used for the treatment of topical skin conditions. Topically administered dosage forms also tend to have more erratic rates and extents of systemic drug absorption. One key challenge for topical drug formulation administration is nonstandardized and subjective drug dosing, which can lead to variability in patient responses. Drug release from topically administered drug products also tends to be less controlled because drug absorption is dependent on the drug release rate from the formulation, the skin penetration rate, and the area of application.

The transdermal route of administration also allows for the controlled delivery of some drug molecules. For many transdermally administered drugs, the rate-limiting step in absorption is the rate of drug permeation through the skin. Specialized transdermal drug delivery systems have been developed as patches to provide more standardization and control over the rate of systemic drug absorption after topical application. The general principle of controlling the rate of drug absorption from these delivery systems is to control the rate of drug release from a fixed surface area for diffusion based on the patch geometry and make it slower than the rate of drug penetration across the skin. Unidirectional absorption through the skin allows the surface area in contact with the skin to be a key determinant in the rate of drug absorption with larger applied surface areas producing a greater magnitude and faster rate of drug absorption. Controlled transdermal patches tend to minimize the effect of physiological or pathological differences on the drug absorption rate. Good candidates for transdermal delivery include potent drugs because the amount of the drug that can be absorbed after administration of these dosage forms is usually very small. Drugs with short half-lives are also suitable for transdermal delivery systems because the slow drug absorption from these delivery systems can achieve relatively constant blood-drug concentration over an extended period of time.

Several formulation strategies have been used to improve the drug penetration across the skin after application of these transdermal patches [3]. This includes skin hydration, which can enhance the drug penetration through the skin, which can be achieved by using occlusive devices and moisturizing additives. Some formulations may include penetration enhancers as additives, which can transiently enhance the permeability of the drug across the skin. Another strategy is the use of prodrugs with better permeability through the skin. However, topical formulation excipients as well as patch adhesives may cause irritation or immunological sensitization. Patients starting transdermal drug regimens should exercise caution before long-term use is undertaken. Specifically, the skin should be evaluated after initial and repeated dose administrations for possible allergic reactions or hypersensitivity.

15.4. OPHTHALMIC DRUG ADMINISTRATION

The eye consists of two spherical pieces joined together with the smaller frontal part known as the cornea and the larger posterior unit known as the sclera. The cornea is curved and completely transparent, and the sclera is white and encloses the ocular structure. The cornea and sclera are connected by a ring known as the limbus. The iris is a circular structure that gives the eye color. Light enters the eye through a central opening in the transparent cornea known as the pupil. The pupil can change in size by contraction or relaxation of the muscles of the iris to regulate the amount of light available for vision. The lens is located toward the rear of the pupil and is connected from above and below to sets of ciliary muscles that are responsible for shaping the lens to focus the light on the retina. The retina is located on the inner surface of the back of the eye and has a pale disk where the optic nerve is attached to the eye. The anterior portion of the eye is filled with aqueous humor that is a clear fluid. The posterior part of the eye is filled with vitreous body that is clear gelatinous material. The conjunctiva is the inner surface of the eyelids and usually covers the outside surface of the cornea. Figure 15.2 shows the general structure of the human eye.

Drug distribution into and out of the eye from the systemic circulation is negligible. Therefore, ocular drug administration is typically used for the treatment of eye conditions. Ophthalmic drug administration is typically a topical application of the drug to the external eye or by intraocular injection to the vitreous body. Although some parenteral drug products can be injected directly into the eye, those clinical circumstances are typically chronic and associated with other medical interventions.

Topical application of ophthalmic drug products is a relatively straightforward route of drug administration. The cornea is made up mainly of the stroma, which is covered externally by the epithelium layer and internally by the endothelium layer. The epithelial

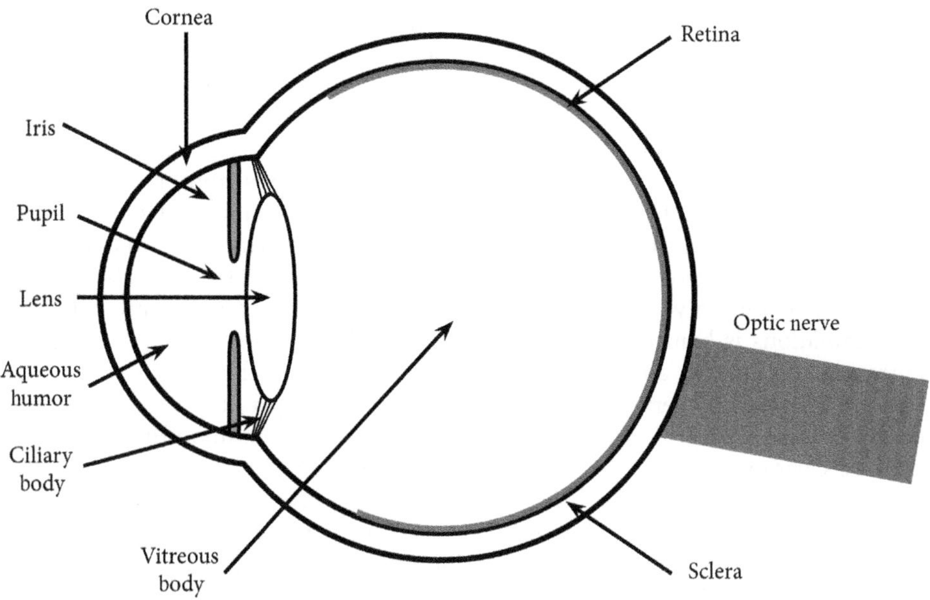

FIGURE 15.2 A diagram showing the general structure of the human eye.

and endothelial layers are permeable to lipophilic compounds, while the stroma is a cellular layer with high water content that makes it permeable to hydrophilic compounds. Compounds that can penetrate the cornea should have balanced hydrophilic/lipophilic properties with partition coefficient in the range of 10–100 [4]. Drug ionization is an important factor in determining corneal penetration of drugs because the unionized form of the drug can penetrate the lipophilic epithelial and endothelial layers of the cornea easier than the ionized form of the drug. When ophthalmic products are administered in the eye, the drug is mixed with tears, and the resulting pH will be influenced by the pH of the formulation for a period of time before the tears return the local pH to the physiological level. Buffering the ophthalmic formulation is an important formulation factor that can be used to optimize ocular drug absorption. Another important factor in determining corneal penetration of drugs is the drug binding to the proteins such as albumin, globulin, and lysozyme, which are present in tears. Bound drugs cannot penetrate the cornea because of the size of the protein molecule. Drug binding to the protein in the conjunctiva decreases the drug available for corneal absorption, and some inflammatory conditions increase the number of proteins in the tears, which increases the drug protein binding. The sclera is another route through which some drugs can penetrate to reach the inner structure of the eye, especially for drugs with low corneal permeability. *In vitro* studies have shown that the main mechanism of scleral penetration is by diffusion across the intercellular aqueous space [5].

The conventional drug products administered to the eye are liquid solutions and suspension as well as ointments. It is critical that ophthalmic drug products be sterile, nonimmunogenic, and pyrogen free to avoid infection, allergic response, or inflammation. Additionally, ophthalmic drug products should be isotonic to avoid eye irritation and stinging.

A major challenge for the ocular route of drug administration is tear production. The tears form a thin layer of fluids that bathe the corneal surface and the conjunctiva to provide nutrition for the cornea, to protect against bacterial infections, and to clear any cell debris and foreign substances. Drugs administered to the eye can be diluted and rapidly cleared from the eye by the tears. Often, this is overcome by frequent drug administration to the eye to maintain adequate pharmacologic effects. A limited number of drug products are also formulated as polymeric inserts under the eyelids or as contact lenses for controlled drug delivery for prolonged periods. However, several additional approaches have been shown to influence the retention of the drug formulation on the eye to counteract this rapid clearance. These factors include proper administration technique, adjustments to the dose volume, the use of preservatives, and formulation strategies such as excipients that alter drug product viscosity or drug release rates [4].

The proper way of administering eye drops should be by gently pulling the lower lid from the eye to form a pocket to receive the drug product. When the eyelid is released, some drug is usually entrapped between the eyelid and the sclera to prolong drug contact time with the sclera. The drug contact time with the eye can be increased further by eyelid closure for a short time and gentle ocular movement. Administration of large ocular drug product volumes also increases the rate of tear formation. Often, administration of small dose volumes (typically a few drops or a short ribbon of ointment) may require concentrated drug products that may then represent tonicity or other formulation challenges. Ophthalmic formulations typically include preservatives to prevent microbial growth in multiple dose containers. The most commonly used preservative in ophthalmic formulations is benzalkonium chloride at a concentration of 0.01% although other preservatives are used. At higher preservative concentrations, irritation and increased tear formation may occur to exacerbate drug clearance.

Ophthalmic liquid drug products cannot typically maintain high local drug concentration and have short contact times with the eye. The contact time of eye drops with the eye can be increased through the addition of polymers that can increase the viscosity, such as methylcellulose and polyvinyl alcohol. Eye ointments are also commonly used ophthalmic formulations, but they are not as acceptable as the eye drops because they may cause blurred vision after application. Ophthalmic ointments are typically used with pediatric patients, for overnight use, and when the eye is covered by a bandage. Eye ointments have the advantage of producing prolonged contact. Other topically applied ophthalmic formulations include aqueous drug suspensions. The particle size of these suspensions is an important factor affecting dose retention on the eye since larger particles can cause irritation and increase the rate of drug removal. Novel sustained-release devices for ocular drug administration have been used to maintain adequate drug concentration for an extended period of time. Soft contact lenses can be used as a drug reservoir that releases a drug in a controlled manner. The drug can be introduced to the lens by soaking the lens in a drug solution before use or by installing drops of drug solution while using the lens. Polymeric inserts have also been formulated to be inserted under the eyelid, where they can dissolve or disintegrate while gradually releasing the drug. These inserts have been used for the ocular delivery of a drug for an extended period of time.

Treatment of intraocular diseases using a topical drug application on the eye or systemic drug administration usually cannot achieve therapeutic drug concentration in the vitreous body. Topically applied drugs are usually removed rapidly by the efficient clearance mechanism of the eye, while systemically administered drugs usually have limited intraocular distribution, which requires the administration of large doses that can increase the drug side effects. Intravitreal injection of drugs is the main route of delivery of drugs for the treatment of ophthalmic conditions that affect the posterior segment of the eye. After intravitreal injection, the drug can diffuse through the vitreous body, where the drug is cleared with the aqueous humor drainage or through the retina by active secretion. Drugs that are mainly cleared from the eye with aqueous humor drainage usually have a residence time of about 20 hours in the eye, whereas drugs mainly cleared through the transretinal route usually have a residence time of 5–10 hours. Since most of the intraocular diseases are usually chronic in nature, repeated intravitreal injections may be required to maintain therapeutic drug concentration in the eye. Alternatively, pharmaceutical formulations such as liposomes and nanoparticles have been developed to increase drug residence time in the eye after intravitreal injection. Parenteral liposomal amphotericin B formulations have been shown to have longer residence time in the eye and less intraocular toxicity compared to the free amphotericin B formulation when administered intravitreally for the treatment of fungal eye infections. Nanoparticles made of erodible polymers provide a potential formulation strategy that can slowly release the drug in the eye, which increases the residence time of the drug in the eye. Intraocular devices or implants that can release the drug at a constant rate over an extended period of time have been developed for the treatment of diseases that require treatment for a long time to avoid the need to repeat intravitreal injections. Vitrasert® is a commercially available sustained-release ganciclovir formulation approved for the treatment of cytomegalovirus infections of the eye.

15.5. AURICULAR (OTIC) DRUG ADMINISTRATION

Drug administration to the ear is very similar to transdermal drug delivery in that the ears are specialized skin and soft-tissue structures. The ear is composed of three parts: the external ear, the middle ear, and the inner ear. The external ear is a skin-covered cartilaginous structure that collects and funnels sounds down the ear canal. The middle ear includes the tympanic membrane and auditory ossicles that transmit sound to the inner ear. The inner ear contains the structures involved in the transfer of fluid sound waves to nerve signals and for balance and the Eustachian tubes that allow auricular communication with the sinuses.

The ear has poor blood perfusion and is unlikely to promote systemic drug absorption following topical instillation of otic drug products. As a result, most drug products intended for auricular administration are for the topical treatment of ear conditions. Common dosage forms include aqueous and oily solutions and suspensions as well as semisolid formulations such as ointments, creams, and lotions. These otic drug products are often formulated in like manner to transdermal products. Auricular drug administration is unlikely to encounter mucous membranes, which limit the concerns regarding formulation tonicity, sterility, immunogenicity, and pyrogenicity due to the low likelihood of systemic drug exposure following ear administration. More variability in drug product formulations and excipients is permissible than for parenteral or ophthalmic preparations. As a result, otic formulations must not be used in the eye. However, ophthalmic drug products may be used in the ear.

15.6. NASAL DRUG ADMINISTRATION

The external openings of the nose are known as nostrils, and the nasal cavity extends backward into the nasopharynx, which then leads to the trachea and esophagus. The nose is a principal entrance of air to the body for respiration. Key nose functions are to filter, warm, and moisten the inspired air. The nasal cavity is covered with a layer of mucous membrane with projections that can remove large particles and debris from inspired air. The blood supply of the nasal cavity helps in warming the inspired air while the fluids secreted by the glands and cells covering the nasal cavity humidify the inspired air. The average pH of the fluid lining the nasal cavity ranges from 6.2 to 6.4 [4].

The nasal cavity epithelium has ciliated microvilli, which increase the surface area available for drug absorption in the nasal cavity. The nasal cavity is also supplied by the lymphatic system, which is also involved in the absorption of drugs after nasal administration. However, the nasal epithelium is covered with a thin layer of mucus, which is renewed every 10 minutes by the secretions of the mucosal cells and glands. The ciliated epithelial cells also facilitate the clearance of deposited particles towards the back of the nasal cavity, where they can be swallowed or forwarded to be expelled by sneezing. The action of the ciliated epithelium and mucous layer can significantly limit drug absorption from the nasal cavity due to nasal drug clearance before the drug can be absorbed [4].

Nasal drug administration can be utilized for systemic drug delivery as well as local drug effects. Drug absorption from the nasal cavity is usually rapid and occurs mainly by passive diffusion or through epithelial pores. However, drug absorption can be variable and erratic. Systemic drug concentrations after nasal administration typically increase rapidly and can achieve relatively high values. Nasal administration bypasses hepatic first-pass metabolism. However, drug removed from the nasal cavity by mucociliary clearance can be ingested and then absorbed from the gastrointestinal tract. Typically, the rate and extent of drug absorption after nasal drug administration are affected by drug retention in the nasal cavity and the significance of nasal drug clearance through mucociliary elimination. Longer drug retention in the nasal cavity can result from appropriate methods of drug administration and specialized formulation design in order to reduce the rate of mucous clearance. Physicochemical and formulation factors such as the volume of the drug solution per drug dose, drug concentration, particle density, solution viscosity, and solution can also affect the rate and extent of drug absorption after nasal administration.

Different dosage forms can be administered to the nose, including solutions, suspensions, emulsions, and dry powders. The appropriate method of drug administration to the nose is product specific based on the formulation and method of application. Some drug products are instilled as liquid drops and require proper head positioning and dropper positioning within the nostrils. Other nasal products are spray pumps, actuators, or dry powder nasal inhalers that require patient coordination with the device orientation and breathing to promote droplet or particle deposition in the nasal cavity. Poor nasal administration technique can lead to poor drug deposition in the nasal cavity epithelium and could promote mucociliary clearance.

Strategies used for improving drug absorption after nasal drug administrations include modification of the formulation pH, use of a penetration enhancer, and prolongation of the nasal residence time [6]. The formulation pH can be adjusted to keep the active drug in the un-ionized form, which can be absorbed better than the ionized form across the nasal mucosa. Penetration enhancers such as bile salts, EDTA, and fatty acids have been utilized to increase paracellular absorption of drugs from the nasal mucosa. Increasing the formulation viscosity or using bioadhesive formulations significantly prolongs the transit time of the drug administered in the nasal cavity, which can lead to increasing the extent of drug absorption.

15.7. PULMONARY DRUG ADMINISTRATION

Pulmonary drug administration and the anatomical features of the lung were explained in detail in

Chapter 10. Briefly, inhaled drugs are administered to the respiratory system through gases, fine liquid droplets, or solid particles. Pulmonary drug administration is also device specific with substantial differences between formulations, devices, and proper administration techniques. The administered drug can deposit in different parts of the respiratory tract, where the drug may exert local effects, or be absorbed into the circulation to produce systemic effects. Formulation and physiological factors are significant influences on ultimate drug deposition patterns. For solid and liquid inhaled particles, the aerosol particle size distribution is an important parameter in evaluating pulmonary drug deposition. Typically, particles with an average aerodynamic size of 1–5 μm have optimal drug deposition in the deep lung. Pulmonary pathological conditions can also affect the deposition patterns.

Pulmonary drug deposition in the deep lungs can lead to very rapid rates of drug absorption due to the extremely large alveolar surface area, thin alveolar epithelial membranes, and complete body blood flow. Although systemic drug absorption will likely take place following inhalation, pulmonary drug administration can be used to minimize systemic drug exposure. For example, inhaled corticosteroids have been used to avoid the side effects of systemically administered corticosteroids. Also, pulmonary drug delivery has been used for the administration of systemically acting drugs. Drugs absorbed from the lungs avoid hepatic first-pass metabolism. During the administration of formulations intended for pulmonary drug delivery, a fraction of the administered dose is often deposited in the mouth and the upper part of the respiratory tract, where it can be swallowed for further systemic absorption from the gastrointestinal system [7].

15.8. ORAL DRUG ADMINISTRATION

The process of oral absorption was discussed in Chapter 14. Briefly, the oral route of drug administration is a very convenient route of administration, with the majority of all manufactured drugs administered by this route. Most orally administered drug products are intended to produce systemic effects following absorption. Drugs can be absorbed from several locations within the gastrointestinal tract, such as the buccal cavity, stomach, small intestine, large intestine (colon), and the rectum. These segments of the gastrointestinal tract have different anatomical and physiological characteristics that can affect drug absorption. Formulation strategies can also be used to design orally administered dosage forms that can target specific segments and optimize the rate and extent of drug absorption as described in Chapter 14.

15.8.1 The Buccal Cavity

The buccal cavity includes the spaces or gaps in the cheek adjacent to the mouth and extends from the lips to the oropharynx. The oral mucosa lines the buccal cavity and consists of a multilayered epithelial lining that includes the basement membrane, the lamina propria, and a layer of connective tissues supplied by blood vessels and nerves. Saliva is continuously secreted in the mouth at a slow rate that increases in the presence or smelling of food. The pH of the saliva ranges from 6.2 to 7.4, and it consists of water, mucus, protein, minerals, and the enzyme amylase. The buccal cavity is a good site for drug absorption due to rich blood supply and substantial lymphatic drainage, which can lead to fast absorption and rapid drug effect [8]. Drugs absorbed into buccal capillaries drain into the jugular vein and escape hepatic first-pass metabolism. For a drug to be absorbed in the buccal cavity, it must dissolve in the saliva and then diffuse through the buccal mucosa. Dissolved or undissolved drugs that are not buccally absorbed will pass into the esophagus for possible absorption from other parts of the gastrointestinal tract.

Several factors can limit the buccal absorption of drugs. Drug absorption through the buccal mucosa is mainly by passive diffusion with little paracellular absorption, active transport, and endocytosis, which is favorable for absorbing lipophilic drugs that are not ionized in the buccal pH. Polar drugs usually have limited buccal absorption, whereas highly lipophilic drugs usually have limited solubility in the saliva and will not be absorbed from the buccal cavity. Also, the small surface area of the buccal cavity and the short transit time through the mouth usually limit drug absorption from the mouth. Furthermore, there are differences in the drug absorption from the different areas in the oral cavity. For example, drug absorption from the sublingual area is usually better than drug absorption from the mucous membrane lining the cheeks and the periodontal area. Drug formulations intended for buccal drug delivery should be designed to be retained in the buccal cavity for optimal drug absorption.

Drug formulations used for buccal drug delivery such as sublingual tablets are rapidly dissolving tablets placed under the tongue to achieve a fast rate of drug absorption. This fast rate of drug absorption makes sublingual tablets suitable for the treatment of acute conditions when fast onset of drug effect is required. Sublingual nitrate tablets have been used for many decades in the treatment of acute angina. Also, medicated chewable formulations can be used to prolong the drug transit time in the buccal cavity and increase drug absorption. The rate of drug release from chewable tablets is dependent on the drug-water solubility, with water-soluble drugs released faster than poorly soluble drugs. Slowly releasing drugs can have a better chance of absorption from the buccal cavity. Chewable formulations can be used for the treatment of dental conditions and also for antifungal therapy. Mucoadhesive dosage forms have been used to retain the formulation in the buccal cavity for prolonged times to increase the extent of drug absorption. These formulations usually utilize polymers that can adhere to the mucosal surface of the buccal cavity and slowly release the drug over an extended period of time. Bioadhesive formulations have been used for nitroglycerin and also for the local anesthetic drug lidocaine [9].

15.8.2 Esophagus

The esophagus is the gastrointestinal tract segment connecting the pharynx to the stomach. It is a muscular tube, approximately 25 cm in length in adults, and has a pH value of approximately 6–7. The typical transit time for most pharmaceutical dosage forms in the esophagus is about 15 seconds. Any drug administered orally must pass through the esophagus when it is swallowed. However, drugs are not typically absorbed from the esophagus because of the short transit time, thick mucosal lining, and limited surface area.

15.8.3 Stomach

The stomach is located in the left upper part of the abdominal cavity and is attached to the esophagus by the cardiac sphincter and the duodenum by the pyloric sphincter. The inner surface of the stomach is a thick, vascular, and glandular mucosa that is covered by a layer of mucus secreted by the epithelial lining. The gastric mucus is principally composed of glycoproteins that lubricate and facilitate the movement of food through the stomach. The gastric epithelium produces approximately 1.5 L of secretions per day that are rich in hydrochloric acid and enzymes. The mucous layer also protects the gastric epithelium from the low pH (approximately 1–3) and proteolytic enzymes present in the stomach [10]. The gastric pH depends on many factors including acid secretion, gastric contents, gender, and age. After one eats, the gastric pH usually increases due to the buffering and neutralizing effects of food, and females usually have slightly higher gastric pH compared to men [11]. Also, older individuals have been shown to have more gastric secretions and lower gastric pH compared to younger individuals [12].

The stomach usually has a limited role in the absorption of orally administered conventional dosage forms because of the small surface area and the relatively short transit time. The gastric transit time is especially short if the dosage form is administered on an empty stomach. The low gastric pH can also impair drug absorption for acid labile drugs and ionizable drug molecules. The rate of drug dissolution is affected by the pH of the gastric contents with basic drugs dissolving faster in the acidic pH of the stomach and getting ready to be absorbed once they leave the stomach and reach the small intestine. Furthermore, the gastric pH affects the ionization of drugs with weak acids usually present in the un-ionized form that can be absorbed better in the acidic pH of the stomach.

The gastric emptying rate is the rate at which stomach contents move from the stomach into the small intestine and is an important factor in determining the rate of drug absorption because the small intestine is a principal site of absorption for many orally administered drugs. In general, the stomach undergoes multiphase cycles, which causes gradual emptying of the gastric contents into the duodenum. When a drug is administered on an empty stomach, the gastric emptying rate is rapid, and the drug reaches the small intestine faster than when the drug is taken with food. Administered drugs are usually mixed with the gastric contents and then emptied from the stomach at the same rate as the gastric contents. Therefore, food usually slows the gastric emptying rate, with the meal consistency, composition, and size usually affecting the gastric emptying rate [13]. Liquids and low-viscosity food are emptied from the stomach faster than solid and high-viscosity foods [14]. Also, meals with higher calories per volume and fat-rich meals slow the rate of gastric emptying. The gastric emptying rate is also affected by drugs and diseases. Narcotic analgesics and drugs with anticholinergic effects can significantly slow the gastric emptying rate, whereas prokinetic drugs can speed the gastric emptying rate. Diseases such as pyloric stenosis, gastroenteritis, and gastroesophageal reflux can also affect the gastric emptying rate and slow the rate of drug absorption. Modifying the gastric emptying rate of the dosage form is one of the strategies that can be used to affect the rate of drug absorption after oral administration.

The rate and extent of drug absorption after oral administration are affected by the acidic environment of the stomach and the gastric contents. Specialized dosage forms can be used to optimize drug absorption, either by protecting the drug from the effect of the acidic gastric secretions or controlling the drug release from the dosage form and hence the rate of drug absorption. Enteric-coated tablets are usually used to protect acid labile drugs from the acidic environment of the stomach and deliver the drug to the small intestine. These tablets are usually coated with an acid-resistant material that keeps the tablet intact while going through the stomach. The tablet coat dissolves in the alkaline medium of the small intestine, and drug absorption starts once the tablet reaches the small intestine. In this case, the onset of drug absorption will be dependent on the gastric emptying rate, which differs depending on whether the drug is administered on an empty stomach or after a meal.

Other dosage forms can be designed to remain in the stomach and gradually release the drug over a prolonged period of time. This approach can be useful when the drug is intended for the treatment of a stomach condition, such as in the treatment of *Helicobacter pylori* infections. Gastric retention of dosage forms can also be used to formulate controlled-release formulations for drugs with site-specific absorption in the upper segment of the small intestine to improve the extent of their absorption. The retention of the dosage forms in the stomach can be achieved through several approaches, including mucoadhesion through incorporation of polymers that adhere to the mucous lining. Mucoadhesion protects the dosage form from emptying with the gastric content into the small intestine, and the drug is slowly released from the dosage form [15]. Floating tablets are low-density formulations that can absorb water and swell once they come in contact with the gastric contents. Because of the low density of the floating formulations, these tablets remain floating on top of the gastric contents and slowly release the drug over a prolonged period of time [16]. Formulations that expand or unfold when they reach the stomach and become too large to exit through the pylorus have been used to prolong the formulation retention in the stomach. The effect of gastric retention of dosage forms in the stomach on the rate and extent of drug absorption depends on the drug's physicochemical characteristics, stability, and the mechanism of drug absorption.

15.8.4 Small Intestine

The small intestine is approximately 6 meters long, and it is abruptly divided into three segments that have different absorption capacities. The first segment that follows the stomach is the duodenum, and it is about 20–30 cm; the following 2.5 meters is called the jejunum; and the last 3.5-meter segment represents the ileum. The small intestine wall is formed of several layers: the outermost layer is the serosa, followed by a layer of longitudinal muscles, and a layer of circular muscles that play an important role in the peristaltic movement of the intestine. These muscular layers are followed by a layer of connective tissues forming the submucosa and then the mucosa, which consists of several layers of cells that end with the epithelium. The epithelium layer consists mainly of a single layer of columnar cells, or the enterocytes, which cover all the inner surface of the small intestine. Other cells in the epithelial layer can secrete mucus and a variety of enzymes, hormones, and peptides. The small intestine has the folds of Kerckring, which extend most of the way into the lumen. The inner surface of the small intestine is covered with finger-like structures known as the villi, and the microvilli, which are small projections on the apical surface of the epithelial cells that are directed to the lumen of the intestine as presented in Figure 15.3. The folds of Kerckring, villi, and microvilli increase the absorptive surface area of the small intestine to be about 600 times that of a cylinder with

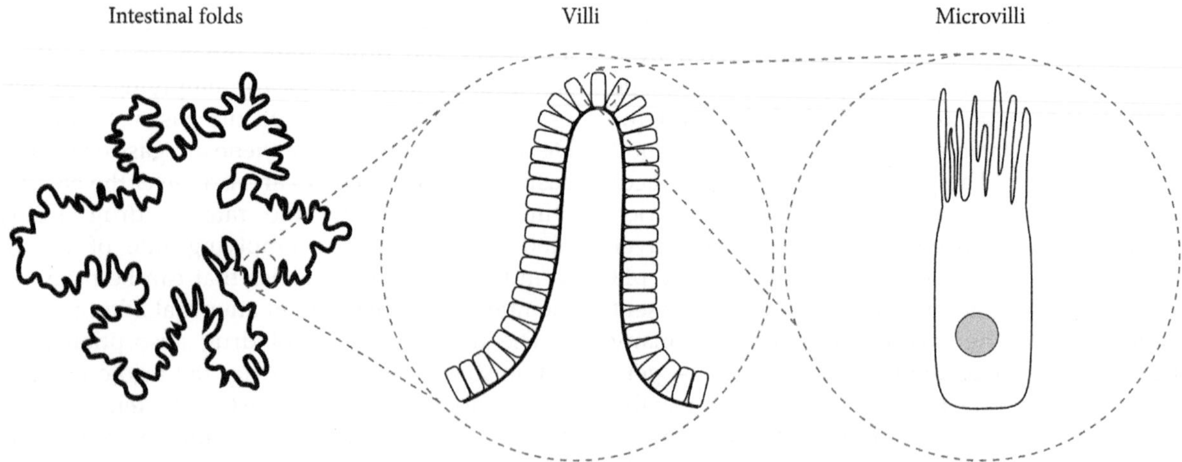

FIGURE 15.3 Intestinal structures that increases the absorption surface area.

the same diameter. This large surface area makes the small intestine the major site of absorption for most orally administered drugs. During the absorption process, the drug is transferred to the blood supply of the small intestine, which drains into the portal vein that passes the blood to the liver. Highly lipophilic compounds and fats can be absorbed from the small intestine by the lymphatic system [4].

The epithelial permeability to small ions and water-soluble molecules is greater in the duodenum and jejunum compared to the ileum. The reason is due to the presence of numerous larger aqueous pores in the upper segment of the small intestine compared to the lower segment. Also, surface area per unit length in the proximal segment of the small intestine is much higher than that of the distal segment, and the proximal segment has more carrier-mediated transport systems [4]. Moreover, more commensal bacteria are present in the ileum compared to the duodenum and jejunum. The pH in the lumen of the different intestinal segments ranges from 6 to 6.5 in the duodenum, and 7 to 8 in the other parts of the small intestine [17]. The microenvironment of the mucosal fluid adjacent to the intestinal epithelium has pH of 4.5–6.0 which allows the absorption of weak acids in the small intestine. This pH causes ionization of weak bases and suggests poor absorption of weak bases in the small intestine, which is not the case.

A fraction of the drug dose may be lost in the gastrointestinal tract lumen during the absorption process by degradation, metabolism, or excretion in the feces, which reduces the amount of the drug available to be absorbed. The gut wall contains a variety of drug-metabolizing enzymes and transporters that allow only a fraction of the drug in the gastrointestinal tract lumen to be absorbed into the portal vein. The drugs in the portal vein are delivered to the liver, where they can be metabolized or excreted in bile, thus allowing only a fraction of the drug absorbed to reach the systemic circulation [18]. The bioavailability of the drug after oral administration is the fraction of the administered dose that escapes degradation or metabolism during the absorption process and reaches the systemic circulation. All orally administered drugs are exposed to the previously mentioned conditions that can cause drug loss during the absorption process before they reach the systemic circulation, which is known as presystemic elimination. The extent of presystemic elimination of different drugs is different depending on the susceptibility of the drugs to the degradation and metabolism before reaching the systemic circulation. It can be minimal, causing a large fraction of the drug dose to reach the systemic circulation, or it can be larger, leading to only a small fraction of the administered dose reaching the systemic circulation. Some drugs are not administered orally due to their extensive presystemic elimination after oral administration.

The enterocytes of the small intestine contain several transport systems that play an important role in drug absorption, such as the p-glycoprotein (P-gp) transport system. The P-gp transport is an efflux transport localized on the apical side of the epithelial cells, which can transport a wide variety of drugs outside the epithelial cell back to the intestinal lumen. The extent of absorption of the drugs that are substrates for the P-gp is usually not complete because this transport system acts as a barrier for their absorption. Since drugs that are substrates for the P-gp can compete for the transport system, drug interaction can result from administration of multiple drugs that are substrates for the same transport system. The small intestine also contains a variety of metabolizing enzymes that can metabolize many drugs, reducing the extent of their absorption. Since the drug-metabolizing enzymes can be inhibited and induced, drug interaction that affects the extent of drug absorption can result from administration of enzyme inhibitors or inducers with drugs that undergo extensive presystemic metabolism [19].

The time the drug spends in the small intestine before it reaches the colon, known as the intestinal transit, is an important factor affecting drug absorption. The average time from drug administration until it reaches the colon is between 6 and 8 hours, and can vary depending on the presence of food, diseases, administration of other drugs, and dosage form characteristics [20]. Dosage forms administered on an empty stomach pass through the small intestine much faster than when administered with food. Conditions such as constipation and intestinal obstruction usually prolong the intestinal transit time, whereas diarrhea and irritable bowel syndrome can shorten the transit time. Drugs such as narcotic analgesics and drugs with anticholinergic activity prolong the intestinal transit time, whereas prokinetic drugs such as metoclopramide shorten the intestinal transit time. Dosage forms designed to release the drug over a period of more than 8 hours have to be retained in the small intestine during the period of drug release, or the drug has to be absorbed in the large intestine to ensure complete absorption.

In general, the absorption of most drugs after administration of conventional dosage forms, including solutions, suspensions, capsules, and tablets, occurs in the small intestine. The drug in solution dosage forms is ready to be absorbed once it reaches the site of its absorption, whereas suspended drugs have to dissolve first before they can be absorbed. Immediate-release solid dosage forms such as capsules and tablets have to disintegrate and then dissolve in the gastrointestinal tract contents before the drug can be absorbed. This makes the general order of drug absorption rate from solution to suspension to capsule to tablets. Modified-release formulations are formulations with a slow rate of drug release, which slows the rate of drug absorption and maintains therapeutic drug concentrations for an extended period of time during multiple drug administration of these formulations. The transit time of the dosage forms in the gastrointestinal tract is an important factor affecting the time over which the drug can be absorbed, indicating that the dosage form characteristics are important in determining the rate and extent of drug absorption.

15.8.5 Large Intestine

The large intestine is the section of the gastrointestinal tract that follows the small intestine, and it consists of the caecum; ascending, transverse, descending, and sigmoid colon; rectum; and anus. It is about 130 cm long and has a larger diameter than that of the small intestine. The mucosa of the large intestine has the same structural features of the small intestine, but it does not have villi and microvilli, which result in much smaller surface area compared with that of the small intestine. The pH of the large intestine contents is approximately 6.5 [21]. The metabolic activity in the wall of the large intestine is very low, but the lumen of the large intestine has many aerobic and anaerobic bacteria that have digestive and metabolic functions and can cause drug degradation. The blood supply to the large intestine, except for the lower part of the rectum, drains into the portal circulation that takes the blood to the liver. Most of the drug absorption from the large intestine is through transmucosal passive diffusion and paracellular with bulk water absorption because there is no documented active transport system in the large intestine. The transit time through the large intestine is very long, which compensates for the small surface area and allows more drug absorption. The average transit time in the large intestine is approximately 14 hours, which can be prolonged by high dietary fiber intake [22]. Other factors that can prolong the large intestine transit time include drugs such as narcotic analgesics and anticholinergic drugs. Drug absorption in the large intestine mainly occurs in the caecum and ascending colon, where the contents are less viscous and contain more water compared to the other parts of the large intestine. The gradual absorption of water makes the contents of the distal sections of the large intestine more viscous, which slows drug solubility and decreases the chance of the drug coming into contact with the absorption surface. Dosage forms intended for colonic drug delivery have to target the proximal part of the colon.

Drug delivery to the colon can be intended to treat local colon disease, such as in the case of treating inflammatory diseases and infections, or to treat systemic disease when the drug can be absorbed from the colon into the systemic circulation. Formulations for colonic delivery have to be protected from the effect of the acidic and alkaline secretions and the digestive enzymes in the stomach and small intestine, and then deliver the drug in the ascending colon. Several strategies have been utilized to deliver the drug to the colon, including the use of acid-resistant coating that keeps the formulation intact in the acidic contents of the stomach. Then, controlling the drug release to start about 4 hours after leaving the stomach can allow release of the drug at approximately the time when the formulation reaches the base of the ascending colon [23]. Other formulations take advantage of the colonic bacteria by including prodrugs that can be hydrolyzed by the colonic bacteria and liberate the active drug in the colon, such as the use of salicylazosulfapyridine for the treatment of inflammatory bowel disease [24]. Additionally, formulations have been coated with polymers that can be hydrolyzed by the colonic bacteria and release the drug when the formulation reaches the colon. The onset of drug absorption after administration of colonic delivery systems is usually delayed and depends on the gastric and intestinal transit times.

15.9. RECTAL DRUG ADMINISTRATION

The rectum is the final segment of the large intestine and can be utilized for drug administration in the form of suppositories or enemas. Suppositories are solid dosage forms that usually melt or dissolve in the rectum to release the drug, whereas enemas are liquid dosage forms in which the drug is dissolved or suspended in the vehicle. Rectal drug administration is a convenient route of administration for elderly, young, and unconscious patients, especially when oral drug administration is not possible and parenteral formulations are not available. Because of the limited fluids available in the rectum, the drug is not diluted after rectal administration, and drug absorption is usually transcellular by passive diffusion or paracellular through the aqueous pores. After rectal administration, the absorbed drug can escape the first-pass hepatic metabolism if the drug is administered to the lower part of the rectum because the venous return from this part of the rectum does not go through the portal circulation [25].

The rate of drug absorption after rectal drug administration is usually dependent on the rate of drug release from the dosage form. Because of the small area of the absorptive surface of the rectum, the relatively short rectal transit time, and the limited spreading of the rectally administered drugs to the colon, rapid drug release from the rectal formulation is preferred. The high concentration of the drug produced in the rectum, due to the rapid drug release from the dosage form and the limited dilution with the rectal contents, produces the driving force of drug absorption after rectal administration because most of the drug absorption in the rectum is by passive diffusion. When the drug is formulated in the form of suppositories, the choice of the base is usually dependent on the drug solubility in the base. Hydrophilic drugs are released faster from lipophilic bases and slower from hydrophilic bases, whereas lipophilic drugs are released faster from hydrophilic bases and slower from lipophilic bases. The reason has to do with the solubility of hydrophilic drugs in hydrophilic bases, and the solubility of lipophilic drugs in lipophilic bases will slow the rate of drug release from the dosage forms [26].

The physicochemical properties of the drug are important factors in determining the drug solubility in the contents of the rectum, and hence the drug absorption. Highly lipophilic drugs have poor solubility in the limited volume of aqueous fluids in the rectum, whereas highly hydrophilic drugs have very limited diffusivity across the biological membranes. So, balanced lipophilic and hydrophilic drug properties are necessary for optimal drug absorption after rectal drug administration. Other factors that can affect rectal drug absorption include the drug particle size, which affects the rate of drug dissolution. Also, the surface properties of the drug particles and the drug load per unit dose can cause particle agglomeration, leading to slower drug dissolution rate and causing unequal drug distribution in the dosage forms. The *in vitro* release of the drug from the dosage forms is useful for quality control purposes, but they have limited predictive value for *in vivo* formulation performance, and the human *in vivo* studies are still the most reliable method for evaluating the rate and extent of drug absorption after rectal administration of dosage forms.

15.10. VAGINAL DRUG ADMINISTRATION

The vagina is a fibromuscular tube that is part of the birth canal in females. The vaginal mucosa is a stratified squamous epithelium with several layers of epithelial cells that are attached together with desmosomes and tight junctions. The mucosa is followed by two layers of longitudinal and circular muscles that are covered with connective tissues supplied by blood vessels, lymph ducts, and nerves. Vaginal secretions vary in viscosity during different phases of the menstrual cycle.

Vaginal drug administration has been used mainly for the treatment of local conditions such as inflammation and infections and also for administration of contraceptive agents. The vagina can be a route for systemic drug delivery due to a permeable and highly vascularized epithelium. However, drug absorption following vaginal administration can be highly variable due to variable epithelial and musculature thicknesses during the different stages of the menstrual cycle. The permeability of steroid hormones through the vaginal mucosa has been shown to be widely variable during the different stages of the menstrual cycle in experimental animals [27]. Other factors that can affect the absorption after vaginal drug administration include secretions, personal hygiene, and the nature of the dosage forms.

Solutions, suspensions, and foams can spread much better than the tablets or capsules when administered to the vagina. Creams, foams, and jellies are the most commonly used formulations for the delivery of topical drug products for local effects but are less appealing due to leakage of the dosage form after application. Tablets and suppositories for vaginal insertion are usually formulated to dissolve or melt after application, thereby releasing the drug. Medicated sponges made of polyester resins have also been used for vaginal drug administration. Polymeric rings have also been formulated for controlled drug delivery to the systemic circulation following vaginal administration. Mucoadhesive tablets and particles have also been used for sustained delivery of drugs for the treatment of local vaginal disorders. Some intrauterine implants and devices have been used for controlled drug delivery.

15.11. CONCLUSIONS

Dosage forms are administered via various available routes of administration, each of which has associated with it certain advantages and disadvantages. All the routes of drug administration need to be understood properly so that the patient receives an effective drug therapy with the greatest compliance. A route of drug administration is determined by taking into account various external factors that may include the physicochemical property of the drug to be administered; the rate of drug release from the dosage form; the rate of adsorption from the site of administration; accuracy and urgency of the drug needed at the site of action; stability factors such as extreme pH conditions, enzyme degradation, and first-pass metabolism; and condition of the patient.

References

[1] Hedaya MA. Basic pharmacokinetics. 2nd ed. Boca Raton: CRC Press; 2012.

[2] Katz M, Poulsen BJ. Absorption of drugs through the skin. In: Brodie BB, Gilette JR, editors. Handbook of experimental pharmacology. Berlin: Springer-Verlag; 1971 [New Series 28 part 1], pp. 28–103.

[3] Ranade VV. Drug delivery systems: 6. Transdermal drug delivery. J Clin Pharmacol 1991;31:401–18.

[4] Washington N, Washington C, Wilson CG. Physiological pharmaceutics, barriers to drug absorption. 2nd ed. New York: Taylor&Francis; 2001.

[5] Ahmed I, Gokhale RD, Shah MV, Patton TF. Physicochemical determinations of drug diffusion across the conjunctiva, sclera and cornea. J Pharm Sci 1987;76:583–6.

[6] Chien YW, Su KSE, Chang S. Nasal systemic drug delivery. In: Chien YW, editor. Drugs and the pharmaceutical sciences. New York: Marcel Dekker; 1989, pp. 39–78.

[7] Walker SR, Evans ME, Richards AJ, Paterson JW. The clinical pharmacology of oral and inhaled salbutamol. Clin Pharmacol Ther 1972;13:861–7.

[8] Squier CA, Johnson NW. Permeability of the oral mucosa. Br Med Bull 1975;31:169–75.

[9] Nagai T, Konishi R. Buccal/gingival drug delivery systems. J Cont Rel 1987;6:353–60.

[10] McLaughlan G, Fullarton GM, Crean GP, McColl KEL. Comparison of gastric body and antral pH: a 24 hour ambulatory study in healthy volunteers. Gut 1989;30:573–8.

[11] Feldman M, Barnett C. Fasting gastric pH and its relationship to true hypochlorhydria in humans. Dig Dis Sci 1991;36:866–9.

[12] Goldschmiedt M, Barnett C, Schwartz BE. Effect of age on gastric acid secretion and serum gastric concentration in healthy men and women. Gastroenterol 1991;101:977–90.

[13] Feldman M, Smith HJ, Simon TR. Gastric emptying of solid radiopaque markers: studies in healthy subjects and diabetes patients. Gastroenterol 1984;87:895–902.

[14] Hunt NJ, Knox MT. A relation between the chain length of fatty acids and the slowing of gastric emptying. J Physiol 1968;194:327–36.

[15] Burton S, Washington N, Steele RJC, Musson R, Feely L. Intragastric distribution of ion-exchange resins: a drug delivery system for the topical treatment of the gastric mucosa. J Pharm Pharmacol 1995;47:901–6.

[16] Ingani HM, Timmermans J, Moes AJ. Concept and *in vivo* investigation of peroral sustained release floating dosage forms with enhanced gastrointestinal transit. Int J Pharmaceut 1987;35:157–64.

[17] Hardy JG, Evans DF, Zaki I, Clark AG, Tennesen HH, Gamst ON. Evaluation of an enteric-coated naproxen tablet using gamma scintigraphy and pH monitoring. Int J Pharmaceut 1987;37:245–50.

[18] Rowland M, Benet LZ, Graham GG. Clearance concepts in pharmacokinetics. J Pharmacokinet Biopharm 1973;1:123–36.

[19] Watkins P. The barrier function of CYP3A4 and P-glycoprotein in the small bowel. Adv Drug Deliv Rev 1997;27:161–70.

[20] Davis SS, Hardy JG, Fara JW. Transit of pharmaceutical dosage forms through the small intestine. Gut 1986;27:886–92.

[21] Evans DF, Pye G, Bramley R, Clark AG, Dyson TJ, Hardcastle JD. Measurement of gastrointestinal pH profiles in normal ambulant human subjects. Gut 1988;29:1035–41.

[22] Metcalf AM, Phillips SF, Zinsmeister AR, MacCarty RL, Beart RW, Wolff BG. Simplified assessment of segmental colonic transit. Gastroenterol 1987;92:40–7.

[23] Dew MJ, Hughes PJ, Lee MG, Evans BK, Rhodes J. An oral preparation to release drugs in the human colon. Br J Clin Pharmacol 1982;14:405–8.

[24] Rubinstein A. Microbially controlled drug delivery to the colon. Biopharm Drug Dispos 1990;11:465–87.

[25] DeBoer AG, Breimer DD, Pronk FJ, Gubbens-Stibbe JM. Rectal bioavailability of lidocaine in rats: absence of significant first-pass elimination. J Pharm Sci 1980;69:804–7.

[26] DeBoer AG, Moolenaar F, deLeede LGJ, Breimer DD. Rectal drug administration: clinical pharmacokinetic considerations. Clin Pharmacokinet 1982;7:285–311.

[27] Richardson JL, Illum L. The vaginal route of peptide and protein drug delivery. Adv Drug Deliv Rev 1992;8:341–66.

CHAPTER

16

Bioavailability and Bioequivalence

Ajit S. Narang[1] *and Ram I. Mahato*[2]

[1]Drug Product Science and Technology, Bristol-Myers Squibb, Co., New Brunswick, NJ, USA [2]Department of Pharmaceutical Sciences, University of Nebraska Medical Center, Omaha, NE, USA

CHAPTER OBJECTIVES

- Define and differentiate between bioavailability and bioequivalence.
- Differentiate between absolute and relative bioavailability.
- Discuss how bioavailability is determined.
- Discuss different dosage form and drug substance–related factors that affect drug bioavailability.
- Describe the role of physiological variables in oral drug absorption.
- Discuss the statistical basis of bioequivalence analysis.
- Discuss important considerations in study design for bioavailability and bioequivalence assessment.

Keywords

- Area Under the Curve (AUC)
- Bioavailability (BA)
- Bioequivalence (BE)
- *In vitro–in vivo* correlation (IVIVC)
- Rate and extent of drug absorption

16.1. INTRODUCTION

A drug must be absorbed in the body for it to elicit its desired pharmacological action. Measures of the amount and rate of drug absorption in the body—bioavailability (BA) and bioequivalence (BE)—play a key role in new drug development as well as in the understanding of certain drug interactions and clinical variation in drug effects. The BA and BE provide important information that ensures safety and efficacy of new and generic medicines. The BA and BE studies also form the basis of regulation for introduction of new drug products to the market. BA studies form the cornerstone of approval of new drugs, whereas BE studies are the foundation of generic drug approvals.

This chapter discusses the background, concepts, and methodology for the assessment of BA. In addition, factors affecting BA related to drug substance characteristics, dosage form factors, and the physiological parameters are discussed, along with their potential interactions. Finally, the concepts of BE, study design, data interpretation, and the criteria for the assessment of BE are discussed.

16.2. BIOAVAILABILITY

The rate and extent of drug entering the systemic circulation or at its site of action, such as a target organ or tissue, is termed *bioavailability (BA)*. Drug availability at its site of action is not readily quantifiable in most cases. Nevertheless, most drugs need to go through the systemic circulation to reach their site of action. For drugs that need to be systemically available for their pharmacological action, drug availability in plasma is typically measured and considered indicative of their target tissue availability.

16.2.1 Estimation of Area Under the Curve (AUC)

Drug availability in the plasma is typically quantified in terms of the total amount of drug in the plasma from the time of drug administration until its complete elimination. Drug plasma concentration is measured at

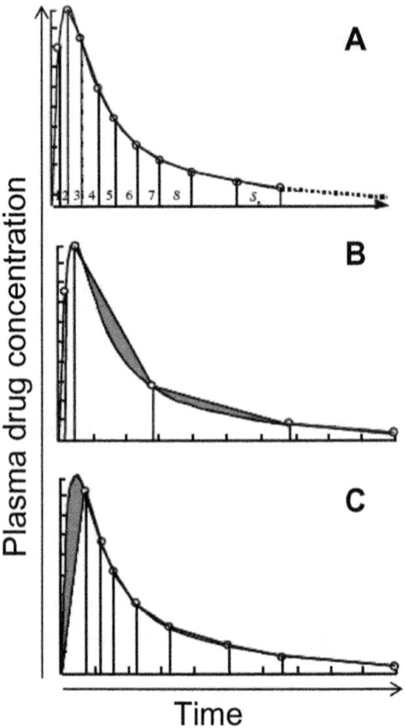

FIGURE 16.1 Plasma concentration-time profile of a drug constructed by measuring drug blood concentrations (plotted on the y-axis) at different points in time after drug administration (plotted on the x-axis). This figure further demonstrates the use of trapezoidal rule for measurement of area under the plasma concentration-time curve (AUC). The accuracy of AUC measurement by the arithmetic trapezoidal rule depends on the sampling design of the study. Thus, while the arithmetic trapezoidal rule may work well for a study with high frequency of sampling time points in the absorption phase and adequate time points in the elimination phase (as exemplified in case **A**), it can underestimate the true area if the sampling is not frequent enough in the absorption phase (as exemplified in case **B**) or overestimate the true area if the sampling is not frequent enough in the elimination phase (as exemplified in case **C**) [1].

several time points after drug administration and used to construct a plasma concentration-time profile (Figure 16.1). The total amount of drug in the plasma is calculated by quantifying the area under the plasma concentration-time profile curve (AUC).

AUC is utilized for the assessment of BA. Typically, the trapezoidal rule is utilized to calculate the AUC by adding together the results of multiplying the mean of plasma concentrations to the time period for each consequent sampling time point. This method of assessing AUC is highly dependent on the sampling design of the study. While the arithmetic trapezoidal rule may work well for a study with high frequency of sampling time points in the absorption phase and adequate time points in the elimination phase (as exemplified in Figure 16.1A), it can underestimate the true area if the sampling is not frequent enough in the absorption phase (as exemplified in Figure 16.1B) or overestimate the true area if the sampling is not frequent enough in the elimination phase (as exemplified in Figure 16.1C) [1].

When concavity of the plasma concentration-time profile is substantial, the log-linear trapezoidal rule may provide a more accurate measure of AUC. The log-linear rule is based on taking geometric rather than arithmetic mean of the plasma concentration. Thus, for all plasma concentrations c_1 and c_2 at all time points t_1 and t_2, the trapezoidal rule would estimate AUC using Eq. 16.1, whereas the log-linear trapezoidal rule would use Eq. 16.2:

$$AUC_{0-t} = \sum_0^t \left(\frac{C_1 + C_2}{2}\right) \times (t_2 - t_1) \tag{16.1}$$

$$AUC_{0-t} = \sum_0^t \left(\sqrt{c_1 \times c_2}\right) \times (t_2 - t_1) \tag{16.2}$$

Nonlinear mixed effects modeling can be used for estimating AUC in populations when samples are not taken at fixed time points for plasma concentration determination. It is also useful in cases of sparse sampling, such as in toxicokinetic studies wherein the number of samples per animal are fairly limited and kinetic analysis often requires pooling of data from multiple animals. Mixed effects modeling partitions variability in the magnitude of plasma concentration between and within animals based on user-specified models, allowing better estimation of typical drug exposures. However, it requires appropriate structural models for the description of pharmacokinetics.

16.2.2 Absolute Bioavailability

By definition, drug administration directly into the systemic circulation by an intravenous injection results in complete (100%) BA. However, when a drug is administered by another route, not all the drug may reach the systemic circulation. The percentage of drug available in the systemic circulation after its administration from a given dosage form and through a selected route of administration as compared to the amount of drug available in plasma after direct intravenous injection is termed *absolute* BA and is designated as $F_{absolute}$. For example, $F_{absolute}$ by the oral route can be defined by Eq. 16.3:

$$F_{absolute} = \frac{\text{AUC}_{\text{per oral}}}{\text{AUC}_{\text{intravenous}}} \times 100 \tag{16.3}$$

Frequently, the drug dose used for oral drug administration is different from that used for intravenous administration. This requires dose normalization to calculate $F_{absolute}$ as in Eq. 16.4:

$$F_{absolute} = \frac{\text{AUC}_{\text{per oral}}}{\text{AUC}_{\text{intravenous}}} \times \frac{\text{Dose}_{\text{intravenous}}}{\text{Dose}_{\text{per oral}}} \times 100 \tag{16.4}$$

16.2.3 Relative Bioavailability

When the BA of a drug (from a given dosage form and through a selected route of administration) is measured as a proportion of a drug's systemic availability through any route other than the intravenous administration, it is termed *relative* BA and is designated as $F_{relative}$. The $F_{relative}$ of one formulation (Formulation A) can be compared to another formulation (Formulation B) through the same or another route of administration. Thus, $F_{relative}$ can be defined by Eqs. 16.5 and 16.6:

$$F_{relative} = \frac{AUC_{\text{formulation A, route 1}}}{AUC_{\text{formulation B, route 1}}} \times 100 \quad (16.5)$$

$$F_{relative} = \frac{AUC_{\text{formulation A, route 1}}}{AUC_{\text{formulation A, route 2}}} \times 100 \quad (16.6)$$

Drug administration by different routes of administration may require different doses. Also, if formulations with significantly different drug release or $F_{absolute}$ are compared, different doses may need to be administered. These scenarios require dose normalization to calculate $F_{relative}$ as in Eqs. 16.7 and 16.8:

$$F_{relative} = \frac{AUC_{\text{formulation A,route1}}}{AUC_{\text{formulation B,route1}}} \times \frac{Dose_{\text{formulation B,route1}}}{Dose_{\text{formulation A,route1}}} \times 100 \quad (16.7)$$

$$F_{relative} = \frac{AUC_{\text{formulationA,route1}}}{AUC_{\text{formulationA,route2}}} \times \frac{Dose_{\text{formulation A,route2}}}{Dose_{\text{formulation A,route1}}} \times 100 \quad (16.8)$$

16.2.4 Measurement of Bioavailability

Estimation of $F_{absolute}$ from a reference formulation (given dosage form and route of administration) is important to appreciate the clinical significance of changes in BA. For example, if any modification, such as change in the dosage form, route of administration, or food effect, changes the BA by 100%, its significance would be much greater for a reference formulation with $F_{absolute}$ of 50% than for a reference formulation with $F_{absolute}$ of 5%. Thus, the anti-arrhythmic compound felodipine has low and variable oral BA, attributable to metabolism by intestinal CYP3A4 enzymes during absorption. Its BA can significantly increase with the co-ingestion of grapefruit, which inhibits intestinal CYP enzyme activity [2]. In addition, intersubject variability may be linked to the variability in the $F_{absolute}$ of drugs. Thus, drugs with low BA generally tend to show high variability (Figure 16.2) [3].

$F_{absolute}$ is typically estimated by quantitating the AUC from time of drug administration ($t = 0$) to the last sampling time point (t) to give $AUC_{0\rightarrow t}$. Extrapolation of the curve to infinite time by estimation of terminal elimination rate constant yields $AUC_{0\rightarrow\infty}$. For prodrugs and drugs that are metabolized into active metabolites, BA assessment may be done only for the active moiety. This assumes complete metabolism during administration or by a first-pass effect, which may not be the case. Therefore, either both administered drug or prodrug and the active moiety may be quantitated or a nonspecific assay (such as a radioactive label) may be utilized for the quantitation of $F_{absolute}$.

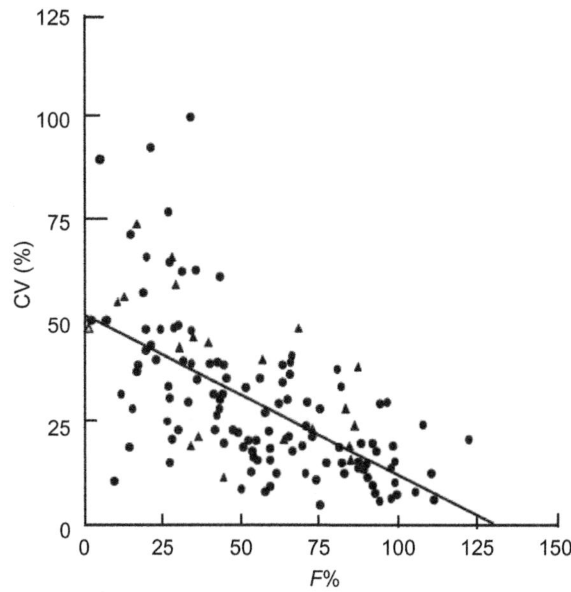

FIGURE 16.2 Plot of absolute bioavailability ($F_{absolute}$, $F\%$) against intersubject variability (% coefficient of variation, CV) for 100 drugs in humans. Drugs with lower $F_{absolute}$ tend to show higher variability [3].

Special modifications to the measurement of BA are sometimes required depending on the underlying factors. For example,

- If plasma drug concentrations are not measurable, drug concentrations in the urine are utilized for an assessment of $F_{absolute}$ by an extravascular (EV) route of administration—if excretion through kidney is the major route of drug elimination. This assumes that the ratio of renal clearance to total drug clearance is the same for the intravenous (IV) and the EV routes of administration.
- Semisimultaneous drug administration may be utilized for drugs with long terminal half-life [4]. In this case, two doses (IV followed by EV, or vice versa) are administered at a short, optimal interval, and mathematical model fitting of the plasma concentration-time profile is utilized to estimate BA.
- If, for any reason, a drug may not be administered IV, measurement of $F_{absolute}$ is possible by measuring the amount of drug eliminated if a drug is eliminated by one or more experimentally accessible routes, such as urine.

- Measurement of $F_{relative}$ between two formulations or two EV routes of administration may also be done under steady-state conditions since the total AUC over a dosing interval at steady state is equal to $AUC_{0\rightarrow\infty}$. This method requires achieving steady state with one formulation and then shifting the formulation to achieve another steady state. This method is useful for drugs with long terminal half-lives and assumes that drug absorption does not continue beyond the dosing interval.

16.2.5 Underlying Assumptions in Bioavailability Assessment

$F_{absolute}$ of a dosage form is the actual percentage of administered dose that reaches the general circulation. In general, the $F_{absolute}$ of a drug administered by the IV route of administration is considered 100%. Therefore, $F_{absolute}$ is typically estimated by measuring the plasma drug concentration after IV and EV drug administration. The EV route of administration requires the step of drug absorption before it becomes available in the systemic circulation. However, the rate of drug absorption may not reflect the rate of drug availability in plasma, such as in cases where drug gets metabolized after absorption. The first-pass effect in the liver or the lung can reduce oral BA of drugs even though they may be well absorbed.

$F_{absolute}$ of drugs administered by the IV route is generally assumed to be 100%, but this may not necessarily be the case. The systemic circulation relevant to the drug concentration at the site of action is the arterial blood concentration. Drugs administered systemically are typically administered intravenously. There could be differences between the venous drug concentration and the drug concentration in the arteries. This difference could be due to, for example, drug metabolism in the lungs since the drugs administered by the IV route must cross the pulmonary circulation before reaching arterial blood. Prostaglandins, for example, are significantly metabolized in the lungs. Also, the BA of a drug after IV administration of its prodrug can sometimes be less than 100%. For example, the BA of methylprednisolone after IV administration of its succinic acid ester prodrug in dogs was about 44% [5].

In addition, measurement of $F_{absolute}$ involves several assumptions. For example, the clearance of a drug by the IV and the EV routes of administration is assumed to be the same. Also, the utilization of a crossover study design (drug administration by one route followed by a washout period, and then another route) assumes no carryover effect. While the washout period takes care of residual drug concentration from the first period of administration to the next, there could be carryover effects by indirect means such as induction or inhibition of metabolizing enzymes after first drug administration. These effects could lead to nonlinearity due to time dependency. Also, determination of $F_{absolute}$ typically requires estimation of terminal half-life of a drug beyond the last sampling time point for measured plasma drug concentration. This estimation may not be robust depending on the sampling design of the study and possible presence of other confounding factors such as continued drug absorption into the elimination phase, which could happen due to, for example, entero-hepatic recycling.

16.3. FACTORS AFFECTING BIOAVAILABILITY

BA of a drug from a dosage form is a result of sequential processes of drug dissolution and absorption. Several drug substance and drug product or dosage form characteristics can affect either of these processes, thus affecting the rate and extent of drug availability in the systemic circulation. In addition, physiological variables such as GI motility, gastric emptying time, pH of the gastric milieu, window of absorption of the drug, and interindividual variations in the content and/or activity of metabolizing enzymes and transporters can influence drug absorption either directly or by interacting with drug or dosage form properties.

16.3.1 Drug Substance Characteristics

Drug substance characteristics that affect the rate and extent of drug release include solubility, surface area, polymorphism, and salt form.

16.3.1.1 Solubility

The solubility of a drug in a given medium represents the concentration of the drug in solution when a thermodynamic equilibrium has been reached between the drug in solution and the solid drug in contact with each other at a fixed temperature. The thermodynamic solubility, however, may not be the biorelevant solubility of a drug. In cases in which the drug dissolution rate is so low that the amount of time and agitation needed to reach thermodynamic solubility is higher than the drug residence time at its site of absorption, such as the gastrointestinal tract (GIT). In these cases, kinetic drug solubility within biorelevant time frames (such as a few hours) may be more important. Also, some drugs tend to self-associate in solution to form dimers, trimers, micelles, or continuous self-association structures. The formation of these structures leads to an increase in the perceived solubility of the drug compared to the monomeric form alone.

Most drugs are weak acids or weak bases. Accordingly, they exhibit pH-dependent solubility. For weak acids, the solubility is higher at basic pH and lower at acidic pH. For weak bases, the solubility is higher at acidic pH and lower at basic pH. The extent of difference in the solubility of a weakly acidic/basic drug with the change in pH depends on the solubility of the un-ionized free acid/free and the ionized form of a drug. The pH-dependent extent of ionization of a drug can be calculated by the modified Henderson–Hasselbalch equation, as shown in Eqs. 16.9 and 16.10:

$$\frac{[\textit{salt of weakly acidic drug}]}{[\textit{free acid}]} = 10^{pH-pKa} \tag{16.9}$$

$$\frac{[\textit{free base}]}{[\textit{salt of weakly basic drug}]} = 10^{pH-pKa} \tag{16.10}$$

where *pKa* represents the negative log of the ionization constant of the drug.

The pH-dependent drug solubility differences can lead to drug solubility changes with pH differences across the GIT for orally administered drugs to affect oral drug BA. Thus, a weakly acidic drug would not dissolve substantially in the stomach but would dissolve rapidly when it reaches the intestines. Only the un-ionized form of the drug rapidly permeates passively through membranes, leading to drug absorption. Thus, although a weakly acidic drug would have a greater proportion of the free acid form of the dissolved drug present in the stomach, the lower surface area of the absorptive surface in the stomach, compared to that of intestines, and lower total amount of dissolved drug is likely to lead to some, but not substantial, drug absorption from the stomach.

For a weakly basic drug, the drug would be predominantly ionized and dissolved in the acidic stomach, while the intestinal pH favors the un-ionized form. Thus, the higher surface area of the intestines combined with the presence of higher proportion of un-ionized form of the drug in solution can lead to higher rate and extent of drug absorption from the intestines. However, the drug dissolved in the stomach may precipitate upon change in pH as it transitions to the intestine. The precipitated form of the drug may be amorphous or crystalline, or admixed with components from the GI milieu, and would need to undergo dissolution again in the intestinal environment for absorption. This rate of re-dissolution may be slow and/or erratic, leading to low and variable oral drug BA. In these cases, the rate of drug precipitation and the ability of the drug to sustain supersaturation (such as by self-association) can affect oral drug absorption.

In addition to pH, the solubility of a drug is also affected by temperature and the physical form of the drug. Solubility should always be determined under isothermal conditions, i.e., at a fixed temperature. The temperature of biorelevant solubility is 37°C, whereas the temperature at which the dosage form is formulated is typically room temperature.

In addition, solubility of a drug can be significantly altered by the preparation of its solvate (e.g., hydrate), salt, or prodrug. Salt forms of drugs typically have higher solubility than the corresponding free acid or the free base form [6]. In terms of the physical form of the drug, the amorphous (noncrystalline) form of a drug typically has higher solubility than the crystalline form. For drugs that exist in more than one crystalline form (polymorphism), solubility differences between the polymorphic forms are commonly observed in addition to differences in melting point, dissolution rate, and physico-chemical stability. Typically, the metastable (physically less stable) form of the drug has higher solubility, which may also translate into higher dissolution rate and BA. For example, chloramphenicol palmitate exists in three polymorphic forms, which differ in solubility and dissolution rates [7], as well as BA [8].

Highly hydrophobic drugs that may have a functional group for conjugation in a manner that can be cleaved *in vivo*, such as for the formation of an ester that can release the parent compound by hydrolysis, can be developed into prodrugs. For example, brivanib alaninate is a higher-solubility ester prodrug of the active moiety brivanib [9]. Prodrug strategies are also utilized for *in vivo* targeting to the site of drug action, such as the targeting of drugs to cancer by developing macromolecular prodrugs that can undergo selective extravasation in the tumor vasculature [10], or delivery to the preferred site of drug action, such as balsalazide for colon-specific delivery of the anti-inflammatory aminosalicylic acid [11].

16.3.1.2 Dissolution Rate

Dissolution rate represents the rate at which a drug dissolves in a given medium. It is a function of the surface area of the drug particles, its solubility, the diffusion coefficient, the amount of drug dissolved, and the hydrodynamic conditions during dissolution—represented by the thickness of an unstirred layer of dissolved drug. These interrelationships are given by the Noyes–Whitney equation (Eq. 16.11):

$$\frac{dQ}{dt} = \frac{D}{h}S(C_s - C) \tag{16.11}$$

where Q is the amount of drug dissolved; t is time; D is the diffusion coefficient of the drug in the dissolving medium; h is the thickness of the stationary, saturated layer of solvent on a solid surface; S is the effective surface area of particles; C_s is the saturation solubility of the drug; and C is the drug concentration in solution.

Particle size and surface area of a solid drug are inversely related to each other. The smaller the drug particle size, the greater is its surface area–to–volume ratio. Since the surface area increases with decreasing particle size, micronization generally leads to higher dissolution rates. For example, micronization of the poorly water-soluble drugs griseofulvin, chloramphenicol, and tetracycline resulted in higher dissolution rates when compared with their nonmicronized forms [12,13]. Micronization has also been used for solubility enhancement of griseofulvin [13], aspirin [14], and several other drugs. The dissolution rate of hydrophobic drugs can be further enhanced by the concomitant use of surfactants (e.g., Tween-80) and hydrophilic polymers [e.g., polyvinyl pyrrolidone (PVP) and polyethylene glycol (PEG)] as wetting agents, to decrease the interfacial tension and displace adsorbed air on the surface of solid particles.

Micronization sometimes leads to the unexpected observation of a decrease in surface area and dissolution rate. This effect is often due to the aggregation of micronized particles, due to high surface energy and/or electrostatic charge, during the micronization process. In such cases, use of excipients during or after micronization is helpful in reducing aggregation. Thus, deposition of a micronized drug on an excipient surface can also lead to an increase in surface area and dissolution. For example, microparticles of nevirapine, a poorly water-soluble drug, were prepared by supercritical antisolvent method and deposited on the surface of excipients such as lactose and microcrystalline cellulose. The nevirapine/excipients mixture showed faster dissolution rate compared to drug microparticles alone or when physically mixed with the excipients [15]. This could be due to the minimization of aggregation in micronized drug particles.

Viscosity-inducing hydrophilic macromolecules such as povidone, carboxymethyl cellulose (CMC), pectin, and gelatin, when incorporated in an intimate mixture with the drug in the dosage form, can minimize the rate of interconversion of one polymorphic form into another. In addition, conversion of drugs to their salt forms can improve their solubility and dissolution rate, thus impacting BA. Furthermore, prodrug strategies are often utilized to maximize drug absorption. Passive transport of a drug across the biological membrane is governed by the proportion of the un-ionized form present, which is governed by the drug's dissociation constant (pKa) and pH at the site of absorption, and lipid solubility of the un-ionized drug. Prodrug strategies that alter the pKa and lipophilicity of drug molecules can impact their absorption.

16.3.1.3 **In Vitro–In Vivo** *Correlation (IVIVC)*

Predictive mathematical correlations describing the relationship between an *in vitro* property of the dosage form, such as the rate and extent of drug release, and an *in vivo* response, such as the rate and extent of drug absorption, are termed *in vitro-in vivo* correlations (IVIVC). These correlations are based on the central premise that the rate of drug release determines the rate of drug absorption. While drug dissolution from the dosage form must precede drug absorption in all cases, the relative rate of drug release and drug absorption determines the feasibility of establishing IVIVC for drug products. For example, while IVIVC may be established for drugs where dissolution from the dosage form is the rate-limiting factor (i.e., rate of drug release < rate of drug absorption), it may not be meaningful for drugs where the rate of drug absorption is rate limiting (i.e., rate of drug absorption < rate of drug release). In line with these considerations, IVIVC is generally more likely to be established for sustained- or controlled-release dosage forms, but not for immediate-release dosage forms.

The value of establishing IVIVC stems from its potential use in allowing *in vitro* drug-release studies to be used as a surrogate for *in vivo* BE or BA studies. Thus, if an IVIVC is established during drug product development, subsequent changes to the drug product, such as formulation composition or the manufacturing process, which might otherwise necessitate a $F_{relative}$ or BE study can be substituted with an *in vitro* drug-release study. A further advantage of establishing IVIVC is to be able to set up realistic specification controls for *in vitro* drug release that are reflective of *in vivo* performance of the drug product. Any dissolution method may be selected for establishing IVIVC, as long as it meets the validation criteria outlined in the compendia.

As per the United States Food and Drug Administration (U.S. FDA) guidance for industry on the application of IVIVC to extended-release dosage forms (available at http://www.fda.gov/cder/guidance/index.htm), IVIVC can be of following different categories or levels:

- *Level A correlation* involves establishing a point-to-point correlation between *in vitro* dissolution and *in vivo* input rate of the drug. The *in vivo* input rate can be interpreted as the fraction of drug dissolved *in vivo* or the fraction of drug absorbed. The latter can be obtained by deconvolution of the plasma concentration-time profile of a drug. Such correlations are usually linear, but could also be nonlinear. In the case of linear correlations, the *in vitro* dissolution and *in vivo* absorption curves may be superimposable with or without the use of a scaling or conversion factor. An alternative approach to generate a level A IVIVC is to convolute the *in vitro* dissolution data to obtain a predicted plasma concentration-time profile, which may then be compared with the *in vivo* data obtained with test formulations. Level A correlations are generally the most difficult to establish because the model should predict good correlation of the entire *in vitro* dissolution-time data with the *in vivo* concentration-time profile.

- *Level B correlation* is the correlation of mean *in vitro* dissolution time to the mean *in vivo* dissolution time or the mean residence time of the drug. Level B correlation is based on statistical moment analysis, and while it utilizes all the *in vitro* and *in vivo* data in establishing a correlation, it is not considered a point-to-point correlation. An example of a level B correlation would be a linear regression model between the mean dissolution time and the mean absorption time of a dosage form. This correlation does not predict exact *in vivo* plasma concentration-time profile of a drug.
- *Level C correlation* establishes a single point relationship between a dissolution parameter and a pharmacokinetic parameter. The parameters used in this correlation could be the time to 50% drug release during dissolution testing with the total exposure, the time to maximum concentration, or the maximum plasma concentration of the drug from the *in vivo* data. An example of a level C correlation would be the linear regression between the fraction of drug dissolved at a given time point and the maximum drug concentration in plasma. Level C correlation uses a single parameter, which usually does not reflect the complete shape of the plasma concentration-time profile. Sometimes multiple level C correlations can be established using different parameters, such as by relating one or more pharmacokinetic parameters of interest to the amount of drug dissolved at various time points in the *in vitro* dissolution profile.

16.3.1.4 In Vitro–In Vivo *Relationship (IVIVR)*

Sometimes only a qualitative relationship can be established between the *in vitro* and the *in vivo* parameters, especially for immediate-release dosage forms. These qualitative relationships can be of the rank-order correlation kind, where, for example, slow rate of drug release is considered indicative of lower total exposure or lower rate of drug absorption. Such cases are termed *in vitro–in vivo* relationships (IVIVR) and have sometimes also been called level D IVIVC. Establishing IVIVR can be of value in determining formulation strategies during drug product development.

16.3.1.5 *Dimensionless Representation of Factors Affecting Drug Absorption*

Establishing IVIVC and the probability of success of delivery strategies in altering the pharmacokinetics of a drug depends largely on the relative rates of drug absorption and dissolution, in the context of drug dose and therapeutic window. These variables are assessed by the use of three dimensionless numbers: the absorption number, the dose number, and the dissolution number.

- *Dissolution number* represents the time required for drug dissolution. It is the ratio of mean residence time of the drug in the intestines to its mean dissolution time. The mean dissolution time, in turn, is a function of the diameter, density, and diffusivity of particles, in addition to the drug's saturation concentration.
- *Dose number* is indicative of drug solubility. It is the ratio of drug concentration in administered volume of 250 mL to the saturation solubility of drug in water.
- *Absorption number* is the ratio of effective permeability of the drug and the gut radius times the residence time of the drug in the small intestine.

Dose number and absorption number represent the inherent properties of the drug and the physiological system that may not be readily altered by the dosage form, except perhaps by the preparation of a prodrug or a complex to alter permeability and/or solubility, or use of a mucoadhesive or gastro-retentive dosage form. Dissolution number, on the other hand, can be more readily influenced by dosage form–related factors, such as by the preparation of extended- or sustained-release dosage forms.

These numbers can be utilized to calculate the absorbable dose of a drug ($D_{absorbable}$). The absorbable dose is the maximum amount of drug that can be absorbed after oral administration, taking into account the transit time of the drug ($T_{intestinal}$), effective drug permeability ($P_{effective}$), saturation concentration of the drug ($C_{saturation}$), and the area of small intestine available for absorption (A). It assumes the presence of saturated concentration of the drug in the solution at the site of absorption. Thus,

$$D_{absorbable} = A \times P_{effective} \times C_{saturation} \times T_{intestinal}$$

16.3.1.6 *Biopharmaceutics Classification System (BCS)*

The relative importance of solubility and permeability in oral drug absorption is reflected in various aspects of drug development, such as the ability to establish an IVIVC, the need and ability to develop an extended- or controlled-release dosage form, and the variability in drug absorption between and among subjects. For the relative assessment of drugs based on their solubility and permeability parameters, Amidon et al. [16] proposed a Biopharmaceutics Classification System (BCS) that categorizes drugs in four classes:

- *BCS Class I* drugs are the drugs with high solubility and high permeability.
- *BCS Class II* drugs are the drugs with low solubility and high permeability.
- *BCS Class III* drugs are the drugs with high solubility and low permeability.
- *BCS Class IV* drugs are the drugs with low solubility and low permeability.

The boundary of what may be considered high or low in terms of solubility and permeability for the BCS is defined in the U.S. FDA guidance for industry on the waiver of *in vivo* BA and BE studies for immediate-release solid oral dosage forms (available at http://www.fda.gov). A highly soluble drug is defined as one whose highest dose is soluble in 250 mL or less of aqueous media across the pH range of 1–7.5. This solubility criterion is based on the administration of 8 fluid ounces of water with drug administration in clinical studies, and the pH range criterion ensures lack of pH-induced precipitation of drug in the gastrointestinal milieu.

The permeability category of a drug is defined based on direct measurement of rate of drug transport across a human intestinal membrane and indirectly by assessing the fraction of dose absorbed after oral administration. A drug that demonstrates 90% or more extent of absorption after oral administration is considered to be highly permeable.

BCS can be utilized in supporting a waiver of *in vivo* BA or BE study for immediate-release oral solid dosage forms once the BA has been initially established and a change in the formulation composition or manufacturing process is made that would otherwise necessitate a BE study. In addition, generic drug products filing an abbreviated new drug application can utilize BCS classification in support of requests for waiver of BE studies against the then-marketed innovator or brand drug product. Typically, drugs that belong to BCS class I have a low risk of variation in BA based on dosage form–related factors.

16.3.1.7 Biopharmaceutics Drug Disposition Classification System (BDDCS)

The Biopharmaceutics Drug Disposition Classification System (BDDCS) was proposed in 2005 as a surrogate for determining the permeability of compounds using the elimination criteria to predict overall drug disposition, including the effect of the route of drug administration, transporters (efflux and absorptive), and food effect [17]. BDDCS is useful in predicting the effect of efflux and uptake transporters on drug absorption. This classification proposes the use of extent of drug metabolism (≥ 90%) to define highly permeable compounds to feed into the BCS classification system. This can provide a robust *in vivo* approach to overcome the difficulties associated with experimentally determining permeability of compounds using *in vitro* cell culture assays using cell lines such as Caco-2 or Pampa, or direct intestinal permeability assessment. The BDDCS proposes that if the major route of elimination of a drug is metabolism, then the drug should be categorized as a highly permeable compound since it must be absorbed to be metabolized.

16.3.2 Dosage Form Factors

A dosage form is utilized more often than not to deliver a drug to its target site of absorption. The dosage form design factors inherently affect the rate and extent of drug release, which can impact BA. The following would exemplify some dosage form–related factors that can affect drug BA.

16.3.2.1 Disintegration and Drug Release

The rate and extent of drug release from the dosage form can impact BA of drugs where disintegration and dissolution are the rate-limiting steps for absorption. For example, increased disintegration time led to reduced BA for the antihelmintic agent praziquantel [18]. Therefore, superdisintegrants, such as croscarmellose sodium, crospovidone, and sodium starch glycolate, are frequently added to immediate-release solid dosage forms for rapid disintegration in the aqueous medium.

In addition, coprocessing, such as the preparation of solid-solid dispersions, is utilized to change drug-release characteristics by preparation of a microcrystalline or amorphous drug-containing matrix. Solid dispersions are prepared by combining two solid ingredients, one of which is the poorly soluble drug and the other is a release-modifying hydrophilic excipient, together in a manner that allows molecular mixing (which leads to solid solutions) or formation of very fine particle size dispersion of one component in the other. These techniques include melt fusion, hot melt extrusion, spray drying, freeze drying, and supercritical fluid precipitation. The hydrophilic excipients typically used are polyvinyl pyrrolidone (PVP) and various derivatives of hydroxypropyl methylcellulose (HPMC) [19–21]. Solid dispersions often lead to improved dissolution rate and BA of drugs [22–25].

Longer duration of drug residence at its site of absorption can help improve the extent of drug absorption. This is typically attempted with the use of mucoadhesive excipients in dosage forms. Thus, coprocessing of a drug with a bioadhesive excipient can lead to longer residence time of the drug at the absorptive surface. For example, freeze drying of a combination of maize starch and Carbopol® 974P, a cross-linked acrylic acid-based polymer, increased the nasal delivery of metoprolol tartrate in rabbits [26].

Sustained-release dosage forms are prepared with an intentional and a controlled rate and/or timing of drug release to produce delayed and/or prolonged plasma drug concentrations. Thus, oral-delayed release dosage forms employ technologies such as enteric coating or colonic delivery that allow the drug to be released only later in the GIT [11]. These drug products are often formulated to release the drug in a bolus when environmental conditions, such as the pH, for drug release are optimum. Other dosage forms, such as drug complexes with ion exchange resins or drugs embedded in an insoluble polymer matrix, can lead to a sustained and/or controlled rate of drug release. The rate of drug release may or may not be pH dependent. This is important since the pH of the GIT varies from acidic in the stomach to increasingly basic in the small intestinal duodenum, jejunum, ileum, and the colon.

Also, depending on the site of drug absorption, dosage forms may be designed to be retained longer at a given site, leading to higher BA. For example, gastroretentive dosage forms can allow higher drug absorption from the duodenum. In addition, change of the route of administration can lead to significant changes in the rate and extent of drug BA, as well as the duration of drug action. For example, use of a parenteral depot formulation can allow prolonged drug absorption over several days or weeks, whereas oral sustained-release formulations can typically extend the duration of drug absorption to no longer than a day.

16.3.2.2 Drug-excipient Interactions

Drug-excipient interactions may affect the stability, release, and/or BA of drugs from their dosage forms. In certain cases, drug-excipient binding interactions affect drug release but not BA. For example, cyclodextrin complexation increased both drug release and oral BA of griseofulvin [27] and spironolactone [28], but not of naproxen [29] and tolbutamide [30]. This difference in whether changes in *in vitro* drug release correspond to changes in *in vivo* BA are dependent on the selection of dissolution method, in addition to the biopharmaceutical characteristics of the drug (e.g., its absorption window), and the strength and extent of binding.

Drug-excipient binding interactions could be specific or nonspecific. Specific binding interactions involve, for example, complexation through a known mechanism. Drug complexation with cyclodextrins is utilized to affect a drug's solubility, dissolution rate, stability, and/or diffusion coefficient. These complexes are expected to be pharmacologically inert and to dissociate readily at the site of absorption. The use of cyclodextrins has resulted in improved BA of several drugs such as griseofulvin [27], ursodeoxycholic acid [31], cinnarizine [32], acyclovir [33], artemisinin [34], glibenclamide [35], ibuprofen [36], nifedipine [37], and theophylline [38].

Drug-excipient complexes that don't readily dissociate at the site of absorption can lead to altered, or reduced, BA of drugs, due to the altered biopharmaceutical properties of the drug, including reduction in partition coefficient and diffusion coefficient (due to the large molecular size of the drug-excipient complex). These cases are illustrated by the complexation of tetracycline with divalent cations [39] and of phenobarbital with PEG 4000 [40]. In both cases, formation of insoluble complexes led to a decrease in drug BA.

Nonspecific drug-excipient binding interactions are exemplified by acid-base pairing of drug and a polymeric excipient in the dosage form, such that the exact site of interaction is not well established. These interactions are commonly utilized in the use of ion exchange resins, e.g., sulfonated and/or carboxylated polystyrenes, for preparing sustained-release dosage forms of amine drugs such as dextromethorphan [41] and phenylpropanolamine [42].

In general, whether drug-excipient binding interactions affect oral drug BA is not well understood. For ionic interactions, disruption of the interaction *in vitro* by physiological salt concentration is considered an indicator of lack of its impact on a drug's BA.

16.3.3 Physiological Factors

GI physiological characteristics often interact with drug substance or dosage form characteristics to impact drug absorption. In addition, interindividual variability in the physiological characteristics can lead to variability in a drug's pharmacokinetic parameters. An understanding of the interaction of physiological variables with drug and dosage form can allow drug product design strategies that may minimize or mitigate variability in drug absorption.

16.3.3.1 GI Motility

Peristaltic motion of the stomach and the intestines carry their contained mass forward to the progressing segments of the GI tract. Normal motility of the GI tract is characterized in terms of transit time through different "compartments" of the GI tract, which are utilized in modeling drug absorption. The transit time is defined as the time taken for a dosage form or its components to pass through a compartment. For example, the following parameters are utilized in the GastroPlus software (Simulations Plus, Inc., Lancaster, CA) for simulation of human drug absorption after oral administration:

- *Stomach:* Gastric emptying time in the fasted state is generally less than half an hour, while a high fat breakfast can increase the gastric emptying time to several hours.
- *Small intestines:* Transit time through different intestinal segments is estimated based on the volume of fluid in each segment. The average small intestinal transit time is considered about 3.3 hours.
- *Caecum:* Transit time for human caecum is 4.5 hours.
- *Colon:* Human colon transit time is generally considered to be 13.5 hours.

The rate of transfer of a drug product from one segment of the GI tract to the next can influence the time period available for drug dissolution or absorption in one particular component. Of all the stages of GI transit, gastric emptying provides the greatest influence on the rate of oral drug absorption because an orally administered dosage form encounters the stomach first. In addition to the emptying of stomach contents, gastric muscles exert mechanical pressure on the dosage form. GI transit times can influence oral drug bioavailability through a multitude of mechanisms, such as the following:

- *Rapid gastric emptying:* Basic drugs that are administered as solid particles or tablets first dissolve in the acidic gastric environment before being transported as drug solutions to the upper intestinal tract, where most of the drug absorption takes place. In some cases, rapid gastric emptying can lead to incomplete drug dissolution in the stomach, leading to transfer of partially undissolved drug particles into the duodenum. This can not only lead to incomplete drug dissolution and absorption, but the undissolved drug particles can serve as nucleation sites for precipitation of dissolved drug in to the duodenum—which can further reduce the extent of drug absorption and also introduce interindividual variability. This phenomenon is the main reason for variability in drug absorption in monkey models for many drugs that exhibit pH-based solubility and supersaturation in the duodenum.
- *Increased intestinal transit rate:* A general increase in intestinal motility can increase the rate of drug transport from one intestinal segment to the next. This can impact the total duration of time a drug has for absorption from the proximal segments of the intestine (such as duodenum), which have a higher surface area than latter segments (such as the ileum and colon). Thus, the effect of GI motility on the extent of drug absorption would depend on the rate of drug absorption and the effective permeability of the compound. The impact can be higher for drugs with a specific and short window of absorption.

GI motility can be affected by several factors, including pharmacological effect of the drug itself. Gastric emptying is affected by a multitude of factors including posture and presence of food.

16.3.3.2 Food and pH Effect

Food intake can affect drug absorption either by directly interacting with the dosage form or by affecting GI physiological parameters relevant to drug absorption. For example, GI fluid volumes are different in the fed and the fasted state, as illustrated in Table 16.1 [43].

Food also influences gastric pH. Thus, while the normal gastric pH is 1–3 in the fasted state, the fed state gastric pH in humans can be 4.3–5.4 [44]. The effect of gastric pH on oral drug absorption can be most predominant for weakly basic compounds that have high solubility at acidic pH and low solubility at the basic pH. The rate and extent of oral bioavailability of these drugs in humans are dependent on their rapid dissolution from an oral solid dosage form in the acidic stomach. Change in gastric pH, due to coadministration of food or other reasons such as the use of antihistaminic drugs, can lead to altered oral drug bioavailability.

In addition to the quantity and type of food (e.g., liquid ingestion versus solid food), fat content in the food can affect GI motility, concentration of bile in upper intestines, and drug-release characteristics from the dosage form. Fat and high calorie meals delay gastric emptying. The presence of surfactants in the intestinal milieu (e.g., from the bile) can lead to solubilization of a drug at the site of absorption (small intestine), leading to supersaturation of the drug. This can prevent precipitation of a weakly basic compound

TABLE 16.1 Gastrointestinal Fluid Volumes in the Fasted and Fed State.

Compartment	Fasted State Volume (mL, mean ± SD)	Fed State Volume (mL, mean ± SD)
Stomach	45 ± 18	686 ± 93
Small intestine	105 ± 72	54 ± 41
Large intestine	13 ± 12	11 ± 26

that dissolved in the low gastric pH and was subsequently transported to the high intestinal pH environment, in which it has low solubility. In cases in which the supersaturation phenomenon contributes to oral drug bioavailability, alterations in bile secretion or other physiological changes in the intestinal fluids can become significant determinants of drug absorption.

16.3.3.3 Window of Absorption

Passive absorption of orally administered drugs is assumed to follow a uniform rate of permeation across the GI tract. The rate of absorption for these drugs, therefore, is a function of the relative area of a GI segment and the residence time of the drug in that segment. Some drugs, however, display significantly high absorption in some specific region of the GI tract, while the absorption rate may be very low in other segments. The high absorption regions for these drugs are termed the "window of absorption." The phenomenon of the window of absorption of a drug can also be related to differential drug solubility and stability in various regions of the GI tract, or the presence of active transporters in certain regions.

The window of absorption of a drug *in vitro* can be ascertained by measuring drug permeability across different sections of the GI tract mounted in an Ussing chamber. *In vivo* assessment, or confirmation of a window of absorption, is generally deductive based on the plasma concentration–time profile of a drug after administration to different regions of the GI tract. Such studies may be carried out using, for example, a radio-frequency-based remote-controlled delivery capsule coupled with real-time visualization of capsule location in the GI tract using gamma scintigraphy. In addition, direct administration of a drug to different intestinal segments using animals that are ported for direct drug administration to such regions of the GI tract (e.g., cynomolgus monkeys can be surgically ported for direct drug administration to the duodenum and ileum) can help elucidate relative absorption rates of the drug from different segments. Significant change in the AUC of the drug after administration to different regions is indicative of a window of absorption.

A window of absorption in the proximal regions of the small intestine, such as the duodenum, can potentially limit the oral bioavailability of drugs and also present an obstacle to the development of controlled-release formulations. Drugs that show higher permeability in the upper intestinal regions include ciprofloxacin, levodopa, furosemide, captopril, acyclovir, and gabapentin. Oral drug absorption from these drugs is sensitive to physiological parameters, such as GI motility. This sensitivity is reflected in the inter- and intrasubject variability in their oral drug absorption. In addition, such drugs are also amenable to dosage form strategies that target to maximize and prolong drug concentration in the upper GI tract—such as gastroretentive dosage forms or bioadhesive microspheres. For example, a prolonged-release gastroretentive dosage form of ciprofloxacin prolonged the exposure of the drug in humans [45].

16.3.3.4 Variability in Metabolizing Enzymes and Efflux Transporters

Several drugs are substrates of drug-metabolizing enzymes in the GI tract, such as the cytochrome P450 (CYP) enzymes in the intestinal mucosa, and efflux transporters, such as the P-glycoprotein (P-gp) family of transporters. CYP enzymes are membrane-bound heme-containing proteins that are responsible for the metabolism of endogenous compounds such as steroids and fatty acids, and are often the metabolizing enzymes of drugs and xenobiotics. Isoform 3A4 of the cytochrome P450–metabolizing enzyme has been recognized as dominant in the gut wall metabolism of drugs. P-gp is the active transporter that secretes drugs back in the GI tract and is located on the mucosal surface of GI epithelial cells. P-gp expression in normal tissues, such as canalicular side of hepatocytes, apical surface of renal proximal tubules, and endothelial cells of the blood-brain barrier, serves to minimize physiological exposure to potentially toxic xenobiotics.

Oral absorption of drugs that are substrates of efflux transporters and metabolizing enzymes is affected by the interindividual expression level and intra-individual distribution of these proteins in the GI tract. The distribution of the P-gp transporter and CYP3A4 metabolizing enzymes differs across regions of the GI tract, which can contribute to variability in oral drug absorption. P-gp transport has been linked to the low and variable oral bioavailability of several compounds, such as propranolol and felodipine [46]. Drugs such as itraconazole and cyclosporin are substrates for both CYP3A4 and P-gp. In addition, drugs whose absorption is affected by transporters and metabolizing enzymes can also be sensitive to certain food effects. For example, grapefruit juice is an inhibitor of CYP3A4 [47], and can thus affect the oral absorption of drugs that are CYP3A4 substrates.

16.4. BIOEQUIVALENCE

BE refers to equivalent rate and extent of drug absorption of a drug from two different formulations or dosage forms when administered in the same molar dose. Two drug products with similar rate and extent of drug absorption are termed bioequivalent. Rate of absorption of a drug influences the maximum plasma concentration reached (C_{max}) and the time to maximum plasma concentration (t_{max}). The extent of drug absorption is indicated by $F_{relative}$ of the two formulations or drug products.

BE to the marketed brand-name drug product is a requirement for granting the marketing authorization of generic drug products by regulatory agencies such as the U.S. FDA and the European Medicines Agency (EMEA) in Europe.

16.4.1 Derived Pharmacokinetic Parameters for Bioequivalence Assessment

When two drug products are administered for the purpose of single-dose BE assessment, the data collected is typically the plasma concentration-time profile for a fixed duration of time, such as 48 hours or 72 hours. Direct comparison of the two profiles becomes difficult and subjective given various aspects of the data that are of importance in identifying their similarity or differences. These aspects include the rate of absorption, intersubject variability in the data, total amount of drug absorbed, peak plasma concentration (C_{max}), and the time to reach the peak plasma concentration (T_{max}). Notably, the rate of elimination is an aspect of the plasma concentration-time profile that typically would not depend on the dosage form. Assessing the similarity of the two profiles becomes difficult when several aspects of the profiles need to be taken into consideration. Parameters that are used for BE assessment include C_{max} and the total amount of drug absorbed. The latter can be inferred from AUC from the time of dose administration ($t = 0$) to the last sampling time point (t) or an infinite time point (∞), which estimates drug concentrations in plasma until very low levels by extrapolating the last time point using a parameter derived from the curve (terminal rate of drug elimination). These AUC parameters are termed $AUC_{0\rightarrow t}$ and $AUC_{0\rightarrow\infty}$, respectively.

BE assessment is carried out using the parameters $AUC_{0\rightarrow t}$, $AUC_{0\rightarrow\infty}$, and C_{max}. The first two of these parameters represent the extent of drug absorption, whereas C_{max} is primarily affected by the rate of drug absorption. Notably, the parameter T_{max}, which also represents the rate of drug absorption, is not used in the BE calculations. The reason is that T_{max} is a discrete measured parameter that depends on the design of the study in terms of sampling time points. Further, the shape of the plasma concentration-time profile can influence T_{max}. For example, the presence of two peaks in the plasma concentration-time profile can lead to a perception of significant differences between two formulations in terms of T_{max} if the two peaks have minor differences in their peak concentration. While these limitations also hold true for C_{max}, the assessment of peak plasma concentration is critical to drug safety because many drugs exhibit concentration-dependent toxicity.

16.4.2 Statistical Basis of Bioequivalence Assessment

Statistically, two drug products are considered bioequivalent if the 90% confidence intervals (CI) for the ratio of the population geometric means between the test (T) and the reference (R) drug products for log-transformed values of parameters representing the rate (C_{max}) and the extent (AUC) of drug absorption fall within the 0.80 to 1.25 range. The 90% CI is based on a two-sided test and is equivalent to two one-sided tests of significance with null hypothesis of bioinequivalence at a significance level (α) of 0.05 [48].

The log-transformed data is analyzed using the analysis of variance (ANOVA), a parametric statistical model, to derive the confidence interval for the difference between formulations. The confidence interval is then back-transformed to obtain the desired confidence interval for the ratio of the two formulations on the original scale. The sources of variation that are usually accounted for in the ANOVA model are sequence, period, and formulation using fixed effects for all terms.

16.4.2.1 Logarithmic Transformation

The logarithmic transformation of data is preferred for clinical and pharmacokinetic reasons [49]. The primary comparison of interest in a BE study is the ratio, rather than the difference of the average pharmacokinetic parameters from the two formulations. Therefore, logarithmic transformation allows the use of a linear statistical model (which utilizes differences between the means) to infer differences between the two means (which are transformed on a log scale). The analyzed data can be back- transformed to derive inferences about the ratio of the two averages on the original scale. This allows comparison between the two formulations on the basis of ratio.

The pharmacokinetic rationale for log transformation of data is to convert the factors responsible for variation in drug plasma levels from a multiplicative to an additive model. This enables the use of linear statistical methods that utilize differences in the comparison of two formulations. For example, the total amount of drug absorbed, $AUC_{0\rightarrow\infty}$, is a function of administered dose (D), fraction absorbed (F), and clearance (CL), as shown in Eq. 16.12:

$$AUC_{0\rightarrow\infty} = \frac{FD}{CL} \tag{16.12}$$

This equation relates the $AUC_{0\rightarrow\infty}$ to subject-factors that influence this parameter using multiplicative terms, which could lead to the effect of the subject not being additive. Logarithmic transformation of data indicates logarithmic transformation of underlying mechanistic terms, which were originally multiplicative, thus allowing their use in additive statistical models. Thus, logarithmic transformation of $AUC_{0\rightarrow\infty}$ yields Eq. 16.13:

$$\ln(AUC_{0\rightarrow\infty}) = \ln(F) + \ln(D) - \ln(CL) \qquad (16.13)$$

16.4.2.2 Range of Confidence Interval

BE study is designed to test differences between two different drug products or formulations made of the same drug substance or active pharmaceutical ingredient (API) at the same dose. The pharmacokinetic parameters and therapeutic window of the API, however, can influence the statistical criteria for BE by affecting variability in the data and the clinical tolerance for such variability. Thus, the recommended range of 90% CI could be different depending on the inherent variability and the therapeutic window of a compound.

The general recommended range of 90% confidence intervals (CIs) for assessing BE is 80%–125% of the ratio of averages for each drug product tested. This ratio represents a multiplicative symmetry for 20% variation since $1.25 = (0.8)^{-1}$. In addition to meeting the BE limit based on these confidence interval boundaries, the point estimate of the geometric mean ratio of pharmacokinetic parameters should fall within this range.

The European Committee for Proprietary Medicinal Products (CPMP) guidance recognizes highly variable drug products as those whose intrasubject variability for a parameter is larger than 30% [50]. For these products, when a wider difference in C_{max} may be considered clinically irrelevant, the C_{max} acceptance criteria may be widened to 69.84%–143.19%. For all other cases (clinically relevant parameters), widening of the acceptable confidence interval range is allowed to different extents based on the intrasubject variability. Thus, the widening of acceptance criteria for the CI requires the study design to involve replicate dosing of the same drug product to demonstrate intrasubject variability. Similarly, for narrow therapeutic index drugs, the acceptance interval for AUC could be tightened to 90.00%–111.11%. These tighter limits could also be applied to C_{max}, where the maximum drug concentration is of particular importance for drug safety.

16.4.3 Bioequivalence Study Design Considerations

The objective of a BE study is to assess variation in mean drug pharmacokinetics based on differences between the two formulations (groups) while separately accounting for intersubject variability (to assess the power of the study). A typical BE study design incorporates several elements, such as the following:

- *Crossover* instead of parallel group design: Crossover design refers to the administration of both formulations to all subjects in the study in a sequential fashion; i.e., each subject undergoes two dosings: the subject receives one of the two formulations in the first dose and the other formulation in the second dose. A parallel group design, on the other hand, would involve different subjects receiving the two different formulations. This approach is not preferred because any inherent pharmacokinetic variation in the subjects chosen between the two groups can introduce bias in the study.
- *Random:* Since each subject undergoes two dosings, the formulation administered in each dosing period is not unique but mixed up. For example, if 12 subjects were to be utilized for BE assessment, both the formulations must be utilized in both dosing periods, and an equal number of subjects should receive each formulation in each dosing period. Each subject is randomly selected to receive either of the two formulations in each dosing period. These aspects are included to avoid any systematic bias in the study design that can alter the affect of the study.
- *Washout period:* Since each subject must undergo two dosings, the dose periods must be separated by adequate time to allow complete elimination of the drug administered in period 1 before the drug is re-administered in period 2. This period of time between the two dosings when the subjects are "rested" is known as the washout period. The minimum duration of time for the washout is based on the elimination half-life of the drug. A minimum time equivalent to five half-lives is preferred to allow complete drug elimination from the system.
- *Double blinded:* BE studies are designed such that none of the study subjects or other participants (including physicians and analysts) are aware of the identity of the formulation given to the subjects. Blinding is carried out by assigning a code to each drug product, which is not revealed until study completion (including sample analysis and statistical interpretation of data). This aspect is designed to avoid any bias from the patients, physicians, or other study participants toward one of the two products.

The blinding requirement places a further burden on the study directors to ensure that both products being administered are organoleptically similar. In other words, if two tablets are administered, the patient or physicians should not be able to make out differences between the two based on their appearance, odor, or any such perceptible feature. This, therefore, requires that both tablets be of similar size and shape, and have the same color and markings (if any). These requirements can become challenging when one of the products being compared is a marketed drug product, which cannot be altered. Often, these requirements are fulfilled by encapsulating both the drug products in hard gelatin capsules.

16.5. CONCLUSIONS

The rate and extent of drug absorption into the systemic circulation can be measured by estimation of the C_{max}, T_{max}, and AUC after drug administration. These measures of BA are also helpful in determining BE of different formulations or dosage forms. Assessment of $F_{relative}$ is important to new drug product development, while assessment of $F_{absolute}$ is important to understand the clinical impact of changes in a drug's BA.

Oral drug BA is determined by the physicochemical characteristics of the drug and the dosage form, and their interactions with GI physiology. Drug properties important to oral drug absorption include its solubility, stability, lipophilicity, and surface activity. The pH-dependent variation in these drug substance properties can lead to their interactions with physiological variations in GI pH, which may affect drug absorption in different regions of the GI tract. In addition, physiological parameters such as the gastric emptying time, intestinal motility, and expression of metabolizing enzymes and transporters can also affect oral drug BA. Dosage form–related factors that affect drug BA include drug-excipient interactions and drug-release characteristics.

The dosage form design can be tailored in certain ways to achieve the desired targeted oral drug absorption profile. Drug product development, therefore, must take into consideration the interaction of drug substance characteristics with physiological parameters to design optimal drug delivery strategies. Drug product design characteristics, such as controlled release formulations or regionally targeted dosage forms, can often be helpful in optimizing drug absorption and BA.

CASE STUDIES

Case 16.1

A brand and a generic product were compared, and the data are as follows:

	Dose (mg)	AUC (mg*hr/mL)
Brand	250	6392
Generic	350	7992

Advise the FDA panel on the relative bioavailability of this generic product.

Approach: The calculated relative bioavailability of the generic product is 89.3%

$$F_{rel} = \frac{\frac{AUC_{Generic}}{Dose_{Generic}}}{\frac{AUC_{Brand}}{Dose_{Brand}}} = \frac{\frac{7992}{350}}{\frac{6392}{250}} = \frac{22.834}{25.568} = 0.893$$

$$F_{rel} = 0.893 \times 100 = 89.3\%$$

Case 16.2

Two dosage forms are available to you. You also have information on their bioavailability and salt factor, as shown here. You have been asked to determine an equivalent dose for the coated tablet in this situation. How will you proceed on this calculation?

Dosage Form	Dose	Salt Factor S	Bioavailability F
Immediate Release (IR) Tablet	500 mg	0.87	0.35
Coated Tablet (CT)	?	0.94	0.70

Approach: The equivalent dose for the coated tablet can be determined as follows, where D represents dose, *IR* represents immediate release, and *CT* represents coated tablets:

$$S_{IR} \times F_{IR} \times D_{IR} = S_{CT} \times F_{CT} \times D_{CT}$$
$$0.87 \times 0.35 \times 500 = 0.94 \times 0.7 \times D_{CT}$$
$$D_{CT} = 231.4 \approx 230\ mg$$

Therefore, your recommendation should be for a coated 230 mg tablet. Note that salt factor refers to the ratio of molecular weight of the free acid/free base of the drug with that of the corresponding salt. This example illustrates calculating the relative dose of two different salt forms of a drug (different salt factors).

References

[1] Toutain PL, Bousquet-Melou A. Bioavailability and its assessment. J Vet Pharmacol Ther 2004;27(6):455–66.

[2] Bailey DG, Dresser GK, Kreeft JH, Munoz C, Freeman DJ, Bend JR. Grapefruit-felodipine interaction: effect of unprocessed fruit and probable active ingredients. Clin Pharmacol Ther 2000;68 (5):468–77.

[3] Hellriegel ET, Bjornsson TD, Hauck WW. Interpatient variability in bioavailability is related to the extent of absorption:

implications for bioavailability and bioequivalence studies. Clin Pharmacol Ther 1996;60(6):601–7.

[4] Karlsson MO, Bredberg U. Bioavailability estimation by semisimultaneous drug administration: a Monte Carlo simulation study. J Pharmacokinet Biopharm 1990;18(2):103–20.

[5] Toutain PL, Koritz GD, Fayolle PM, Alvinerie M. Pharmacokinetics of methylprednisolone, methylprednisolone sodium succinate, and methylprednisolone acetate in dogs. J Pharm Sci 1986;75(3):251–5.

[6] Serajuddin AT. Salt formation to improve drug solubility. Adv Drug Deliv Rev 2007;59(7):603–16.

[7] Aguiar AJ, Zelmer JE. Dissolution behavior of polymorphs of chloramphenicol palmitate and mefenamic acid. J Pharm Sci 1969;58(8):983–7.

[8] Maeda T, Takenaka H, Yamahira Y, Noguchi T. Use of rabbits for absorption studies on polymorphs of chloramphenicol palmitate. Chem Pharm Bull 1980;28(2):431–6.

[9] Cai ZW, Zhang Y, Borzilleri RM, Qian L, Barbosa S, Wei D, et al. Discovery of brivanib alaninate ((S)-((R)-1-(4-(4-fluoro-2-methyl-1H-indol-5-yloxy)-5-methylpyrrolo[2,1-f] [1,2,4]triazin-6-yloxy)propan-2-yl)2-aminopropanoate), a novel prodrug of dual vascular endothelial growth factor receptor-2 and fibroblast growth factor receptor-1 kinase inhibitor (BMS-540215). J Med Chem 2008;51(6):1976–80.

[10] Narang AS, Desai DD. Anticancer drug development: unique aspects of pharmaceutical development. In: Mahato RI, Lu Y, editors. Pharmaceutical perspectives of cancer therapeutics. New York, NY: AAPS-Springer Publishing Program; 2009.

[11] Narang AS, Mahato RI. Targeting colon and kidney: pathophysiological determinants of design strategy. In: Narang AS, Mahato RI, editors. Targeted delivery of small and macromolecular drugs. New York, N.Y.: CRC Press; 2010. p. 351–70.

[12] Chaumeil JC. Micronization: a method of improving the bioavailability of poorly soluble drugs. Methods Find Exp Clin Pharmacol 1998;20(3):211–5.

[13] Reverchon E, Della Porta G, Spada A, Antonacci A. Griseofulvin micronization and dissolution rate improvement by supercritical assisted atomization. J Pharm Pharmacol 2004;56(11):1379–87.

[14] Hammond RB, Pencheva K, Roberts KJ, Auffret T. Quantifying solubility enhancement due to particle size reduction and crystal habit modification: case study of acetyl salicylic acid. J Pharm Sci 2007;96(8):1967–73.

[15] Sanganwar GP, Sathigari S, Babu RJ, Gupta RB. Simultaneous production and co-mixing of microparticles of nevirapine with excipients by supercritical antisolvent method for dissolution enhancement. Eur J Pharm Sci 2010;39(1–3):164–74.

[16] Amidon GL, Lennernas H, Shah VP, Crison JR. A theoretical basis for a biopharmaceutic drug classification: the correlation of *in vitro* drug product dissolution and *in vivo* bioavailability. Pharm Res 1995;12(3):413–20.

[17] Wu CY, Benet LZ. Predicting drug disposition via application of BCS: transport/absorption/ elimination interplay and development of a biopharmaceutics drug disposition classification system. Pharm Res 2005;22(1):11–23.

[18] Kaojarern S, Nathakarnkikool S, Suvanakoot U. Comparative bioavailability of praziquantel tablets. Dicp 1989;23(1):29–32.

[19] Clarke JM, Ramsay LE, Shelton JR, Tidd MJ, Murray S, Palmer RF. Factors influencing comparative bioavailability of spironolactone tablets. J Pharm Sci 1977;66(10):1429–32.

[20] Owusu-Ababio G, Ebube NK, Reams R, Habib M. Comparative dissolution studies for mefenamic acid-polyethylene glycol solid dispersion systems and tablets. Pharm Dev Tech 1998;3 (3):405–12.

[21] Chowdary KPR, Suresh Babu KVV. Dissolution, bioavailability and ulcerogenic studies on solid dispersions of indomethacin in water soluble cellulose polymers. Drug Dev Ind Pharm 1994;20:799–813.

[22] Janssens S, De Zeure A, Paudel A, Van Humbeeck J, Rombaut P, Van den Mooter G. Influence of preparation methods on solid state supersaturation of amorphous solid dispersions: a case study with itraconazole and eudragit e100. Pharm Res 2010;27(5):775–85.

[23] Liu X, Lu M, Guo Z, Huang L, Feng X, Wu C. Improving the chemical stability of amorphous solid dispersion with cocrystal technique by hot melt extrusion. Pharm Res 2012;29 (3):806–17.

[24] Marsac PJ, Konno H, Rumondor AC, Taylor LS. Recrystallization of nifedipine and felodipine from amorphous molecular level solid dispersions containing poly(vinylpyrrolidone) and sorbed water. Pharm Res 2008;25(3):647–56.

[25] Shimpi SL, Chauhan B, Mahadik KR, Paradkar A. Stabilization and improved *in vivo* performance of amorphous etoricoxib using Gelucire 50/13. Pharm Res 2005;22(10):1727–34.

[26] Coucke D, Vervaet C, Foreman P, Adriaensens P, Carleer R, Remon JP. Effect on the nasal bioavailability of co-processing drug and bioadhesive carrier via spray-drying. Int J Pharm 2009;379(1):67–71.

[27] Dhanaraju MD, Kumaran KS, Baskaran T, Moorthy MS. Enhancement of bioavailability of griseofulvin by its complexation with beta-cyclodextrin. Drug Dev Ind Pharm 1998;24(6):583–7.

[28] Kaukonen AM, Lennernas H, Mannermaa JP. Water-soluble beta-cyclodextrins in paediatric oral solutions of spironolactone: preclinical evaluation of spironolactone bioavailability from solutions of beta-cyclodextrin derivatives in rats. J Pharm Pharmacol 1998;50(6):611–9.

[29] Otero-Espinar FJ, Anguiano-Igea S, GarcÃa-Gonzalez N, Vila-Jato JL, Blanco-MÃndez J. Oral bioavailability of naproxen-Î²-cyclodextrin inclusion compound. Int J Pharm 1991;75(1):37–44.

[30] Kedzierewicz F, Zinutti C, Hoffman M, Maincent P. Bioavailability study of tolbutamide Î²-cyclodextrin inclusion compounds, solid dispersions and bulk powder. Int J Pharm 1993;94(1–3):69–74.

[31] Panini R, Vandelli MA, Forni F, Pradelli JM, Salvioli G. Improvement of ursodeoxycholic acid bioavailability by 2-hydroxypropyl-beta-cyclodextrin complexation in healthy volunteers. Pharmacol Res 1995;31(3–4):205–9.

[32] Jarvinen T, Jarvinen K, Schwarting N, Stella VJ. Beta-cyclodextrin derivatives, SBE4-beta-CD and HP-beta-CD, increase the oral bioavailability of cinnarizine in beagle dogs. J Pharm Sci 1995;84(3):295–9.

[33] Luengo J, Aranguiz T, Sepulveda J, Hernandez L, Von Plessing C. Preliminary pharmacokinetic study of different preparations of acyclovir with beta-cyclodextrin. J Pharm Sci 2002;91 (12):2593–8.

[34] Wong JW, Yuen KH. Improved oral bioavailability of artemisinin through inclusion complexation with beta- and gamma-cyclodextrins. Int J Pharms 2001;227(1–2):177–85.

[35] Savolainen J, Jarvinen K, Taipale H, Jarho P, Loftsson T, Jarvinen T. Co-administration of a water-soluble polymer increases the usefulness of cyclodextrins in solid oral dosage forms. Pharm Res 1998;15(11):1696–701.

[36] Nambu N, Shimoda M, Takahashi Y, Ueda H, Nagai T. Bioavailability of powdered inclusion compounds of nonsteroidal antiinflammatory drugs with beta-cyclodextrin in rabbits and dogs. Chem Pharm Bull 1978;26(10):2952–6.

[37] Emara LH, Badr RM, Elbary AA. Improving the dissolution and bioavailability of nifedipine using solid dispersions and solubilizers. Drug Dev Ind Pharm 2002;28(7):795–807.

[38] Ammar HO, Ghorab M, El-nahhas SA, Omar SM, Ghorab MM. Improvement of some pharmaceutical properties of drugs by cyclodextrin complexation. 5. Theophylline. Pharmazie 1996;51 (1):42–6.

[39] Shargel L, Susanna W-P, Andrew BCY. *Applied biopharmaceutics & pharmacokinetics*. 5th ed. Appleton & Lange Reviews/ McGraw-Hill, Medical Pub. Division; 2005.

[40] Singh P, Guillory JK, Sokoloski TD, Benet LZ, Bhatia VN. Effect of inert tablet ingredients on drug absorption. I. Effect of polyethylene glycol 4000 on the intestinal absorption of four barbiturates. J Pharm Sci 1966;55(1):63–8.

[41] Jeong SH, Park K. Drug loading and release properties of ion-exchange resin complexes as a drug delivery matrix. Int J Pharm 2008;361(1–2):26–32.

[42] Raghunathan Y, Amsel L, Hinsvark O, Bryant W. Sustained-release drug delivery system I: Coated ion-exchange resin system for phenylpropanolamine and other drugs. J Pharm Sci 1981;70 (4):379–84.

[43] Schiller C, Frohlich C-P, Giessmann T, Siegmund W, Monnikes H, Hosten N, et al. Intestinal fluid volumes and transit of dosage forms as assessed by magnetic resonance imaging. Alimentary Pharmacol Ther 2005;22(10):971–9.

[44] Chiou WL, Buehler PW. Comparison of oral absorption and bioavailablity of drugs between monkey and human. Pharm Res 2002;19(6):868–74.

[45] Mostafavi A, Emami J, Varshosaz J, Davies NM, Rezazadeh M. Development of a prolonged-release gastroretentive tablet formulation of ciprofloxacin hydrochloride: pharmacokinetic characterization in healthy human volunteers. Int J Pharm 2011;409 (1–2):128–36.

[46] Siegmund W, Ludwig K, Engel G, Zschiesche M, Franke G, Hoffmann A, et al. Variability of intestinal expression of P-glycoprotein in healthy volunteers as described by absorption of talinolol from four bioequivalent tablets. J Pharm Sci 2003;92 (3):604–10.

[47] Kakar SM, Paine MF, Stewart PW, Watkins PB. 6′7′-Dihydroxybergamottin contributes to the grapefruit juice effect. Clin Pharmacol Ther 2004;75(6):569–79.

[48] Mahato RI, Narang AS. Pharmaceutical dosage forms and drug delivery. 2nd ed. Boca Raton, FL: CRC Press; 2012.

[49] Center for Drug Evaluation and Research, US Food and Drug Administration. Guidance for industry: statistical approaches to establishing bioequivalence. Available from <http://www.fda.gov/cder/guidance/index.htm>; 2001.

[50] Committee for Medicinal Products for Human Use, European Medical Agency. Guideline on the investigation of bioequivalence. Available from <http://www.ema.europa.eu>.

Index

Note: Page numbers followed by "*f*" and "*t*" refer to figures and tables, respectively.

D

E

Q

R